D0744393

Clinical Management of Thyroid Disease

Clinical Management of Thyroid Disease

Edited by

Fredric E. Wondisford, MD
Professor and Director, Metabolism Division
Departments of Pediatrics, Medicine, and Physiology
Director, Diabetes Research and Training Center
Johns Hopkins University School of Medicine
Baltimore, Maryland

Sally Radovick, MD
Lawson Wilkins Professor of Pediatrics
Director, Division of Endocrinology
Department of Pediatrics
Johns Hopkins University School of Medicine
Baltimore, Maryland

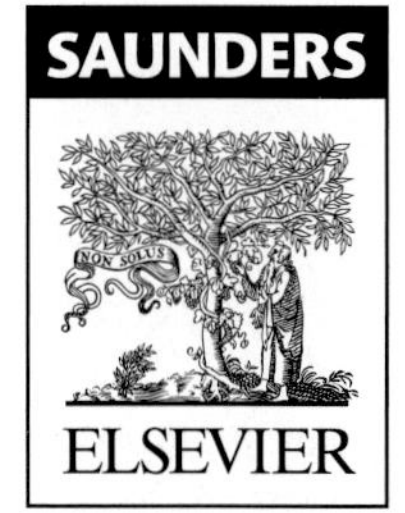

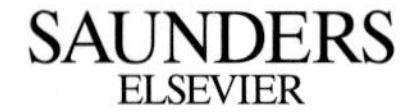

1600 John F. Kennedy Blvd.
Suite 1800
Philadelphia, PA 19103

CLINICAL MANAGEMENT OF THYROID DISEASE

ISBN: 978-1-4160-4745-2

Notice

Knowledge and best practice in this field are constantly changing. As new research and experience broaden our knowledge, changes in practice, treatment and drug therapy may become necessary or appropriate. Readers are advised to check the most current information provided (i) on procedures featured or (ii) by the manufacturer of each product to be administered, to verify the recommended dose or formula, the method and duration of administration, and contraindications. It is the responsibility of the practitioner, relying on their own experience and knowledge of the patient, to make diagnoses, to determine dosages and the best treatment for each individual patient, and to take all appropriate safety precautions. To the fullest extent of the law, neither the Publisher nor the Editors assumes any liability for any injury and/or damage to persons or property arising out of or related to any use of the material contained in this book.

The Publisher

Library of Congress Cataloging-in-Publication Data
Clinical management of thyroid disease/[edited by] Fredric E. Wondisford; associate editor, Sally Radovick—1st ed.
p. ; cm
ISBN 978-1-4160-4752-2
1. Thyroid gland—Diseases—Textbooks. I. Wondisford, Fredric E. II. Radovick, Sally.
[DNLM: 1. Thyroid Diseases—therapy. 2. Thyroid Diseases— physiopathology. WK 200 C641 2009]
RC655.C63 2009
616.4'4—dc22 2009001594

Acquisitions Editor: Pamela Hetherington
Publishing Services Manager: Frank Polizzano
Senior Project Manager: Robin E. Hayward
Design Direction: Louis Forgione

Printed in China.
Last digit is the print number: 9 8 7 6 5 4 3 2 1

Contributors

Suzanne Myers Adler, MD
Assistant Clinical Professor, George Washington University School of Medicine; Division of Endocrinology, George Washington University Hospital, Washington, DC
Chronic Thyroiditis

Kenneth B. Ain, MD
Professor of Medicine and Thyroid Oncology Program Director, Division of Endocrinology and Molecular Medicine, Department of Internal Medicine, University of Kentucky; Director, Thyroid Cancer Research Laboratory, Veterans Affairs Medical Center, Lexington, Kentucky
Follicular Carcinoma

Douglas W. Ball, MD
Associate Professor of Medicine and Oncology, Johns Hopkins University School of Medicine; Staff, Division of Endocrinology and Metabolism, Johns Hopkins Hospital, Baltimore, Maryland
Medullary Thyroid Cancer

Paolo Beck-Peccoz, MD
Professor of Endocrinology, University of Milan; Department of Medical Sciences, Endocrinology and Diabetology Unit, Fondazione Ospedale Maggiore IRCCS, Milan, Italy
Thyroid-Stimulating Hormone–Induced Hyperfunction

Antonio C. Bianco, MD, PhD
Professor of Medicine, Chief, Division of Endocrinology, Diabetes, and Metabolism, Miller School of Medicine, University of Miami, Miami, Florida
Thyroid Hormone Metabolism

Gregory Brent, MD
Professor of Medicine and Physiology, David Geffen School of Medicine at UCLA; Chief, Division of Endocrinology and Diabetes, VA Greater Los Angeles Healthcare System, Los Angeles, California
Pregnancy

Kenneth D. Burman, MD
Chief, Endocrine Section, Washington Hospital Center, Washington, DC
Chronic Thyroiditis

Naifa L. Busaidy, MD
Assistant Professor, Division of Internal Medicine, Department of Endocrine Neoplasia and Hormonal Disorders, University of Texas M. D. Anderson Cancer Center, Houston, Texas
Papillary Thyroid Carcinoma

Patrizio Caturegli, MD, MPH
Associate Professor of Pathology, Endocrinology, and Immunology, Johns Hopkins University School of Medicine and School of Public Health, Baltimore, Maryland
Anatomy of the Hypothalamic-Pituitary-Thyroid Axis

Ronald N. Cohen, MD
Associate Professor of Medicine, Section of Endocrinology, Diabetes, and Metabolism, The University of Chicago, Chicago, Illinois
Drugs

Terry F. Davies, MD
Florence and Theodore Baumritter Professor of Medicine, Mount Sinai School of Medicine; Attending Physician, Mount Sinai Hospital; Director, Endocrinology and Metabolism, James J. Peters VA Medical Center, New York, New York
Graves' Disease

Mario De Felice, MD
Professor of Pathology, Department of Molecular Biology and Pathology, University of Naples, Federico II, Naples, Italy; Scientific Coordinator, Biogem scarl, Ariano Irpino, Italy
Thyroid Development

Roberto Di Lauro, MD
Professor of Human Genetics, Department of Cellular and Molecular Biology and Pathology, University of Naples, Federico II, President, Stazione Zoologica Anton Dohrn, Naples, Italy
Thyroid Development

Alexandra M. Dumitrescu, MD, PhD
Resident, Department of Medicine, The University of Chicago, Chicago, Illinois
Cell Transport Defects

Thomas P. Foley, Jr., MD
Professor Emeritus, Department of Pediatrics, Division of Endocrinology, University of Pittsburgh School of Medicine; Director Emeritus, Division of Pediatric Endocrinology, Children's Hospital of Pittsburgh, Pittsburgh, Pennsylvania
Hypothyroidism

Stéphanie Gaillard, MD, PhD
Resident, Internal Medicine, Johns Hopkins University, Baltimore, Maryland
Thyroid-Stimulating Hormone and Thyroid-Stimulating Hormone Receptor

Annette Grueters-Kieslich, Prof, Dr
Professor and Dean, Charité University Medicine, Humboldt and Free University, Berlin, Germany
Screening for Congenital Disease

Koshi Hashimoto, MD, PhD
Assistant Professor, Department of Medicine and Molecular Science, Gunma University Graduate School of Medicine, Maebashi, Gunma, Japan
Thyroiditis

Bryan R. Haugen, MD
Professor of Medicine and Pathology, University of Colorado School of Medicine, Denver, Colorado
Solitary Thyroid Nodule

Jerome M. Hershman, MD
Distinguished Professor of Medicine, David Geffen School of Medicine at UCLA; Associate Chief, Endocrinology and Diabetes Division, VA Greater Los Angeles Healthcare System, Los Angeles, California
Hyperthyroidism and Trophoblastic Disease

Jason M. Hollander, MD
Princeton Endocrinology, Princeton, New Jersey
Graves' Disease

Anthony N. Hollenberg, MD
Associate Professor, Harvard Medical School; Chief, Thyroid Unit, Beth Israel Deaconess Medical Center, Boston, Massachusetts
Role of Thyroid-Releasing Hormone in the Regulation of the Thyroid Axis

Brian W. Kim, MD
Assistant Professor, Division of Endocrinology, Diabetes, and Metabolism, Miller School of Medicine, University of Miami, Miami, Florida
Thyroid Hormone Metabolism

Richard T. Kloos, MD
Co-Director, The Ohio State University Thyroid Cancer Unit, Divisions of Endocrinology and Nuclear Medicine; Secretary and Chief Operating Officer, The American Thyroid Association, Columbus, Ohio
Papillary Thyroid Carcinoma

Ronald J. Koenig, MD, PhD
Professor of Internal Medicine, Division of Metabolism, Endocrinology, and Diabetes, University of Michigan; University of Michigan Hospitals, Ann Arbor, Michigan
Nonthyroidal Illness Syndrome

Peter Kopp, MD
Associate Professor and Interim Director, Center for Genetic Medicine, Division of Endocrinology, Metabolism, and Molecular Medicine, Northwestern University, Chicago, Illinois
Thyroid Hormone Synthesis

Paul W. Ladenson, MD
John Eager Howard Professor of Endocrinology and Metabolism and Professor of Medicine, Pathology, Oncology, Radiology, and Radiological Sciences; Director, Division of Endocrinology and Metabolism, Johns Hopkins University School of Medicine, Baltimore, Maryland
Toxic Nodular Goiter: Toxic Adenoma and Toxic Multinodular Goiter

Melissa Landek
Department of Pathology, Johns Hopkins University School of Medicine; Department of Molecular Microbiology and Immunology, Johns Hopkins University School of Public Health, Baltimore, Maryland
Anatomy of the Hypothalamic-Pituitary-Thyroid Axis

Juliane Léger, MD
Professor of Pediatrics, Paris 7 University; Professor of Pediatrics, Pediatric Endocrinology Unit and Reference Center for Endocrine Growth Disease, Hospital Robert Debre, Paris, France
Hyperthyroidism

Meranda Nakhla, MD
Assistant Professor and Pediatric Endocrinologist, Division of Endocrinology and Metabolism, Children's Hospital of Eastern Ontario, Ottawa, Ontario, Canada
Hypothyroidism

Joanna M. Peloquin, MD
Resident, Department of Medicine, Johns Hopkins University School of Medicine, Baltimore, Maryland
Nontoxic Diffuse and Nodular Goiter

Luca Persani, MD
Associate Professor of Endocrinology, University of Milan; Department of Medical Sciences, Endocrinology and Diabetology Unit, Fondazione Ospedale Maggiore IRCCS, Milan, Italy
Thyroid-Stimulating Hormone–Induced Hyperfunction

Samuel Refetoff, MD
Frederick H. Rawson Professor, Departments of Medicine and Pediatrics, The University of Chicago, Chicago, Illinois
Syndromes of Resistance to Thyroid Hormone; Cell Transport Defects

Joanne F. Rovet, PhD
Professor of Pediatrics and Psychology, University of Toronto Medical School; Senior Scientist, Neuroscience and Mental Health Program, The Hospital for Sick Children, Toronto, Ontario, Canada
Hypothyroidism

Amin Sabet, MD
Instructor in Pediatrics and Medicine, Johns Hopkins University School of Medicine, Baltimore, Maryland
Thyroid Hormone Action

Sherif Said, MD, PhD
Associate Professor of Pathology, University of Colorado, Denver, School of Medicine; Attending Pathologist and Director, Head and Neck Pathology, University of Colorado Hospital, Aurora, Colorado
Solitary Thyroid Nodule

Tetsuro Satoh, MD, PhD
Assistant Professor, Department of Medicine and Molecular Science, Gunma University Graduate School of Medicine, Maebashi, Gunma, Japan
Thyroiditis

Pamela R. Schroeder, MD, PhD
Assistant Professor of Medicine, Johns Hopkins University School of Medicine, Baltimore, Maryland
Toxic Nodular Goiter: Toxic Adenoma and Toxic Multinodular Goiter

Aniket Sidhaye, MD
Instructor, Johns Hopkins University School of Medicine, Department of Endocrinology and Metabolism, Baltimore, Maryland
Central Hypothyroidism

Juan Carlos Solis-S, MD
Assistant Professor, Universidad Autónoma de Querétaro, Querétaro, Qro, Mexico
Thyroid Hormone Synthesis

Emily J. Tan, MD
Staff Endocrinologist, Southern California Permanente Medical Group, Kaiser Permanente, Garden Grove, California
Hyperthyroidism and Trophoblastic Disease

Neil Tran, MD
Endocrinology Fellow, Department of Medicine, David Geffen School of Medicine at UCLA; Division of Endocrinology and Diabetes, VA Greater Los Angeles Healthcare System, Los Angeles, California
Pregnancy

Guy Van Vliet, MD
Professor of Pediatrics, University of Montreal Medical School; Chief, Endocrinology Service, Centre Hospitalier Universitaire Sainte-Justine, Montreal, Quebec, Canada
Genetics and Epigenetics of Congenital Hypothyroidism

Roy E. Weiss, MD, PhD
Rabbi Morris I. Esformes Endowed Professor and Chief, Departments of Medicine and Pediatrics, The University of Chicago, Chicago, Illinois
Syndromes of Resistance to Thyroid Hormone

Fredric E. Wondisford, MD
Professor and Director, Metabolism Division, Departments of Pediatrics, Medicine, and Physiology; Director, Diabetes Research and Training Center, Johns Hopkins University School of Medicine, Baltimore, Maryland
Thyroid-Stimulating Hormone and Thyroid-Stimulating Hormone Receptor; Nontoxic Diffuse and Nodular Goiter

Masanobu Yamada, MD, PhD
Associate Professor of Medicine and Molecular Science, Gunma University Graduate School of Medicine, Maebashi, Gunma, Japan
Thyroiditis

Paul M. Yen, MD
Associate Professor of Medicine and Pharmacology, Johns Hopkins University School of Medicine, Baltimore, Maryland
Thyroid Hormone Action

Contents

Part III Adult Thyroid Disease

Section A—Hyperfunction

Section B—Hypofunction

Part IV Conditions with Variable Effects

Part V Structural Lesions

Section A—Follicular Cell Thyroid Cancer

Section B—Medullary Thyroid Cancer

PART I

Normal Thyroid Axis

Section A

ANATOMY

Anatomy of the Hypothalamic-Pituitary-Thyroid Axis

Chapter 1

*Melissa Landek and Patrizio Caturegli**

Key Points

- The thyroid is regulated mainly by pituitary TSH and hypothalamic TRH.
- The thyroid is the largest endocrine gland and is made of a collection of follicles that synthesize and store thyroid hormones.

The thyroid has the longest phylogenetic history of all endocrine glands, being present not only in all vertebrates but also in protochordates (e.g., the lancelet) and ascidians (e.g., the sea squirt). In humans and most vertebrates, the thyroid gland is situated in the neck, but its gross morphologic arrangement varies among species. For example, in teleost fish such as the tuna, thyroid follicles aggregate along blood vessels and occasionally can be found far away from the neck, even in the kidney.

The main goal of the thyroid is to produce and store thyroid hormones, which are involved in numerous fundamental processes ranging from body growth, differentiation, and metamorphosis to thermogenesis. Thyroid hormone synthesis is regulated by a complex interplay involving the thyroid-stimulating hormone (TSH, thyrotropin), secreted by the anterior hypophysis, and the thyrotropin-releasing hormone (TRH), secreted by the hypothalamus, as well as other factors. This chapter will discuss the key anatomic features of the hypothalamic-pituitary thyroid axis.

*Supported by grant DK55670 from the National Institutes of Health.

HYPOTHALAMUS AND PITUITARY

Hypothalamic Thyrotropin-Releasing Hormone Neurons

The neurons that produce TRH and are involved in the regulation of the thyroid gland via the anterior hypophysis (hypophysiotropic TRH neurons) are located in the paraventricular nucleus of the hypothalamus. This is an intricate structure adjacent to the third ventricle composed of two major parts, a lateral part containing magnocellular neurons and a medial part with parvocellular neurons. Each part has numerous subdivisions; the hypophysiotropic TRH neurons are in the medial and periventricular parvocellular subdivisions.[1] These neurons project their processes to the median eminence, where they release TRH, a tripeptide hormone synthesized from a large precursor of 242 amino acids that contains six copies of TRH. TRH then diffuses to the anterior pituitary through the portal circulation, and binds to a specific G protein– coupled receptor present on the plasma membrane of the thyrotrophs.[2] The binding initiates a cascade of intracellular events that leads to the prompt secretion and glycosylation of TSH.

The synthesis of TRH by hypophysiotropic neurons is inhibited by fasting and restored to normal by feeding or the administration of leptin.[3] The action of leptin occurs mainly through the arcuate nucleus of the hypothalamus,[4] but also through other regions of the brain, such as the brainstem, fourth ventricle, and dorsal vagal complex, which all innervate the paraventricular nucleus by monosynaptic or multisynaptic projections.

TRH-producing neurons are also located in the anterior subdivision of the parvocellular neurons. Although similarly regulated by fasting, they are anatomically and functionally distinct from the hypophysiotropic neurons described. Their role is poorly known. They remind us that TRH, in addition to its control of the hypothalamic-pituitary thyroid axis, exerts other effects on the central nervous system centered on food intake and thermoregulation.

Pituitary Thyrotrophs

The cells of the anterior pituitary that produce TSH (thyrotrophs) are the least abundant cell type, comprising less than 5% of the total adenohypophyseal cell population. They are located in isolation or in small clusters in the anteromedial portion of the pituitary gland. Thyrotrophs are basophilic (a shade of blue color) when stained by conventional dyes such as hematoxylin and eosin, and contain periodic acid–Schiff (PAS) material, but can only be identified with certainty by immunohistochemistry using an antibody specific for the beta subunit of TSH. Thyrotrophs are medium to large elongated angular cells, with a central nucleus, abundant cytoplasm, and cytoplasmic processes. The secretory granules of thyrotrophs are small, 100 to 200 nm, round, electron-dense, and often positioned near the plasma membrane.

Thyrotrophs are constant throughout life and similar in both genders. Their cytologic appearance, however, is affected by the secretion of TSH. In cases of hyperthyroidism, secretion of TSH is suppressed, the thyrotrophs become small, and their immunoreactivity for TSH-β is greatly diminished or almost absent.[5] When patients with hyperthyroidism are treated, thyrotrophs return to their original size and TSH-β immunoreactivity returns to normal.[5] In patients with long-standing hypothyroidism, the thyrotrophs undergo hypertrophy and hyperplasia.[6] The thyrotroph area within the anterior pituitary enlarges and the thyrotrophs extend to other regions of the anterior pituitary. These changes are caused by the loss of the negative feedback of thyroid hormones. These chronically stimulated cells are known as thyroidectomy cells; they have an eccentric nucleus and abundant cytoplasm containing dilated rough endoplasmic reticulum, a prominent Golgi apparatus, large lysosomes, and few secretory granules.[6,7] This hyperplasia and hypertrophy secondary to hypothyroidism can cause a radiologically detectable enlargement of the pituitary gland and mimic a pituitary tumor. The distinction between the two entities is critical for the patient because the pituitary enlargement caused by thyrotroph hyperplasia and hypertrophy does not require surgery and is reversible on thyroid hormone replacement.

TSH is a 28-kD glycoprotein hormone composed of two subunits, alpha and beta. The alpha subunit is shared among follicle-stimulating hormone, luteinizing hormone, and human chorionic gonadotropin; the beta subunit, instead, is specific for TSH. TSH binds to a specific G protein–coupled receptor, located on the basolateral membrane of thyroid follicular cells, and is the master regulator of thyroid gland function.

THYROID GLAND

The thyroid gland develops from a diverticulum of the pharynx, similarly to the adenohypophysis, parathyroid glands, and thymus. It originates at the base of the tongue (as evidenced by the foramen cecum) and migrates downward along the midline to its final location by the trachea. The course of this migration is indicated by the thyroglossal duct, remnants of which become apparent in adult life when they give rise to mucus-filled cysts.

The thyroid is composed of two pear-shaped lobes, bordering the right and left sides of the trachea and held together by an isthmus, giving overall the appearance of a Greek shield. It is the largest endocrine gland, weighing about 2 g at birth and 15 g in adults. In about 50% of the population, a third lobe, called the pyramidal lobe, emerges upward from the isthmus, most commonly from its left part.[8] Its presence is not reliably diagnosed by scintigraphic or ultrasound imaging; the anterior cervical region should be investigated carefully during surgery so as not to leave residual thyroid tissue when total thyroidectomy is indicated.[8]

The thyroid gland has a rich blood flow of approximately 5 mL/g/min, supplied by the superior, inferior, and lowest accessory thyroid arteries. There is significant variation in the anatomy of these arteries, both among races and within individuals of the same race.[9] This is a critical consideration during imaging of the parathyroid glands and en bloc transplantation of larynx and thyroid. In Graves' disease or other hyperthyroid states, the blood flow is markedly increased, so that a thrilling vibration can be felt when palpating the gland. Venous drainage occurs via the superior, lateral, and inferior veins and lymphatic drainage is into the cervical lymph nodes, which are frequently involved in metastatic papillary thyroid cancer.

The thyroid makes contact with two important structures, which can be damaged by an inexperienced surgeon during thyroidectomy. The parathyroid glands, usually four in humans, are often located behind the thyroid lobes, but their location is extremely variable, so that extreme care must be taken during surgery to preserve their integrity.

The inferior laryngeal nerve, better known as the recurrent nerve, is a branch of the vagus nerve that supplies motor function and sensation to the larynx. It follows a tortuous route because it descends down into the thorax and then ascends back up in the neck, running between the trachea and esophagus behind the thyroid gland. The left recurrent nerve loops under and around the arch of the aorta before ascending, whereas the right one loops around the right subclavian artery. These nerves can be damaged during thyroidectomy and cause dysphonia and less efficient coughing.

The superior laryngeal nerve can also be injured during thyroidectomy, although its lesion usually goes unrecognized because it is clinically subtle. The lesion was publicized by the operatic soprano Amelita Galli-Curci, who underwent thyroidectomy in 1935 for a large (170-g) nontoxic multinodular goiter and was apparently incapable of reaching the high notes afterward, although a report has discredited the story.[10]

The thyroid gland is attached loosely to neighboring structures, especially in the posterior and inferior sides, so that a thyroid enlargement (goiter) will most commonly extend backward and downward, or even below the sternum. The thyroid is encapsulated by a fine connective tissue, which invaginates into the gland to form smaller lobules. Each lobule is composed of about 30 follicles, which represent the functional unit of the gland. There are approximately 3 million follicles in an adult thyroid. Each follicle can be compared to a watermelon, with the red, largest inner part corresponding to the colloid and the green thin capsule representing the thyroid epithelium. The follicles are relatively uniform in size and shape but have different orientations, so that the plane of section gives the impression on histologic slides that large follicles are interspersed with small ones.[11] The follicles are lined by a single layer of epithelial cells, whose height varies with the functional activity of the gland. They become thin and flat in hypothyroid states, and much taller and columnar in hyperthyroidism. Thyroid follicular cells (thyrocytes) have a clear polarity—their apex is oriented toward the colloid-filled lumen of the follicle, whereas their base is toward the interfollicular space.[12] The apex is densely populated by microvilli that project into the central colloid, and the base is separated from the interfollicular space by a basement membrane approximately 400 Å thick. Thyrocyte activity is stimulated by TSH and also by factors that mimic TSH action, such as the antibodies against the TSH receptor found in patients with Graves' disease.

In the interfollicular space, fenestrated capillaries and collagen fibers are found, and occasionally one or two circulating lymphocytes. Dietary iodine enters the thyrocytes at this basolateral surface through the action of the sodium iodide symporter.[13] It then moves through the thyrocyte, reaching the apex, where it is incorporated by thyroperoxidase onto specific tyrosines of the large thyroglobulin molecule. Thyroglobulin is the most abundant protein of the thyroid gland, representing about 20% of the total thyroid weight. Thyroglobulin is found in the colloid and inside the thyrocytes (Fig. 1-1). When thyroid hormones are needed, portions of colloid are engulfed at the apex by pseudopodia, enclosed in vacuoles within the thyrocytes and hydrolyzed to release thyroxine and also triiodothyronine into the bloodstream.

This follicular structure, with a central depot area, renders the thyroid unique among endocrine glands because it is the only gland in which hormones are stored in an extracellular location. It has probably evolved in response to the uncertain and scarce availability of iodine in the environment. Iodine is the key component of thyroid hormones, which have a simple chemical structure (two modified tyrosines) and yet are fundamental in numerous processes, from brain development to body growth and thermoregulation.

In addition to the thyrocytes, the thyroid gland also contains parafollicular cells, or C cells. These are neuroendocrine cells that originate from the ultimobranchial body, which develops from the fourth pharyngeal pouch and then migrates into the thyroid gland to give rise to the C cells. They constitute only about 0.1% of the thyroid mass, and are difficult to identify with standard hematoxylin and eosin staining. They are located in the interfollicular stroma, sometimes bordering and inserting in between follicular cells, either as individual or small groups of cells.[14] C cells are larger than thyrocytes and have

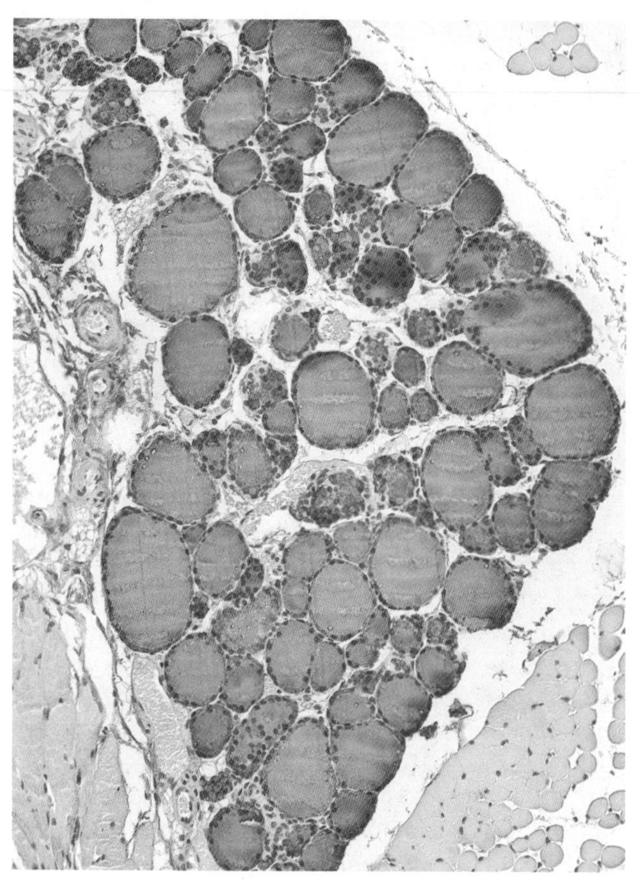

Figure 1–1 Section of a normal, adult mouse thyroid. The section was incubated with an antibody directed against thyroglobulin (dark red staining) and then counterstained with hematoxylin (blue staining). Note the intense red color filling the follicles. The thyroid follicular cells are cuboidal, with a clear nucleus (blue color) and a cytoplasm containing thyroglobulin (red color).

a granular cytoplasm, but their identification usually requires immunostaining for calcitonin. C cells are the source of calcitonin, the 32–amino acid hormone that lowers the serum calcium level by inhibiting osteoclast-mediated bone resorption. However, they secrete many other factors, such as calcitonin gene-related peptide, somatostatin, and other peptides, usually referred to as autocrine or paracrine factors.[15] More recently, TRH has also been found to be expressed in C cells, implicating a possible role of C cells in thyroid homeostasis.[16]

References

1. Segerson TP, Kauer J, Wolfe HC, et al: Thyroid hormone regulates TRH biosynthesis in the paraventricular nucleus of the rat hypothalamus. Science 238:78-80, 1987.
2. Yu R, Ashworth R, Hinkle PM. Receptors for thyrotropin-releasing hormone on rat lactotropes and thyrotropes. Thyroid 8:887-894, 1998.
3. Légrádi G, Emerson CH, Ahima RS, et al. Leptin prevents fasting-induced suppression of prothyrotropinreleasing hormone messenger ribonucleic acid in neurons of the hypothalamic paraventricular nucleus. Endocrinology 138:2569-2576, 1997.
4. Ahima RS, Flier JS. Leptin. Annu Rev Physiol 62: 413-437, 2000.
5. Scheithauer BW, Kovacs KT, Young WF Jr., Randall RV: The pituitary gland in hyperthyroidism. Mayo Clin Proc 67:22-26, 1992.
6. Alkhani AM, Cusimano M, Kovacs K, et al: Cytology of pituitary thyrotroph hyperplasia in protracted primary hypothyroidism. Pituitary 1:291-295, 1999.
7. Pioro EP, Scheithauer BW, Laws ER Jr., et al: Combined thyrotroph and lactotroph cell hyperplasia simulating prolactin-secreting pituitary adenoma in long-standing primary hypothyroidism. Surg Neurol 29:218-226, 1988.
8. Braun EM, Windisch G, Wolf G, et al: The pyramidal lobe: Clinical anatomy and its importance in thyroid surgery. Surg Radiol Anat 29:21-27, 2007.
9. Toni R, Della Casa C, Mosca S, et al: Anthropological variations in the anatomy of the human thyroid arteries. Thyroid 13:183-192, 2003.
10. Crookes PF, Recabaren JA: Injury to the superior laryngeal branch of the vagus during thyroidectomy: lesson or myth? Ann Surg 233:588-593, 2001.
11. Sugiyama S: Histological studies of the human thyroid gland observed from the viewpoint of its postnatal development. Ergeb Anat Entwicklungsgesch 39:1-71, 1967.
12. Nitsch L, Tramontano D, Ambesi-Impiombato FS, et al: Morphological and functional polarity of an epithelial thyroid cell line. Eur J Cell Biol 38:57-66, 1985.
13. Dohan O, Carrasco N: Advances in Na^+/I^- symporter (NIS) research in the thyroid and beyond. Mol Cell Endocrinol 213:59-70, 2003.
14. Borda A, Berger N, Turcu M, et al. The C-cells: Current concepts on normal histology and hyperplasia. Rom J Morphol Embryol 45:53-61, 1999.
15. Sawicki B. Evaluation of the role of mammalian thyroid parafollicular cells. Acta Histochem 97:389-399, 1995.
16. De Miguel M, Fernández-Santos JM, Utrilla JC, et al. Thyrotropin-releasing hormone receptor expression in thyroid follicular cells: A new paracrine role of C-cells? Histol Histopathol 20:713-718, 2005.

Chapter 2

Thyroid Development

*Mario De Felice and Roberto Di Lauro**

Key Points

- Thyroid follicular cells derive from a few endodermal cells of the primitive pharynx.
- In humans thyroid precursor cells are evident by the third week of gestation. At week 7 the developing thyroid reaches its final position in front of the trachea and becomes a bilobed organ. At week 10 thyroid hormone synthesis begins.
- Studies in animal models have identified a number of transcription factors expressed in thyroid cells indispensable in controlling thyroid development. Mutations in these genes are associated with thyroid dysgenesis in humans.

The thyroid gland consists of two elongated lobes connected by an isthmus and located anterior to the trachea at the base of the neck. In adult mammals, the thyroid is composed of two distinct endocrine cell types—the thyroid follicular cells (TFCs), the most abundant, and the parafollicular or C cells, scattered in the interfollicular space. TFCs are organized in particular spheroid structures, known as follicles and express a number of specific proteins required to produce and export thyroid hormones. Parafollicular C cells express the peptide hormone calcitonin-related polypeptide alpha, also known as calcitonin. Follicular and C cells derive from different embryonic structures. The thyroid anlage, a small group of endodermal cells of the primitive pharynx, is the site of origin of the TFCs. C cells derive from ultimobranchial bodies (UBBs), transient embryonic structures budded off from the fourth pharyngeal pouch. During embryonic life, the thyroid anlage and the UBBs migrate from their original sites and fuse to form the definitive thyroid gland.

Both the organogenesis of the thyroid gland and the functional differentiation of follicular and parafollicular cells occur through processes not yet fully elucidated. In humans, thyroid development initiates around the third week of gestation and terminates around the tenth week of gestation. Data on thyroid organogenesis in humans are scarce. However, the morphogenesis and differentiation of the thyroid have been extensively studied in animal models, mostly in mice, in which thyroid development starts around embryonic day (E) 8 to 8.5 and is completed by E17.5 to 18 at the end of gestation.

This chapter will focus on the genes and mechanisms controlling thyroid development, which have been discovered mainly through the study of murine models. This information can plausibly be extended to other species, including humans, because it is likely that thyroid development follows the same pathways in all mammals.

MORPHOLOGIC ASPECTS

In mammals, by the end of gastrulation, the endoderm germline is transformed in a primitive gut tube, whose anterior portion is called the foregut, which runs along the anteroposterior axis of the embryo. The tube initially appears as a homogeneous epithelial tube surrounded by mesoderm. Shortly thereafter, through the effects of signaling molecules and specific transcription factors, the gut tube begins to be patterned along its anteroposterior axis. As development proceeds, different districts are defined that subsequently undergo differential development and eventually give rise to different organ primordia, including that of the thyroid.[1-3]

Thyroid anlage, the presumptive thyroid-forming district, is evident by E8 to 8.5 as a midline thickening of the endodermal epithelium in the ventral wall of the primitive pharynx.[4] At this

*This work was supported in part by Telethon, Grant GGPO5161, Molecular Genetics of Thyroid Dysgenesis.

stage, the bud appears as an outpouching of the endoderm apposed to the aortic sac and localized caudal to the tuberculum impar, the region of the first branchial arch that gives rise to the median portion of the tongue. By E9, the bud evaginates from the floor of the pharynx and, maintaining a close association with the aortic sac,[5] invades the surrounding mesenchyma. One day later, the thyroid bud appears as an elongated structure, caudally migrating but still connected to the pharynx by a transient, narrow, endodermal-lined channel, the thyroglossal duct. At E11.5, the thyroglossal duct disappears and the thyroid primordium loses any contact with the floor of the pharynx. At early stages of morphogenesis, the growth of the thyroid primordium does not seem to be affected by the proliferation of cells of the primitive thyroid anlage because of the low proliferation rate of the cells in the thyroid primordium. Other cells from the pharyngeal endoderm could have been recruited into the developing thyroid, thus contributing to the expansion of the thyroid bud.[5]

By E12 to 12.5, the thyroid bud continues its downward migration and begins to expand laterally. At this stage, intense cell proliferation is detectable in the thyroid primordium. At E13 to 14, the developing thyroid reaches its definitive pretracheal position and joins with the UBBs which, in turn, have completed their ventrocaudal migration from the fourth pharyngeal pouch. The two rudimentary paratracheal lobes expand by E15 to 16 and the thyroid gland assumes its definitive shape; at the same time, TFCs start organizing into cords of cells, forming small rudimentary follicles. In late fetal life (E17 to 18), the thyroid increases in size and its parenchyma is organized into small follicles, surrounded by a capillary network, and enclosing thyroglobulin in their lumen.

In humans, thyroid morphogenesis follows essentially the same patterns as in mice (Table 2-1).[6] A thickening of the floor of the pharynx, revealing the thyroid anlage, is evident by the third week of gestation. By week 4, a migrating primordium, connected to the pharynx by the thyroglossal duct, is visible. After a few days, the developing thyroid loses any connection with the pharynx and becomes a bilobed organ, which merges with the UBBs and reaches its final position in front of the trachea at week 7. By this time, TFCs begin to form the first follicular structures although the follicular organization is accomplished only by weeks 10 to 12. In humans, the thyroid continues to grow until birth; in addition, the hypothalamic-pituitary-thyroid axis starts functioning at midgestation. On the contrary, in mice, the hypothalamic-pituitary axis is fully active only after birth.

Table 2–1 Chronology of Thyroid Organogenesis in Humans and Mice

Event	EMBRYONIC DAY (E)	
	Humans	Mice
Thyroid anlage appears	20-22	8.5
Thyroid primordium buds from floor of pharynx and begins to migrate	26-28	9.5-10
Thyroglossal duct starts to break	32-34	11-11.5
Median primordium appears as bilobed structure	34-38	12.5-13
Median primordium fuses with ultimobranchial bodies	44-46	14
Thyroid migration complete	46-50	14.5
First follicles containing colloid become visible; beginning of thyroid hormone synthesis	70-80	16-16.5

DIFFERENTIATION OF THYROID FOLLICULAR CELLS

Origin and Specification

As noted, the adult thyroid gland in mammals is assembled from two different embryologic structures, the thyroid anlage and UBBs. This double origin reflects the composite cell population of the gland.[7] According to this picture, TFCs are endodermal cells derived from the thyroid anlage and C cells originate from neural crest cells that have colonized UBBs.[8,9]

The different lineage of the endocrine thyroid cells can be considered reasonably proved in fish and birds, in which thyroxine- and calcitonin-producing cells are found in separate gland organs. Studies of chick quail chimeras[9] have demonstrated that avian C-cell precursors originate from the neural crest and which have colonized UBBs; in addition, lineage studies in zebrafish have shown that all TCFs derive from endodermal cells of the thyroid anlage.[10] These assumptions have not yet been proved in mice and humans, in whom thyroid primordium and UBBs merge in the definitive gland. The ectodermal origin of C cells in mice has been recently questioned[11] and it has been proposed that these cells can be derived from the endodermal epithelium of the fourth pharyngeal pouch. Furthermore, although it is clear that TFCs derive mostly from the thyroid anlage, some evidenced has suggested that the epithelial cells of UBBs can also contribute to the follicular cells. As an example, in mutant murine models in which UBBs fail to fuse with the thyroid bud (persistent UBB), the size of the thyroid appears smaller than would be expected if only C cells were missing.[12-14,15]

The differentiation of thyroid follicular cells is initiated when a group of endodermal cells, acquiring specific signatures that distinguish them from their neighbors, are recruited to establish the thyroid anlage. This process, called thyroid specification, is a consequence of the foregut regionalization. The specific genes required to induce thyroid fate are unknown and murine models are not useful for the study of this process. The inactivation of genes involved in foregut patterning generally causes the death of the embryos at stages that preclude assessment of thyroid specification. However, evidence obtained from other models could be valuable for the study of the early steps of thyroid development.

Although in zebrafish the morphology of the thyroid gland differs from that in mice or humans, fish and mammals probably use the same molecular mechanisms to accomplish the differentiation of the TCFs.[16] It is possible to hypothesize that H proteins such as Nodal, members of the Gata, Fgf, or Sox family, which are involved in the regionalization of the foregut, could be required for the formation of the thyroid anlage. In zebrafish, Bon and Gata5, two transcription factors downstream of Nodal signaling, both seem to be specifically required for thyroid bud specification because in the absence of either of these, thyroid cells are never detected.[17]

Undifferentiated endodermal cells could be specified toward their thyroid fate as a result of short-range inductive signals from the mesenchyma or adjacent cardiac mesoderm, or from the endothelial lining of the adjacent aortic sac. Signals from the cardiac mesoderm are relevant to the development of endodermal organs, such as the liver and lung[18]; in addition, foregut defects can be secondary to an impaired heart development.[19] In mice, the thyroid anlage forms in the primitive pharynx adjacent to the heart mesoderm.[5] This spatial correlation is conserved also in zebrafish.[20] In this species it has been demonstrated that the expression in the cardiac mesoderm of the transcription factor *han* is required for thyroid development.[21] This finding suggests a central role of heart development in thyroid specification. Interestingly, in humans, DiGeorge syndrome is characterized by congenital heart defects and an increased risk of congenital hypothyroidism.[22] In addition, cardiac malformations represent the most frequent birth defects associated with thyroid dysgenesis.[23]

Early Events in Thyroid Cell Differentiation

From E8.5 in mice and E32 in humans, the endodermal cells present in the thyroid anlage can be already considered as the precursors of the TFCs. A specific molecular signature, the coexpression of four transcription factors—*Hhex*,[24] *Titf1/Nkx2-1*,[25] *Pax8*[25] and *Foxe1*[26]—distinguishes these cells from the other cells of the primitive pharynx. It is worth noting that each of these transcription factors is also expressed in other tissues, but such a combination is a unique hallmark of differentiated thyroid follicular cells and their precursors.[7,27] Their expression is downregulated only after transformation of TFCs.[28] Studies of animal models and patients affected by thyroid dysgenesis have indicated that these factors are essential for the development of the thyroid.[7] In the absence of Titf1/Nkx2-1, Hhex, Pax8, or Foxe1, the thyroid anlage is correctly formed but the subsequent thyroid morphogenesis is severely impaired.[29] The presence of Titf1/Nkx2-1,[30,31] Hhex,[32] and Pax8[33] is required for the survival of the TFC precursors, whereas in the absence of Foxe1, the thyroid primordium disappears or remains in an ectopic sublingual position.[34] Although much evidence has suggested that these transcription factors play individual roles in the organogenesis of the gland, a complex network of reciprocal regulatory interactions among Titf1/Nkx2-1, Hhex, and Pax8 has been demonstrated in the developing thyroid. Each controls the maintenance of expression of the other factors. In addition, the simultaneous presence of Titf1/Nkx2-1, Hhex, and Pax8 is required for the expression of *Foxe1*, suggesting that Foxe1 is located downstream in the thyroid regulatory network.[29] These findings are consistent with data obtained in studies of the developing human thyroid. In humans, TFC precursors are identified by the presence of both TITF1/NKX2-1 and PAX8 at E32, and FOXE1 appears 1day later.[35]

Shortly after specification, the thyroid primordium begins to migrate to reach the sublaryngeal position.[4] Budding and translocation from the gut tube is a developmental process shared by many endoderm-derived organs.[36] In the case of the thyroid, this process mostly involves active migration of the precursors.[29] However, other morphogenetic events occurring in the neck region and in the mouth could also contribute to thyroid translocation.[37] Foxe1 plays a crucial role in the active migration of TFC precursors because the presence of this factor in the thyroid bud is absolutely required to allow the cells to move.[7,29] Foxe1 probably controls the expression of key molecules required for migration. Cell migration is a phenomenon observed in many relevant events during embryogenesis, such as gastrulation, neural crest migration, and heart formation. In these cases, the cells, during the process of migration, undergo a phenomenon called epithelial-mesenchymal transition (EMT).[38] They lose their epithelial phenotype, as shown by a downregulation of E-cadherin, and acquire mesenchymal features, characterized by an increased expression of N-cadherin. However, it should be stressed that EMT has never been reported in the case of migration of TFC precursors. TFC precursors maintain an epithelial phenotype throughout the entire translocation process and never acquire a mesenchymal identity.[39]

Late Events in Thyroid Cell Differentiation

From E14 in mice and week 7 in humans, the last phase of thyroid development is initiated. This phase will be completed at birth in mice and at about week 10 in humans. During this time, the gland expands and acquires its definitive shape, two lobes connected by an isthmus. In addition, TFC precursors, completing their differentiation, become functional follicular cells. These processes begin after the thyroid primordium has reached the sublaryngeal position. However, the finding that ectopic thyroids are functional in mice and in humans indicates that the correct location of the developing thyroid is not a prerequisite for the final differentiation of TCF precursors.[34]

The molecular mechanisms leading to the formation of the two lateral lobes of the gland (lobulation) are now beginning to be understood. In mouse embryos deprived of the Sonic hedgehog gene *(Shh),* a key regulator of embryogenesis, the correct patterning of the vessels is disturbed and the developing thyroid appears as a single midline tissue mass located laterally to the trachea.[40] It is most likely that the impaired thyroid morphogenesis is secondary to Shh-dependent defective patterning of vessels. This hypothesis seems to be confirmed by analyzing the phenotype of *Tbx* null embryos, which also display impaired lobulation of thyroid.[41] In these mutant embryos, as a consequence of the absence of caudal pharyngeal arch arteries, the thyroid primordium is enclosed by the mesenchyme and is never in close contact with vessels. It is worth noting that both *Shh* and *Tbx* are expressed in the tissues surrounding the developing thyroid and are never detectable in the thyroid itself. Hence, thyroid lobulation is a non–cell autonomous process controlled by inductive signals originating from adjacent structures, mainly the vessels located close to the thyroid tissue. This hypothesis is consistent with the finding that impaired thyroid morphogenesis has been reported in human diseases such as DiGeorge syndrome[22] and truncus arteriosus syndrome, characterized by congenital anomalies of the heart and great vessels.[42]

The fully functional differentiation of TFCs, hallmarked by the synthesis of thyroxine, is achieved through a differentiative program characterized by the expression of a number of genes, such as thyroglobulin (*Tg*), thyroid-stimulating hormone receptor (*Tshr*), thyroid peroxidase (*TPO*), sodium-iodide symporter (*NIS*), thyroid reduced nicotinamide adenine dinucleotide phosphate (NADPH), oxidase (*Duox*), and pendrin (*PDS*) genes. These genes are not activated simultaneously but follow a precise temporal pattern that begins with the expression of *Tg* and *Thsr* at E14 and week 7 in mice[25] and humans,[6] respectively. The expression of *TPO* and *NIS*, the two key enzymes involved in the process of Tg iodination, follows the expression of *Tg* and *Tshr*. A possible mechanism for the delayed expression of *TPO* and *Nis* is their dependence on the pathway activated by the binding of TSH to its receptor, Tshr.[43] As expected, Tshr is not necessary for the onset of Tg.[43] Duox appears at E15.5 but its expression is not dependent on TSH-Tshr signals.[44] The differentiative program is completed in 3 days in mice (thyroxine is present at E16.5 and in 3 weeks in humans), in which thyroxine has been detected at about week 10.[6]

In the last stages of thyroid organogenesis, E17 to 18 in mice, the gland expands, probably because of the high proliferation of TCFs. At the same time, small follicles that are accumulating thyroglobulin in the lumen, and surrounded by a capillary network, appear.[5] In humans, follicular organization is evident after 10 to 11 weeks of gestation[6] and the thyroid continues to grow until birth.

The growth of the thyroid continues after birth. In both humans and mice, TSH-Tshr signaling controls the growth of the adult thyroid. Conversely, at least in mice, signals triggered by TSH do not seem to be relevant for the expansion of the fetal thyroid.[46] The mechanisms controlling the growth of fetal TCFs are still unknown.

MOLECULAR GENETICS

In the early 1990s, two transcription factors, Titf1/Nkx2-1 and Pax8, whose expression is restricted to the developing thyroid and a few other tissues, were identified for the first time. This discovery made it possible to begin the study of the molecular genetics of thyroid development. In the last few years, a number of genes involved in thyroid morphogenesis have been identified, mainly because of the availability of genetically modified mice. Furthermore, the study of patients affected by thyroid dysgenesis is also offering additional insights into the molecular mechanisms involved in normal thyroid development. Here we will describe

Table 2–2 Chromosomal Localization and Expression Patterns of Genes Encoding Thyroid-Specific Transcription Factors

GENE		CHROMOSOME		EXPRESSION PATTERN IN EMBRYOS	
Humans	Mice	Humans	Mice	Humans	Mice
TITF1/NKX2-1	*Titf1/Nkx2-1*	14q13	12	Thyroid, lungs, diencephalon	Thyroid, lungs, diencephalon, fourth pharyngeal pouch, C cells
PAX8	*Pax8*	2q12-14	2	Thyroid, myelencephalon and spinal cord, otic vesicle, fourth pharyngeal pouch, nephrogenic cord, mesonephric tubules, ureteric bud	Thyroid, myelencephalon and spinal cord, otic vesicle, nephrogenic cord, mesonephric tubules
FOXE1	*Foxe1*	9q22	4	Thyroid, thymus, hair follicles, esophagus	Thyroid, foregut, palate, choanae, hair follicles, esophagus

only those genes that are particularly relevant to the development and differentiation of the thyroid.

Hhex

The *Hhex* gene is located on chromosome 19 in mice[47] and on chromosome 10q23.32 in humans.[48] The gene encodes a 270–amino acid transcription factor containing a homeodomain. At early stages of mouse development, *Hhex* is detected in the primitive and then in the definitive endoderm. At later stages, it is expressed in the developing blood islands, endothelium of the developing vasculature and heart, and primordia of several organs derived from the foregut endoderm, including the thyroid anlage.[24]

Hhex has a crucial role in the morphogenesis of the liver, forebrain, heart, and thyroid, as demonstrated from the analysis of the *Hhex* null mouse embryos.[32] In these mutant embryos, TFC precursors are present and express *Titf1/Nkx2-1, Pax8,* and *Foxe1* until E9. However, 1 day later, the developing thyroid appears as a hypoplastic bud composed of a few cells, which do not express *Titf1/Nkx2-1, Pax8,* or *Foxe1* mRNA, and then TFC precursors are found to disappear.[29] Hence, Hhex guarantees the survival of TFC precursors and maintains the expression of other thyroid-specific transcription factors. However, we cannot state definitively that the absence of these factors is the direct cause of the thyroid phenotype displayed by $Hhex^{-/-}$ embryos.

No *Hhex* mutations associated with thyroid diseases have been described so far in humans.

Titf1/Nkx2-1

Titf1/Nkx2-1 was formerly called TTF-1, for thyroid transcription factor-1, or T/EBP, thyroid-specific enhancer-binding protein. It is a homeodomain containing transcription factor that belongs to the Nkx-2 family of transcription factors. In mice, Titf1/Nkx2-1 is encoded by a gene located on chromosome 12, whereas the human orthologue, *TITF1/NKX2-1,* is located on chromosome 14q13.[49] Multiple transcripts have been identified of which the major transcripts, 2.3 and 2.5 kb, encode proteins 401 and 371 amino acids long, respectively.[50] The most abundant protein is the shorter isoform that is phosphorylated in several serine residues. As described for other transcription factors, the phosphorylation could be a regulatory mechanism to modulate its binding and transactivating properties. Mutated mice in which phosphorylated serine residues have been replaced by alanine residues show impaired differentiation of both thyroid and lung, thus confirming the relevant role of post-translation modifications of Titf1/Nkx2-1.[51]

In the mouse embryo, *Titf1/Nkx2-1* is expressed in the thyroid primordium and in the epithelial cells of the developing trachea, lungs, and brain.[25] *Titf1/Nkx2-1* is expressed in the brain in some areas of the developing diencephalon, such as the hypothalamic areas and the infundibulum, from which the neurohypophysis develops.[25] In the developing thyroid, Titf1/Nkx2-1 is detectable in TCF precursors and also in other cells—C cells[52] and epithelial cells of the ultimobranchial body[33]—which merge with the thyroid anlage to assemble the definitive thyroid gland. In the adult thyroid, *Titf1/Nkx2-1* maintains its expression in follicular and parafollicular cells. The expression pattern of *TITF1/NKX2-1* in humans does not appear different from that described in mice (Table 2-2), except that *TITF1/NKX2-1* is not expressed in humans in the fourth pharyngeal pouches from which the ultimobranchial body develops.[35]

Table 2–3 Consequence of Loss-of-Function Mutations in Genes Encoding Thyroid Specific Transcription Factors

Defective Gene	HETEROZYGOUS THYROID PHENOTYPE		HOMOZYGOUS THYROID PHENOTYPE	
	Humans	Mice	Humans	Mice
Titf1/Nkx2-1	Variable, ranging from a normal-sized gland to athyreosis	Slight hyperthyrotropinemia	Not reported	Athyreosis
Pax8	Variable, ranging from a normal-sized gland to a severe hypoplasia	Normal	Not reported	Athyreosis
Foxe1	Normal	Normal	Athyreosis or hypoplasia of thyroid	Athyreosis or ectopic thyroid

The functions of Titf1/Nkx2-1 in vivo have been studied in mice, in which the corresponding gene has been disrupted by homologous recombination. Because mice die at birth in the absence of Titf1/Nkx2-1, its role can be elucidated only during embryonic life. *Titf1/Nkx2-1*$^{-/-}$ embryos show an impaired morphogenesis of all the structures that normally express the factor, suggesting that Titf1/Nkx2-1 is essential for the correct development of the thyroid, lungs, and brain.[30] Until E9, the development of the thyroid anlage is not affected by the absence of Titf1/Nkx2-1; at E10, in the mutants, the thyroid bud appears hypoplastic and TFC precursors show reduced or lack of expression of *Pax8, Foxe1,* and *Hhex.*[29] At E11, the thyroid bud disappears, probably through apoptosis.[31] Calcitonin-producing cells and epithelial cells of the ultimobranchial body follow the same fate of TFCs; ultimobranchial bodies form but degenerate by E12.[53] Thus, Titf1/Nkx2-1 is not required for the specification of cell types that will form the thyroid but, in its absence, neither the follicular nor parafollicular cells develop. This could be why no thyroid rudiment is visible in *Titf1/Nkx2-1* null newborns. In the case of the lung, Titf1/Nkx2-1 does not seem to be required for the initial specification because the lung bud as well as lung lobar bronchi are visible in *Titf1/Nkx2-1* null embryos. However, the branching process of bronchi, which starts by E12.5, is impaired and, as a result, the lungs develop as dilated saclike structures, without normal pulmonary parenchyma.[30] In *Titf1/Nkx2-1* null embryos, in addition to the lung defects, the absence of Titf1/Nkx2-1 causes two peculiar alterations in trachea development—the number of cartilage rings of the trachea is reduced and this structure is not separated from the esophagus, but a shared tube is visible.[54]

The consequences of the absence of Titf1/Nkx2-1 on brain development are rather complex. *Titf1/Nkx2-1* null embryos show evident alterations in the ventral region of the forebrain. The development of the pallidal structures is impaired and the pallidal primordium appears as a striatum-like structure.[55] In addition, *Titf1/Nkx2-1* null embryos have neither pituitary nor adrenal glands. In the absence of Titf1/Nkx2-1 in the infundibulum of the diencephalon, the development of neurohypophysis is blocked, causing the regression of Rathke's pouch, which normally gives rise to the anterior hypophysis. Finally, the lack of endocrine signals from the pituitary could affect the morphogenesis of adrenal glands.[30]

TITF1/NKX2-1 AND CONGENITAL HYPOTHYROIDISM

Heterozygous point mutations or chromosomal deletions in the *TITF1/NKX2-1* locus have been reported in subjects with thyroid affections associated with respiratory distress and neurologic problems.[56-62] In these patients, choreoathetosis is the most frequent neurologic defect. In accordance with this finding, numerous data point to the identification of *TITF1/NKX2-1* as the candidate gene in benign hereditary chorea, an autosomal dominant movement disorder.[63] Homozygous *TITF1/NKX2-1* mutations have not been reported in humans. Although loss of function of a single allele in humans produces an overt phenotype, the *Titf1/Nkx2-1*$^{+/-}$ mice (Table 2-3) show mild neurologic defects and a slight hyperthyrotropinemia.[60] The mechanisms explaining the dominant effect of *TITF1/NKX2-1* have not yet been delineated. The reduction of levels of functional TITF1/NKX2-1 protein remains the most likely mechanism that causes the disease. *TITF1/NKX2-1*$^{+/-}$ subjects display a highly variable thyroid phenotype. This variability could be caused by other modifier genes that contribute to the phenotype. There is no clear correlation between the phenotype severity and the type of mutations; in addition, a variable phenotype has also been reported in the same familial cluster.

Pax8

Pax8 belongs to the Pax family of transcription factors. In mice, Pax8 is encoded by a gene located on chromosome 2, whereas the human orthologue, *PAX8,* is located on chromosome 2q12-q14.[64] The gene is split into 12 exons[65]; alternative splicing produces transcripts that differ in their carboxy-terminal regions. At least six different Pax8 variants have been identified in mice and five in humans. The longest isoform is composed of 457 and 450 amino acids in mice[66] and humans,[67] respectively. It has been demonstrated that the expression of different isoforms is temporally and spatially regulated during early mouse development. Furthermore, Pax8 isoforms display different transactivating activities when tested in cell lines.

Pax8 is expressed in the thyroid, kidneys, and nervous system.[66] In the thyroid anlage, it is expressed only in TFCs precursors. In the developing kidney, Pax8 is expressed in the nephrogenic cord and mesonephric tubules and, by E13, in epithelial structures generated on induction by the nephric duct and ureter. In the nervous system, Pax8 is expressed in the myelencephalon, developing spinal cord, otic vesicle, and at the midbrain-hindbrain boundary, but is no longer detected by E12.5.[66] The pattern of *PAX8* expression in human embryos is similar to that in mouse embryos (see Table 2-2); *PAX8* is detected in the developing thyroid, kidneys, otic vesicle, and central nervous system at E32.[35]

In vitro studies have indicated that TSH-induced signals can regulate Pax8 expression in TFCs. However, it is worth noting that the TSH control on Pax8 expression seems to be effective only in adult TFCs, because in the developing thyroid of mice harboring severe alterations in TSH/Tshr signaling, the presence of Pax8 expression is not affected.[43]

The study of the phenotype of Pax8 null mice suggests that the absence of Pax8 apparently affects only the thyroid. These mutant mice are born without any apparent brain or kidney defects.[33] It has been proposed that kidney organogenesis is normal in Pax8 null mice because of the presence of Pax2. Pax8 and Pax2 share many biochemical features and could have redundant functions during morphogenesis of the kidneys.[68] On the contrary, thyroid development is impaired in the absence of Pax8. At birth, the gland appears as a rudimentary structure composed only of C cells, whereas TFCs are undetectable. Consistent with a severe hypothyroid phenotype, the pups show growth retardation and die after weaning. The administration of thyroxine to these mice leads to their survival, confirming that severe hypothyroidism has caused their death. An exhaustive analysis of thyroid development in Pax8 null embryos offers some insights into the functional role of this factor. At E9, the thyroid anlage is correctly formed in its proper position and begins to migrate but, at E11, both the morphologic and molecular phenotypes of the developing thyroid change. The thyroid bud is much smaller, the expression of *Foxe1* and *Hhex* is strongly downregulated and, finally, by E12.5, TFC precursors are still not detected.[29] This indicates that in the developing thyroid, Pax8 is involved in the control of survival and/or expansion of TFC precursors, although we do not know the target genes that execute this program. In addition, Pax8 has a specific upper role in the genetic network that maintains the expression of other thyroid-enriched transcription factors. In TFC precursors, *Foxe1* is tightly regulated by Pax8, which is necessary for the onset of its expression. This indicates that *Foxe1* can be a transcriptional target of Pax8.[29]

PAX8 AND CONGENITAL HYPOTHYROIDISM

In humans, heterozygous mutations in *PAX8* have been reported in sporadic and familial cases of congenital hypothyroidism with thyroid dysgenesis. All affected individuals are heterozygous for the mutations and the familial cases show an autosomal dominant transmission of the disease. This indicates that in humans, loss of function of a single allele is sufficient to produce the disease (see Table 2-3). This feature is evident in humans only, because $Pax8^{+/-}$ mice do not show any phenotype. The reason for the dominant effect caused by *PAX8* mutations is unknown. A pathogenic role of the reduced dosage of the gene product (haploinsufficiency) has been proposed, but allele-specific regulation has been also suggested. The thyroid phenotype is variable, ranging from a normal-sized gland to a severe hypoplasia. Because the phenotype shows discrepancy, even in familial cases in which related individuals carry the same mutation, effects of other modifier genes could be hypothesized. In two patients, renal hemiagenesis has been reported.[69] However, in these subjects, additional gene defects could not be excluded. Pax8-deficient mice show renal malformations only if they harbor a concomitant heterozygous null mutation for Pax2 gene.[68]

Foxe1

Foxe1, formerly called TTF-2, thyroid transcription factor-2, is encoded by a gene located on chromosome 4 in mice.[26] The human orthologue, *FOXE1,* is located on chromosome 9q22.[70] Foxe1 is a phosphorylated 42-kD protein[71] that is a member of the winged helix–forkhead family of transcription factors. The most frequent allele, in humans, contains 14 alanine residues and is 371 amino acids long.[72]

Foxe1 is widely expressed in mouse embryos. It is detected early in the thyroid anlage, in the endodermal layer of the primitive pharynx and pharyngeal arches and in Rathke's pouch.[26] At E15, *Foxe1* is expressed in tissues that have developed from the pharynx and pharyngeal arches, the thyroid, tongue, epiglottis, palate, choanae, and esophagus. Foxe1 is also present in ectoderm derivatives such as whiskers and hair follicles.[71] In humans, in addition to the thyroid and foregut, *FOXE1* expression (see Table 2-2) is also found in the embryonic thymus,[35] outer follicular hair sheath, and seminiferous tubules of the prepubertal testis.[73] The expression of *Foxe1* is subjected to spatial regulation; *Foxe1* is tightly regulated in the thyroid bud by Pax8 and in the pharyngeal cells by Shh.

The generation of mice with *Foxe1* disrupted by homologous recombination has been a tool for studying the role of this factor in vivo.[34] In mutant mouse embryos, the thyroid anlage is correctly specified at E8.5, but it still remains on the pharyngeal floor. At E11to 11.5, the normal thyroid primordium is close to the aortic arch. At the same stage, in the absence of Foxe1, the nonmigrating phenotype is more evident, with the developing thyroid in the form of a group of cells attached to the pharyngeal floor. The phenotype is variable at E15.5, showing either the presence of a severely hypoplastic thyroid, located in a sublingual position, or the absence of the thyroid bud itself. This finding suggests that Foxe1 is involved not only in the translocation of TFC precursors but also in the survival of TFCs.[29,34]

FOXE1 AND CONGENITAL HYPOTHYROIDISM

In humans, the homozygous loss-of-function mutation *FOXE1* gene was first reported[74] in two siblings affected by syndromic congenital hypothyroidism characterized by athyreosis, cleft palate, bilateral choanal atresia, and spiky hair (Bamfort-Lazarus syndrome[75]). The phenotype is consistent with the expression domain of *FOXE1* and partially overlaps that displayed by *Foxe1* null mice (see Table 2-3).

After this report, a different mutation in *FOXE1* was recorded in two siblings with athyreosis and a less severe extrathyroidal phenotype.[76] Recently, a third loss-of-function mutation within the *FOXE1* forkhead domain was described[77] in a child displaying extrathyroidal defects (cleft palate, bilateral choanal atresia, and spiky hair) and congenital hypothyroidism but not athyreosis; actually, the patient presented with eutopic thyroid tissue. The variable thyroid phenotype displayed by patients carrying *FOXE1* mutations could be the result of different effects of the various mutations. Another possibility is the role of modifier genes in making the phenotype manifest.

Tshr

Tshr (thyroid-stimulating hormone receptor) is a member of the glycoprotein hormone receptor family.[78] The *Tshr* gene is located on chromosome 12 in mice[79] and the human orthologue, *TSHR*, is located on chromosome 14q31.[80] The gene, made up of 10 exons, is translated in a protein 765 amino acids long, expressed on the basolateral membrane of TFCs. In the mouse embryo, *Tshr* is detected in TFC precursors by E14 to 14.5.[25,81] At later stages of development, *Tshr* expression increases and remains expressed in adult life.

The role of TSH/Tshr signaling during embryonic life has been studied in genetically modified mice, in which the *Tshr* gene has been disrupted by homologous recombination ($Tshr^{-/-}$),[82] and in spontaneous mutant mice carrying a loss-of-function mutation in the *Tshr* gene ($Tshr^{hyt/hyt}$).[83] E16 mouse embryos deprived of TSH/Tshr signaling do not show defects in the morphology of the gland, which displays a normal size and follicular structure. However, both TPO and NIS are undetectable in TFCs; this finding demonstrates that the TSH pathway is absolutely required for the differentiation process of the thyroid.[43] It is worth noting that although the Tshr pathway becomes active by E15, when the expansion of the fetal thyroid also begins, this signaling is not relevant for the growth of the gland. This is in contrast with the role of TSH/Tshr signals in differentiated TFC, in which the TSH-induced cAMP pathway is the main regulator of thyroid growth. Both $Tshr^{-/-}$ and $Tshr^{hyt/hyt}$ mice display a severe hypoplastic adult thyroid,[43,82] whereas at birth the gland appears normal. However the requirements for the development of a normal-sized thyroid gland seem to be different between mice and humans; in the latter, the role of TSH/Tshr signaling for the growth of the thyroid is also relevant during fetal life.[46]

TSHR AND CONGENITAL HYPOTHYROIDISM

Loss-of-function mutations in the *TSHR* gene are responsible for a syndrome characterized by elevated levels of TSH in serum, a normal or hypoplastic gland, and variable levels of thyroid hormones.[84] Notably, several years ago, before *TSHR* was cloned and identified, Stanbury and colleagues[85] suggested that an impaired response to TSH could be responsible for congenital hypothyroidism in the absence of goiter. *TSHR* mutations have been identified in a number of families. Individuals carrying heterozygous loss-of-function mutations are euthyroid, even though most of them present with borderline elevations of TSH. Subjects homozygous or compound heterozygous for the mutation are affected; the disease is transmitted as an autosomal recessive trait displaying a variable phenotype, ranging from hyperthyrotropinemia associated with a normal gland to severe hypothyroidism with a hypoplastic gland.[86] The residual functional activity of the mutant TSHR could be responsible for the differing severity of the phenotype.

CONCLUSIONS

Over the past 15 years, the efforts of many research groups have led to the elucidation of many of the steps involved in thyroid development, even if crucial issues of this process are still unknown.

1. It is worth noting that many genes relevant for thyroid development have been identified; mutations in some of these genes are associated with thyroid dysgenesis (TD) in mice and humans. This finding indicates that TD is caused by inheritable genetic defects, albeit in only a small fraction of human patients.
2. However, in most patients, the genetic defects underlying TD are yet to be discovered. In addition, the discordance for TD, occurring in 12 of 13 monozygotic twins,[87] suggests that nonmendelian events must be considered as responsible for most cases of the disease.[88]
3. Despite the fact that Titf1/Nkx2-1, Hhex, Pax8, and Foxe1 are detected in the developing thyroid by E8.5, their absence does not affect the specification process. The prime mover of the initial specification of the thyroid anlage is obscure—candidate genes may be those still unidentified encoding factors responsible for the onset of *Titf1/Nkx2-1*, *Pax8*, and *Hhex* expression in the thyroid bud.
4. Titf1/Nkx2-1, Hhex, Pax8, and Foxe1 are transcription factors that control the expression of downstream genes that execute the differentiating program of the thyroid gland. Most of these target genes have not yet been identified.
5. The mechanisms regulating the shape and position of the gland are still a matter of debate. Recent evidence has suggested that the determination of the final shape of the thyroid gland requires autonomous events, restricted to the thyroid follicular cells, that must interact with an appropriate cellular environment.

Defects in several genes have been demonstrated to impair the development of the thyroid in animal models (Table 2-4). In humans, 85% of cases of congenital hypothyroidism are caused by thyroid dysgenesis,[89] which is a consequence of disturbances during thyroid organogenesis. The identification of new genes and mechanisms involved in thyroid development will be valuable to elucidate the molecular pathology of thyroid dysgenesis.

Table 2–4 Mouse Models of Thyroid Dysgenesis

Gene Symbol	Thyroid Phenotype in Mouse Embryos Homozygous for Null Mutations
Hhex	Athyreosis
Titf1	
Pax8	
Fgfr2	
Fgf10	
Foxe1	Athyreosis or ectopia
Hoxa3	Hypoplasia
Eya 1	
Edn-1	
Pax3	
Tbx1	Hypoplasia and impaired lobulation
Shh	
Tshr	Hypoplasia and defects in functional differentiation
Hoxa5	Defects in functional differentiation

References

1. Fukuda KY, Kikuchi Y: Endoderm development in vertebrates: Fate mapping, induction and regional specification. Dev Growth Differ 47:343-355, 2005.
2. Grapin-Botton A, Melton M: Endoderm development: From patterning to organogenesis. Trends Genet 16:124-130, 2000.
3. Shivdasani RA: Molecular regulation of vertebrate early endoderm development. Dev Biol 249:191-203, 2002.
4. Kaufman MH, Bard J: The thyroid. In Kaufman MH, Bard J (eds): The Anatomic Basis of Mouse Development. San Diego, Calif, Academic Press, 1999, pp 165-166.
5. Fagman H, Andersson L, Nilsson M: The developing mouse thyroid: Embryonic vessel contacts and parenchymal growth pattern during specification, budding, migration, and lobulation. Dev Dyn 235:444-455, 2006.
6. Polak M, Sura-Trueba S, Chauty A, et al: Molecular mechanisms of thyroid dysgenesis. Horm Res 62:14-21, 2004.

7. De Felice M, Di Lauro R: Thyroid development and its disorders: Genetics and molecular mechanisms. Endocr Rev 25:722-746, 2004.
8. Fontaine J: Multistep migration of calcitonine cell precursors during ontogeny of the mouse pharynx. Gen Comp Endocrinol 37:81-92, 1979.
9. Le Douarin N, Fontaine J, LeLievre C: New studies on the neural crest origin of the avian ultimobranchial glandular cells. Interspecific combinations and cytochemical characterization of C cells based on the uptake of biogenic amine precursors. Histochemie 38:297-305, 1974.
10. Alt B, Reibe S, Feitosa NM, et al: Analysis of origin and growth of the thyroid gland in zebrafish. Dev Dyn 235:1872-1883, 2006.
11. Kameda Y, Nishimaki T, Chisaka O, et al: Expression of the epithelial marker E-cadherin by thyroid C cells and their precursors during murine development. Histochem Cytochem 55:1075-1088, 2007.
12. Chisaka O, Musci TS, Capecchi MR: Developmental defects of the ear, cranial nerves and hindbrain resulting from targeted disruption of the mouse homeobox gene Hox-1.6. Nature 355:516-520, 1992.
13. Manley NR, Capecchi M: The role of Hoxa-3 in mouse thymus and thyroid development. Development 121:1989-2003, 1995.
14. Manley NR, Capecchi M: Hox group 3 paralogs regulate the development and migration of the thymus, thyroid, and parathyroid glands. Dev Biol 195:1-15, 1998.
15. Xu PX, Zheng W, Laclef C, et al: Eya1 is required for the morphogenesis of mammalian thymus, parathyroid and thyroid. Development 129:1033-1044, 2002.
16. Wendl T, Lun K, Mione M, et al: Pax2.1 is required for the development of thyroid follicles in zebrafish. Development 129:3751-3760, 2002.
17. Elsalini OA, von Gartzen J, Cramer M, Rohr KB: Zebrafish hhex, nk2.1a, and pax2.1 regulate thyroid growth and differentiation downstream of Nodal-dependent transcription factors. Dev Biol 263:67-80, 2003.
18. Lammert E, Cleaver O, Melton D: Role of endothelial cells in early pancreas and liver development. Mech Dev 120:35-43, 2003.
19. Cai CL, Liang X, Shi Y, et al: Isl1 identifies a cardiac progenitor population that proliferates prior to differentiation and contributes a majority of cells to the heart. Dev Cell 5:877-889, 2003.
20. Alt B, Elsalini OA, Schrumpf P, et al: Arteries define the position of the thyroid gland during its developmental relocalisation. Development 133:3797-3804, 2006.
21. Wendl T, Adzic D, Schoenebeck JJ, et al: Early developmental specification of the thyroid gland depends on han-expressing surrounding tissue and on FGF signals. Development 134:2871-2879, 2007.
22. Burke BA, Johnson D, Gilbert EF, et al: Thyrocalcitonin-containing cells in the DiGeorge anomaly. Hum Pathol 4:355-360, 1987.
23. Olivieri A, Stazi MA, Mastroiacovo P, et al: A population-based study on the frequency of additional congenital malformations in infants with congenital hypothyroidism: Data from the Italian Registry for Congenital Hypothyroidism (1991-1998). J Clin Endocrinol Metab 87:557-562, 2002.
24. Thomas PQ, Brown A, Beddington R: Hex: A homeobox gene revealing peri-implantation asymmetry in the mouse embryo and an early transient marker of endothelial cell precursors. Development 125:85-95, 1998.
25. Lazzaro D, Price M, De Felice M, Di Lauro R: The transcription factor TTF-1 is expressed at the onset of thyroid and lung morphogenesis and in restricted regions of the foetal brain. Development 113:1093-1104, 1991.
26. Zannini MV, Avantaggiato E, Biffali M, et al: TTF-2, a new forkhead protein, shows a temporal expression in the developing thyroid which is consistent with a role in controlling the onset of differentiation. EMBO J 16:3185-3197, 1997.
27. Damante G, Tell G, Di Lauro R: A unique combination of transcription factors controls differentiation of thyroid cells. Prog Nucleic Acid Res Mol Biol 66:307-356, 2001.
28. Francis-Lang H, Zannini MS, De Felice M, et al: Multiple mechanisms of interference between transformation and differentiation in thyroid cells. Mol Cell Biol 12:5793-5800, 1992.
29. Parlato R, Rosica A, Rodriguez-Mallon A, et al: An integrated regulatory network controlling survival and migration in thyroid organogenesis. Dev Biol 276:464-475, 2004.
30. Kimura S, Hara Y, Pineau T, et al: The T/ebp null mouse: Thyroid-specific enhancer-binding protein is essential for the organogenesis of the thyroid, lung, ventral forebrain, and pituitary. Genes Dev 10:60-69, 1996.
31. Kimura S, Ward JD, Minoo P: Thyroid-specific enhancer-binding protein/transcription factor 1 is not required for the initial specification of the thyroid and lung primordia. Biochemie 81:321-328, 1999.
32. Martinez Barbera JP, Clements M, et al: The homeobox gene Hex is required in definitive endodermal tissues for normal forebrain, liver and thyroid formation. Development 127:2433-2445, 2000.
33. Mansouri A, Chowdhury K, Gruss P: Follicular cells of the thyroid gland require Pax8 gene function. Nat Genet 19:87-90, 1998.
34. De Felice M, Ovitt C, Biffali E, et al: A mouse model for hereditary thyroid dysgenesis and cleft palate. Nat Genet 19:395-398, 1998.
35. Trueba SS, Auge J, Mattei G, et al: PAX8, TITF1 and FOXE1 gene expression patterns during human development: New insights into human thyroid development and thyroid dysgenesis associated malformations. J Clin Endocrinol Metab 90:455-462, 2004.
36. Hogan B, Zaret K: Development of the endoderm and its tissue derivatives. In Rossant J, Tam PP (eds): Mouse Development: Patterning, Morphogenesis, and Organogenesis. New York, 2002, pp 301-310.

37. Hilfer SR, Brown JW: The development of pharyngeal endocrine organs in mouse and chick embryos. Scan Electron Microsc 4:2009-2022, 1984.
38. Thiery JP, Sleeman J: Complex networks orchestrate epithelial-mesenchymal transitions. Nat Rev Mol Cell Bio 7:131-142, 2006.
39. Fagman H, Grande M, Edsbagge J, et al: Expression of classical cadherins in thyroid development: Maintenance of an epithelial phenotype throughout organogenesis. Endocrinology 144:3618-3624, 2003.
40. Fagman H, Grande M, Gritli-Linde A, Nilsson M: Genetic deletion of sonic hedgehog causes hemiagenesis and ectopic development of the thyroid in mouse. Am J Pathol 164:1865-1872, 2004.
41. Fagman H, Liao J, Westerlund J, et al: The 22q11 deletion syndrome candidate gene Tbx1 determines thyroid size and positioning. Hum Mol Genet 16:276-285, 2007.
42. Gamallo C, Garcia M, Palacios J, Rodriguez J: Decrease in calcitonin-containing cells in truncus arterious. Am J Med Genet 46:149-153, 1993.
43. Postiglione MP, Parlato R, Rodriguez-Mallon A, et al: Role of the thyroid-stimulating hormone receptor signalling in development and differentiation of the thyroid gland. Proc Natl Acad Sci U S A 99:15462-15467, 2002.
44. Milenkovic M, De Deken X, Jin L, et al: Duox expression and related H2O2 measurement in mouse thyroid: Onset in embryonic development and regulation by TSH in adult. J Endocrinol 192:615-626, 2007.
45. Meunier D, Aubin J, Jeannotte L: Perturbed thyroid morphology and transient hypothyroidism symptoms in Hoxa5 mutant mice. Dev Dyn 227:367-378, 2003.
46. De Felice M, Postiglione MP, Di Lauro R: Minireview: Thyrotropin receptor signalling in development and differentiation of the thyroid gland: Insights from mouse models and human diseases. Endocrinology 145:4062-4067, 2004.
47. Ghosh B, Jacobs HC, Wiedemann LM, et al: Genomic structure, cDNA mapping, and chromosomal localization of the mouse homeobox gene, Hex. Mamm Genome 10:1023-1025, 1999.
48. Hromas R, Radich J, Collins S: PCR cloning of an orphan homeobox gene (PRH) preferentially expressed in myeloid and liver cells. Biochem Biophys Res Commun 195:976-983, 1993.
49. Guazzi S, Price M, De Felice M, et al: Thyroid nuclear factor 1 (TTF-1) contains a homeodomain and displays a novel DNA binding specificity. EMBO J 9:3631-3639, 1990.
50. Li C, Cai J, Pan Q, Minoo M: Two functionally distinct forms of NKX2.1 protein are expressed in the pulmonary epithelium. Biochem Biophys Res Commun 270:462-468, 2000.
51. De Felice M, Silberschmidt D, DiLauro R, et al: TTF-1 phosphorylation is required for peripheral lung morphogenesis, perinatal survival, and tissue-specific gene expression. J Biol Chem 278:35574-35583, 2003.
52. Suzuki K, Kobayashi Y, Katoh R, et al: Identification of thyroid transcription factor-1 in C cells and parathyroid cells. Endocrinology 139:3014-3017, 1998.
53. Kusakabe T, Hoshi N, Kimura S: Origin of the ultimobranchial body cyst: T/ebp/Nkx2.1 expression is required for development and fusion of the ultimobranchial body to the thyroid. Dev Dyn 235:1300-1309, 2006.
54. Minoo P, Su G, Drum H, et al: Defects in tracheoesophageal and lung morphogenesis in Nkx2.1 (-/-) mouse embryos. Devel Biol 209:60-71, 1999.
55. Sussel L, Marin O, Kimura S, Rubenstein J: Loss of Nkx2.1 homeobox gene function results in a ventral to dorsal molecular respecification within the basal telencephalon: Evidence for a transformation of the pallidum into the striatum. Development 126:3359-3370, 1999.
56. Devriendt K, Vanhole C, Matthijs G, De Zegher F: Deletion of thyroid transcription factor-1 gene in an infant with neonatal thyroid dysfunction and respiratory failure. N Engl J Med 338:1317-1318, 1998.
57. Doyle DA, Gonzalez I, Thomas B, Scavina M: Autosomal dominant transmission of congenital hypothyroidism, neonatal respiratory distress, and ataxia caused by a mutation of NKX2-1. J Pediatr 145:190-193, 2004.
58. Iwatani N, Mabe H, Devriendt K, et al: Deletion of NKX2.1 gene encoding thyroid transcription factor-1 in two siblings with hypothyroidism and respiratory failure. J Pediatr 137:272-276, 2000.
59. Krude H, Schutz B, Biebermann H, et al: Choreoathetosis, hypothyroidism, and pulmonary alterations due to human NKX2-1 haploinsufficiency. J Clin Invest 109:475-480, 2002.
60. Moeller LC, Kimura S, Kusakabe T, et al: Hypothyroidism in thyroid transcription factor 1 haploinsufficiency is caused by reduced expression of the thyroid-stimulating hormone receptor. Mol Endocrinol 17:2295-2302, 2003.
61. Moya CM, Perez de Nanclares G, Castano L, et al: Functional study of a novel single deletion in the TITF1/NKX2.1 homeobox gene that produces congenital hypothyroidism and benign chorea but not pulmonary distress. Clin Endocrinol Metab 91:1832-1841, 2006.
62. Pohlenz J, Dumitrescu A, Zundel D, et al: Partial deficiency of thyroid transcription factor 1 produces predominantly neurologic defects in humans and mice. J Clin Invest 109:469-473, 2002.
63. Breedveld GJ, van Dongen JW, Danesino C, et al: Mutations in TITF-1 are associated with benign hereditary chorea. Hum Mol Genet 11:971-979, 2002.
64. Stapleton P, Weith A, Urbanek P, et al: Chromosomal localization of 7 Pax genes and cloning of a novel family member, Pax-9. Nat Genet 3:292-298, 1993.
65. Okladnova O, Poleev A, Fantes J, et al: The genomic organization of the murine Pax 8 gene and characterization of its basal promoter. Genomics 15:452-461, 1997.

66. Plachov D, Chowdhury K, Walther C, et al: Pax8, a murine paired box gene expressed in the developing excretory system and thyroid gland. Development 110:643-651, 1990.
67. Poleev A, Wendler F, Fickenscher H, et al: Distinct functional properties of three human paired-box-protein, PAX8, isoforms generated by alternative splicing in thyroid, kidney and Wilms' tumors. Eur J Biochem 228:899-911, 1995.
68. Bouchard M, Souabni A, Mandler M, et al: Nephric lineage specification by Pax2 and Pax8. Genes Dev 16:2958-2970, 2002.
69. Meeus L, Gilbert B, Rydlewski C, et al: Characterization of a novel loss of function mutation of PAX8 in a familial case of congenital hypothyroidism with in-place, normal-sized thyroid. J Clin Endocrinol Metab 89:4285-4291, 2004.
70. Chadwick BP, Obermayr F, Frischau A: FKHL15, a new human member of the forkhead gene family located on chromosome 9q22. Genomics 41:390-396, 1997.
71. Dathan N, Parlato R, Rosica A, et al: Distribution of the titf2/foxe1 gene product is consistent with an important role in the development of foregut endoderm, palate, and hair. Dev Dyn 224:450-456, 2002.
72. Macchia PE, Mattei MG, Lapi P, et al: Cloning, chromosomal localization and identification of polymorphisms in the human thyroid transcription factor 2 gene (TITF2). Biochimie 81:433-440, 1999.
73. Sequeira M, Al-Khafaji F, Park S, et al: Production and application of polyclonal antibody to human thyroid transcription factor 2 reveals thyroid transcription factor 2 protein expression in adult thyroid and hair follicles and prepubertal testis. Thyroid 13:927-932, 2003.
74. Clifton-Bligh RJ, Wentworth JM, Heinz P, et al: Mutation of the gene encoding human TTF-2 associated with thyroid agenesis, cleft palate and choanal atresia. Nat Genet 19:399-401, 1998.
75. Bamforth JS, Hughes IA, Lazarus JH, et al: Congenital hypothyroidism, spiky hair, and cleft palate. J Med Genet 26:49-60, 1989.
76. Castanet M, Park SM, Smith A, et al: Novel loss-of-function mutation in TTF-2 is associated with congenital hypothyroidism, thyroid agenesis and cleft palate. Hum Mol Genet 11:2051-2059, 2002.
77. Baris I, Arisoy AE, Smith A, et al: A novel missense mutation in human TTF-2 (FKHL15) gene associated with congenital hypothyroidism but not athyreosis. J Clin Endocrinol Metab 91:4183-4187, 2006.
78. Parmentier M, Libert F, Maenhaut C, et al: Molecular cloning of the thyrotropin receptor. Science 246:1620-1622, 1989.
79. Taylor BA, Grieco D, Kohn L: Localization of gene encoding the thyroid-stimulating hormone receptor (Tshr) on mouse chromosome 12. Mamm Genome 7:626-628, 1996.
80. Rousseau-Merck MF, Misrahi M, Loosfelt H, et al: Assignment of the human thyroid stimulating hormone receptor (TSHR) gene to chromosome 14q31. Genomics 8:233-236, 1990.
81. Brown RS, Shalhoub V, Coulter S, et al: Developmental regulation of thyrotropin receptor gene expression in the fetal and neonatal rat thyroid: Relation to thyroid morphology and to thyroid-specific gene expression. Endocrinology 141:340-345, 2000.
82. Marians RC, Ng L, Blair HC, et al: Defining thyrotropin-dependent and -independent steps of thyroid hormone synthesis by using thyrotropin receptor-null mice. Proc Natl Acad Sci U S A 99:15776-15781, 2002.
83. Stuart A, Oates E, Hall C, et al: Identification of a point mutation in the thyrotropin receptor of the hyt/hyt hypothyroid mouse. Mol Endocrinol 8:129-138, 1994.
84. Refetoff S: Resistance to thyrotropin. J Endocrinol Invest 26:770-779, 2003.
85. Stanbury JB, Rocmans P, Buhler UK, Ochi Y: Congenital hypothyroidism with impaired thyroid response to thyrotropin. N Engl J Med 279:1132-1136, 1968.
86. Park SM, Chatterjee VK: Genetics of congenital hypothyroidism. J Med Genet 42:379-389, 2005.
87. Perry R, Heinrichs C, Bourdoux P, et al: Discordance of monozygotic twins for thyroid dysgenesis: Implications for screening and for molecular pathophysiology. J Clin Endocrinol Metab 87:4072-4077, 2002.
88. Vassart G, Dumont JE: Thyroid dysgenesis: Multigenic or epigenetic... or both. Endocrinology 146:5035-5037, 2005.
89. Klett M: Epidemiology of congenital hypothyroidism. Exp Clin Endocrinol Diabetes 105:19-23, 1997.

Section B

THYROID HORMONE

Chapter 3

Thyroid Hormone Synthesis

*Peter Kopp and Juan Carlos Solis-S**

Key Points

- Normal thyroid hormone synthesis requires a normally developed thyroid gland, a series of highly regulated biochemical steps, and an adequate nutritional iodide intake.
- After iodide uptake in thyrocytes by the sodium-iodide symporter (NIS), it is transported at the apical membrane into the follicular lumen, partly by pendrin, then oxidized by thyroperoxidase (TPO) and incorporated into selected tyrosyl residues of thyroglobulin (TG). This results in formation of mono- and diiodotyrosines.
- Iodotyrosines are subsequently coupled by TPO to form thyroxine (T_4) and triiodothyronine (T_3). After pinocytosis of TG into thyrocytes, it is hydrolyzed in lysosomes and T_4, T_3 are released into the bloodstream.
- Defects in all major steps in thyroid hormone synthesis have been identified. Clinical defects in thyroid hormonogenesis typically result in goiter development if the condition is not recognized early because of thyroid gland stimulation by thyrotropin. The severity of the defects varies and results in a clinical spectrum from severe congenital hypothyroidism to a euthyroid metabolic state with an enlarged thyroid.
- Usually, defective hormonogenesis requires biallelic mutations in the involved gene products (autosomal recessive inheritance). Therefore, hormone synthesis defects are more commonly found in inbred families and populations; monoallelic mutations in the dual oxidase DUOX2 are associated with transient hypothyroidism.

The synthesis of thyroid hormones requires a normally developed thyroid gland, a normal iodide intake, and a series of regulated biochemical steps.[1-3] At the basolateral membrane, iodide is actively transported into thyroid follicular cells by the sodium-iodide symporter (NIS; Fig. 3-1). The function of NIS is dependent on the electrochemical gradient generated by the Na^+,K^+-ATPase. Iodide then reaches the apical membrane, where it is transported into the follicular lumen. Compared to the mechanism controlling iodide uptake, the efflux of iodide is less well understood. Iodide efflux is, at least in part, mediated by pendrin (PDS/SLC26A4). Within the follicular lumen, iodide is then oxidized by the membrane-bound enzyme thyroperoxidase (TPO). The oxidation of iodide by TPO requires the presence of hydrogen peroxide (H_2O_2). H_2O_2 generation is catalyzed by the dual oxidase DUOX2, an enzyme that requires a specific maturation factor, DUOXA2. The large glycoprotein thyroglobulin (TG) serves as a matrix for the synthesis of thyroxine (T_4) and triiodothyronine (T_3) in the follicular lumen. First, TPO iodinates selected tyrosyl residues on TG (organification or iodination). This results in the formation of monoiodotyrosines (MITs)

*This work has been supported by 1R01DK63024-01 from NIH/NIDDK and by David Wiener.

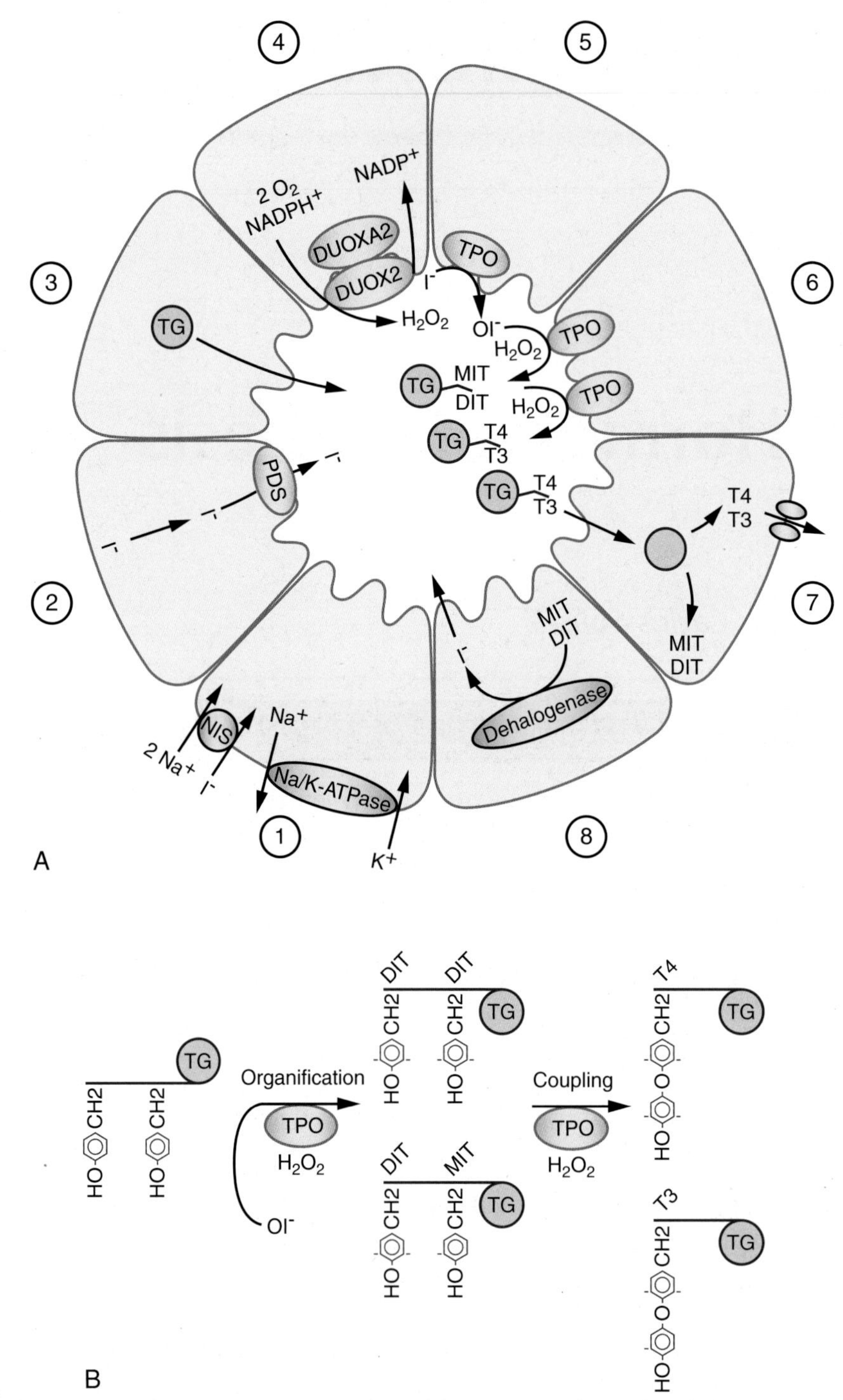

Figure 3–1 Thyroid hormone synthesis. **A,** Key steps in thyroid hormone synthesis. 1. Iodide is transported into the cell by the sodium-iodide symporter (NIS). This step is dependent on the generation of an electrochemical gradient generated by the Na^+,K^+-ATPase. 2. Iodide is transported into the follicular lumen, at least in part by pendrin (PDS/SLC26A4). 3. Thyroglobulin (TG) is secreted into the follicular lumen, where it serves as the matrix for the synthesis of thyroxine (T_4) and triiodothyronine (T_3). 4. The oxidation of iodide requires the generation of hydrogen peroxide (H_2O_2) by the dual oxidase DUOX2, an enzyme that requires a specific maturation factor, DUOXA2. 5. Iodide is oxidized by the enzyme thyroperoxidase (TPO). 6. TPO iodinates selected tyrosyl residues on TG (organification or iodination), which results in the formation of mono- and diiodotyrosines (MIT, DIT). The iodotyrosines are then coupled (coupling reaction) by TPO to form T_4 or T_3. 7. Iodinated TG is then internalized by micro- and macropinocytosis and digested in lysosomes, and T_4 and T_3 are secreted into the bloodstream through unidentified channels. 8. MIT and DIT are deiodinated in the cytosol by the iodotyrosine dehalogenase DEHAL1, and the released iodide is recycled for hormone synthesis. **B,** Detailed schematic representation of the organification and the coupling reactions.

and diiodotyrosines (DITs). Next, iodotyrosines are coupled (coupling reaction) by TPO to form T_4 or T_3. Iodinated TG is primarily internalized into the follicular cell by micro- and macropinocytosis. Within the cell, it is digested in lysosomes. T_4 (approximately 80%) and T_3 (approximately 20%) are then released into the bloodstream through unidentified channels. MITs and DITs are deiodinated in the cytosol by the iodotyrosine dehalogenase DEHAL1, and the released iodide is recycled for hormone synthesis.

Genetic defects in all steps involved in thyroid hormonogenesis have been described. If untreated, they typically result in the development of a goiter caused by the chronic stimulation of the thyroid gland by thyrotropin (TSH). The severity of the defects varies and the phenotype encompasses a spectrum from severe congenital hypothyroidism to a euthyroid metabolic state with a compensatory goiter.

IODIDE UPTAKE BY THE SODIUM-IODIDE SYMPORTER

The uptake of iodide at the basolateral membrane requires a sodium gradient, which is generated by Na^+,K^+-ATPase.[4-6] Active iodide transport is mediated by NIS, which transports two sodium ions and one iodide ion into the cell.[6,7] This results in a iodide concentration in the thyrocyte that is up to 40-fold higher compared with plasma.[4]

Sodium-Iodide Symporter Gene and Protein Structure

The rat NIS cDNA was isolated in 1996 using an expression cloning strategy.[7] This was promptly followed by cloning of the human NIS cDNA using

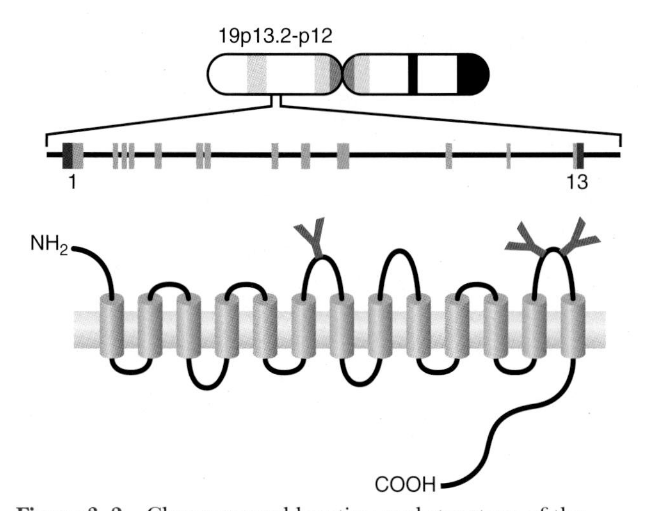

Figure 3–2 Chromosomal location and structure of the *NIS/SLC5A* gene and current model of the secondary structure of the sodium-iodide symporter (NIS) protein. The 5′ and 3′ untranslated regions of the gene are shown in red and the coding region in blue. In the secondary protein structure, the green symbols depict glycosylation sites.

primers complementary to rNIS.[8] Human NIS, officially designated as solute carrier 5A (SLC5A), is encoded by a single-copy gene with 15 exons that is located on chromosome 19p13 (Fig. 3-2).[9] The SLC5 family members rely on an electrochemical sodium gradient as the driving force for solute transport. Human NIS is a 643–amino acid glycoprotein with presumably 13 transmembrane domains.[10,11] The amino terminus is located extracellularly and the carboxy terminus is located in the cytosol.

Sodium-Iodide Symporter Function, Inhibition by Competitors, and Perchlorate Test

The Michaelis-Menten constant (K_m) of NIS is approximately 36 μM.[7,12] Electrophysiologic studies in oocytes have demonstrated that NIS is electrogenic because of the influx of sodium with a stoichiometric ratio of sodium to iodide of 2:1.[13] NIS is blocked by several anions, in particular perchlorate and thiocyanate, by competitive inhibition.[14,15] Although there was some controversy in the past as to whether perchlorate is a substrate for NIS, recent evidence has indicated that it is actively transported by NIS.[16,17] In contrast to the transport of iodide, the transport of perchlorate is electroneutral, indicating that NIS translocates different substrates with different stoichiometries.

Perchlorate is used for the so-called perchlorate test, which permits determination of the extent of iodide organification.[15] Under normal conditions, iodide is transported very rapidly into thyroid cells by NIS, released into the follicular lumen by pendrin and one or several other anion channel(s), and then organified on tyrosyl residues of TG by TPO. After the inhibition of NIS by perchlorate, any intrathyroidal iodide that has not been incorporated into TG is rapidly released into the bloodstream at the basolateral membrane and cannot be transported back into thyrocytes. In the standard perchlorate test, the thyroidal counts are measured at frequent intervals after the administration of radioiodine to determine the uptake into the thyroid gland. One hour later, 1 g of $KClO_4$ or $NaClO_4$ is administered, and the amount of intrathyroidal radioiodine is monitored longitudinally. In individuals with normal iodide organification, there is no decrease in intrathyroidal counts because the iodide has been incorporated into TG. In contrast, a loss of 10% or more indicates an organification defect; common causes include thyroiditis and congenital defects with abnormal efflux of iodide into the follicular lumen, such as Pendred's syndrome, defects of DUOX and DUOXA2, or dysfunction of TPO.[18-20] In the case of a complete organification defect (total iodide organification defect [TIOD]), such as in patients with complete inactivation of TPO, there is no meaningful organification and the tracer is completely released from the gland. In the situation of a partial iodide organification defect (PIOD), such as in Pendred's syndrome or partially inactivating TPO mutations, the fraction of the tracer that has not been incorporated is released from the gland.

Regulation of Sodium-Iodide Symporter and Iodide Uptake

Iodide uptake is stimulated by TSH through the cyclic adenosine monophosphate–protein kinase A (cAMP-PKA) pathway and by iodide. Exposure to TSH results in increased NIS gene expression and posttranscriptional activation of NIS.[21-23] TSH upregulates NIS mRNA and protein expression in vivo and in vitro.[10,24-26] In the presence of TSH, the half-life of NIS in FRTL-5 cells is approximately 5 days; in its absence, it decreases to approximately 3 days.[27] TSH also regulates the subcellular distribution of NIS, specifically the targeting to and retention of NIS in the basolateral membrane. In the absence of TSH, NIS is redistributed from the plasma membrane to intracellular compartments.[6]

Iodide accumulation and organification are also directly regulated by iodide itself.[28-30] Moderate doses of nutritional iodide result in the negative regulation of NIS mRNA expression.[26,31] High doses of iodide block thyroid hormone synthesis acutely through inhibition of the organification process, the so-called Wolff-Chaikoff effect. This inhibition is transient and dependent on the intracellular iodide concentration. Because the inhibition results in a decrease in iodide uptake, the intracellular concentrations decrease and the inhibitory effect disappears, a phenomenon referred to as escape from the acute Wolff-Chaikoff effect.[31] At the molecular level, an iodide-induced downregulation of NIS expression, possibly an increase in NIS protein turnover, and a decrease in NIS activity contribute to this autoregulation.[32,33-35]

Interestingly, high concentrations of extracellular TG downregulate NIS transcription.[36,37] In cell culture, final TG concentrations of 1 to 10 mg/mL are effective in altering gene expression in experiments using rat thyroid FRTL-5 cells.[37,38] This is thought to represent the lower range of intrafollicular TG concentrations, which vary from 0.1 to 250 mg/mL. TG decreases the mRNA expression of thyroid-restricted transcription factors such as PAX8 and thyroid-restricted transcription factors TTF-1 and TTF-2.[37-40] In addition, TG is a suppressor of its own mRNA expression, as well as of the *TSHR, NIS,* and *TPO* genes. This may in part be the consequence of the repression of TTF-1, TTF-2, and PAX8 expression. In contrast, *PDS* mRNA is upregulated by TG.[39]

Suppression of NIS expression by TG decreases iodide uptake in vitro, and the accumulation of TG in the follicular lumen correlates with low iodide uptake in vivo.[37] The inverse relationship between the amount of follicular TG and uptake of radioiodine in vivo, which is the consequence of differential gene regulation within thyroid follicular cells, appears to be of importance in the regulation of follicular function under conditions of constant TSH levels.[40]

IODIDE EFFLUX

Iodide efflux at the apical membrane is less well characterized. After exposure to TSH, iodide efflux increases rapidly in the poorly polarized FRTL-5 rat thyroid cells,[41] as well as in polarized porcine thyrocytes.[42,43] In primary porcine thyrocytes grown in a bicameral system, TSH stimulates iodide efflux at the apical membrane while leaving efflux in the basal direction unchanged, thus facilitating the vectorial transport of iodide into the follicular lumen. Based on electrophysiologic studies performed with inverted plasma membrane vesicles, it is assumed that iodide efflux can be mediated by two apical iodide channels with different affinities (K_m of approximately 70 and 33 μM, respectively).[44] However, identity of these channels has not been established at the molecular level. The demonstration of iodide transport by the anion channel pendrin, together with the clinical phenotype in patients with Pendred's syndrome, suggests that pendrin could correspond to one of the channels.[45-49] It had been proposed that SLC5A8, a homologue of NIS, initially called human apical iodide transporter (hAIT), is also involved in apical iodide efflux.[50] However, functional studies in oocytes and polarized MDCK cells did not show any evidence for iodide translocation by SLC5A8.[51]

Pendrin (PDS/SLC26A4) Gene and Pendred's Syndrome

Pendred's syndrome is an autosomal recessive disorder defined by the triad of sensorineural deafness, goiter, and impaired iodide organification.[52-55] The *PDS* gene, now officially designated as *SLC26A4* (solute carrier 26A4), was cloned in 1997, encompasses 21 exons, and contains an open reading frame of 2343 base pairs (bp) (Fig. 3-3).[45] The SLC26A family contains several anion transporters and the motor protein prestin (SLC26A5), which is expressed in outer hair cells.[56-58] The *PDS/SLC26A4, DRA/CLD/SLC26A3* (downregulated in adenoma and congenital chloride diarrhea), and *prestin/SCLC26A5* genes are located in close proximity on chromosome 7q21-31 and have a very similar genomic structure, suggesting a common ancestral gene.

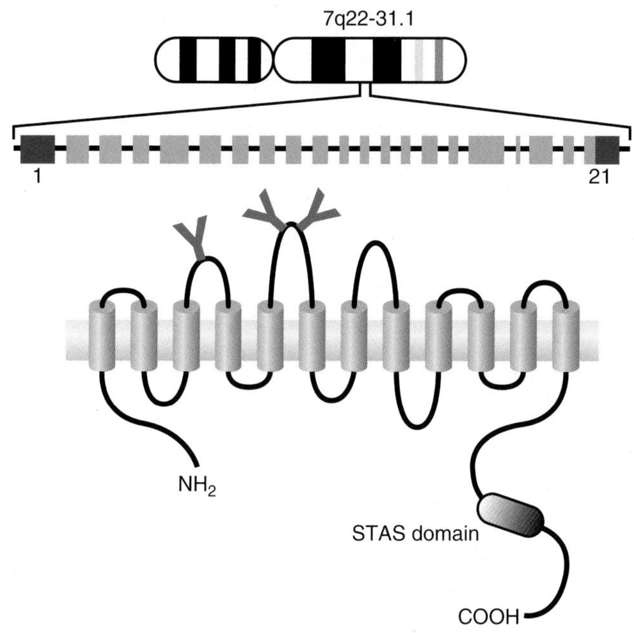

Figure 3–3 Chromosomal location and structure of the *PDS/SLC26A4* gene and current model of the secondary structure of the PDS protein. The 5′ and 3′ untranslated regions of the gene are shown in red and the coding region in blue. In the secondary protein structure, the green symbols depict putative glycosylation sites. The intracellular carboxyterminus contains a STAS (sulfate transporter and antisigma factor antagonist) domain, which may be of importance for the interaction with other proteins.

PROTEIN STRUCTURE OF PENDRIN

Pendrin is a highly hydrophobic membrane protein consisting of 780 amino acids (see Fig. 3-3).[45] It is thought to have 12 transmembrane domains with an intracellular amino- and carboxy-terminus,[39,49] and it has three putative extracellular *N*-glycosylation sites.[59] Pendrin contains a so-called STAS (sulfate transporter and antisigma factor antagonist) domain in its intracellular carboxyterminus.[60] It has been suggested that the STAS domain of SLC26 members, including pendrin, can interact with the regulatory domain of CFTR (cystic fibrosis transmembrane conductance regulator) in some epithelial cells.[61-63]

EXPRESSION PATTERN AND REGULATION OF PDS

PDS/SLC26A4 mRNA and protein expression are found in thyroid follicular cells,[45,64] the endolymphatic system of the inner ear,[65,66] type B intercalated cell of the renal cortical collecting duct,[67-69] and syncytiotrophoblast cells of the placenta,[70] endometrium,[71] and mammary glands of pregnant and lactating mice.[72] Very low levels of *PDS/SLC26A4* mRNA expression of unknown physiologic relevance have also been reported in tissues such as lung, breast, prostate, and testis.[73] In thyroid follicular cells, pendrin is located at the apical membrane.[39,64] Immunostaining for pendrin is more abundant in thyroid tissue from patients with Graves' disease, suggesting a possible correlation of protein abundance with increased iodide organification.[74]

Whether *SLC26A4* mRNA levels are regulated by TSH in FRTL-5 cells is controversial.[39,75] TTF-1 appears to be involved in the positive regulation of the rat and human *SLC26A4* gene promoter.[75,76] Exposure of FRTL-5 cells to TG results in a significant upregulation of *SLC26A4* mRNA, which contrasts with the downregulation of thyroid-restricted genes such as *TSHR, NIS, TPO, TG, PAX8, TTF-1,* and *TTF-2*.[37-40,77] Iodide does not have a major effect on *SLC26A4* gene expression in vitro. Exposure of rat thyroid PCCL3 cells transfected with *SLC26A4* promoter constructs to TG results in a significant upregulation of transcriptional activity, and this induction is thyroid-specific.[78]

Remarkably, exposure of rat PCCL3 cells to TSH leads to a rapid increase in pendrin protein abundance in the membrane.[79] This results in a pendrin-mediated increase in iodide efflux (L. Pesce and P. Kopp, personal communication, 2008), which may explain the rapid increase in iodide observed in FRTL-5 and porcine thyroid cell efflux in response to TSH.[41-43]

PDS/SLC26A4 mRNA levels are similar in hyperfunctioning adenomas compared with normal tissue, but protein expression, determined by immunohistochemistry and immunoblotting, appears to be higher in most follicular cells.[64,80] In contrast, *PDS/SLC26A4* mRNA and total pendrin protein expression are not increased in follicular adenomas.[59] In hypofunctioning adenomas, *PDS/SLC26A4* mRNA expression is similar compared with normal thyroid tissue, and pendrin immunostaining is highly variable or decreased.

In differentiated thyroid carcinomas, *PDS* mRNA and pendrin protein expression are significantly decreased,[59,64,74,81-83] and the expression of pendrin protein does not correlate with NIS expression. *PDS/SLC26A4* mRNA is also scarce in thyroid cancer cell lines.[39] Consistent with this low or absent expression of the *PDS/SLC26A4* gene in thyroid cancer, hypermethylation of the *PDS/SLC26A4* promoter was found in most thyroid cancers.[84]

FUNCTIONAL CHARACTERIZATION OF PENDRIN

Using *Xenopus* oocytes, pendrin was first shown to mediate the uptake of chloride and iodide in a sodium-independent manner.[46] The demonstration of iodide transport, the impaired organification of iodide in patients with Pendred's syndrome, and the apical localization of pendrin in thyroid follicular cells[39,64] have suggested a possible role in iodide transport into the follicle.[56] Functional studies in transfected cells have subsequently demonstrated that pendrin can mediate iodide efflux.[47,48] Further evidence for pendrin-mediated apical iodide efflux was obtained in a model system with polarized Madin-Darby canine kidney (MDCK) cells expressing NIS and pendrin.[49] Consistent with the partial organification defect observed in patients with Pendred's syndrome, naturally occurring mutations of pendrin lead to a loss of function in terms of iodide transport.[85]

PENDRIN IN THE KIDNEY

In addition to its expression in the thyroid and inner ear, *SLC26A4* mRNA is readily found in the kidney,[45] in particular in the renal cortex, and nephron segment reverse transcriptase–polymerase chain reaction (RT-PCR) assays have led to the detection of positive signals in the cortical collecting duct.[67] In the cortical collecting duct, pendrin localizes to the apical brush border membrane in type B, and in non-A, non-B intercalated cells.[68] Type B intercalated cells secrete hydroxide, whereas type A intercalated cells are hydrogen-secreting cells.[86]

Functionally, pendrin was found to act as an exchanger of chloride for bicarbonate, hydroxide, and formate.[67,87] Renal tubules isolated from alkali-loaded wild-type mice secrete bicarbonate, whereas tubules from alkali-loaded *Pds* −/− mice fail to secrete bicarbonate, confirming that pendrin is a chloride-base exchanger.[68] Acid loading of mice results in reduction of pendrin protein expression in the cortical collecting duct cells, and pendrin is relocalized from the apical membrane to the cytosol; this observation further corroborates a physiologic role of pendrin in bicarbonate secretion.[88,89] In contrast, bicarbonate loading results in upregulation of pendrin protein expression and increased membrane insertion. In mice, pendrin is upregulated after treatment with aldosterone analogues and with chloride restriction.[90,91] Remarkably, *Slc26a4* knockout mice do not develop weight gain and hypertension after treatment with deoxycorticosterone pivalate (DOCP), an aldosterone analogue.

PENDRIN IN THE INNER EAR

In the developing mouse, *Slc26a4* mRNA is predominantly detectable in the endolymphatic duct and sac, in areas of the utricule and saccule, and in the external cochlear sulcus region by in situ hybridization.[65] This expression pattern involves several regions for endolymphatic fluid resorption. This, and the typical enlargement of the endolymphatic system in patients with Pendred's syndrome and the *Pds* null mouse, strongly suggest that pendrin is involved in anion and fluid transport and maintenance of the endocochlear potential in the inner ear.[66,92,93] More recent studies have revealed that *Slc26a4* −/− mice lack the endocochlear potential, which is normally generated by the basolateral potassium channel KCNJ10 located in intermediate cells, because they do not express this channel.[94,95] In addition, the endolymphatic calcium concentration is elevated in the *Slc26a4* −/− mouse through inactivation of two apical calcium channels, TRPV5 and TRPV6.[96]

Controversies Concerning the Role of Pendrin in Apical Iodide Efflux

Studies performed with thyroid cell membrane vesicles have suggested that iodide crosses the apical membrane through two anion channels or transporters,[44] but their molecular identity remains uncertain. The results of functional studies performed in polarized cells cultured in a bicameral system are consistent with a role of pendrin as an apical iodide transporter.[49,55] However, the fact that individuals with biallelic mutations in the *SLC26A4* gene and a sufficiently high iodide intake have no or only a mild thyroidal phenotype[97] indicates that iodide crosses the apical membrane independently of pendrin through another iodide channel or unspecific channels. Very high iodide intake can even mitigate the phenotype in patients homozygous for completely inactivating NIS mutations.[6] Although *Pds* knockout mice do not have an overt thyroid phenotype,[93] it is currently unknown whether the phenotype could become apparent under conditions of scarce iodide intake.[98] It has also been argued that the distinct functional roles for pendrin in the thyroid, kidney, and inner ear are not readily acceptable. It should be noted, however, that many SLC26A family members transport several anions. Moreover, pendrin may interact with other proteins, which could lead to variable anion selectivity.

THYROGLOBULIN

Thyroglobulin serves as the matrix for the synthesis of T_4 and T_3 and the storage of thyroid hormone and iodide. On demand for thyroid hormone, TG reenters the cell to be digested in lysosomes, and T_4 and T_3 are secreted into the bloodstream (see Fig. 3-1).

Structure of the Thyroglobulin Gene

TG is encoded by a large 270-kb gene that consists of 48 exons (Fig. 3-4).[99-101] It is located on chromosome 8q24.2-8q24.3.[102-104] The TG promoter, which has remarkable structural similarity with the TPO promoter, is regulated by the transcription factors TTF1, TTF2, and PAX 8.[105,106] The open reading frame consists of 8307 bp and encodes a protein of 2768

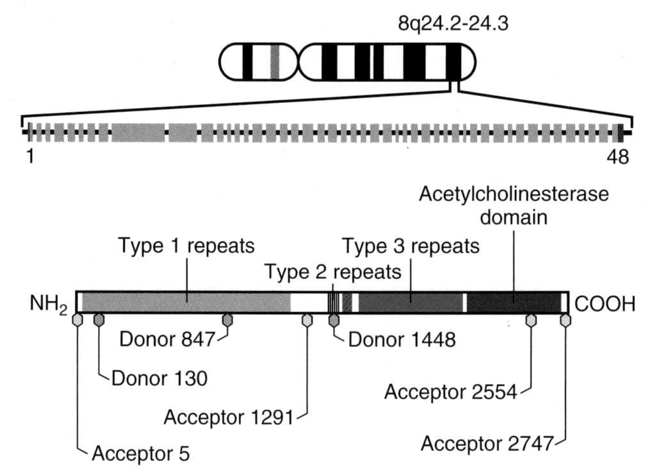

Figure 3–4 Chromosomal location and structure of the *TG* gene and current model of the secondary structure of the TG protein. The 5′ and 3′ untranslated regions of the gene are shown in red and the coding region in blue. In the secondary protein structure, the TG protein has been divided into three regions that contain repetitive elements and the carboxyterminus shares high homology with acetylcholinesterase. The main acceptor and donor tyrosyls are shown in yellow and light blue. The major acceptor site is at tyrosyl number 5 and the major donor site is at tyrosyl number 130 (numbering after cleavage of the signal peptide).

amino acids.[107,108] Alternative splicing generates various transcripts and subsequently a heterogeneous population of TG polypeptides.[109] Moreover, the *TG* genes contain multiple synonymous and nonsynonymous single-nucleotide polymorphisms (SNPs).

Thyroglobulin Protein Structure

The monomer of TG is composed of a 19–amino acid signal peptide followed by 2749 residues.[108] After translation of the mRNA, the 19–amino acid signal peptide conducts the TG molecule into the endoplasmic reticulum (ER), where the TG polypeptide is submitted to folding and dimerization. From the Golgi apparatus, glycosylated TG migrates to the apical membrane and is secreted into follicular lumen in a tightly regulated process.[110,111] In the follicular lumen, TG is present as a 19S dimeric glycoprotein of 660 kD.[112]

The TG protein has been divided into four major regions based on internal homology (see Fig. 3-4). The type 1 repetitive region contains 11 type 1 motifs formed by a cysteine-rich consensus sequence CWCV(D), a module found in a large family of proteins.[113-115] Type 1 repeats may bind and inhibit cysteine proteases, a feature that could play a role in the processing and degradation of TG. The carboxyterminal part of the TG monomer (residues 2192 to 2716) shares remarkable homology with acetylcholinesterase.[116] These structural characteristics suggest that the *TG* gene emerged from the fusion of two ancestral genes.[117]

Properly folded TG dimers migrate to the Golgi apparatus, where they are glycosylated.[112] About 10% of the molecular weight is accounted for by carbohydrates. Among the 20 potential glycosylation sites of the TG monomer, 16 are known to be glycosylated.[118] Other secondary modifications of TG include sulfation and phosphorylation.[119,120] It has been suggested that tyrosine sulfation may play a role in the hormonogenic process.[121]

From the Golgi apparatus, glycosylated TG migrates to the apical membrane in small secretory vesicles and is secreted into the follicular lumen,[110,111] where selected tyrosyl residues of the TG polypeptide are iodinated.[1] This organification reaction results in the generation of MITs and DITs (see Fig. 3-1).[2] The coupling reaction then leads to the formation of T_4 from two DIT residues, or T_3 from one DIT and one MIT.[2] During the coupling reaction, a tyrosyl residue donates its iodinated phenyl group to become the outer ring of the iodothyronine amino acid at an acceptor site, leaving dehydroalanine at the donor position. In human TG, the four main hormonogenic acceptor sites are localized at positions 5, 1291, 2554, 2568, and 2747 (see Fig. 3-4).[112,122] Donor sites are located at tyrosines 130, 847, and 1448. The most important T_4-forming sites are the acceptor tyrosine 5 and the donor tyrosine 130 (see Fig. 3-4).[123]

To generate T_4 and T_3 for release into the bloodstream, TG is internalized predominantly by micropinocytosis.[124,125] The TG-containing vesicles fuse with lysosomes, where TG is digested, resulting in the release of thyroid hormones.[3] Intact TG can also be transported from the apical to basolateral membrane, where it is released into the bloodstream.[126,127] This transepithelial transport, also referred to as transcytosis, is initiated by the interaction of TG with megalin, a receptor located on the apical membrane of the thyroid follicular cells.

Expression and Regulation of Thyroglobulin

The *TG* gene is expressed exclusively in thyroid follicular cells, which defines it as a specific and sensitive tumor marker for papillary and follicular thyroid cancer. In cell culture, TSH and insulin-like growth factor I (or insulin) need to be present concomitantly to induce expression of the *TG* gene.[128] In contrast, expression of the *TPO* gene can occur independently by the two growth factors.[129] The human *TG* gene promoter has similarities with the *TPO* promoter and contains, among others, binding sites for PAX8 and TTF2.[105] The PAX8 and TTF1 sites are overlapping and, in vitro, the binding of the two transcription factors to DNA is mutually exclusive.[130] PAX8 and TTF-1 interact directly through protein-protein interaction and synergistically activate the *TG* gene promoter.[131]

HYDROGEN PEROXIDE GENERATING SYSTEM

Hydrogen peroxide (H_2O_2) is essential for the oxidation of iodide, its organification, and the coupling reaction (see Fig. 3-1).[132] As shown through cytochemical studies, the H_2O_2 generating system is localized at the apical membrane[133,134] and involves the oxidation of reduced nicotinamide adenine dinucleotide phosphate (NADPH) by an NADPH oxidase.[135-138] It then became apparent that this enzyme system contains a membrane-bound flavoprotein using flavine adenine dinucleotide (FAD) as a cofactor,[139,140] and that it requires micromolar concentrations of calcium for its activity.[134,136,141-143] A functional NADPH oxidase, generating H_2O_2 in a Ca^{2+}-dependent manner, was finally solubilized from porcine plasma membranes, and sequence information derived from this protein led to cloning of a partial cDNA of DUOX2 (see later) by RT-PCR.[144] Subsequently, two cDNAs encoding thyroidal NADPH oxidases have been cloned using a strategy assuming a homology between the NADPH oxidase systems in thyroid follicular cells and neutrophil granulocytes.[145] These two oxidases, initially referred to as THOX1 and THOX2 for thyroid oxidase, are now officially designated as dual oxidases, DUOX1 and DUOX2. This nomenclature is based on the fact that these oxidases contain an NADPH oxidase domain and peroxidase activity.[146] DUOX2 has also been detected as an abundant transcript in thyroid cells using serial analysis of gene expression (SAGE).[147]

DUOX Gene and Protein Structure

The two *DUOX* genes are closely linked and located on chromosome 15q15 (Fig. 3-5).[144,148] They both consist of 33 exons; the *DUOX1* gene spans about 36 kb and the *DUOX2* gene encompasses about 22 kb. Human DUOX1 has an open reading frame of 1551 amino acids, and DUOX2 has 1548 residues.

The *DUOX* genes encode two highly related proteins with a similarity of 83%. They are related to several other oxidases (NOX2, MOX1).[145,149,150] Secondary structure analysis has predicted seven putative transmembrane domains, two everted finger (EF) motifs in the first intracellular loop, four NADPH binding sites, and one FAD binding site (see Fig. 3-5).[144] The intracellular location of the calcium-binding EF domains is consistent with the activation of the H_2O_2 generation system by cytosolic Ca^{2+} in thyroid membranes,[138,141] intact follicles,[134] and thyroid slices.[132,151]

Western blots have detected two proteins with a molecular weight of approximately 180 to 190 kD caused by glycosylation of five putative glycosylation sites.[145,148] Only the 190-kD form is resistant to endoglycosidase hydrogen digestion, suggesting that it is the completely processed form. After complete deglycosylation, the protein size is reduced to approximately 160 kD.

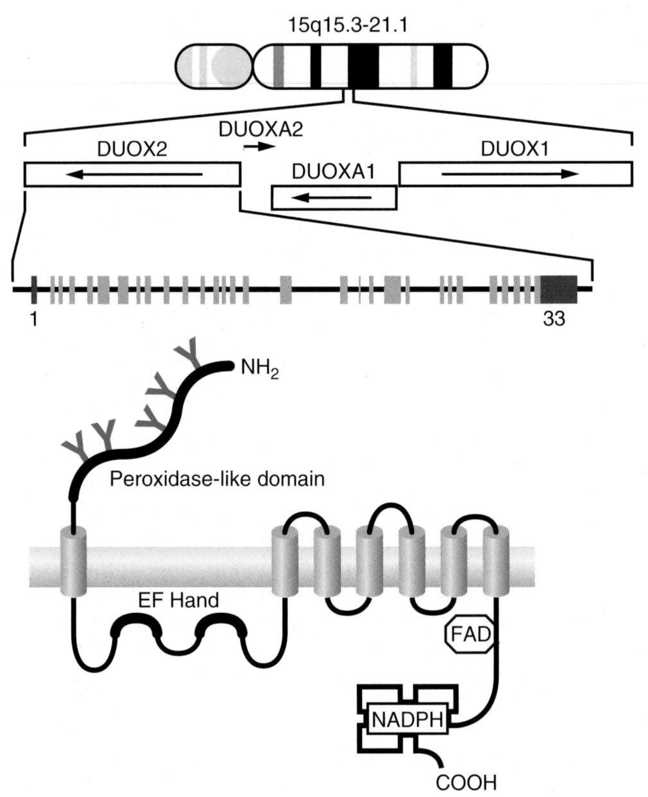

Figure 3–5 Chromosomal location and structure of the *DUOX2* and *DUOX1* genes and the genes encoding the specific maturation factors DUOXA2 and DUOXA1, which are essential for trafficking of the enzymes. The 5′ and 3′ untranslated regions of the gene are shown in red and the coding region in blue. In the secondary protein structure, the green symbols depict glycosylation sites. The DUOX proteins contain two putative Ca^{2+}-binding everted finger motifs in the first intracellular loop, and cytosolic FAD and NADPH binding sites. The extracellular amino terminus contains a peroxidase-like domain whose function awaits further characterization.

Intriguingly, the amino termini of both DUOX proteins have a homology of approximately 43% with TPO, and this domain of DUOX1 and its *Caenorhabditis elegans* homologue displays peroxidase activity.[146]

EXPRESSION AND REGULATION OF DUOX

DUOX1 and DUOX2 mRNA expression is almost exclusively detected in thyroid tissue using Northern blot analysis.[144,145] Only very weak signals for DUOX2 mRNA have been reported in the stomach and trachea.[152] Using RT-PCR assay, DUOX2 transcripts have also been reported in the intestinal tract (duodenum, small intestine, colon) of the adult rat.[153] An expressed sequence tag (EST) for DUOX2 has also been reported in a pancreas library.[147]

The expression of DUOX1 and DUOX2 mRNA levels is rapidly stimulated through the cAMP pathway in human, porcine, canine, and rat thyroid cells in vitro.[144,145,153] Treatment of thyroid cells with iodide inhibits H_2O_2 generation and NADPH activity in vitro.[143,154] Treatment of porcine thyroid follicles with iodide downregulates NIS and TPO mRNA levels, but does not affect the abundance of DUOX2 transcripts.[155] Exposure to iodide antagonizes the cAMP-induced glycosylation of DUOX2 to its mature form, and may explain the decrease in H_2O_2 generation. This phenomenon may contribute to the mechanisms underlying the Wolff-Chaikoff effect. In rats treated with methimazole, DUOX2 mRNA levels are reduced, but this is not the case in cultured thyroid cells.

In benign and malignant human thyroid tissue, the mRNA expression of the two *DUOX* genes is variable.[152,156] Protein expression determined by immunostaining is higher in thyroid tissue from patients with hypothyroidism, there are no significant differences between normal tissue and multinodular goiters, and only few positive cells in thyroid tissue are obtained from patients with Graves' disease. Immunopositivity for NIS and DUOX expression shows an inverse relationship.

Membrane insertion of DUOX2 is dependent on a specific maturation factor, DUOXA2. DUOX proteins are located at the apical membrane of thyroid follicular cells and colocalize with TPO.[145,152] As for TPO,[157] the fraction of DUOX proteins reaching the membrane is modest.[148] It has been proposed that this could serve as a regulatory mechanism of the cell to limit the generation of oxidative agents. In nonthyroidal cells transfected with DUOX1 and DUOX2 cDNAs, the expressed proteins reside predominantly in intracellular compartments and are only present as a 180-kD form.

Recent findings have revealed that the DUOX2 protein requires a specific maturation factor, referred to as DUOXA2, for proper processing of the protein.[158] DUOXA2 was identified by data mining that analyzed tissue-specific transcripts. It is arranged head to head with the DUOX2 gene (see Fig. 3-5). DUOXA2 is coexpressed with DUOX2 and permits transition of the protein from the endoplasmic reticulum to the Golgi apparatus, maturation, and translocation to the plasma membrane. DUOX2 is therefore dependent on the presence of DUOXA2 to achieve normal function. This has recently been corroborated by the finding of biallelic inactivating mutations in DUOXA2 in a patient with congenital hypothyroidism.[159] The expression of DUOX1, whose physiologic role remains to be determined, is dependent on its own paralog, DUOXA1.

FUNCTIONAL ANALYSES OF DUOX2 AND GENERATION OF HYDROGEN PEROXIDE

Initial attempts to reconstitute an H_2O_2-generating system through transfection of DUOX cDNAs, alone or in combination with components required for other oxidases, failed.[148] These findings suggested a need for additional components for achieving proper membrane targeting and enzymatic activity. As noted, membrane insertion of the DUOX proteins is dependent on the presence of their specific maturation factors, and coexpression of DUOX2 and DUOXA2 permits to reconstitute an H_2O_2-generating enzyme in heterologous cells.[158]

The biochemical mechanisms resulting in H_2O_2 generation remain controversial. It is currently unclear whether H_2O_2 is formed directly or through a process that includes the formation of O_2^- as an intermediate step.[1,2] A more recent model has proposed that O_2 is directly converted into H_2O_2 by a complex Ca^{2+}-dependent NADPH oxidase system containing a flavoprotein.[139,160-163] The secondary structure of the DUOX proteins is consistent with these predicted functions,[144,145] and the successful reconstitution of an H_2O_2-generating system through coexpression of DUOX2 and DUOXA2 will now permit clarification of this question.

REGULATION OF HYDROGEN PEROXIDE ACTIVITY

The generation of H_2O_2 is Ca^{2+}-dependent and can be acutely stimulated through the phosphatidylinositol pathway.[134,142,154,164,165] TSH also modulates the production of H_2O_2 through the protein kinase A pathway. Studies performed in canine and porcine cells have documented a stimulatory role of TSH and stimulators of the cAMP pathway on H_2O_2 generation,[143,162] whereas chronic exposure to TSH decreases H_2O_2 production in pig and FRTL-4 cells.

H_2O_2 generation is regulated by iodide. High concentrations of iodide inhibit H_2O_2 production,[151,154] possibly through the intermediary product 2-iodohexadecanal,[166,167] whereas low concentrations stimulate H_2O_2 generation in thyroid tissue slices.[168] This inverse regulation of H_2O_2 generation is one of the mechanisms that results in efficient hormone synthesis under conditions of low iodine intake and in downregulating hormone production when iodide intake is high or excessive.

Thyroperoxidase

Iodide must be oxidized to a higher oxidation state before it can serve as an iodinating agent. This oxidation of iodide requires the presence of H_2O_2 and is catalyzed by TPO.[2,169] TPO is a membrane-bound glycoprotein with a prosthetic heme group,

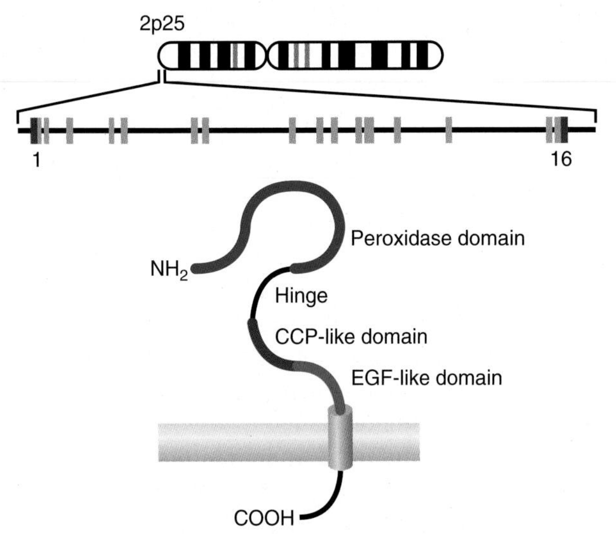

Figure 3–6 Chromosomal location and structure of the *TPO* gene and current model of the secondary structure of the TPO protein. The 5′ and 3′ untranslated regions of the gene are shown in red and the coding region in blue. The catalytic site of the enzyme faces the follicular lumen. The protein contains a region with high homology to the complement control protein (CCP) and the epidermal growth factor (EGF).

located in the follicular lumen (Fig. 3-6). In addition to catalyzing the oxidation of iodide, which results in the iodination of selected tyrosyl residues, TPO is also required for the coupling of iodotyrosines to generate T_4 and T_3 (see Fig. 3-1).

THYROPEROXIDASE GENE AND PROTEIN STRUCTURE

The human *TPO* gene is located on chromosome 2pter-p12,[170,171] spans about 150 kb, and consists of 17 exons (see Fig. 3-6).[172] The full-length human TPO cDNA encodes a protein of 933 amino acids (TPO1). Several shorter transcripts of unknown biologic relevance have also been identified.[173,174] The most abundant alternative transcript is lacking 171 nucleotides secondary to deletion of exon 10 encoding codons 533-590 (TPO2), which lacks enzymatic activity.[175]

EXPRESSION AND REGULATION OF THYROPEROXIDASE

The activity of TPO is enhanced by TSH in vivo through increased TPO protein expression.[176-178] In cultured thyroid cells, TSH and pharmacologic stimulators of the cAMP pathway increase TPO mRNA abundance.[128,129,179-181] In FRTL-5 cells, the increase in TPO mRNA levels seems to be the consequence of enhanced mRNA stability, whereas transcriptional stimulation of the *TPO* gene has been implicated in canine thyroid cells.[182]

TSH and forskolin rapidly upregulate TPO promoter activity.[183] This direct effect does not require protein synthesis and correlates with an increase in TTF2 binding activity.[184] It does not involve stimulation of a CRE (cAMP response element) or TTF-1.[105,185]

The human *TPO* gene promoter contains three binding sites for TTF1 and a binding site for PAX8 and TTF2 in the region between −170 to +1 bp relative to the transcriptional start site.[105] The PAX8 and TTF1 sites overlap and, in vitro, the binding of the two transcription factors to DNA is mutually exclusive.[130] PAX8 and TTF1 interact synergistically, possibly through interactions between enhancer and promoter.[186] The CCAAT-binding transcription factor CTF/NF-1, which is inducible by cAMP and insulin, cooperates with TTF2 in TPO promoter regulation.[187] PAX8 also interacts with the nuclear coactivator p300 to enhance *TPO* gene transcription.[188] Expression of the human *TPO* gene is, in part, regulated by a thyroid-specific enhancer located 5.5 kb upstream of the transcriptional start site.[105,189] One region of the enhancer has overlapping binding sites for TTF1 and PAX8 that seem to be mutually exclusive.[190,191]

As noted, follicular TG, acting in a counterregulatory fashion to the stimulatory effect of TSH, downregulates the expression of TTF1, TTF2, and PAX8, a mechanism that leads to a decrease in NIS, TPO, TG, and TSH receptor expression.[36,37] Phorbol esters, interferon-gamma, and interleukin-1α (IL-1α) and IL-1β downregulate TSH-induced TPO mRNA expression in human thyroid cell cultures.[192-194]

In immunoblot analyses, TPO appears as a doublet of 110 and 105 kDa, a phenomenon that is not explained by the translation of TPO2.[195] The amino terminus of TPO is located extracellularly and the extracellular region forms a loop that is created by two intramolecular disulfide bonds in the case of human TPO.[196-198] The single membrane-spanning domain is in close proximity to its carboxy terminus (see Fig. 3-6). Human TPO has five potential glycosylation sites and about 10% of its weight stems from the addition of carbohydrates, but the location of the *N*-linked glycosylation sites have only been determined for porcine TPO.[2,199]

The prosthetic heme group is covalently bound to glutamine 399 and aspartate 238 of the apoprotein. It is distinct from the heme b (protoporphyrin IX) found in many other hemoproteins and is composed of a *bis*-hydroxylated heme b. Amino acids directly coordinated to the iron atom or positioned in its immediate proximity are critical for modulating enzyme reactivity and specificity.[200-202]

All mammalian peroxidases belong to a single gene family.[202] TPO displays a high degree of sequence similarity with myeloperoxidase (MPO)[203-206] and other mammalian peroxidases.[207-209] The first 735 amino acids of TPO display a 42% sequence identity with MPO[210] and the polypeptide region interacting with the heme group is 74% homologous between TPO and MPO. The structure of MPO has initially been solved at 3 Å resolution[211] and, more recently, at a resolution of 1,8 Å.[212,213] Based on this structure, theoretical three-dimensional structures have been derived for other mammalian peroxidases,[201] but the three-dimensional structure of TPO has not been modeled.[2]

Immunohistochemical studies localize TPO at the apical membrane,[214] but abundant immunopositivity is also found in the cytoplasm.[215] Acute stimulation with TSH increases the abundance of TPO at the apical membrane and results in enhanced enzymatic activity.[216,217] These observations indicate that TPO is brought to the plasma membrane through the secretory pathway. Interestingly, the sorting and trafficking of TPO are cell type–dependent and, in stable transfected heterologous cell systems, TPO is often largely retained in intracellular compartments.[218-221] In contrast, TPO reaches the plasma membrane efficiently in transiently transfected Chinese hamster ovary (CHO) cells and stably transfected rat PCCl3 thyroid cells. These findings suggest that membrane insertion of TPO requires the presence of thyroid-specific factors.

FUNCTIONAL CHARACTERIZATION OF THYROPEROXIDASE

Catalytically active TPO was first successfully purified by solubilizing thyroid membrane fractions and by immunoaffinity chromatography.[196,197,222,223] The catalytic activity of these preparations was characterized with different biochemical assays such as guaiacol oxidation, iodide oxidation, iodination of albumin, and coupling of DIT within TG to T_4. After the molecular cloning of TPO cDNAs, recombinant protein has been successfully expressed using several mammalian and nonmammalian expression systems.[224] Remarkably, many of the recombinant TPO preparations have been particularly useful for immunologic studies, but display modest catalytic activity.[2,225] Eukaryotic cells may be more suitable as an expression system for obtaining a functional and soluble recombinant TPO, possibly because of their ability to glycosylate the protein.

The chemical nature of the oxidizing iodide is not known with certainty.[2] More recent studies have suggested that iodide is oxidized in a two-electron reaction that may result in the formation of hypoiodite (OI^-), hypoiodous acid (HOI), or iodinium (I^+).[226-234]

OXIDATION OF THYROPEROXIDASE TO COMPOUND I AND COMPOUND II

In native peroxidase, the heme is in the ferric (iron III) form (Fe^{3+}). The reaction of TPO and other peroxidases with H_2O_2 is a two-electron reaction, resulting in the reduction of H_2O_2 to H_2O and oxidation of the enzyme; the reaction product is referred to as compound I (E-O or TPO-O).[235] A one-electron reduction of compound I generates compound II, and a second one-electron reduction brings the enzyme back to its native state.

In the iodination reaction, only a subset of the 132 tyrosyl residues of the TG dimer are iodinated, resulting in the formation of MIT and DIT.[112,122,236,237] In the coupling reaction, which results in the formation of T_4 or T_3, a tyrosyl residue donates its iodinated phenyl group to become the outer ring of the iodothyronine amino acid at an acceptor site, leaving dehydroalanine at the donor position.[238,239] In the formation of T_4, the outer ring stems from a DIT residue and in the formation of T_3 it stems from MIT.

Hormonogenic sites are conserved in various species and must be defined by their location in the three-dimensional structure of TG.[3,112,122,237,240] The main hormonogenic acceptor sites in human TG have been localized at positions 5, 1291, 2554, 2568, and 2747 (see Fig. 3-4). Donor sites include tyrosines 130, 847, and 1448. The most important T_4-forming site is located at tyrosine 5 and tyrosine 130 is the dominant donor site.[123]

Cellular Uptake and Proteolysis of Thyroglobulin

Iodinated TG, carrying T_4, T_3, DIT, and MIT, is stored as colloid in the follicular lumen. The release of thyroid hormone requires uptake of iodinated TG into the thyroid follicular cell, subsequent digestion in lysosomes, and transport of the thyronines T_4 and T_3 into the bloodstream (see Fig. 3-1). For a detailed review, see Dunn[3] and Dunn and Dunn.[112]. Uptake of TG occurs predominantly through micropinocytosis, which is initiated by nonselective fluid phase uptake and by receptor-mediated endocytosis.[124,241,242] Digestion of thyroglobulin is dependent on several endopeptidases, including the cathepsins D, B, L, and H.[243,244] After cleavage of TG by endopeptidases, it undergoes further degradation by several exopeptidases. In vitro, digestion of TG with lysosomal extracts results in the preferential release of hormone-rich fractions,[245] and digestion with the endopeptidase cathepsin B and the exopeptidase lysosomal dipeptidase I results first in the release of the dipeptide

T_4 glutamine, corresponding to the amino terminal hormonogenic site 5 and glutamine at position 6, and subsequent release of T_4.[246] After degradation of TG in the lysosomal pathway, T_4 and T_3 are secreted into the bloodstream at the basolateral membrane. As of yet, the channel(s) mediating the transport of thyroid hormone across the basolateral membrane have not been identified. The thyroid hormone transporter MCT8, which is also expressed at the basolateral membrane of thyrocytes, is a potential candidate.[247]

Dehalogenation of Monoiodotyrosine and Diiodotyrosine

The iodotyrosines MIT and DIT are much more abundant within the TG molecule, but they are only released in minute amounts into the circulation. A thyroidal iodotyrosine dehalogenase had already been identified in 1952 , and was shown to deiodinate MIT and DIT efficiently, but not T_4.[248] Importantly, it was also shown that the released iodide is reused for hormone synthesis. Formal identification of the gene encoding this enzyme has only been obtained very recently.[249,250] The dehalogenase was known to be a flavin mononucleotide (FMN)–dependent enzyme.[251] Using the SAGE technique, several thyroid-restricted genes were isolated and one of them was postulated to be the long-sought iodotyrosine dehalogenase.[147] The predicted protein, referred to as dehalogenase 1 (DEHAL1), contains a nitroreductase domain and a flavin mononucleotide domain, a finding consistent with the previously obtained biochemical data (Fig. 3-7).[252] However, functional or genetic proof that DEHAL1 corresponds to the iodotyrosine deiodinase was pending until patients with congenital hypothyroidism and mutations in the *DEHAL1* gene could be identified (see later). Patients with DEHAL1 mutations spill MIT and DIT into the bloodstream, which ultimately leads to the urinary loss of iodide. Under conditions of scarce iodide intake, this is associated with insufficient synthesis of thyroid hormone, severe hypothyroidism, and goiter development. These findings illustrate that thyroid follicular cells have developed an intricate system to reduce the loss of the hormonally inactive iodotyrosines to recycle iodide, an element that is usually scarce.[253] A more detailed characterization of DEHAL1 is still pending.

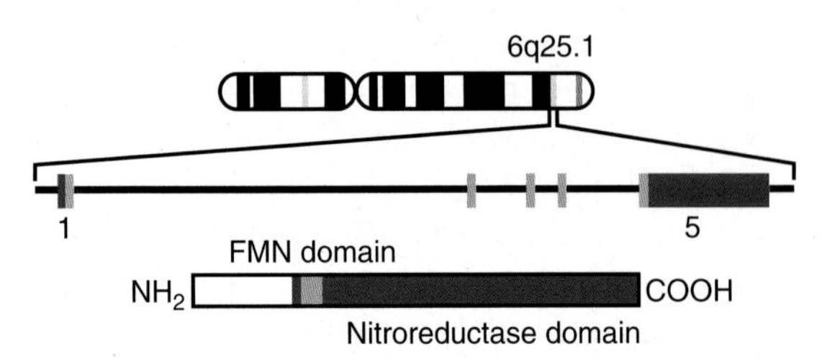

Figure 3–7 Chromosomal location and structure of the *DEHAL1* gene and current model of the secondary structure of the DEHAL1 protein. The 5′ and 3′ untranslated regions of the gene are shown in red and the coding region in blue. The protein contains a flavin mononucleotide (FMN) binding domain and a nitroreductase-like domain.

DEFECTS IN THYROID HORMONE SYNTHESIS

Congenital hypothyroidism can be caused by developmental defects of the thyroid (approximately 85%), thyroid dysgenesis, or inborn errors of metabolism in one of the steps required for thyroid hormone synthesis, dyshormonogenesis (approximately 10% to 15%).[18,254-256] Defects in thyroid hormone synthesis have been identified in all steps discussed earlier (see Fig. 3-1) and are briefly summarized here. If these conditions are not recognized and treated with levothyroxine, patients with defects in thyroid hormone synthesis usually develop a goiter because of the chronic stimulation with TSH.

Gene Mutations

MUTATIONS IN THE NIS GENE

A small subset of patients with dyshormonogenesis have an iodide trapping defect (ITD).[257] These patients have a low or absent uptake of radioiodide in scintigraphic studies, and a decreased saliva-to-serum radioiodide ratio. After the cloning of the *NIS* gene, several cases of hypothyroidism resulting from ITD have been characterized at the molecular level.[5,258-260] These individuals are homozygous or compound heterozygous for inactivating mutations in the *NIS* gene. Certain mutations affect NIS function by substituting key functional residues,[261] and others lead to misfolding and retention in intracellular compartments.[262]

MUTATIONS IN THE SLC26A4/PDS GENE AND PENDRED'S SYNDROME

Pendred's syndrome is an autosomal recessive disorder defined by sensorineural deafness, goiter, and a positive perchlorate test that indicates a PIOD.[52,55,56,263,264] The thyroid phenotype varies and depends on the nutritional iodide uptake. Despite the PIOD, most individuals with Pendred's syndrome are clinically and biochemically euthyroid under conditions of normal iodide intake,[53-55] and goiter development may be absent if the iodide consumption is high.[97] Individuals with Pendred's syndrome are homozygous or compound heterozygous for mutations in the *SLC26A4/PDS* gene.[45] Mutations in the *SLC26A4/PDS* gene display impressive allelic heterogeneity and more than 150 mutations have been documented.[45,265-270] (More information can be found at http://www.healthcare.uiowa.edu/laboratories/pendredandbor/slcMutations.htm.)

Some *SLC26A4/PDS* mutations result in retention of the protein in intracellular compartments. Others are inserted into the membrane, but display impaired or abolished ability to mediate iodide efflux.[47,49,271] Pendred's syndrome is probably the most common form of syndromic deafness and accounts for about 10% of all cases with hereditary deafness.[263,272]

MUTATIONS IN THE TG GENE

Biallelic mutations in the *TG* gene result in a wide phenotypic spectrum that ranges from euthyroid goiter to severe congenital hypothyroidism.[109,273,274] In patients who are not treated with levothyroxine, goiters are often remarkably large and display continuous growth. The radioiodine uptake is elevated, indicating an activation of the iodine concentration mechanism caused by chronic TSH stimulation. Because the organification process itself is not affected, the perchlorate test is usually normal. Serum TG levels are usually very low, or in the low-normal range.[275] In many cases, the affected individuals have related parents and are homozygous for inactivating mutations in the *TG* gene.[276] More rarely, affected patients are compound heterozygous for inactivating mutations in the *TG* gene.[277] Molecular analyses have indicated that most of the mutations are retained in the endoplasmic reticulum.[278-280] The maturation of TG is controlled by several molecular chaperones. Misfolded TG that accumulates in the ER is translocated back into the cytoplasm and undergoes degradation by the proteasome system, a process referred to as endoplasmic reticulum–associated degradation (ERAD).

MUTATIONS IN THE TPO GENE

Biallelic mutations in the *TPO* gene are a relatively frequent cause of defective thyroid hormone synthesis associated with congenital hypothyroidism.[281-284] Patients with TPO mutations have a PIOD or TIOD, and *TPO* gene defects are the most common cause of TIOD.

DEFECTS IN THE DUOX2 GENE

Monoallelic and biallelic mutations in the *DUOX2* gene result in transient or permanent congenital hypothyroidism.[19] Biallelic mutations result in a severe phenotype and a TIOD. In contrast, inactivation of a single allele causes transient congenital hypothyroidism and a PIOD. The documentation of a TIOD in patients with biallelic DUOX2 mutations has provided evidence that it is essential for the normal synthesis of H_2O_2 and thyroid hormone synthesis. Of note, no mutations have been found in the *DUOX1* gene, and DUOX1 is unable to compensate for the deficiency in DUOX2. This suggests that the enzymes have distinct functional roles. Coexpression of DUOX2 mutations with its specific maturation factor, DUOXA2, indicates that the mutations are retained by the quality control system within the endoplasmic reticulum or reduced surface expression.[159] Oxidative folding of DUOX2 in the endoplasmic reticulum appears to be the rate-limiting step in the maturation of the enzyme, but is not facilitated by DUOXA2. Folded DUOX2 is dependent on DUOXA2 for exit from the endoplasmic reticulum, whereas misfolded DUOX2 mutations are directed toward degradation.

MUTATIONS IN THE DUOXA2 GENE

As noted, DUOXA2 is necessary for the exit of folded wild-type DUOX2 from the endoplasmic reticulum, and the maturation factor is necessary and sufficient for expression of a functional enzyme.[158] In retrospect, this finding explains why it was not possible to reconstitute active DUOX enzymes in the past using heterologous cell systems. Further proof for the essential role of DUOXA2 has recently been provided by the identification of a patient homozygous for a *DUOXA2* gene mutation and congenital hypothyroidism.[20] The mutation leads to a complete loss of function caused by a truncation of the DUOXA2 protein and thus results in an inability to escort DUOX2 from the endoplasmic reticulum.

MUTATIONS IN THE DEHAL1 GENE

Patients with a defective thyroid dehalogenase system were identified more than 5 decades ago.[285,286] MIT and DIT leak into the circulation and are excreted in the urine. This leads to a significant loss of iodide and, under conditions of scarce iodine intake, severe hypothyroidism and goiter develop.[287] Remarkably, the TSH levels at neonatal screening may be normal, and the phenotype only becomes apparent later in infancy or childhood. Recently, mutations in the *DEHAL1* gene were identified in four individuals[250]; all were homozygous for inactivating mutations in the *DEHAL1* gene. All mutations disrupt the nitroreductase domain of the enzyme (see Fig. 3-7) and one of them also affects the FMN-binding domain. Functional characterization of the mutations revealed absent or severely impaired enzymatic activity to deiodinate iodotyrosines and an abolished or reduced induction in response to FMN. These findings have provided definitive evidence that DEHAL1 is the enzyme responsible for the deiodination of iodotyrosines, and that this mechanism is essential for thyroidal iodide metabolism. From a clinical perspective, it is important to note that neonatal screening may not detect those individuals with primary hypothyroidism.[253] In these patients, the onset of hypothyroidism varied significantly and could be confounded with common acquired hypothyroidism. As in patients with mutations in *NIS* or *SLC26A3*, it is likely that the expression of the phenotype is dependent on the nutritional iodide intake.

References

1. Kopp P: Thyroid hormone synthesis: Thyroid iodine metabolism. In Braverman L, Utiger R(eds): Werner and Ingbar's The Thyroid: A Fundamental and Clinical Text. Philadelphia, Lippincott, Williams & Wilkins, 2005, pp 52-76.
2. Taurog A: Hormone synthesis: Thyroid iodine metabolism. In Braverman L, Utiger R (eds): Werner and Ingbar's The Thyroid: A Fundamental and Clinical Text. Philadelphia, Lippincott, Williams & Wilkins, 2005, pp 61-85.
3. Dunn J: Biosynthesis and secretion of thyroid hormones. In De Groot L, Jameson J (eds): Endocrinology. Philadelphia, WB Saunders, 2001, pp 1290-1300.
4. Wolff J: Transport of iodide and other anions in the thyroid gland. Physiol Rev 44:45-90, 1964.
5. De La Vieja A, Dohan O, Levy O, Carrasco N: Molecular analysis of the sodium/iodide symporter: Impact on thyroid and extrathyroid pathophysiology. Physiol Rev 80:1083-1105, 2000.
6. Dohan O, De la Vieja A, Paroder V, et al: The sodium/iodide symporter (NIS): Characterization, regulation, and medical significance. Endocr Rev 24:48-77, 2003.
7. Dai G, Levy O, Carrasco N: Cloning and characterization of the thyroid iodide transporter. Nature 379:458-460, 1996.
8. Smanik PA, Liu Q, Furminger TL, et al: Cloning of the human sodium iodide symporter. Biochem Biophys Res Commun 226:339-345, 1996.
9. Smanik PA, Ryu KY, Theil KS, et al: Expression, exon-intron organization, and chromosome mapping of the human sodium iodide symporter. Endocrinology 138:3555-3558, 1997.
10. Levy O, Dai G, Riedel C, et al: Characterization of the thyroid Na^+/I^- symporter with an anti-COOH terminus antibody. Proc Natl Acad Sci U S A 94:5568-5573, 1997.
11. Levy O, De la Vieja A, Ginter CS, et al: N-linked glycosylation of the thyroid Na^+/I^- symporter (NIS). Implications for its secondary structure model. J Biol Chem 273:22657-22663, 1998.
12. Weiss SJ, Philp NJ, Grollman EF: Iodide transport in a continuous line of cultured cells from rat thyroid. Endocrinology 114:1090-1098, 1984.
13. Eskandari S, Loo DD, Dai G, et al: Thyroid Na^+/I^- symporter. Mechanism, stoichiometry, and specificity. J Biol Chem 272:27230-27238, 1997.
14. Barker HM: The blood cyanates in the treatment of hypertension. JAMA 106:762-767, 1936.
15. Hilditch TE, Horton PW, McCruden DC, et al: Defects in intrathyroid binding of iodine and the perchlorate discharge test. Acta Endocrinol (Copenh) 100:237-244, 1982.
16. Van Sande J, Massart C, Beauwens R, et al: Anion selectivity by the sodium iodide symporter. Endocrinology 144:247-252, 2003.
17. Dohan O, Portulano C, Basquin C, et al: The Na^+/I symporter (NIS) mediates electroneutral active transport of the environmental pollutant perchlorate. Proc Natl Acad Sci U S A 104:20250-20255, 2007.
18. Kopp P: Perspective: Genetic defects in the etiology of congenital hypothyroidism. Endocrinology 143:2019-2024, 2002.
19. Moreno JC, Bikker H, Kempers MJ, et al: Inactivating mutations in the gene for thyroid oxidase 2 (THOX2) and congenital hypothyroidism. N Engl J Med 347:95-102, 2002.
20. Zamproni I, Grasberger H, Cortinovis F, et al: Biallelic Inactivation of the Dual Oxidase Maturation Factor 2 (DUOXA2) gene as a novel cause of congenital hypothyroidism. J Clin Endocrinol Metab 93:605-610, 2008.
21. Weiss SJ, Philp NJ, Ambesi-Impiombato FS, Grollman EF: Thyrotropin-stimulated iodide transport mediated by adenosine 3′,5′-monophosphate and dependent on protein synthesis. Endocrinology 114:1099-1107, 1984.
22. Vassart G, Dumont JE: The thyrotropin receptor and the regulation of thyrocyte function and growth. Endocr Rev 13:596-611, 1992.
23. Vassart G, Parma J, van Sande, J, Dumont, JE: The thyrotropin receptor and the regulation of thyrocyte function and growth: Update 1994. In Braverman LE, Refetoff S (eds): Endocrine Review Monographs. Bethesda, Md, Endocrine Society, 1994, pp 77-80.
24. Kogai T, Endo T, Saito T, et al: Regulation by thyroid-stimulating hormone of sodium/iodide symporter gene expression and protein levels in FRTL-5 cells. Endocrinology 138:2227-2232, 1997.
25. Saito T, Endo T, Kawaguchi A, et al: Increased expression of the Na^+/I^- symporter in cultured human thyroid cells exposed to thyrotropin and in Graves' thyroid tissue. J Clin Endocrinol Metab 82:3331-3336, 1997.
26. Kogai T, Curcio F, Hyman S, et al: Induction of follicle formation in long-term cultured normal human thyroid cells treated with thyrotropin stimulates iodide uptake but not sodium/iodide symporter messenger RNA and protein expression. J Endocrinol 167:125-135, 2000.

27. Riedel C, Levy O, Carrasco N: Post-transcriptional regulation of the sodium/iodide symporter by thyrotropin. J Biol Chem 276:21458-21463, 2001.
28. Wolff J, Chaikoff I: Plasma inorganic iodide as homeostatic regulator of thyroid function. J Biol Chem 174:555-564, 1948.
29. Wolff J, Chaikoff I, Goldberg R, Meier J: The temporary nature of the inhibitory action of excess iodide on organic iodide synthesis in the normal thyroid. Endocrinology 45:504-513, 1949.
30. Grollman EF, Smolar A, Ommaya A, et al: Iodine suppression of iodide uptake in FRTL-5 thyroid cells. Endocrinology 118:2477-2482, 1986.
31. Braverman LE, Ingbar SH: Changes in thyroidal function during adaptation to large doses of iodide. J Clin Invest 42:1216-1231, 1963.
32. Uyttersprot N, Pelgrims N, Carrasco N, et al: Moderate doses of iodide in vivo inhibit cell proliferation and the expression of thyroperoxidase and Na^+/I^- symporter mRNAs in dog thyroid. Mol Cell Endocrinol 131:195-203, 1997.
33. Spitzweg C, Joba W, Morris JC, Heufelder AE: Regulation of sodium iodide symporter gene expression in FRTL-5 rat thyroid cells. Thyroid 9:821-830, 1999.
34. Eng PH, Cardona GR, Fang SL, et al: Escape from the acute Wolff-Chaikoff effect is associated with a decrease in thyroid sodium/iodide symporter messenger ribonucleic acid and protein. Endocrinology 140:3404-3410, 1999.
35. Eng PH, Cardona GR, Previti MC, et al: Regulation of the sodium iodide symporter by iodide in FRTL-5 cells. Eur J Endocrinol 144:139-144, 2001.
36. Suzuki K, Lavaroni S, Mori A, et al: Autoregulation of thyroid-specific gene transcription by thyroglobulin. Proc Natl Acad Sci U S A 95:8251-8256, 1998.
37. Suzuki K, Mori A, Saito J, et al: Follicular thyroglobulin suppresses iodide uptake by suppressing expression of the sodium/iodide symporter gene. Endocrinology 140:5422-5430, 1999.
38. Suzuki K, Mori A, Lavaroni S, et al: In vivo expression of thyroid transcription factor-1 RNA and its relation to thyroid function and follicular heterogeneity: Identification of follicular thyroglobulin as a feedback suppressor of thyroid transcription factor-1 RNA levels and thyroglobulin synthesis. Thyroid 9:319-331, 1999.
39. Royaux IE, Suzuki K, Mori A, et al: Pendrin, the protein encoded by the Pendred's syndrome gene (PDS), is an apical porter of iodide in the thyroid and is regulated by thyroglobulin in FRTL-5 cells. Endocrinology 141:839-845, 2000.
40. Suzuki K, Kohn LD: Differential regulation of apical and basal iodide transporters in the thyroid by thyroglobulin. J Endocrinol 189:247-255, 2006.
41. Weiss SJ, Philp NJ, Grollman EF: Effect of thyrotropin on iodide efflux in FRTL-5 cells mediated by Ca^{2+}. Endocrinology 114:1108-1113, 1984.
42. Nilsson M, Bjorkman U, Ekholm R, Ericson LE: Iodide transport in primary cultured thyroid follicle cells: Evidence of a TSH-regulated channel mediating iodide efflux selectively across the apical domain of the plasma membrane. Eur J Cell Biol 52:270-281, 1990.
43. Nilsson M, Bjorkman U, Ekholm R, Ericson LE: Polarized efflux of iodide in porcine thyrocytes occurs via a cAMP-regulated iodide channel in the apical plasma membrane. Acta Endocrinol (Copenh) 126:67-74, 1992.
44. Golstein P, Abramow M, Dumont JE, Beauwens R: The iodide channel of the thyroid: A plasma membrane vesicle study. Am J Physiol 263:C590-597, 1992.
45. Everett LA, Glaser B, Beck JC, et al: Pendred's syndrome is caused by mutations in a putative sulphate transporter gene (PDS). Nat Genet 17:411-422, 1997.
46. Scott DA, Wang R, Kreman TM, et al: The Pendred's syndrome gene encodes a chloride-iodide transport protein. Nature Genet 21:440-443, 1999.
47. Taylor JP, Metcalfe RA, Watson PF, et al: Mutations of the *PDS* gene, encoding pendrin, are associated with protein mislocalization and loss of iodide efflux: Implications for thyroid dysfunction in Pendred's syndrome. J Clin Endocrinol Metabol 87:1778-1784, 2002.
48. Yoshida A, Taniguchi S, Hisatome I, et al: Pendrin is an iodide-specific apical porter responsible for iodide efflux from thyroid cells. J Clin Endocrinol Metabol 87:3356-3361, 2002.
49. Gillam MP, Sidhaye A, Lee EJ, et al: Functional characterization of pendrin in a polarized cell system: Evidence for pendrin-mediated apical iodide efflux. J Biol Chem 279:13004-13010, 2004.
50. Rodriguez AM, Perron B, Lacroix L, et al: Identification and characterization of a putative human iodide transporter located at the apical membrane of thyrocytes. J Clin Endocrinol Metab 87:3500-3503, 2002.
51. Paroder V, Spencer SR, Paroder M, et al: Na(+)/monocarboxylate transport (SMCT) protein expression correlates with survival in colon cancer: Molecular characterization of SMCT. Proc Natl Acad Sci U S A 103:7270-7275, 2006.
52. Fraser GR, Morgans ME, Trotter WR: The syndrome of sporadic goitre and congenital deafness. Q J Med 29:279-295, 1960.
53. Medeiros-Neto G, Stanbury JB: Pendred's syndrome: Association of congenital deafness with sporadic goiter. In Medeiros-Neto G, Stanbury JB (eds): Inherited Disorders of the Thyroid System. Boca Raton, Fla, CRC Press, 1994, pp 81-105.
54. Kopp P: Pendred's syndrome and genetic defects in thyroid hormone synthesis. Rev Endocrinol Metab Dis 1/2:109-121, 2000.
55. Kopp P, Pesce L: Solis-S J: Pendred's syndrome and iodide transport in the thyroid. Trends Endocrinol 19:260-268, 2008.

56. Everett LA, Green ED: A family of mammalian anion transporters and their involvement in human genetic diseases. Hum Mol Genet 8:1883-1891, 1999.
57. Zheng J, Shen W, He DZ, et al: Prestin is the motor protein of cochlear outer hair cells. Nature 405:149-155, 2000.
58. Liu XZ, Ouyang XM, Xia XJ, et al: Prestin, a cochlear motor protein, is defective in non-syndromic hearing loss. Hum Mol Genet 12:1155-1162, 2003.
59. Porra V, Bernier-Valentin F, Trouttet-Masson S, et al: Characterization and semiquantitative analyses of pendrin expressed in normal and tumoral human thyroid tissues. J Clin Endocrinol Metab 87:1700-1707, 2002.
60. Aravind L, Koonin EV: The STAS domain—a link between anion transporters and antisigma-factor antagonists. Curr Biol 10:R53-R55, 2001.
61. Ko SB, Shcheynikov N, Choi JY, et al: A molecular mechanism for aberrant CFTR-dependent HCO(3)(-) transport in cystic fibrosis. EMBO J 21:5662-5672, 2002.
62. Ko SB, Zeng W, Dorwart MR, et al: Gating of CFTR by the STAS domain of SLC26 transporters. Nat Cell Biol 6:343-350, 2004.
63. Shcheynikov N, Ko SB, Zeng W, et al: Regulatory interaction between CFTR and the SLC26 transporters. Novartis Found Symp 273:177-186, 2006.
64. Bidart JM, Mian C, Lazar V, et al: Expression of pendrin and the Pendred's syndrome (PDS) gene in human thyroid tissues. J Clin Endocrinol Metab 85:2028-2033, 2000.
65. Everett LA, Morsli H, Wu DK, Green ED: Expression pattern of the mouse ortholog of the Pendred's syndrome gene (Pds) suggests a key role for pendrin in the inner ear. Proc Natl Acad Sci 96:9727-9732, 1999.
66. Royaux IE, Belyantseva IA, Wu T, et al: Localization and functional studies of pendrin in the mouse inner ear provide insight about the etiology of deafness in Pendred's syndrome. J Assoc Res Otolaryngol 4:394-404, 2003.
67. Soleimani M, Greeley T, Petrovic S, et al: Pendrin: An apical $Cl^-/OH^-/HCO_3^-$ exchanger in the kidney cortex. Am J Physiol Renal Physiol 280:F356-F364. 2001.
68. Royaux IE, Wall SM, Karniski LP, et al: Pendrin, encoded by the Pendred's syndrome gene, resides in the apical region of renal intercalated cells and mediates bicarbonate secretion. Proc Natl Acad Sci U S A 98:4221-4226, 2001.
69. Wall SM, Hassell KA, Royaux IE, et al: Localization of pendrin in mouse kidney. Am J Physiol Renal Physiol 284:F229-241, 2003.
70. Bidart JM, Lacroix L, Evain-Brion D, et al: Expression of Na^+/I^- symporter and Pendred's syndrome genes in trophoblast cells. J Clin Endocrinol Metab 85:4367-4372, 2000.
71. Suzuki K, Royaux IE, Everett LA, et al: Expression of PDS/Pds, the Pendred's syndrome gene, in endometrium. J Clin Endocrinol Metab 87:938, 2002.
72. Rillema JA, Hill MA: Prolactin regulation of the pendrin-iodide transporter in the mammary gland. Am J Physiol Endocrinol Metab 284:E25-28, 2003.
73. Lacroix L, Mian C, Caillou B, et al: Na^+/I^- symporter and Pendred's syndrome gene and protein expressions in human extra-thyroidal tissues. Eur J Endocrinol 144:297-302, 2001.
74. Mian C, Lacroix L, Alzieu L, et al: Sodium iodide symporter and pendrin expression in human thyroid tissues. Thyroid 11:825-830, 2001.
75. Dentice M, Luongo C, Elefante A, et al: Pendrin is a novel in vivo downstream target gene of the TTF-1/Nkx-2.1 homeodomain transcription factor in differentiated thyroid cells. Mol Cell Biol 25:10171-10182, 2005.
76. Solis-S J, Schnyder S, Chen L, Kopp P: Synergistic stimulation of the human PDS/SLC26A4 promoter by PAX8 and TTF-1. Presented at the 77th Annual Meeting of the American Thyroid Association. Phoenix, Ariz, October 2006.
77. Suzuki K, Mori A, Ishii KJ, et al: Activation of target-tissue immune-recognition molecules by double-stranded polynucleotides. Proc Natl Acad Sci U S A 96:2285-2290, 1999.
78. Solis-S J, Schnyder S, Chen L, Kopp P: Regulation of thyroidal transcripts and the human PDS/SLC26A4 promoter by thyroglobulin. Presented at the 78th Annual Meeting of the American Thyroid Association. New York, October 2007.
79. Pesce L, Kopp P: Thyrotropin rapidly regulates pendrin membrane abundance via PKA dependent and PKC independent pathways in rat thyroid cells. Presented at the 78th Annual Meeting of the American Thyroid Association. New York, October 2007.
80. Russo D, Bulotta S, Bruno R, et al: Sodium/iodide symporter (NIS) and pendrin are expressed differently in hot and cold nodules of thyroid toxic multinodular goiter. Eur J Endocrinol 145:591-597, 2001.
81. Arturi F, Russo D, Bidart JM, et al: Expression pattern of the pendrin and sodium/iodide symporter genes in human thyroid carcinoma cell lines and human thyroid tumors. Eur J Endocrinol 145:129-135, 2001.
82. Kondo T, Nakamura N, Suzuki K, et al: Expression of human pendrin in diseased thyroids. J Histochem Cytochem 51:167-173, 2003.
83. Gerard AC, Daumerie C, Mestdagh C, et al: Correlation between the loss of thyroglobulin iodination and the expression of thyroid-specific proteins involved in iodine metabolism in thyroid carcinomas. J Clin Endocrinol Metab 88:4977-4983, 2003.
84. Xing M, Tokumaru Y, Wu G, et al: Hypermethylation of the Pendred's syndrome gene SLC26A4 is an early event in thyroid tumorigenesis. Cancer Res 63:2312-2315, 2003.
85. Scott DA, Wang R, Kreman TM, et al: Functional differences of the PDS gene product are associated with phenotypic variation in patients with Pendred's syndrome and non-syndromic hearing loss (DFNB4). Hum Mol Genet 9:1709-1715, 2000.

86. Wall SM: Recent advances in our understanding of intercalated cells. Curr Opin Nephrol Hypertens 14:480-484, 2005.
87. Scott DA, Karniski LP: Human pendrin expressed in *Xenopus laevis* oocytes mediates chloride/formate exchange. Am J Cell Physiol 278:C207-C211, 2000.
88. Petrovic S, Wang Z, Ma L, Soleimani M: Regulation of the apical Cl^- /HCO_3^- exchanger pendrin in rat cortical collecting duct in metabolic acidosis. Am J Physiol Renal Physiol 284:F103-112, 2003.
89. Wagner CA, Finberg KE, Stehberger PA, et al: Regulation of the expression of the Cl^-/anion exchanger pendrin in mouse kidney by acid-base status. Kidney Int 62:2109-2117, 2002.
90. Verlander JW, Hassell KA, Royaux IE, et al: Deoxycorticosterone upregulates PDS (Slc26a4) in mouse kidney: Role of pendrin in mineralocorticoid-induced hypertension. Hypertension 42:356-362, 2003.
91. Verlander JW, Kim YH, Shin W, et al: Dietary Cl^- restriction upregulates pendrin expression within the apical plasma membrane of type B intercalated cells. Am J Physiol Renal Physiol 291:F833-F839, 2006.
92. Reardon W, OMahoney CF, Trembath R, et al: Enlarged vestibular aqueduct: A radiological marker of Pendred's syndrome, and mutation of the PDS gene. QJM 93:99-104, 2000.
93. Everett LA, Belyantseva IA, Noben-Trauth K, et al: Targeted disruption of mouse Pds provides insight about the inner-ear defects encountered in Pendred's syndrome. Hum Mol Genet 10:153-161, 2001.
94. Wangemann P, Itza EM, Albrecht B, et al: Loss of KCNJ10 protein expression abolishes endocochlear potential and causes deafness in Pendred's syndrome mouse model. BMC Med 2:30, 2004.
95. Wangemann P, Nakaya K, Wu T, et al: Loss of cochlear HCO_3^- secretion causes deafness via endolymphatic acidification and inhibition of Ca^{2+} reabsorption in a Pendred's syndrome mouse model. Am J Physiol Renal Physiol 292:F1345-1353, 2007.
96. Nakaya K, Harbidge DG, Wangemann P, et al: Lack of pendrin $HCO3^-$ transport elevates vestibular endolymphatic [Ca^{2+}] by inhibition of acid-sensitive TRPV5 and TRPV6 channels. Am J Physiol Renal Physiol 292:F1314-1321, 2007.
97. Sato E, Nakashima T, Miura Y, et al: Phenotypes associated with replacement of His by Arg in the Pendred's syndrome gene. Eur J Endocrinol 145:697-703, 2001.
98. Wolff J: What is the role of pendrin? Thyroid 15:346-348, 2005.
99. Mendive FM, Rivolta CM, Moya CM, et al: Genomic organization of the human thyroglobulin gene: The complete intron-exon structure. Eur J Endocrinol 145:485-496, 2001.
100. Mendive FM, Rivolta CM, Vassart G, Targovnik HM: Genomic organization of the 3′ region of the human thyroglobulin gene. Thyroid 9:903-912, 1999.
101. Moya CM, Mendive FM, Rivolta CM, et al: Genomic organization of the 5′ region of the human thyroglobulin gene. Eur J Endocrinol 143:789-798, 2000.
102. Baas F, Bikker H, Geurts van Kessel A, et al: The human thyroglobulin gene: A polymorphic marker localized distal to C-MYC on chromosome 8 band q24. Hum Genet 69:138-143, 1985.
103. Rabin M, Barker PE, Ruddle FH, et al: Proximity of thyroglobulin and c-myc genes on human chromosome 8. Somat Cell Mol Genet 11:397-402, 1985.
104. Berge-Lefranc JL, Cartouzou G, Mattei MG, et al: Localization of the thyroglobulin gene by in situ hybridization to human chromosomes. Hum Genet 69:28-31, 1985.
105. Damante G, Di Lauro R: Thyroid-specific gene expression. Biochim Biophys Acta 1218:255-266, 1994.
106. Kambe F, Seo H: Thyroid-specific transcription factors. Endocr J 44:775-784, 1997.
107. Malthiery Y, Lissitzky S: Primary structure of human thyroglobulin deduced from the sequence of its 8448-base complementary DNA. Eur J Biochem 165:491-498, 1987.
108. van de Graaf SA, Pauws E, de Vijlder JJ, Ris-Stalpers CR: The revised 8307 base pair coding sequence of human thyroglobulin transiently expressed in eukaryotic cells. Eur J Endocrinol 136:508-515, 1997.
109. van de Graaf SA, Ris-Stalpers C, Pauws E, et al: Up to date with human thyroglobulin. J Endocrinol 170:307-321, 2001.
110. Kim PS, Arvan P: Hormonal regulation of thyroglobulin export from the endoplasmic reticulum of cultured thyrocytes. J Biol Chem 268:4873-4879, 1993.
111. Arvan P, Kim PS, Kuliawat R, et al: Intracellular protein transport to the thyrocyte plasma membrane: Potential implications for thyroid physiology. Thyroid 7:89-105, 1997.
112. Dunn JT, Dunn AD: Thyroglobulin: Chemistry, biosynthesis, and proteolysis. In Braverman L, Utiger R(eds): Werner and Ingbar's The Thyroid: A Fundamental and Clinical Text. Philadelphia, Lippincott, Williams & Wilkins, 2005, pp 91-104.
113. Molina F, Bouanani M, Pau B, Granier C: Characterization of the type-1 repeat from thyroglobulin, a cysteine-rich module found in proteins from different families. Eur J Biochem 240:125-133, 1996.
114. Yamashita M, Konagaya S: A novel cysteine protease inhibitor of the egg of chum salmon, containing a cysteine-rich thyroglobulin-like motif. J Biol Chem 271:1282-1284, 1996.
115. Mercken L, Simons MJ, De Martynoff G, et al: Presence of hormonogenic and repetitive domains in the first 930 amino acids of bovine thyroglobulin as deduced from the cDNA sequence. Eur J Biochem 147:59-64, 1985.
116. Swillens S, Ludgate M, Mercken L, et al: Analysis of sequence and structure homologies between thyroglobulin and acetylcholinesterase: Possible functional and clinical significance. Biochem Biophys Res Commun 137:142-148, 1986.

117. Parma J, Christophe D, Pohl V, Vassart G: Structural organization of the 5′ region of the thyroglobulin gene. Evidence for intron loss and "exonization" during evolution. J Mol Biol 196:769-779, 1987.
118. Yang SX, Pollock HG, Rawitch AB: Glycosylation in human thyroglobulin: Location of the N-linked oligosaccharide units and comparison with bovine thyroglobulin. Arch Biochem Biophys 327:61-70, 1996.
119. Sakurai S, Fogelfeld L, Schneider AB: Anionic carbohydrate groups of human thyroglobulin containing both phosphate and sulfate. Endocrinology 129:915-920, 1991.
120. Blode H, Heinrich T, Diringe H: A quantitative assay for tyrosine sulfation and tyrosine phosphorylation in peptides. Biol Chem Hoppe Seyler 371:145-151, 1990.
121. Venot N, Nlend MC, Cauvi D, Chabaud O: The hormonogenic tyrosine 5 of porcine thyroglobulin is sulfated. Biochem Biophys Res Commun 298:193-197, 2002.
122. Lamas L, Anderson PC, Fox JW, Dunn JT: Consensus sequences for early iodination and hormonogenesis in human thyroglobulin. J Biol Chem 264:13541-13545, 1989.
123. Dunn AD, Corsi CM, Myers HE, Dunn JT: Tyrosine 130 is an important outer ring donor for thyroxine formation in thyroglobulin. J Biol Chem 273:25223-25229, 1998.
124. Marino M, McCluskey RT: Role of thyroglobulin endocytic pathways in the control of thyroid hormone release. Am J Physiol Cell Physiol 279:C1295-1306, 2000.
125. Marino M, Pinchera A, McCluskey RT, Chiovato L: Megalin in thyroid physiology and pathology. Thyroid 11:47-56, 2001.
126. Herzog V: Transcytosis in thyroid follicle cells. J Cell Biol 97:607-617, 1983.
127. Druetta L, Bornet H, Sassolas G, Rousset B: Identification of thyroid hormone residues on serum thyroglobulin: A clue to the source of circulating thyroglobulin in thyroid diseases. Eur J Endocrinol 140:457-467, 1999.
128. Isozaki O, Kohn LD, Kozak CA, Kimura S: Thyroid peroxidase: Rat cDNA sequence, chromosomal localization in mouse, and regulation of gene expression by comparison to thyroglobulin in rat FRTL-5 cells. Mol Endocrinol 3:1681-1692, 1989.
129. Gerard CM, Lefort A, Libert F, et al: Transcriptional regulation of the thyroperoxydase gene by thyrotropin and forskolin. Mol Cell Endocrinol 60:239-242, 1988.
130. Zannini M, Francis-Lang H, Plachov D, Di Lauro R: Pax-8, a paired domain-containing protein, binds to a sequence overlapping the recognition site of a homeodomain and activates transcription from two thyroid-specific promoters. Mol Cell Biol 12:4230-4241, 1992.
131. Di Palma T, Nitsch R, Mascia A, et al: The paired domain-containing factor Pax8 and the homeodomain-containing factor TTF-1 directly interact and synergistically activate transcription. J Biol Chem 278:3395-3402, 2003.
132. Corvilain B, van Sande J, Laurent E, Dumont JE: The H_2O_2 generating system modulates protein iodination and the activity of the pentose phosphate pathway in dog thyroid. Endocrinology 128:779-785, 1991.
133. Ekholm R: Iodination of thyroglobulin. An intracellular or extracellular process? Mol Cell Endocrinol 24:141-163, 1981.
134. Bjorkman U, Ekholm R: Generation of H_2O_2 in isolated porcine thyroid follicles. Endocrinology 115:392-398, 1984.
135. Virion A, Michot JL, Deme D, et al: NADPH-dependent H_2O_2 generation and peroxidase activity in thyroid particular fraction. Mol Cell Endocrinol 36:95-105, 1984.
136. Nakamura Y, Ogihara S, Ohtaki S: Activation by ATP of calcium-dependent NADPH-oxidase generating hydrogen peroxide in thyroid plasma membranes. J Biochem 102:1121-1132, 1987.
137. Dupuy C, Kaniewski J, Deme D, et al: NADPH-dependent H_2O_2 generation catalyzed by thyroid plasma membranes. Studies with electron scavengers. Eur J Biochem 185:597-603, 1989.
138. Leseney AM, Deme D, Legue O, et al: Biochemical characterization of a Ca^{2+}/NAD(P)H-dependent H_2O_2 generator in human thyroid tissue. Biochimie 81:373-380, 1999.
139. Dème D, Doussiere J, De Sandro V, et al: The Ca^{2+}/NADPH-dependent H_2O_2 generator in thyroid plasma membrane: Inhibition by diphenyleneiodonium. Biochem J 301:75-81, 1994.
140. Gorin Y, Ohayon R, Carvalho DP, et al: Solubilization and characterization of a thyroid Ca^{2+}-dependent and NADPH-dependent $K_3Fe(CN)_6$ reductase. Relationship with the NADPH-dependent H_2O_2-generating system. Eur J Biochem 240:807-814, 1996.
141. Dème D, Virion A, Hammou NA, Pommier J: NADPH-dependent generation of H_2O_2 in a thyroid particulate fraction requires Ca^{2+}. FEBS Lett 186:107-110, 1985.
142. Raspé E, Laurent E, Corvilain B, et al: Control of the intracellular Ca^{2+}-concentration and the inositol phosphate accumulation in dog thyrocyte primary culture: Evidence for different kinetics of Ca^{2+}-phosphatidylinositol cascade activation and for involvement in the regulation of H_2O_2 production. J Cell Physiol 146:242-250, 1991.
143. Raspé E, Dumont JE: Tonic modulation of dog thyrocyte H_2O_2 generation and I^- uptake by thyrotropin through the cyclic adenosine 3′,5′-monophosphate cascade. Endocrinology 136:965-973, 1995.
144. Dupuy C, Ohayon R, Valent A, et al: Purification of a novel flavoprotein involved in the thyroid NADPH oxidase. Cloning of the porcine and human cDNAs. J Biol Chem 274:37265-37269, 1999.
145. De Deken X, Wang D, Many MC, et al: Cloning of two human thyroid cDNAs encoding new members of the NADPH oxidase family. J Biol Chem 275:23227-23233, 2000.

146. Edens WA, Sharling L, Cheng G, et al: Tyrosine cross-linking of extracellular matrix is catalyzed by Duox, a multidomain oxidase/peroxidase with homology to the phagocyte oxidase subunit gp91phox. J Cell Biol 154:879-891, 2001.
147. Moreno JC, Pauws E, van Kampen AH, et al: Cloning of tissue-specific genes using serial analysis of gene expression and a novel computational substraction approach. Genomics 75:70-76, 2001.
148. De Deken X, Wang D, Dumont JE, Miot F: Characterization of ThOX proteins as components of the thyroid H_2O_2-generating system. Exp Cell Res 273:187-196, 2002.
149. Yu L, Quinn MT, Cross AR, Dinauer MC: Gp91(phox) is the heme binding subunit of the superoxide-generating NADPH oxidase. Proc Natl Acad Sci U S A 95:7993-7998, 1998.
150. Suh YA, Arnold RS, Lassegue B, et al: Cell transformation by the superoxide-generating oxidase Mox1. Nature 401:79-82, 1999.
151. Corvilain B, Laurent E, Lecomte M, et al: Role of the cyclic adenosine 3′,5′ -monophosphate and the phosphatidylinositol-Ca^{2+} cascades in mediating the effects of thyrotropin and iodide on hormone synthesis and secretion in human thyroid slices. J Clin Endocrinol Metab 79:152-159, 1994.
152. Caillou B, Dupuy C, Lacroix L, et al: Expression of reduced nicotinamide adenine dinucleotide phosphate oxidase (ThoX, LNOX, Duox) genes and proteins in human thyroid tissues. J Clin Endocrinol Metab 86:3351-3358, 2001.
153. Dupuy C, Pomerance M, Ohayon R, et al: Thyroid oxidase (THOX2) gene expression in the rat thyroid cell line FRTL-5. Biochem Biophys Res Commun 277:287-292, 2000.
154. Corvilain B, Van Sande J, Dumont JE: Inhibition by iodide of iodide binding to proteins: The "Wolff-Chaikoff" effect is caused by inhibition of H_2O_2 generation. Biochem Biophys Res Commun 154:1287-1292, 1988.
155. Morand S, Chaaraoui M, Kaniewski J, et al: Effect of iodide on nicotinamide adenine dinucleotide phosphate oxidase activity and Duox2 protein expression in isolated porcine thyroid follicles. Endocrinology 144:1241-1248, 2003.
156. Lacroix L, Nocera M, Mian C, et al: Expression of nicotinamide adenine dinucleotide phosphate oxidase flavoprotein DUOX genes and proteins in human papillary and follicular thyroid carcinomas. Thyroid 11:1017-1023, 2001.
157. Kuliawat R, Lisanti MP, Arvan P: Polarized distribution and delivery of plasma membrane proteins in thyroid follicular epithelial cells. J Biol Chem 270:2478-2482, 1995.
158. Grasberger H, Refetoff S: Identification of the maturation factor for dual oxidase. Evolution of an eukaryotic operon equivalent. J Biol Chem 281:18269-18272, 2006.
159. Grasberger H, De Deken X, Miot F, et al: Missense mutations of dual oxidase 2 (DUOX2) implicated in congenital hypothyroidism have impaired trafficking in cells reconstituted with DUOX2 maturation factor. Mol Endocrinol 21:1408-1421, 2007.
160. Dupuy C, Deme D, Kaniewski J, et al: Ca^{2+} regulation of thyroid NADPH-dependent H_2O_2 generation. FEBS Lett 233:74-78, 1988.
161. Dupuy C, Virion A, Ohayon R, et al: Mechanism of hydrogen peroxide formation catalyzed by NADPH oxidase in thyroid plasma membrane. J Biol Chem 266:3739-3743, 1991.
162. Carvalho DP, Dupuy C, Gorin Y, et al: The Ca^{2+}- and reduced nicotinamide adenine dinucleotide phosphate-dependent hydrogen peroxide generating system is induced by thyrotropin in porcine thyroid cells. Endocrinology 137:1007-1012, 1996.
163. Gorin Y, Leseney AM, Ohayon R, et al: Regulation of the thyroid NADPH-dependent H_2O_2 generator by Ca^{2+}: Studies with phenylarsine oxide in thyroid plasma membrane. Biochem J 321:383-388, 1997.
164. Bjorkman U, Ekholm R: Accelerated exocytosis and H_2O_2 generation in isolated thyroid follicles enhance protein iodination. Endocrinology 122:488-494, 1988.
165. Bjorkman U, Ekholm R: Hydrogen peroxide generation and its regulation in FRTL-5 and porcine thyroid cells. Endocrinology 130:393-399, 1992.
166. Ohayon R, Boeynaems JM, Braekman JC, et al: Inhibition of thyroid NADPH-oxidase by 2-iodohexadecanal in a cell-free system. Mol Cell Endocrinol 99:133-141, 1994.
167. Panneels V, Van den Bergen H, Jacoby C, et al: Inhibition of H_2O_2 production by iodoaldehydes in cultured dog thyroid cells. Mol Cell Endocrinol 102:167-176, 1994.
168. Corvilain B, Collyn L, van Sande J, Dumont JE: Stimulation by iodide of H_2O_2 generation in thyroid slices from several species. Am J Physiol Endocrinol Metab 278:E692-699, 2000.
169. Taurog A: Hormone synthesis: Thyroid iodine metabolism. In Braverman L, Utiger R (eds) : Werner and Ingbar's The Thyroid: A Fundamental and Clinical Text. Philadelphia, Lippincott-Raven, 1996, pp 47-81.
170. Kimura S, Kotani T, McBride OW, et al: Human thyroid peroxidase: Complete cDNA and protein sequence, chromosome mapping, and identification of two alternately spliced mRNAs. Proc Natl Acad Sci U S A 84:5555-5559, 1987.
171. de Vijlder JJ, Dinsart C, Libert F, et al: Regional localization of the gene for thyroid peroxidase to human chromosome 2pter-p12. Cytogenet Cell Genet 47:170-172, 1988.
172. Kimura S, Hong YS, Kotani T, et al: Structure of the human thyroid peroxidase gene: Comparison and relationship to the human myeloperoxidase gene. Biochemistry 28:4481-4489, 1989.

173. Nagayama Y, Seto P, Rapoport B: Characterization, by molecular cloning, of smaller forms of thyroid peroxidase messenger ribonucleic acid in human thyroid cells as alternatively spliced transcripts. J Clin Endocrinol Metab 71:384-390, 1990.
174. Ferrand M, Le Fourn V, Franc JL: Increasing diversity of human thyroperoxidase generated by alternative splicing characterized by molecular cloning of new transcripts with single- and multispliced mRNAs. J Biol Chem 278:3793-3800, 2003.
175. Niccoli P, Fayadat L, Panneels V, et al: Human thyroperoxidase in its alternatively spliced form (TPO2) is enzymatically inactive and exhibits changes in intracellular processing and trafficking. J Biol Chem 272:29487-29492, 1997.
176. Nagataki S, Uchimura H, Masuyama Y, Nakao K: Thyrotropin and thyroidal peroxidase activity. Endocrinology 92:363-371, 1973.
177. Yamamoto K, DeGroot LJ: Peroxidase and NADPH-cytochrome C reductase activity during thyroid hyperplasia and involution. Endocrinology 95:606-612, 1974.
178. Nagasaka A, Hidaka H: Quantitative modulation of thyroid iodide peroxidase by thyroid stimulating hormone. Biochem Biophys Res Commun 96:1143-1149, 1980.
179. Chazenbalk G, Magnusson RP, Rapoport B: Thyrotropin stimulation of cultured thyroid cells increases steady state levels of the messenger ribonucleic acid for thyroid peroxidase. Mol Endocrinol 1:913-917, 1987.
180. Damante G, Chazenbalk G, Russo D, et al: Thyrotropin regulation of thyroid peroxidase messenger ribonucleic acid levels in cultured rat thyroid cells: Evidence for the involvement of a nontranscriptional mechanism. Endocrinology 124:2889-2894, 1989.
181. Nagayama Y, Yamashita S, Hirayu H, et al: Regulation of thyroid peroxidase and thyroglobulin gene expression by thyrotropin in cultured human thyroid cells. J Clin Endocrinol Metab 68:1155-1159, 1989.
182. Gerard CM, Lefort A, Christophe D, et al: Control of thyroperoxidase and thyroglobulin transcription by cAMP: Evidence for distinct regulatory mechanisms. Mol Endocrinol 3:2110-2118, 1989.
183. Abramowicz MJ, Vassart G, Christophe D: Thyroid peroxidase gene promoter confers TSH responsiveness to heterologous reporter genes in transfection experiments. Biochem Biophys Res Commun 166:1257-1264, 1990.
184. Aza-Blanc P, Di Lauro R, Santisteban P: Identification of a cis-regulatory element and a thyroid-specific nuclear factor mediating the hormonal regulation of rat thyroid peroxidase promoter activity. Mol Endocrinol 7:1297-1306, 1993.
185. Abramowicz MJ, Vassart G, Christophe D: Functional study of the human thyroid peroxidase gene promoter. Eur J Biochem 203:467-473, 1992.
186. Miccadei S, De Leo R, Zammarchi E, et al: The synergistic activity of thyroid transcription factor 1 and Pax 8 relies on the promoter/enhancer interplay. Mol Endocrinol 16:837-846, 2002.
187. Ortiz L, Aza-Blanc P, Zannini M, et al: The interaction between the forkhead thyroid transcription factor TTF-2 and the constitutive factor CTF/NF-1 is required for efficient hormonal regulation of the thyroperoxidase gene transcription. J Biol Chem 274:15213-15221, 1999.
188. De Leo R, Miccadei S, Zammarchi E, Civitareale D: Role for p300 in Pax 8 induction of thyroperoxidase gene expression. J Biol Chem 275:34100-34105, 2000.
189. Kikkawa F, Gonzalez FJ, Kimura S: Characterization of a thyroid-specific enhancer located 5.5 kilobase pairs upstream of the human thyroid peroxidase gene. Mol Cell Biol 10:6216-6224, 1990.
190. Mizuno K, Gonzalez FJ, Kimura S: Thyroid-specific enhancer-binding protein (T/EBP): cDNA cloning, functional characterization, and structural identity with thyroid transcription factor TTF-1. Mol Cell Biol 11:4927-4933, 1991.
191. Esposito C, Miccadei S, Saiardi A, Civitareale D: PAX 8 activates the enhancer of the human thyroperoxidase gene. Biochem J 331:37-40, 1998.
192. Collison KS, Banga JP, Barnett PS, et al: Activation of the thyroid peroxidase gene in human thyroid cells: Effect of thyrotrophin, forskolin and phorbol ester. J Mol Endocrinol 3:1-5, 1989.
193. Ashizawa K, Yamashita S, Nagayama Y, et al: Interferon-gamma inhibits thyrotropin-induced thyroidal peroxidase gene expression in cultured human thyrocytes. J Clin Endocrinol Metab 69:475-477, 1989.
194. Ashizawa K, Yamashita S, Tobinaga T, et al: Inhibition of human thyroid peroxidase gene expression by interleukin 1. Acta Endocrinol (Copenh) 121:465-469, 1989.
195. Cetani F, Costagliola S, Tonacchera M, et al: The thyroperoxidase doublet is not produced by alternative splicing. Mol Cell Endocrinol 115:125-132, 1995.
196. Taurog A, Dorris ML, Yokoyama N, Slaughter C: Purification and characterization of a large, tryptic fragment of human thyroid peroxidase with high catalytic activity. Arch Biochem Biophys 278:333-341, 1990.
197. Yokoyama N, Taurog A: Porcine thyroid peroxidase: Relationship between the native enzyme and an active, highly purified tryptic fragment. Mol Endocrinol 2:838-844, 1988.
198. Foti D, Kaufman KD, Chazenbalk GD, Rapoport B: Generation of a biologically active, secreted form of human thyroid peroxidase by site-directed mutagenesis. Mol Endocrinol 4:786-791, 1990.
199. Rawitch AB, Pollock HG, Yang SX: Thyroglobulin glycosylation: Location and nature of the N-linked oligosaccharide units in bovine thyroglobulin. Arch Biochem Biophys 300:271-279, 1993.
200. Taurog A, Wall M: Proximal and distal histidines in thyroid peroxidase: Relation to the alternatively spliced form, TPO-2. Thyroid 8:185-191, 1998.

201. De Gioia L, Ghibaudi E, Laurenti E, et al: A theoretical three-dimensional model for lactoperoxidase and eosinophil peroxidase, built on the scaffold of the myeloperoxidase X-ray structure. J Biol Inorg Chem 1:476-485, 1996.
202. Taurog A: Molecular evolution of thyroid peroxidase. Biochimie 81:557-562, 1999.
203. Magnusson RP, Gestautas J, Taurog A, Rapoport B: Molecular cloning of the structural gene for porcine thyroid peroxidase. J Biol Chem 262:13885-13888, 1987.
204. Johnson KR, Nauseef WM, Care A, et al: Characterization of cDNA clones for human myeloperoxidase: Predicted amino acid sequence and evidence for multiple mRNA species. Nucleic Acids Res 15:2013-2028, 1987.
205. Morishita K, Kubota N, Asano S, et al: Molecular cloning and characterization of cDNA for human myeloperoxidase. J Biol Chem 262:3844-3851, 1987.
206. Kimura S, Ikeda-Saito M: Human myeloperoxidase and thyroid peroxidase, two enzymes with separate and distinct physiological functions, are evolutionarily related members of the same gene family. Proteins 3:113-120, 1988.
207. Dull TJ, Uyeda C, Strosberg AD, et al: Molecular cloning of cDNAs encoding bovine and human lactoperoxidase. DNA Cell Biol 9:499-509, 1990.
208. Kiser C, Caterina CK, Engle JA, et al: Cloning and sequence analysis of the human salivary peroxidase-encoding cDNA. Gene 173:261-264, 1996.
209. Sakamaki K, Tomonaga M, Tsukui K, Nagata S: Molecular cloning and characterization of a chromosomal gene for human eosinophil peroxidase. J Biol Chem 264:16828-16836, 1989.
210. Libert F, Ruel J, Ludgate M, et al: Thyroperoxidase, an auto-antigen with a mosaic structure made of nuclear and mitochondrial gene modules. Embo J 6:4193-4196, 1987.
211. Zeng J, Fenna RE: X-ray crystal structure of canine myeloperoxidase at 3 Å resolution. J Mol Biol 226:185-207, 1992.
212. Fiedler TJ, Davey CA, Fenna RE: X-ray crystal structure and characterization of halide-binding sites of human myeloperoxidase at 1.8 Å resolution. J Biol Chem 275:11964-11971, 2000.
213. Blair-Johnson M, Fiedler T, Fenna R: Human myeloperoxidase: structure of a cyanide complex and its interaction with bromide and thiocyanate substrates at 1.9 A resolution. Biochemistry 40:13990-13997, 2001.
214. Nilsson M, Molne J, Karlsson FA, Ericson LE: Immunoelectron microscopic studies on the cell surface location of the thyroid microsomal antigen. Mol Cell Endocrinol 53:177-186, 1987.
215. Pinchera A, Mariotti S, Chiovato L, et al: Cellular localization of the microsomal antigen and the thyroid peroxidase antigen. Acta Endocrinol 281:57-62, 1987.
216. Bjorkman U, Ekholm R, Ericson LE: Effects of thyrotropin on thyroglobulin exocytosis and iodination in the rat thyroid gland. Endocrinology 102:460-470, 1978.
217. Chiovato L, Vitti P, Lombardi A, et al: Expression of the microsomal antigen on the surface of continuously cultured rat thyroid cells is modulated by thyrotropin. J Clin Endocrinol Metab 61:12-16, 1985.
218. Zhang X, Arvan P: Cell type-dependent differences in thyroid peroxidase cell surface expression. J Biol Chem 275:31946-31953, 2000.
219. Penel C, Gruffat D, Alquier C, et al: Thyrotropin chronically regulates the pool of thyroperoxidase and its intracellular distribution: A quantitative confocal microscopic study. J Cell Physiol 174:160-169, 1998.
220. Fayadat L, Niccoli-Sire P, Lanet J, Franc JL: Human thyroperoxidase is largely retained and rapidly degraded in the endoplasmic reticulum. Its N-glycans are required for folding and intracellular trafficking. Endocrinology 139:4277-4285, 1998.
221. Fayadat L, Siffroi-Fernandez S, Lanet J, Franc JL: Degradation of human thyroperoxidase in the endoplasmic reticulum involves two different pathways depending on the folding state of the protein. J Biol Chem 275:15948-15954, 2000.
222. Nakagawa H, Kotani T, Ohtaki S, et al: Purification of thyroid peroxidase by monoclonal antibody-assisted immunoaffinity chromatography. Biochem Biophys Res Commun 127:8-14, 1985.
223. Ohtaki S, Kotani T, Nakamura Y: Characterization of human thyroid peroxidase purified by monoclonal antibody-assisted chromatography. J Clin Endocrinol Metab 63:570-576, 1986.
224. McLachlan SM, Rapoport B: The molecular biology of thyroid peroxidase: Cloning, expression and role as autoantigen in autoimmune thyroid disease. Endocr Rev 13:192-206, 1992.
225. Guo J, McLachlan SM, Hutchison S, Rapoport B: The greater glycan content of recombinant human thyroid peroxidase of mammalian than of insect cell origin facilitates purification to homogeneity of enzymatically protein remaining soluble at high concentration. Endocrinology 139:999-1005, 1998.
226. Morrison M, Schonbaum GR: Peroxidase-catalyzed halogenation. Annu Rev Biochem 45: 861-888, 1976.
227. Magnusson RP, Taurog A, Dorris ML: Mechanisms of thyroid peroxidase- and lactoperoxidase-catalyzed reactions involving iodide. J Biol Chem 259:13783-13790, 1984.
228. Magnusson RP, Taurog A, Dorris ML: Mechanism of iodide-dependent catalatic activity of thyroid peroxidase and lactoperoxidase. J Biol Chem 259:197-205, 1984.
229. Dunford HB, Ralston IM: On the mechanism of iodination of tyrosine. Biochem Biophys Res Commun 116:639-643, 1983.
230. Sun W, Dunford HB: Kinetics and mechanism of the peroxidase-catalyzed iodination of tyrosine. Biochemistry 32:1324-1331, 1993.
231. Morris DR, Hager LP: Mechanism of the inhibition of enzymatic halogenation by antithyroid agents. J Biol Chem 241:3582-3589, 1966.

232. Ohtaki S, Nakagawa H, Kimura S, Yamazaki I: Analyses of catalytic intermediates of hog thyroid peroxidase during its iodinating reaction. J Biol Chem 256:805-810, 1981.
233. Nakamura M, Yamazaki I, Nakagawa H, Ohtaki S: Steady state kinetics and regulation of thyroid peroxidase-catalyzed iodination. J Biol Chem 258:3837-3842, 1983.
234. Ohtaki S, Nakagawa H, Nakamura M, Kotani T: Thyroid peroxidase: Experimental and clinical integration. Endocr J 43:1-14, 1996.
235. Dawson JH: Probing structure-function relations in heme-containing oxygenases and peroxidases. Science 240:433-439, 1988.
236. Malthiery Y, Marriq C, Berge-Lefranc JL, et al: Thyroglobulin structure and function: Recent advances. Biochimie 71:195-209, 1989.
237. Xiao S, Dorris ML, Rawitch AB, Taurog A: Selectivity in tyrosyl iodination sites in human thyroglobulin. Arch Biochem Biophys 334:284-294, 1996.
238. Taurog A, Dorris ML, Doerge DR: Mechanism of simultaneous iodination and coupling catalyzed by thyroid peroxidase. Arch Biochem Biophys 330:24-32, 1996.
239. Gavaret JM, Nunez J, Cahnmann HJ: Formation of dehydroalanine residues during thyroid hormone synthesis in thyroglobulin. J Biol Chem 255:5281-5285, 1980.
240. Kim PS, Dunn JT, Kaiser DL: Similar hormone-rich peptides from thyroglobulins of five vertebrate classes. Endocrinology 114:369-374, 1984.
241. Bernier-Valentin F, Kostrouch Z, Rabilloud R, et al: Coated vesicles from thyroid cells carry iodinated thyroglobulin molecules. First indication for an internalization of the thyroid prohormone via a mechanism of receptor-mediated endocytosis. J Biol Chem 265:17373-17380, 1990.
242. Kostrouch Z, Bernier-Valentin F, Munari-Silem Y, et al: Thyroglobulin molecules internalized by thyrocytes are sorted in early endosomes and partially recycled back to the follicular lumen. Endocrinology 132:2645-2653, 1993.
243. Dunn AD, Crutchfield HE, Dunn JT: Thyroglobulin processing by thyroidal proteases. Major sites of cleavage by cathepsins B, D, and L. J Biol Chem 266:20198-20204, 1991.
244. Dunn AD, Crutchfield HE, Dunn JT: Proteolytic processing of thyroglobulin by extracts of thyroid lysosomes. Endocrinology 128:3073-3080, 1991.
245. Tokuyama T, Yoshinari M, Rawitch AB, Taurog A: Digestion of thyroglobulin with purified thyroid lysosomes: Preferential release of iodoamino acids. Endocrinology 121:714-721, 1987.
246. Dunn AD, Myers HE, Dunn JT: The combined action of two thyroidal proteases releases T4 from the dominant hormone-forming site of thyroglobulin. Endocrinology 137:3279-3285, 1996.
247. Visser W, Friesema E, Jansen J, Visser T: Thyroid hormone transport in and out of cells. Trends Endocrinol Metab 19:50-56, 2008.
248. Roche J, Michel R, Michel O, Lissitzky S: Sur la déshalgénation enzymatique des iodotyrosines par le corps thyroïde et sur son role physiologique. [Enzymatic dehalogenation of iodotyrosine by thyroid tissue on its physiological role.] Biochim Biophys Acta 9:161-169, 1952.
249. Moreno JC: Identification of novel genes involved in congenital hypothyroidism using serial analysis of gene expression. Horm Res 60:96-102, 2003.
250. Moreno JC, Klootwijk W, van Toor H, et al: Mutations in the iodotyrosine deiodinase gene and hypothyroidism. N Engl J Med 358:1856-1859, 2008.
251. Rosenberg IN, Goswami A: Purification and characterization of a flavoprotein from bovine thyroid with iodotyrosine deiodinase activity. J Biol Chem 254:12318-12325, 1979.
252. Rosenberg IN: Purification of iodotyrosine deiodinase from bovine thyroid. Metabolism 19:785-798, 1970.
253. Kopp P: Reduce, recycle, reuse—iodotyrosine deiodinase in thyroid iodide metabolism. N Engl J Med 358:1856-1859, 2008.
254. Gillam MP, Kopp P: Genetic regulation of thyroid development. Curr Opin Pediatr 13:358-363, 2001.
255. Van Vliet G: Development of the thyroid gland: Lessons from congenitally hypothyroid mice and men. Clin Genet 63:445-455, 2003.
256. De Felice M, Di Lauro R: Thyroid development and its disorders: Genetics and molecular mechanisms. Endocr Rev 25:722-746, 2004.
257. Wolff J: Congenital goiter with defective iodide transport. Endocr Rev 4:240-254, 1983.
258. Fujiwara H, Tatsumi K, Miki K, et al: Congenital hypothyroidism caused by a mutation in the Na^+/I^- symporter. Nat Genet 16:124-125, 1997.
259. Dohan O, Baloch Z, Banrevi Z, et al: Predominant intracellular overexpression of the Na^+/I^- symporter (NIS) in a large sampling of thyroid cancer cases. J Clin Endocrinol Metab 86:2697-2700, 2001.
260. Reed-Tsur MD, De la Vieja A, Ginter CS, Carrasco N: Molecular characterization of V59E NIS, a Na^+/I^- symporter mutant that causes congenital I^- transport defect. Endocrinology 149:3077-3084, 2008.
261. Levy O, Ginter CS, De la Vieja A, et al: Identification of a structural requirement for thyroid Na^+/I^- symporter (NIS) function from analysis of a mutation that causes human congenital hypothyroidism. FEBS Lett 429:36-40, 1998.
262. Pohlenz J, Duprez L, Weiss RE, et al: Failure of membrane targeting causes the functional defect of two mutant sodium iodide symporters. J Clin Endocrinol Metab 85:2366-2369, 2000.
263. Fraser GR: Association of congenital deafness with goitre (Pendred's syndrome). Ann Hum Genet 28:201-249, 1965.
264. Morgans ME, Trotter WR: Association of congenital deafness with goitre: The nature of the thyroid defect. Lancet 1:607-609, 1958.

265. Coyle B, Reardon W, Herbrick JA, et al: Molecular analysis of the PDS gene in Pendred's syndrome (sensorineural hearing loss and goitre). Hum Mol Genet 7:1105-1112, 1998.
266. Van Hauwe P, Everett LA, Coucke P, et al: Two frequent missense mutations in Pendred's syndrome. Hum Mol Genet 7:1099-1104, 1998.
267. Fugazzola L, Mannavola D, Cerutti N, et al: Molecular analysis of the Pendred's syndrome gene and magnetic resonance imaging studies of the inner ear are essential for the diagnosis of true Pendred's syndrome. J Clin Endocrinol Metab 85:2469-2475, 2000.
268. Gonzalez Trevino O, Karamanoglu Arseven O, Ceballos C, et al: Clinical and molecular analysis of three Mexican families with Pendred's syndrome. Europ J Endocrinol 144:1-9, 2001.
269. Park H-J, Shaukat S, Liu X-Z, et al: Origins and frequencies of SLC26A4 (PDS) mutations in east and south Asians: Global implications for the epidemiology of deafness. J Med Genet 40:242-248, 2003.
270. Tsukamoto K, Suzuki H, Harada D, et al: Distribution and frequencies of PDS (SLC26A4) mutations in Pendred's syndrome and nonsyndromic hearing loss associated with enlarged vestibular aqueduct: A unique spectrum of mutations in Japanese. Eur J Hum Genet 24:24, 2003.
271. Rotman-Pikielny P, Hirschberg K, Maruvada P, et al: Retention of pendrin in the endoplasmic reticulum is a major mechanism for Pendred's syndrome. Hum Mol Genet 11:2625-2633, 2002.
272. Nilsson LR, Borgfors N, Gamstorp I, et al: Non-endemic goitre and deafness. Acta Paed 53:117-131, 1964.
273. Ieiri T, Cochaux P, Targovnik HM, et al: A 3′ splice site mutation in the thyroglobulin gene responsible for congenital goiter with hypothyroidism. J Clin Invest 88:1901-1905, 1991.
274. Vono-Toniolo J, Rivolta CM, Targovnik HM, et al: Naturally occurring mutations in the thyroglobulin gene. Thyroid 15:1021-1033, 2005.
275. Medeiros-Neto G, Targovnik HM, Vassart G: Defective thyroglobulin synthesis and secretion causing goiter and hypothyroidism. Endocr Rev 14:165-183, 1993.
276. Hishinuma A, Fukata S, Nishiyama S, et al: Haplotype analysis reveals founder effects of thyroglobulin gene mutations C1058R and C1977S in Japan. J Clin Endocrinol Metab 91:3100-3104, 2006.
277. Caron P, Moya CM, Malet D, et al: Compound heterozygous mutations in the thyroglobulin gene (1143delC and 6725G>A [R2223H]) resulting in fetal goitrous hypothyroidism. J Clin Endocrinol Metab 88:3546-3553, 2003.
278. Kim PS, Arvan P: Endocrinopathies in the family of endoplasmic reticulum (ER) storage diseases: Disorders of protein trafficking and the role of ER molecular chaperones. Endocr Rev 19:173-202, 1998.
279. Targovnik HM, Vono J, Billerbeck AE, et al: A 138-nucleotide deletion in the thyroglobulin ribonucleic acid messenger in a congenital goiter with defective thyroglobulin synthesis. J Clin Endocrinol Metab 80:3356-3360, 1995.
280. Medeiros-Neto G, Kim PS, Yoo SE, et al: Congenital hypothyroid goiter with deficient thyroglobulin. Identification of an endoplasmic reticulum storage disease with induction of molecular chaperones. J Clin Invest 98:2838-2844, 1996.
281. Abramowicz MJ, Targovnik HM, Varela V, et al: Identification of a mutation in the coding sequence of the human thyroid peroxidase gene causing congenital goiter. J Clin Invest 90:1200-1204, 1992.
282. Bikker H, Vulsma T, Baas F, de Vijlder JJ: Identification of five novel inactivating mutations in the thyroid peroxidase gene by denaturing gradient gel electrophoresis. Human Mutation 6:9-16, 1995.
283. Pannain S, Weiss RE, Jackson CE, et al: Two different mutations in the thyroid peroxidase gene of a large inbred Amish kindred: Power and limits of homozygosity mapping. J Clin Endocrinol Metab 84:1061-1071, 1999.
284. Bakker B, Bikker H, Vulsma T, et al: Two decades of screening for congenital hypothyroidism in the Netherlands: TPO gene mutations in total iodide organification defects (an update). J Clin Endocrinol Metab 85:3708-3712, 2000.
285. McGirr EM, Hutchison JH: Radioactive-iodine studies in non-endemic goitrous cretinism. Lancet 1:1117-1120, 1953.
286. Stanbury JB, Kassenaar AA, Meijer JW, Terpstra J: The occurrence of mono- and di-iodotyrosine in the blood of a patient with congenital goiter. J Clin Endocrinol Metab 15:1216-1227, 1955.
287. Medeiros-Neto G, Stanbury JB: The iodotyrosine deiodinase defect. In Medeiros-Neto G, Stanbury JB (eds): Inherited Disorders of the Thyroid System. Boca Raton, Fla, CRC Press, 1994, pp 139-159 .

Chapter 4

Thyroid Hormone Action

Amin Sabet and Paul M. Yen

Key Points

- At the cellular level in target tissues, thyroid hormone availability and activity are ultimately governed by intracellular hormone transport, metabolism, and availability of nuclear receptors as well as associated cofactors.
- In addition to direct transcriptional effects mediated by nuclear thyroid hormone receptors (TRs) on thyroid hormone response elements (TREs), thyroid hormones exert direct effects on extranuclear proteins.
- Thyroid hormone analogues are being developed and studied as potential therapies for obesity, hypercholesterolemia, heart failure, and other conditions.

Thyroid hormones have a critical role in differentiation, growth, and metabolism. Early clinical observations correlating thyroid function with the syndromes of myxedema and hyperthyroidism established that thyroid hormones have profound effects on almost all tissues. In his *Principles and Practice of Medicine*, Osler referred to the effects of thyroid hormone replacement therapy as "astounding—unparalleled by anything in the whole range of curative measures."[1] The mechanisms by which thyroid hormones exert their diverse actions have long been the subject of study. Physiology studies from the 1930s and 1940s demonstrated major effects of thyroid hormone on oxygen consumption and metabolic rate. In the introduction to his 1951 review, Barker[2] stated the following:

> The extreme variety of effects is generally interpreted as indicating a single primary action of the thyroid hormone, probably on energy metabolism, with all of the others representing a secondary dependence upon integrity of energy pathways. In contradistinction to this is the thesis advanced by some biologists that the thyroid has a specific developmental function independent of any effect on energy transformations. Sided to support this view is such evidence as a lack of increase in metabolic rate during some stages of amphibian metamorphosis, although the thyroid gland stimulates both processes.

During the past 40 years, we have learned that most thyroid hormone effects are mediated by direct transcriptional effects of thyroid hormone bound to nuclear thyroid hormone receptors (TRs). In the 1960s, Tata and coworkers proposed that thyroid hormones might be involved in transcriptional regulation of target genes.[3,4] They showed that L-triiodothyronine (T_3) treatment stimulated RNA synthesis in the liver of hypothyroid rats and that these effects preceded protein synthesis and mitochondrial oxidation.[3,4] Subsequently, research studies demonstrated high-affinity nuclear binding sites for radiolabeled T_3 in different T_3-sensitive tissues, suggesting that transcriptional regulation by T_3 might involve nuclear thyroid hormone receptors (TRs).[5,6] Photoaffinity labeling of nuclear extracts yielded different-sized receptors, raising the possibility of multiple TR isoforms.[7,8] Meanwhile, studies of the induction of the rat growth hormone (GH) gene by T_3 suggested that TRs recognized enhancer sequences, or TR response elements (TREs), similar to steroid hormone receptors.[9-12] The glucocorticoid receptor was cloned in 1985 and found to have surprising homology with a known viral oncogene product, v-*erbA*, which in conjunction with v-*erbB* can cause erythroblastosis in chicks.[13] Subsequent cloning of the estrogen receptor suggested that there is a family of nuclear hormone receptors.[14] The following year, researchers cloned two different TR isoforms and demonstrated that they are the cellular homologues of v-*erbA*.[15,16] Since then, more than 20 years ago, we have learned much regarding the molecular mechanisms of thyroid hormone action. We now know that there are multiple TR isoforms that bind to TREs with variable orientation, spacing, and sequences. It has been shown that TRs interact with other nuclear proteins, including corepressors and coactivators, to form complexes that interact with and regulate the basal transcriptional machinery.

In contrast to this classic nuclear mode of thyroid hormone action, several mechanisms of thyroid hormone action have been identified, which occur at the plasma membrane or in the cytosol. These so-called nongenomic effects of thyroid hormones are mediated by rapid effects on extranuclear proteins. The term *nongenomic* may be somewhat misleading, given that some of these extranuclear actions of thyroid hormones have downstream effects on target gene transcription. Here, nongenomic will be used to distinguish those actions that are not mediated by direct transcriptional effects of thyroid hormone bound to TRs. This chapter will discuss what is known about the molecular mechanisms of thyroid hormone action, with a focus on direct transcriptional regulation by thyroid hormones.

THYROID HORMONE METABOLISM AND TRANSPORT

The ultimate availability and activity of intracellular thyroid hormone are regulated at many levels. The factors controlling thyroidal synthesis and release, as well as plasma transport of thyroid hormones, are covered elsewhere (see Chapter 3). At the cellular level in target tissues, thyroid hormone availability is governed by intracellular transport, metabolism, and availability of nuclear receptors, as well as associated cofactors (Fig. 4-1).

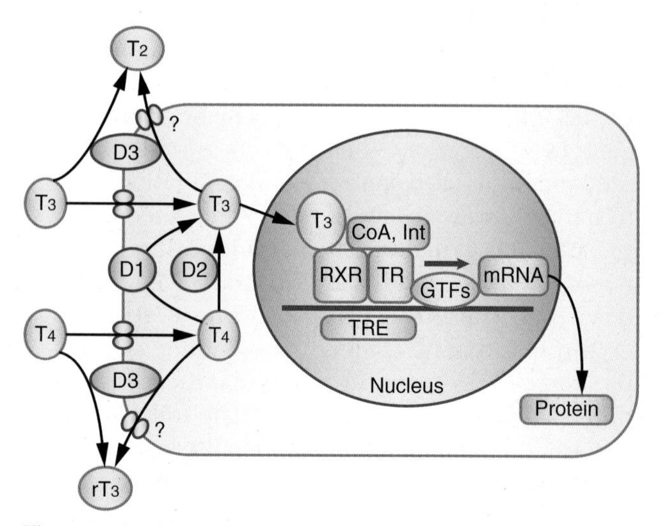

Figure 4–1 Cellular transport and metabolism of thyroid hormones. CoA, coactivators; GTFs, general transcription factors; Int, integrators; rT_3, reverse L-triiodothyronine; T_3, L-triiodothyronine; T_4, thyroxine.

Although both thyroxine (T_4) and T_3 are synthesized by the thyroid gland, T_4 is the principal secreted hormone. However, because T_4 is tightly bound to carrier proteins, plasma free levels of T_3 and T_4 are similar. Although it was previously thought that thyroid hormones enter the cell by simple diffusion, more recent work has established that T_3 and T_4 enter the cell via a number of transporters, including the iodothyronine-specific transporters monocarboxylate transporter 8 (MCT8) and the organic anion transporting polypeptide 1C1 (OATP1C1). OATP1C1 is expressed almost exclusively in brain capillaries and may be necessary for T_4 transport across the blood-brain barrier. MCT8, encoded by a gene on chromosome Xq13.2, is expressed in a wide variety of tissues, including liver, kidney, pituitary, and thyroid. Mutations in MCT8 have been implicated in a familial X-linked syndrome of psychomotor retardation and resistance to thyroid hormone, the pathogenesis of which is believed to involve a defect in the neuronal entry of T_3.[17]

Intracellularly, T_3 is the more potent hormone, binding to TRs with 10-fold greater affinity than T_4. Production of circulating T_3 occurs mainly via 5′ deiodination of the outer ring of T_4 by a class of selenoproteins known as deiodinases.[18] Type I deiodinase, found in peripheral tissues such as liver and kidney, converts circulating T_4 to T_3. Type II deiodinase is found primarily in the pituitary gland, brain, and brown fat, where it contributes to peripheral and intracellular conversion of T_4 to T_3. Tissues that contain type II deiodinase can potentially modulate their response to a given circulating concentration of T_4 by intracellular conversion to T_3. Type III deiodinase is found mainly in the placenta, brain, and skin. Together with type I deiodinase, type III deiodinase converts T_4 to reverse T_3 (rT_3), which is an inactive thyroid hormone metabolite.[19]

Unlike related steroid hormone receptors, TRs are found primarily in the nucleus, whether thyroid hormone (TH) is present or absent.[20,21] Moreover, TRs are tightly associated with chromatin, in keeping with their proposed role as DNA binding proteins that regulate gene expression.[22-24] Nuclear TRs are approximately 50% saturated with thyroid hormone in the liver and kidney and 75% saturated with thyroid hormone in the brain and pituitary.

THYROID HORMONE RECEPTORS

In 1986, researchers independently reported the cloning of cDNAs encoding two different TRs from embryonal chicken and human placental cDNA libraries.[15,16] By amino acid sequence comparison, it was shown that TRs are the cellular homologues of the viral oncogene product v-*erbA*. It was soon noted

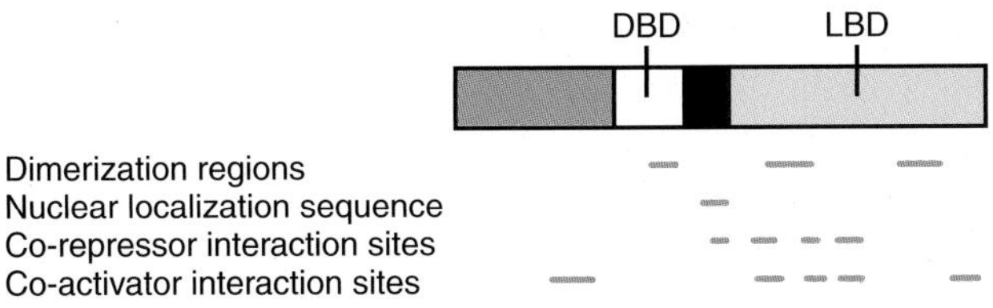

Figure 4–2 Organization of major thyroid hormone receptor domains and functional subregions. DBD, DNA-binding domain; LBD, ligand-binding domain.

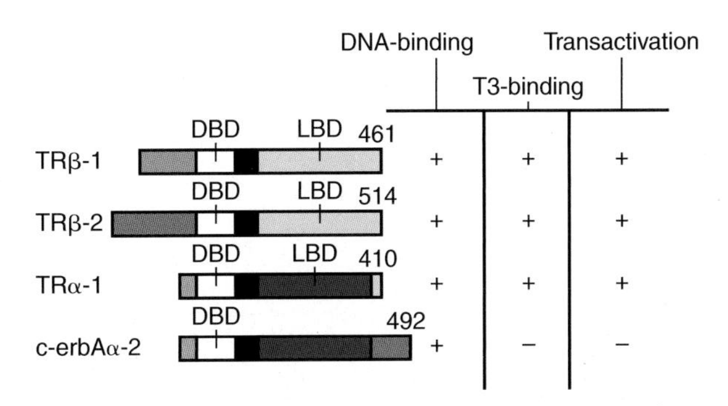

Figure 4–3 Comparison of amino acid homologies and functional properties of thyroid hormone receptor (TR) isoforms. The amino acid length of each TR isoform is indicated just above its diagram. DBD, DNA-binding domain; LBD, ligand-binding domain.

that TRs have amino acid sequence homology with steroid hormone receptors. This was surprising at the time, because T_3 and cholesterol-derived steroids are structurally distinct ligands. However, it has since been demonstrated that TRs belong to a superfamily of nuclear hormone receptors, including the steroid, vitamin D, peroxisomal proliferator, and retinoic acid receptors, in addition to orphan receptors, which lack known ligands.

TR structural domains resemble those of other family members. They have a central DNA binding domain (DBD) containing two zinc fingers, which intercalate with the major and minor grooves of TRE nucleotide sequences, and a carboxy-terminal ligand-binding domain (LBD) (Fig. 4-2). Located in between these two domains, the hinge region contains a stretch of multiple lysine residues that are required for nuclear translocation of the receptor.[25,26] X-ray crystallographic studies of the liganded rat TRα and human TRβ have shown that thyroid hormone nests inside a hydrophobic pocket within the LBD,[27,28] made up of 12 amphipathic helices. Helices 3, 5, 6, and 12 interact with coactivators, whereas helices 3, 4, 5, and 6 interact with corepressors.[29-32] Binding of T_3 induces major confrontational changes within the LBD, particularly in helix 12, affecting TR interactions with coactivators and corepressors.

The *Thra* and *Thrb* genes, located on human chromosomes 17 and 3, respectively, encode the major TR isoforms, TRα-1, TRβ-1, and TRβ-2 (Fig. 4-3). Each of these receptor isoforms binds T_3 with similar affinity and mediates thyroid hormone–regulated gene transcription. Mammalian TR isoforms range from 400 to slightly more than 500 amino acids in length and feature highly conserved DBDs and LBDs.

The *Thra* gene encodes two proteins, TRα-1 and c-erbAα-2, generated by alternative splicing of TRα mRNA. In the rat and human, these proteins are identical from amino acid residues 1 to 370, varying greatly thereafter. In contrast to TRα-1, c-erbAα-2 cannot bind T_3, binds TREs weakly, and is unable to transactivate thyroid hormone responsive genes. On certain target genes, c-erbAα-2 may act as a dominant inhibitor of thyroid hormone action by competing for binding to TREs.[33,34] Furthermore, the dominant negative activity of c-erbAα-2 may be regulated by its phosphorylation state.[35] Another gene product, rev-erbA, is generated from the opposite strand of the TRα gene. Rev-erbA, also an orphan member of the NR superfamily, is expressed in muscle and adipocytes, where it can help promote adipogenesis.[36]

The *Thrb* gene contains two promoters, which encode transcripts for two major TRβ isoforms, TRβ-1 and TRβ-2, through their alternate use.[37,38] These two isoforms are identical, with the exception of their amino termini (see Fig. 4-3). Both contain DBDs and LBDs with high homology to those of TRα-1.

TRα-1 and TRβ-1 are expressed in almost all tissues.[39] In rats, TRα-1 expression is highest in skeletal muscle and brown fat, whereas TRβ-1 expression is highest in brain, liver, and kidney. In contrast to other TR isoforms, TRβ-2 expression is largely restricted to the anterior pituitary gland, hypothalamus, developing brain, and inner ear.[39-42] In the chick and mouse, TRβ-2 is also expressed in the developing retina.[43] Expression of c-erbAα-2 is highest in the testis and brain. Several short forms of TRα and TRβ generated by the use of internal start sites or alternate splicing are expressed in embryonic stem cells and fetal bone cells, where some of them may exert dominant negative activity, blocking wild-type TR transcriptional activity.[44,45]

TR isoforms are highly conserved across mammalian species. In addition, distinct phenotypes are noted in the case of specific TR isoform deletion in animals, suggesting that TRs may exhibit isoform-specific transcriptional effects on particular target genes. Recently, it has been suggested that TRβ-1 may specifically regulate the TRH and myelin basic protein genes, whereas TRβ-2 may differentially regulate the thyroid-stimulating hormone β (TSHβ) and GH genes.[46-49] However, cDNA microarray studies performed in TR isoform knockout mice have suggested that TRα and TRβ provide compensatory regulation

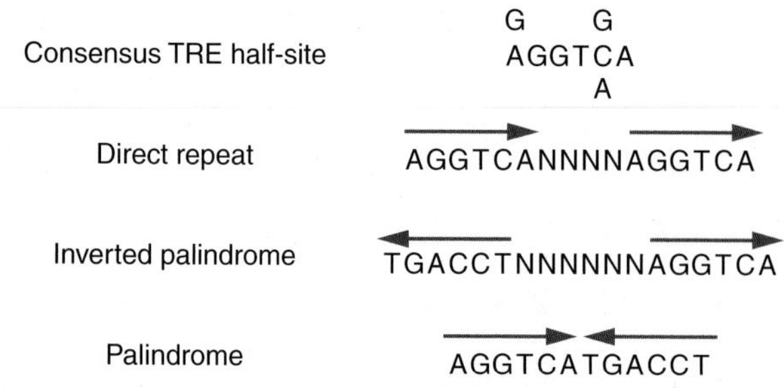

Figure 4–4 Half-site orientation and optimal spacing within thyroid hormone response elements (TREs). Arrows show direction of half-sites on the sense strand.

of target genes in the liver.[50] Thus, total TR expression in specific cells, rather than expression of specific TR isoforms, may be the principal determinant of target gene activity.

THYROID HORMONE RESPONSE ELEMENTS

TRs bind to TREs, which are generally located in the upstream promoter regions of target genes, although in certain cases they may be found in 3′ flanking regions downstream from the coding region. In target genes, which are positively regulated by T_3, TREs generally contain two or more hexamer half-site sequences of AGGT(C/A)A arranged in tandem. Significant degeneracy exists in the primary nucleotide sequences of half-sites.[51] In addition, TRs can bind to half-sites, which are arranged as direct repeats, inverted palindromes, and palindromes containing optimal spacings of four, six, or zero nucleotides between half-sites, respectively (Fig. 4-4). Among the approximately 30 natural TREs that have been described, direct repeats occur most frequently, followed by inverted palindromes.[25]

RXR proteins are the most important heterodimeric partners for TRs.[51] TRE half-site sequence, spacing, orientation, and sequence context determine specificity and affinity for the TR/RXR heterodimer. TR/RXR activates direct repeats spaced by four base pairs, whereas vitamin D receptor/RXR and RXR/RXR activate direct repeats spaced by three and five base pairs, respectively (the proposed 3-4-5 rule).[52,53] In direct repeat TREs, RXR binds to the upstream half-site and TR binds to the downstream half-site.[54-56] Whereas the DBDs interact with the major grooves of the half-sites on the same face of DNA, the carboxy-terminal of the TR DBD forms an α-helical structure that interacts with the spacer region in the DNA minor groove between the two half-sites.[57] Protein-protein contacts between the TR and RXR DBDs contribute to heterodimerization and determine half-site spacing specificity. However, the most critical interaction sites for heterodimerization are thought to be located in their LBDs.[58,59] Helices 10 and 11 of the TR LBD appear to contain residues necessary for heterodimerization.[27]

TRs can form monomers, homodimers, and heterodimers on TREs in electrophoretic mobility shift assays (EMSAs),[38] but the role of TR monomers and homodimers in regulating transcription is not well understood. In contrast to steroid hormone receptors, with which ligand enhances homodimer binding to hormone response elements (HREs), TRs bind predominantly as heterodimers in the presence of ligand.[25] It is therefore likely that TR/RXR heterodimers have a major role in T_3-mediated gene activation. Unliganded TRs can bind as homodimers or as heterodimers to TREs in vitro.[25] Unliganded TR homodimers bind better than unliganded TR heterodimers with corepressors in vitro,[60-63] suggesting that the TR homodimer may mediate gene repression in the absence of thyroid hormone.

Transcriptional Repression by Thyroid Hormone Receptors

In the absence of T_3, TRs bind to TREs and repress basal transcription of positively regulated target genes in cotransfection studies. This characteristic of TRs contrasts with steroid hormone receptors, which are transcriptionally inactive in the absence of ligand.[26] Two major TR-interacting proteins, nuclear receptor corepressor (NCoR) and silencing mediator for RAR and TR (SMRT), have been shown to play important roles in mediating basal repression.[64-66] NCoR and SMRT are 270-kD proteins, which preferentially interact with unliganded TR and RAR. They serve as key components of transcription complexes that repress basal transcription of target genes in the absence of ligand. These corepressors contain three transferable repression domains in addition to two carboxy-terminal α-helical interaction domains. Consensus LXXI/HIXXXI/L sequences, where X represents any amino acid, within the interaction domains resemble the LXXLL sequences that enable coactivators to interact with nuclear hormone receptors.[67] These sequences allow both corepressors and coactivators to interact with similar amino acid residues on helices 3, 5, and 6 of the TR ligand-binding domain. It is now known that NCoR possesses a third nuclear receptor interacting domain, characterized by an altered helical structure that preferentially recognizes the TR homodimer.[68] This third interacting domain appears to interact only with the TR and not other nuclear receptors.[69,70] Currently, it is not known whether TR homo- or heterodimers are the preferred interaction partner with corepressors. Differences in the length and specific sequences of the corepressor and coactivator interaction sites, combined with ligand-induced conformational changes in the conserved AF-2 region of helix 12, help determine whether a corepressor or coactivator binds to TR.[67] In addition, helix 12 of RXR masks a corepressor binding site in RXR, which becomes available for corepressor binding after heterodimerization with TR.[71]

Corepressors can form a larger complex with other repressors, such as Sin 3 and histone deacetylase 3, which are mammalian homologues of well-characterized yeast transcriptional repressors RPD1 and RPD3,[25,26,67] as well as transducin beta-like protein 1 (Fig. 4-5). This complex induces histone deacetylation near the TREs of target genes, resulting in a chromatin structural state that shuts down basal transcription. Studies of TRβA promoter in a *Xenopus* oocyte system have demonstrated that simultaneous chromatin assembly and TR/RXR binding are necessary for basal repression of transcription.[72] Addition of T_3 relieves this repression and also causes chromatin remodeling. It is therefore likely that histone deacetylation, and acetylation on the addition of ligand, modulate the chromatin structure and nucleosome positioning that are critical for target gene transcription. In addition, methyl CpG-binding proteins can associate with a corepressor complex containing Sin 3 and histone deacetylase, suggesting that DNA methylation may play a role in basal repression.[73] Finally, unliganded TR may promote silencing in some cases through direct interaction with the basal transcription factor TFIIB.[74,75]

In addition to enzymes that deacetylate histones, TR-mediated gene repression in vitro has been recently demonstrated to require ATP-dependent chromatin remodeling enzymes.[76] These remodeling enzymes use ATP hydrolysis to alter the structure of chromatin by disrupting DNA-histone interactions.[77] The imitation switch (ISWI) family of ATPases is a heterogeneous group of chromatin remodeling enzymes distinguished by the presence of a highly conserved ISWI catalytic core and C-terminus SANT (SW13, ADA2, N-CoR, and TFIIB) domains.[78] The mammalian ISWI ATPase SNF2H has been shown to interact with unacetylated N-terminus histone H4 tails and mediate gene repression in an integrated TR-responsive reporter gene.[76]

The fact that TR alters the level of gene transcription in the absence and presence of ligand has important implications for thyroid hormone action. In the hypothyroid state, in which hormone concentrations are low, the unliganded receptor is predicted

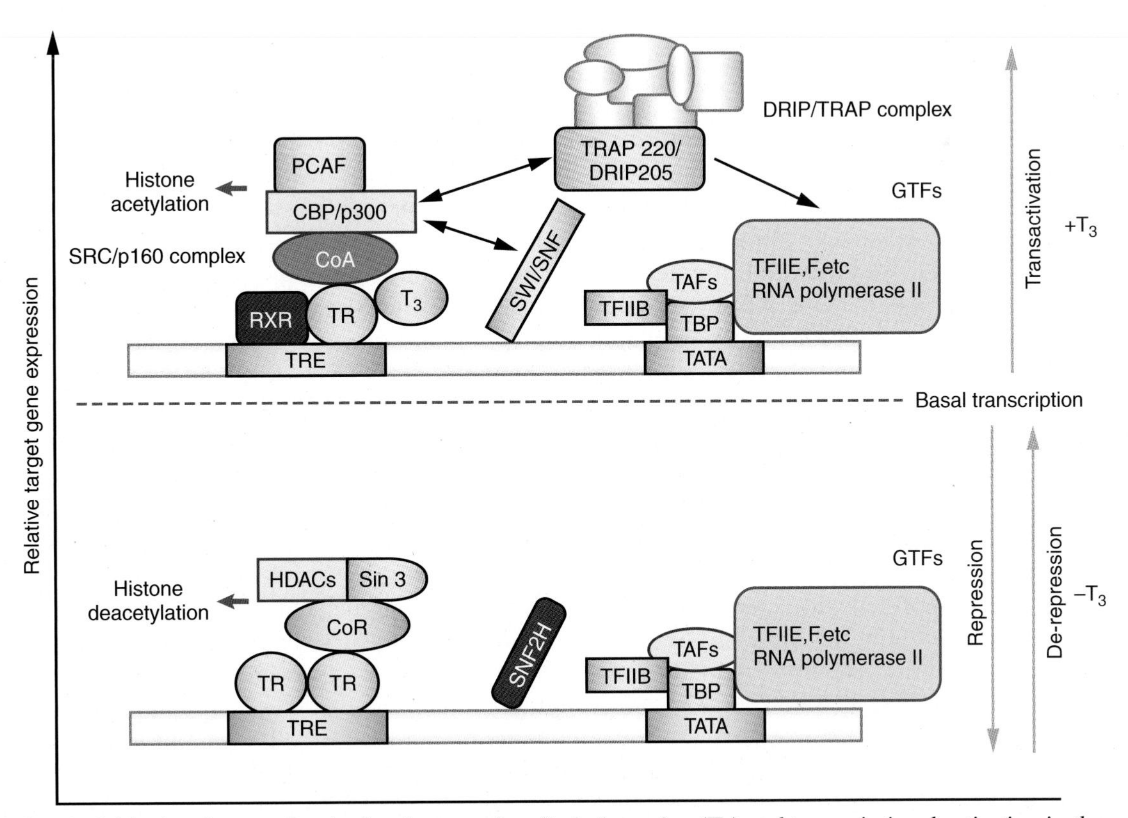

Figure 4–5 Model for basal repression in the absence of L-triiodothyronine (T_3) and transcriptional activation in the presence of T_3 in a positively regulated gene. PCAF, p300-CBP-associated factor; CBP, cAMP response element binding (CREB)-binding protein; CoA, coactivator; GTFs, general transcription factors; TAFs, TATA binding protein (TBP)-associated factors; HDACs, histone deacetylases; CoR, corepressor. See text for details.

to repress expression rather than to simply exist as an inactive receptor. This model is supported by data from the targeted deletion of TRα and TRβ genes. The phenotypes of these knockout mice are, for the most part, milder than the clinical features of congenital hypothyroidism.[79,80] This milder phenotype observed in the setting of TR deletion may be explained by the absence of the receptor-mediated gene repression, which normally accompanies the hypothyroid state.

Transcriptional Activation by Thyroid Hormone Receptors

Although many cofactors have been shown to interact with liganded nuclear hormone receptors and enhance transcriptional activation,[25,81] there appear to be at least two major complexes involved in ligand-dependent transcriptional activation of nuclear hormone receptors—the steroid receptor coactivator (SRC) complex and the vitamin D receptor interacting protein–TR-associated protein (DRIP-TRAP) complex (see Fig. 4-5). Using the yeast two-hybrid system, Oñate and coworkers have identified the first member of the SRC family, SRC-1.[82] This 160-kD protein directly interacts with TRs and other nuclear hormone receptors, enhancing their ligand-dependent transcriptional activity. Subsequent work has shown at least two other members of the SRC family, SRC-2 and SRC-3, which also can enhance transcription by liganded nuclear hormone receptors.[81] The SRCs have multiple nuclear hormone receptor interaction sites, each of which contains a signature LXXLL sequence motif, where X represents any amino acid. This sequence is important for coactivator binding to coactivator interaction sequences within the TR LBD (helices 3, 5, 6, and 12).[83,84] SRCs also interact with the cAMP response element binding (CREB)-binding protein (CBP), the coactivator for cAMP-stimulated transcription, as well as the related protein p300, which interacts with the viral coactivator E1A.[81] As coactivators for CREB, p53, AP-1, and nuclear factor-kappa B (NF-κB), CBP and p300 may function as integrator molecules for multiple cell signaling pathways.[85]

CBP-p300 also interacts with PCAF (p300-CBP–associated factor), the mammalian homologue of a yeast transcriptional activator, general control nonrepressed protein 5 (GCN5).[81,85] PCAF has intrinsic histone acetyltransferase (HAT) activity directed primarily toward H3 and H4 histones. PCAF itself is part of a preformed complex containing TATA binding protein (TBP)–associated factors (TAFs), which can interact with SRC-1 and SRC-3. CBP, which also has HAT activity, is found as part of a stable complex with RNA polymerase II (RNA pol II).[86] Thus, PCAF and CBP possess dual roles, serving both as adaptors of nuclear receptors to the basal transcriptional machinery and as enzymes that can alter chromatin structure (HAT activity).

The DRIP-TRAP complex contains approximately 15 subunits, varying from 70 to 230 kD, that directly or indirectly interact with liganded vitamin D receptors (VDRs) and TRs.[87,88] DRIP205-TRAP220, which contains a LXXLL motif similar to that found in SRCs, is a critical subunit within the coactivator complex, apparently functioning to anchor the rest of the proteins in the complex to the nuclear hormone receptor. Of note, none of the DRIP-TRAP subunits are members of the SRC family or their associated proteins. Additionally, the DRIP-TRAP complex does not appear to possess intrinsic HAT activity. However, several DRIP-TRAP components are mammalian homologues of the yeast mediator complex, which associates with RNA Pol II.[87,88] This suggests that TR recruitment of the DRIP-TRAP complex may help recruit or stabilize RNA Pol II holoenzyme.

TR-binding protein (TRBP) is another coactivator that has been shown to interact with TR via an LXXLL motif.[89] TRBP can also interact with CBP-p300 and DRIP130 as well as a DNA-dependent protein kinase (DNA-PK).[90] Interestingly, DNA-PK subunits Ku70 and Ku86 can interact with the NCoR-SMRT co-repressor complexes and may enhance histone deacetylase (HDAC) activity through phosphorylation of HDAC3.[91] The precise interplay among TRBP, DNA-PK, and the other major coactivator and corepressor complexes is not currently known.

Whereas the ISWI family of chromatin remodeling enzymes has been implicated in transcriptional repression by TR, mammalian homologues of Swi and Snf have been shown to associate with nuclear hormone receptors and activate transcription in vitro.[92] Activation by TR is associated with promoter targeting of SWI-SNF followed by chromatin remodeling with altered DNA topology. p300 appears to direct targeting of SWI-SNF to chromatin, a process facilitated by histone acetylation from CBP-p300.[93]

Chromatin immunoprecipitation assays of proteins bound to HREs have suggested that the recruitment of receptor and coactivator complexes to response elements may occur in a cyclical fashion,[94-97] leading to increased histone acetylation of the promoters of positively regulated target genes. In addition, it has been shown that glucocorticoid and progesterone receptors can recruit different SRC coactivators on the MMTV promoter.[98] Thus, the temporal recruitment pattern of coactivators and the particular coactivators recruited may be two key determinants of transcriptional activation on a given target gene. Additionally, there has been evidence that histone methylation and demethylation may play an important role in gene activation by TRs and other nuclear receptors because demethylation of H3K9 and H3K4 has been associated with transcriptional activation.[98a,98b] Thus, histone demethylation of specific sites, as well as histone acetylation of specific sites—notably H3K9—may be involved in positive regulation of transcription.[98a]

Negative Regulation by Thyroid Hormone Receptors

In contrast to positively regulated target genes, negatively regulated genes are characterized by transcriptional activation in the absence, and repression in the presence, of THs. Negative regulation of TRH and the TSHβ and TSHα subunit genes has been studied extensively because these are critical control points for feedback control of the hypothalamic-pituitary-thyroid (HPT) axis (HPT). Negative regulation of the HPT axis is mediated by the β isoform of the TR.[99-103] The T_3-responsive elements of these negatively regulated genes have been localized to their proximal promoter regions.[104,105] However, TRs bind weakly to the putative TREs of these promoters, so it is not known whether regulation occurs through direct TR binding to negative thyroid response elements (nTREs; on-DNA model of TR action) or via protein-protein interactions between TRs and other cofactors (off-DNA model). As an example of an off-DNA mechanism, TR can inhibit the activity of AP-1, a heterodimeric transcription factor composed of Jun and Fos. T_3-mediated repression of the prolactin promoter has been proposed to occur by the prevention of AP-1 binding.[106] TRs have also been shown to interact with several other classes of transcription factors, including NF-1, Oct-1, Sp-1, p53, Pit-1, and CTCF.[25,107] However, TRB knock-in mice expressing a P-box mutation within the DNA-binding domain that severely impaired its ability to bind DNA had inappropriately elevated TSH levels, despite high circulating thyroid hormone levels, suggesting that direct DNA binding by TR is necessary for negative regulation of the HPT axis by thyroid hormone.[108]

The precise changes in histone acetylation and resultant alterations in chromatin structure that occur during T_3 negative regulation have not been well characterized. Corepressors increase basal transcription of the TSH and TRH genes,[105,109] whereas coactivators may, in some cases, be paradoxically involved in T_3-dependent repression of negatively regulated genes. Both SRC-1 knockout mice and helix 12 mutant knock-in mice, which have mutant TR that cannot interact with co activators, exhibit defective negative regulation of TSH.[110,111] We recently have shown that T_3 can induce histone acetylation on the TSHα subunit promoter (Yen, unpublished results). On the other hand, HDACs can be recruited by TRs during ligand-dependent negative regulation in some cases.[112] Finally, there may be TR isoform-specific functions in the negative regulation of some target genes.[101,113]

MicroRNA Effects on TR Function

MicroRNAs (miRNAs) are small, noncoding, endogenous RNAs that are believed to suppress gene transcription by pairing with specific mRNAs to inhibit translation or promote mRNA degradation.[114] Hundreds of miRNAs have been identified, and more than one third of human genes are predicted targets for miRNA antagonism.[114,115] A cardiac-specific miRNA (miR-208) encoded by an intron of the alpha myosin heavychain (α-MHC) gene has recently been implicated in the regulation of β-MHC expression in response to stress and hypothyroidism.[116] In the mammalian cardiac myocyte, α-MHC and β-MHC are antithetically regulated by thyroid hormone. Whereas T_3 signaling occurs via a positive TRE to stimulate α-MHC transcription, the mechanism whereby T_3 mediates the repression of β-MHC remains incompletely understood.[117] Deletion of miR-208 in mice prevented the upregulation of β-MHC normally seen with propylthiouracil (PTU)-induced hypothyroidism. Thyroid hormone receptor–associated protein 1 (THRAP1), a component of the TR-associated protein (TRAP) complex, is negatively regulated by miR-208, and it has been suggested that an increase in THRAP1 resulting from the absence of miR-208 may enhance TR repression on a negative TRE in the β-MHC gene.[116,118]

Small interfering RNA molecules (siRNAs), which exploit the endogenous processing of miRNAs, have been used with great success in the study of selected genes in various biologic processes in vitro. Although introduction of siRNAs in vivo has been technically challenging, recent studies using adenoviral delivery and direct administration of synthesized siRNA duplexes have demonstrated the feasibility of gene silencing using these methods in animal models.[115] Although off-target effects are of great concern in the therapeutic application of RNA interference in humans, there may be a future clinical role for siRNA delivery in modulating TR-mediated processes. Furthermore, therapeutic targeting of miRNAs may provide yet another means by which to exert specific control over thyroid hormone action.

NONGENOMIC EFFECTS OF THYROID HORMONES

The direct transcriptional regulation of target genes by nuclear TRs was discussed earlier in this chapter, and represents the "classic" concept of thyroid hormone action (see Fig. 4-1). We now know that in addition to these effects, mediated by nuclear TRs on TREs, thyroid hormones exert direct effects on extranuclear proteins.[119] Evidence for these so-called nongenomic actions of thyroid hormones include the lack of dependence on nuclear TRs, structure-function relationships of thyroid hormone analogues that are different than their affinities for TRs, rapid onset of action (typically, seconds to minutes), occurrence in the presence of transcriptional blockade, and use of membrane-signaling pathways. Some of these effects may involve TR, particularly TR located outside the nucleus. Others may use additional thyroid hormone–binding proteins, such as the integrin αVβ3.[120] Some of these extranuclear actions of thyroid hormone may have genomic effects through the initiation of signal transduction cascades, with downstream effectors affecting gene transcription. Figure 4-6 depicts an overview of select TR-dependent and TR-independent extranuclear actions of thyroid hormones.

TR-mediated, nontranscriptional thyroid hormone actions can take place anywhere in the cell. Although primarily located in the nucleus, up to 10% of TRs are located in the cytoplasm.[121] At the plasma membrane, thyroid hormones stimulate phosphoinositide 3-kinase (PI3K) and rac activity, which in turn stimulates voltage-activated potassium channels encoded by the ether-a-go-go gene *KCNH2* in a rat pituitary cell line.[122] Increasing *KCNH2* activity results in reduced excitability and hormone secretion. TRβ was found to interact with the regulatory subunit p85α of PI3K and inhibit PI3K activity;

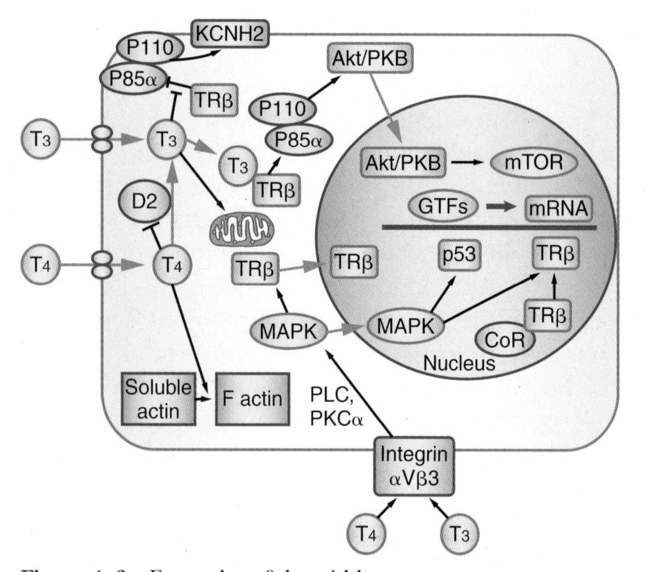

Figure 4–6 Examples of thyroid hormone receptor (TR)-dependent and TR-independent extranuclear actions of thyroid hormones. Gray arrows denote movement. GTFs, general transcription factors; CoR, corepressor. See text for details.

T_3 decreased this interaction. Interestingly, a T337 deletion in the TRβ gene of a patient with resistance to thyroid hormone (RTH) blocked *KCNH2* stimulation by T_3. This finding illustrates a potential nontranscriptional mechanism whereby a mutant TR may mediate some of the neurologic features of RTH.

Activation of the PI3K cascade is critical for cell processes such as cellular proliferation, inflammation, and glucose uptake. It has recently been observed that in cultured human skin fibroblasts, TRβ1 binds to the p85α regulatory subunit of PI3K and activates the PI3K-Akt/PKB-mTOR-$p70^{S6K}$ pathway, which in turn stimulates the translation of ZAKI-4.[123] It is not clear why the mechanism of liganded TR activation of PI3K signaling differs in this setting from that described in rat pituitary cells. Potential reasons include differences in posttranslational modifications of TRβ and p85 in the cytoplasm versus plasma membrane, differences in receptor-enzyme complex formation at these subcellular locations, and perhaps cell-specific effects.

TRα1 has also been shown to interact with p85 in a T_3-dependent manner and modulate the activity of endothelial nitric oxide synthase (eNOS), another downstream target of Akt/PKB.[124] It is possible that eNOS mediates thyroid hormone effects on systemic vascular resistance, arterial blood pressure, renal sodium reabsorption, and blood volume.[125] All these effects contribute to an increase in cardiac output, which is a prominent feature of hyperthyroidism. PI3K activation by T_3 also leads to a direct increase in the transcription of hypoxia-inducible factor 1 (HIF-1) and indirect increases in the transcription of glucose transporter 1 (GLUT1), platelet-type phosphofructokinase (PFKP), and the monocarboxylate transporter 4 (MCT4).[126]

In addition to actions at the plasma membrane and within the cytosol, thyroid hormones may have direct effects on mitochondria, which are established target organelles for regulation of the cellular energy state. Two truncated isoforms related to TRα-1, p43 and p28, have been described in mitochondria. Neither of these is detected in the nucleus. p43 binds T_3 with similar affinity to that reported for TRα-1, interacts with mitochondrial DNA response elements, and induces early stimulation of organelle transcription after the addition of T_3.[127,128] p28 also binds T_3 but lacks a DNA-binding domain because it is initiated at an internal methionine within the hinge region of TRα. In response to T_3, p28 is imported into the mitochondrial inner membrane, where it interacts with adenine nuclear translocase and uncoupling proteins, which in turn may generate a rapid thermogenic response. The interaction with p28 may thus represent a direct mechanism whereby T_3 can stimulate oxidative phosphorylation.

A number of thyroid hormone actions have been reported to occur in the absence of thyroid hormone binding to TRs. Davis and Davis have identified integrin αVβ3 as a plasma membrane binding site for thyroid hormone.[119] They previously had shown that both T_4 and T_3 activates mitogen-activated protein kinase (MAPK) signaling, leading to MAPK translocation into the nucleus, serine phosphorylation of TRβ, and corepressor release from TRβ.[129] Two independent laboratories have found that addition of thyroid hormone also results in prompt translocation of TRβ to the nucleus.[121,130] Purified radiolabeled T_4 and T_3 specifically and reversibly bind to integrin αVβ3. Moreover, siRNA knockdown of either the αV or β3 integrin subunit blocks MAPK activation by thyroid hormone in CV-1 cells. These data provide strong evidence that thyroid hormone binding to a membrane receptor, integrin αVβ3, leads to activation of the MAPK cascade. Using a chick chorioallantoic membrane (CAM) model, Davis and Davis[119] have shown that both T_4 and T_3 promote angiogenesis via activation of MAPK. Activation of MAPK by T_4 also causes rapid phosphorylation of p53 via a complex containing TRβ, p53, and MAPK.[131] This phosphorylation of p53 results in a decrease in its transcriptional activity.

T_4, but not T_3, promotes actin polymerization in astrocytes[132,133] and may influence the downregulation of type II deiodinase activity, a process that depends on an intact actin cytoskeleton.[134,135] Regulation of actin polymerization may contribute to thyroid hormone effects on neuronal arborization, axonal transport, and cell-cell contacts during central nervous system development. Thyroid hormone also binds to an endoplasmic reticulum–associated protein, prolyl hydroxylase, as well as to the monomeric subunit of pyruvate kinase.[136-138] The functional significance of these interactions has not been well characterized.

THYROID HORMONE ANALOGUES

Whereas beneficial effects of thyroid hormones include weight loss, a reduction in serum cholesterol, and improved cardiac output, excess thyroid hormone is associated with undesirable effect on bone, skeletal muscle, and the heart. Novel thyroid hormone analogues that attempt to minimize these untoward effects are being developed as potential therapies for obesity, hypercholesterolemia, and heart failure.[139]

Because the TRα isoform predominates in cardiac tissues, TRβ isoform–specific compounds have been used to avoid the tachycardic and arrhythmogenic effects of thyroid hormone excess. In several animal models, the TRβ-specific agonist KB-141 promoted weight loss and increased Vo_2 without increasing the heart rate.[140] Thyroid hormone analogues designed for cholesterol reduction have exploited several mechanisms to achieve selective action in the liver, including hepatic first-pass uptake, tissue-selective uptake, and TRβ specificity. In a recent phase II randomized controlled trial, one such thyroid hormone mimetic compound designed for liver-specific uptake and TRβ specificity, KB2115 (3-[[3,5-dibromo-4-[4-hydroxy-3-(1-methylethyl)-phenoxy]-phenyl]-amino]-3-oxopropanoic acid), was shown to induce a 40% reduction in serum cholesterol over a 2-week period without detectable effects on the cardiovascular system.[141]

3,5-Diiodothyropropionic acid (DITPA) is a thyroid hormone–related compound with low affinity for nuclear TRs and modest effects on metabolic activity. DITPA has been shown to bind αVβ3 and activate MAPK.[142] In a pilot clinical study of patients with moderate to severe (New York Heart Association Class II or III) congestive heart failure, DITPA treatment was associated with an improved cardiac index, decreased systemic vascular resistance index, decreased isovolumetric relaxation time, and reduced serum cholesterol and triglyceride levels.[143] Further clinical trials of DITPA in congestive heart failure are ongoing.

Other thyroid hormone analogues that act via TR-independent extranuclear pathways have been described. 3-Iodothyronamine (T_1AM) and thyronamine (T_0AM) are naturally occurring byproducts of thyroid hormone that do not bind TRs but are agonists of trace amine–associated receptor (TAAR1), a G protein–coupled receptor.[144] A single injection of T_1AM or T_0AM induced transient hypothermia and reduced infarct size when given after experimental stroke in mice.[145]

In addition to the aforementioned applications, thyroid hormone analogues may prove useful in providing TSH suppressive therapy for thyroid cancer patients. Also, the development of analogues that antagonize TR-mediated thyroid hormone action may be of therapeutic value in selected cases of thyrotoxicosis, such as those associated with the use of amiodarone.

CONCLUSIONS

We have learned a great deal about the mechanisms whereby nuclear TRs regulate transcriptional activity of target genes, particularly those that are positively regulated by thyroid hormone. Recent studies have broadened our appreciation for the scope of thyroid hormone action to include TR-dependent and TR-independent effects on extranuclear cellular proteins and their downstream signaling pathways. It is hoped that future research will provide a better understanding of the mechanisms of disease caused by abnormalities in thyroid hormone action, as well as lead to the development of therapies that target specific sites of thyroid hormone-mediated processes.

References

1. Osler W: Principles and Practice of Medicine, 4th ed. New York, Appleton-Century, 1901.
2. Barker SB: Mechanism of action of the thyroid hormone. Physiol Rev 31:205-243, 1951.
3. Tata JR, Ernster L, Lindberg O, et al: The action of thyroid hormones at the cell level. Biochem J 86:408-428, 1963.
4. Tata JR, Widnell CC: Ribonucleic acid synthesis during the early action of thyroid hormones. Biochem J 98:604-620, 1966.
5. Samuels HH, Tsai JS: Thyroid hormone action in cell culture: Demonstration of nuclear receptors in intact cells and isolated nuclei. Proc Natl Acad Sci U S A 70:3488-3492, 1973.
6. Oppenheimer JH, Koerner D, Schwartz HL, Surks MI: Specific nuclear triiodothyronine binding sites in rat liver and kidney. J Clin Endocrinol Metab 35:330-333, 1972.
7. Pascual A, Casanova J, Samuels HH: Photoaffinity labeling of thyroid hormone nuclear receptors in intact cells. J Biol Chem 257:9640-9647, 1982.
8. Dozin B, Cahnmann HJ, Nikodem VM: Identification of thyroid hormone receptors in rat liver nuclei by photoaffinity labeling with L-thyroxine and triiodo-L-thyronine. Biochemistry 24:5197-5202, 1985.
9. Crew MD, Spindler SR: Thyroid hormone regulation of the transfected rat growth hormone promoter. J Biol Chem 261:5018-5022, 1986.
10. Larsen PR, Harney JW, Moore DD: Sequences required for cell-type specific thyroid hormone regulation of rat growth hormone promoter activity. J Biol Chem 261:14373-14376, 1986.
11. Lavin TN, Baxter JD, Horita S: The thyroid hormone receptor binds to multiple domains of the rat growth hormone 5′-flanking sequence. J Biol Chem 263:9418-9426, 1988.
12. Samuels HH, Forman BM, Horowitz ZD, Ye ZS: Regulation of gene expression by thyroid hormone. J Clin Invest 81:957-967, 1988.
13. Hollenberg SM, Weinberger C, Ong ES, et al: Primary structure and expression of a functional human glucocorticoid receptor cDNA. Nature 318:635-641, 1985.
14. Green S, Walter P, Kumar V, et al: Human oestrogen receptor cDNA: Sequence, expression and homology to v-erb-A. Nature 320:134-139, 1986.
15. Sap J, Muñoz A, Damm K, et al: The c-erb-A protein is a high-affinity receptor for thyroid hormone. Nature 324:635-640, 1986.
16. Weinberger C, Thompson CC, Ong ES, et al: The c-erb-A gene encodes a thyroid hormone receptor. Nature 324:641-646, 1986.
17. Friesema EC, Jansen J, Heuer H, et al: Mechanisms of disease: Psychomotor retardation and high T3 levels caused by mutations in monocarboxylate transporter 8. Nat Clin Pract Endocrinol Metab 2:512-523, 2006.
18. Kohrle J: The selenoenzyme family of deiodinase isozymes controls local thyroid hormone availability. Rev Endocr Metab Disord 1:49-58, 2000.
19. Bianco AC, Kim BW: Deiodinases: Implications of the local control of thyroid hormone action. J Clin Invest 116:2571-2579, 2006.
20. Jorgensen EC: Stereochemistry of thyroxine and analogues. Mayo Clin Proc 39:560-568, 1964.
21. Cody V: Triiodothyronine: Molecular structure and biologic function. Monogr Endocrinol 18:15-57, 1981.
22. Perlman AJ, Stanley F, Samuels HH: Thyroid hormone nuclear receptor. Evidence for multimeric organization in chromatin. J Biol Chem 257:930-938, 1982.
23. Jump DB, Seelig S, Schwartz HL, Oppenheimer JH: Association of the thyroid hormone receptor with rat liver chromatin. Biochemistry 20:6781-6789, 1981.
24. MacLeod KM, Baxter JD: Chromatin receptors for thyroid hormones. Interactions of the solubilized proteins with DNA. J Biol Chem 251:7380-737, 1976.
25. Yen PM: Physiological and molecular basis of thyroid hormone action. Physiol Rev 81:1097-1142, 2001.
26. Zhang J, Lazar MA: The mechanism of action of thyroid hormones. Annu Rev Physiol 62:439-466, 2000.
27. Wagner RL, Apriletti JW, McGrath ME, et al: A structural role for hormone in the thyroid hormone receptor. Nature 378:690-697, 1995.
28. Ribeiro RC, Feng W, Wagner RL, et al: Definition of the surface in the thyroid hormone receptor ligand binding domain for association as homodimers and heterodimers with retinoid X receptor. J Biol Chem 276:14987-14995, 2001.
29. Perissi V, Staszewski LM, McInerney EM, et al: Molecular determinants of nuclear receptor-corepressor interaction. Genes Dev 13:3198-3208, 1999.
30. Nagy L, Kao HY, Love JD, et al: Mechanism of corepressor binding and release from nuclear hormone receptors. Genes Dev 13:3209-3216, 1999.
31. Feng W, Ribeiro RC, Wagner RL, et al: Hormone-dependent coactivator binding to a hydrophobic cleft on nuclear receptors. Science 280:1747-1749, 1998.
32. Hu X, Lazar MA: The CoRNR motif controls the recruitment of corepressors by nuclear hormone receptors. Nature 402:93-96, 1999.

33. Koenig RJ, Lazar MA, Hodin RA, et al: Inhibition of thyroid hormone action by a non-hormone binding c-erbA protein generated by alternative mRNA splicing. Nature 337:659-661, 1989.
34. Lazar MA, Hodin RA, Chin WW: Human carboxyl-terminal variant of alpha-type c-erbA inhibits transactivation by thyroid hormone receptors without binding thyroid hormone. Proc Natl Acad Sci U S A 86:7771-7774, 1989.
35. Katz D, Reginato MJ, Lazar MA: Functional regulation of thyroid hormone receptor variant TR alpha 2 by phosphorylation. Mol Cell Biol 15:2341-2348, 1995.
36. Chawla A, Lazar MA: Induction of Rev-ErbA alpha, an orphan receptor encoded on the opposite strand of the alpha-thyroid hormone receptor gene, during adipocyte differentiation. J Biol Chem 268:16265-16269, 1993.
37. Hodin RA, Lazar MA, Wintman BI, et al: Identification of a thyroid hormone receptor that is pituitary-specific. Science 244:76-79, 1989.
38. Lazar MA: Thyroid hormone receptors: Multiple forms, multiple possibilities. Endocr Rev 14:184-193, 1993.
39. Hodin RA, Lazar MA, Chin WW: Differential and tissue-specific regulation of the multiple rat c-erbA messenger RNA species by thyroid hormone. J Clin Invest 85:101-105, 1990.
40. Yen PM, Sunday ME, Darling DS, Chin WW: Isoform-specific thyroid hormone receptor antibodies detect multiple thyroid hormone receptors in rat and human pituitaries. Endocrinology 130:1539-1546, 1992.
41. Bradley DJ, Towle HC, Young WS 3rd: Alpha and beta thyroid hormone receptor (TR) gene expression during auditory neurogenesis: Evidence for TR isoform-specific transcriptional regulation in vivo. Proc Natl Acad Sci U S A 91:439-443, 1994.
42. Cook CB, Kakucska I, Lechan RM, Koenig RJ: Expression of thyroid hormone receptor beta 2 in rat hypothalamus. Endocrinology 130:1077-1079, 1992.
43. Sjoberg M, Vennstrom B, Forrest D: Thyroid hormone receptors in chick retinal development: Differential expression of mRNAs for alpha and N-terminal variant beta receptors. Development 114:39-47, 1992.
44. Chassande O, Fraichard A, Gauthier K, et al: Identification of transcripts initiated from an internal promoter in the c-erbA alpha locus that encode inhibitors of retinoic acid receptor-alpha and triiodothyronine receptor activities. Mol Endocrinol 11:1278-1290, 1997.
45. Williams GR: Cloning and characterization of two novel thyroid hormone receptor beta isoforms. Mol Cell Biol 20:8329-8342, 2000.
46. Farsetti A, Desvergne B, Hallenbeck P, et al: Characterization of myelin basic protein thyroid hormone response element and its function in the context of native and heterologous promoter. J Biol Chem 267:15784-15788, 1992.
47. Lezoualc'h F, Hassan AH, Giraud P, et al: Assignment of the beta-thyroid hormone receptor to 3,5,3′-triiodothyronine-dependent inhibition of transcription from the thyrotropin-releasing hormone promoter in chick hypothalamic neurons. Mol Endocrinol 6:1797-1804, 1992.
48. Hollenberg AN, Monden T, Wondisford FE: Ligand-independent and -dependent functions of thyroid hormone receptor isoforms depend upon their distinct amino termini. J Biol Chem 270:14274-14280, 1995.
49. Abel ED, Kaulbach HC, Campos-Barros A, et al: Novel insight from transgenic mice into thyroid hormone resistance and the regulation of thyrotropin. J Clin Invest 103:271-279, 1999.
50. Yen PM, Feng X, Flamant F, et al: Effects of ligand and thyroid hormone receptor isoforms on hepatic gene expression profiles of thyroid hormone receptor knockout mice. EMBO Rep 4:581-587, 2003.
51. Glass CK: Differential recognition of target genes by nuclear receptor monomers, dimers, and heterodimers. Endocr Rev 15:391-407, 1994.
52. Umesono K, Murakami KK, Thompson CC, Evans RM: Direct repeats as selective response elements for the thyroid hormone, retinoic acid, and vitamin D_3 receptors. Cell 65:1255-1266, 1991.
53. Näär AM, Boutin JM, Lipkin SM, et al: The orientation and spacing of core DNA-binding motifs dictate selective transcriptional responses to three nuclear receptors. Cell 65:1267-1279, 1991.
54. Kurokawa R, Söderström M, Hörlein A, et al: Polarity-specific activities of retinoic acid receptors determined by a co-repressor. Nature 377:451-454, 1995.
55. Perlmann T, Rangarajan PN, Umesono K, Evans RM: Determinants for selective RAR and TR recognition of direct repeat HREs. Genes Dev 7:1411-1422, 1993.
56. Yen PM, Ikeda M, Wilcox EC, et al: Half-site arrangement of hybrid glucocorticoid and thyroid hormone response elements specifies thyroid hormone receptor complex binding to DNA and transcriptional activity. J Biol Chem 269:12704-12709, 1994.
57. Rastinejad F, Perlmann T, Evans RM, Sigler PB: Structural determinants of nuclear receptor assembly on DNA direct repeats. Nature 375:203-211, 1995.
58. Nagaya T, Jameson JL: Distinct dimerization domains provide antagonist pathways for thyroid hormone receptor action. J Biol Chem 268:24278-24282, 1993.
59. Au-Fliegner M, Helmer E, Casanova J, et al: The conserved ninth C-terminal heptad in thyroid hormone and retinoic acid receptors mediates diverse responses by affecting heterodimer but not homodimer formation. Mol Cell Biol 13:5725-5737, 1993.

60. Hollenberg AN, Monden T, Madura JP, et al: Function of nuclear co-repressor protein on thyroid hormone response elements is regulated by the receptor A/B domain. J Biol Chem 271:28516-28520, 1996.
61. Liu Y, Takeshita A, Misiti S, et al: Lack of coactivator interaction can be a mechanism for dominant negative activity by mutant thyroid hormone receptors. Endocrinology 139:4197-4204, 1998.
62. Yoh SM, Privalsky ML: Transcriptional repression by thyroid hormone receptors. A role for receptor homodimers in the recruitment of SMRT corepressor. J Biol Chem 276:16857-16867, 2001.
63. Cohen RN, Putney A, Wondisford FE, Hollenberg AN: The nuclear corepressors recognize distinct nuclear receptor complexes. Mol Endocrinol 14:900-914, 2000.
64. Hörlein AJ, Näär AM, Heinzel T, et al: Ligand-independent repression by the thyroid hormone receptor mediated by a nuclear co-repressor. Nature 377:397-404, 1995.
65. Chen JD, Evans RM: A transcriptional co-repressor that interacts with nuclear hormone receptors. Nature 377:454-457, 1995.
66. Seol W, Choi HS, Moore DD: Isolation of proteins that interact specifically with the retinoid X receptor: Two novel orphan receptors. Mol Endocrinol 9:72-85, 1995.
67. Hu I, Lazar MA: Transcriptional repression by nuclear hormone receptors. Trends Endocrinol Metab 11:6-10, 2000.
68. Makowski A, Brzostek S, Cohen RN, Hollenberg AN: Determination of nuclear receptor corepressor interactions with the thyroid hormone receptor. Mol Endocrinol 17:273-286, 2003.
69. Cohen RN, Brzostek S, Kim B, et al: The specificity of interactions between nuclear hormone receptors and corepressors is mediated by distinct amino acid sequences within the interacting domains. Mol Endocrinol 15:1049-1061, 2001.
70. Webb P, Anderson CM, Valentine C, et al: The nuclear receptor corepressor (N-CoR) contains three isoleucine motifs (I/LXXII) that serve as receptor interaction domains (IDs). Mol Endocrinol 14:1976-1985, 2000.
71. Zhang J, Hu X, Lazar MA: A novel role for helix 12 of retinoid X receptor in regulating repression. Mol Cell Biol 19:6448-6457, 1999.
72. Wong J, Shi YB, Wolffe AP: A role for nucleosome assembly in both silencing and activation of the xenopus TR beta A gene by the thyroid hormone receptor. Genes Dev 9:2696-2711, 1996.
73. Anderson GW, Larson RJ, Oas DR, et al: Chicken ovalbumin upstream promoter-transcription factor (COUP-TF) modulates expression of the Purkinje cell protein-2 gene. A potential role for COUP-TF in repressing premature thyroid hormone action in the developing brain. J Biol Chem 273:16391-16399, 1998.
74. Baniahmad A, Ha I, Reinberg D, et al: Interaction of human thyroid hormone receptor beta with transcription factor TFIIB may mediate target gene derepression and activation by thyroid hormone. Proc Natl Acad Sci U S A 90:8832-8836, 1993.
75. Hadzic E, Desai-Yajnik V, Helmer E, et al: A 10-amino-acid sequence in the N-terminal A/B domain of thyroid hormone receptor alpha is essential for transcriptional activation and interaction with the general transcription factor TFIIB. Mol Cell Biol 15:4507-4517, 1995.
76. Alenghat T, Yu J, Lazar MA: The N-CoR complex enables chromatin remodeler SNF2H to enhance repression by thyroid hormone receptor. EMBO J 25:3966-3974, 2006.
77. Johnson CN, Adkins NL, Georgel P: Chromatin remodeling complexes: ATP-dependent machines in action. Biochem Cell Biol 83:405-417, 2005.
78. Chen J, Kinyamu HK, Archer TK: Changes in attitude, changes in latitude: Nuclear receptors remodeling chromatin to regulate transcription. Mol Endocrinol 20:1-13, 2006.
79. Flamant F, Samarut J: Thyroid hormone receptor: Lessons from knockout and knock-in mice. Trends Endocrinol Metab 14:85-90, 2003.
80. Forrest D, Vennstrom B: Functions of thyroid hormone receptors in mice. Thyroid 10:41-52, 2000.
81. McKenna NJ, Lanz RB, O'Malley BW: Nuclear receptor coregulators: Cellular and molecular biology. Endocr Rev 20:321-344, 1999.
82. Oñate SA, Tsai SY, Tsai MJ: O'Malley BW: Sequence and characterization of a coactivator for the steroid hormone receptor superfamily. Science 270:1354-1357, 1995.
83. McInerney EM, Rose DW, Flynn SE, et al: Determinants of coactivator LXXLL motif specificity in nuclear receptor transcriptional activation. Genes Dev 12:3357-3368, 1998.
84. Heery DM, Kalkhoven E, Hoare S, Parker MG: A signature motif in transcriptional co-activators mediates binding to nuclear receptors. Nature 387:733-736, 1997.
85. Torchia J, Glass C, Rosenfeld MG: Co-activators and co-repressors in the integration of transcriptional responses. Curr Opin Cell Biol 10:373-383, 1998.
86. Nakajima T, Uchida C, Anderson SF, et al: RNA helicase A mediates association of CBP with RNA polymerase II. Cell 90:1107-1112, 1997.
87. Ito M, Roeder RG: The TRAP/SMCC/Mediator complex and thyroid hormone receptor function. Trends Endocrinol Metab 12:127-134, 2001.
88. Rachez C, Freedman LP: Mediator complexes and transcription. Curr Opin Cell Biol 13:274-280, 2001.
89. Ko L, Cardona GR, Chin WW: Thyroid hormone receptor-binding protein, an LXXLL motif-containing protein, functions as a general coactivator. Proc Natl Acad Sci U S A 97:6212-6217, 2000.
90. Ko L, Chin WW: Nuclear receptor coactivator thyroid hormone receptor-binding protein (TRBP) interacts with and stimulates its associated DNA-dependent protein kinase. J Biol Chem 278:11471-11479, 2003.

91. Jeyakumar M, Liu XF, Erdjument-Bromage H, et al: Phosphorylation of thyroid hormone receptor-associated NCoR corepressor holocomplex by the DNA-dependent protein kinase enhances its histone deacetylase activity. J Biol Chem 282:9312-9322, 2007.
92. DiRenzo J, Shang Y, Phelan M, et al: BRG-1 is recruited to estrogen-responsive promoters and cooperates with factors involved in histone acetylation. Mol Cell Biol 20:7541-7549, 2000.
93. Huang ZQ, Li J, Sachs LM, et al: A role for cofactor-cofactor and cofactor-histone interactions in targeting p300, SWI/SNF and mediator for transcription. EMBO J 22:2146-2155, 2003.
94. Sharma D, Fondell JD: Ordered recruitment of histone acetyltransferases and the TRAP/Mediator complex to thyroid hormone-responsive promoters in vivo. Proc Natl Acad Sci U S A 99:7934-7939, 2002.
95. Shang Y, Hu X, DiRenzo J, et al: Cofactor dynamics and sufficiency in estrogen receptor-regulated transcription. Cell 103:843-852, 2000.
96. Reid G, Hübner MR, Métivier R, et al: Cyclic, proteasome-mediated turnover of unliganded and liganded ERalpha on responsive promoters is an integral feature of estrogen signaling. Mol Cell 11:695-707, 2003.
97. Liu Y, Xia X, Fondell JD, Yen PM: Thyroid hormone-regulated target genes have distinct patterns of coactivator recruitment and histone acetylation. Mol Endocrinol 20:483-490, 2006.
98. Li X, Wong J, Tsai SY, et al: Progesterone and glucocorticoid receptors recruit distinct coactivator complexes and promote distinct patterns of local chromatin modification. Mol Cell Biol 23:3763-3773, 2003.
98a. Li U, Lin Q, Yoon HG, et al. Involvement of histone methylation and phosphorylation in regulation of transcription by thyroid hormone receptor. Mol Cell Biol 22:5688-5697, 2002.
98b. Garcia-Bassets, Kwon YS, Telese F, et al: Histone methylation-dependent mechanisms impose ligand dependency for gene activation by nuclear receptors. Cell 128:505-518, 2007.
99. Forrest D, Erway LC, Ng L, et al: Thyroid hormone receptor beta is essential for development of auditory function. Nat Genet 13:354-357, 1996.
100. Weiss RE, Forrest D, Pohlenz J, et al: Thyrotropin regulation by thyroid hormone in thyroid hormone receptor beta-deficient mice. Endocrinology 138:3624-3629, 1997.
101. Abel ED, Boers ME, Pazos-Moura C, et al: Divergent roles for thyroid hormone receptor beta isoforms in the endocrine axis and auditory system. J Clin Invest 104:291-300, 1999.
102. Gauthier K, Chassande O, Plateroti M, et al: Different functions for the thyroid hormone receptors TRalpha and TRbeta in the control of thyroid hormone production and post-natal development. EMBO J 18:623-631, 1999.
103. Abel ED, Ahima RS, Boers ME, et al: Critical role for thyroid hormone receptor β2 in the regulation of paraventricular thyrotropin-releasing hormone neurons. J Clin Invest 107:1017-1023, 2001.
104. Bodenner DL, Mroczynski MA, Weintraub BD, et al: A detailed functional and structural analysis of a major thyroid hormone inhibitory element in the human thyrotropin beta-subunit gene. J Biol Chem 266:21666-21673, 1991.
105. Hollenberg AN, Monden T, Flynn TR, et al: The human thyrotropin-releasing hormone gene is regulated by thyroid hormone through two distinct classes of negative thyroid hormone response elements. Mol Endocrinol 9:540-550, 1995.
106. Pernasetti F, Caccavelli L, Van de Weerdt C, et al: Thyroid hormone inhibits the human prolactin gene promoter by interfering with activating protein-1 and estrogen stimulations. Mol Endocrinol 11:986-996, 1997.
107. Bassett JH, Harvey CB, Williams GR: Mechanisms of thyroid hormone receptor-specific nuclear and extra nuclear actions. Mol Cell Endocrinol 213:1-11, 2003.
108. Shibusawa N, Hashimoto K, Nikrodhanond AA, et al: Thyroid hormone action in the absence of thyroid hormone receptor DNA-binding in vivo. J Clin Invest 112:588-597, 2003.
109. Tagami T, Madison LD, Nagaya T, Jameson JL: Nuclear receptor corepressors activate rather than suppress basal transcription of genes that are negatively regulated by thyroid hormone. Mol Cell Biol 17:2642-2648, 1997.
110. Weiss RE, Xu J, Ning G, et al: Mice deficient in the steroid receptor co-activator 1 (SRC-1) are resistant to thyroid hormone. EMBO J 18:1900-1904, 1999.
111. Ortiga-Carvalho TM, Shibusawa N, Nikrodhanond A, et al: Negative regulation by thyroid hormone receptor requires an intact coactivator-binding surface. J Clin Invest 115:2517-2523, 2005.
112. Sasaki S, Lesoon-Wood LA, Dey A, et al: Ligand-induced recruitment of a histone deacetylase in the negative-feedback regulation of the thyrotropin beta gene. EMBO J 18:5389-5398, 1999.
113. Safer JD, Langlois MF, Cohen R, et al: Isoform variable action among thyroid hormone receptor mutants provides insight into pituitary resistance to thyroid hormone. Mol Endocrinol 11:16-26, 1997.
114. Liu J: Control of protein synthesis and mRNA degradation by microRNAs. Curr Opin Cell Biol 20:214-221, 2008.
115. Kolfschoten IG, Regazzi R: Technology insight: Small, noncoding RNA molecules as tools to study and treat endocrine diseases. Nat Clin Pract Endocrinol Metab 3:827-834, 2007.
116. van Rooij E, Sutherland LB, Qi X, et al: Control of stress-dependent cardiac growth and gene expression by a microRNA. Science 316:575-579, 2007.
117. Danzi S, Klein I: Posttranscriptional regulation of myosin heavy chain expression in the heart by triiodothyronine. Am J Physiol Heart Circ Physiol 288:H455-H460, 2005.

118. van Rooij E, Liu N, Olson EN: MicroRNAs flex their muscles. Trends Genet 24:159-166, 2008.
119. Davis PJ, Davis FB: Nongenomic actions of thyroid hormone. Thyroid 6:497-504, 1996.
120. Bergh JJ, Lin HY, Lansing L, et al: Integrin alpha(V)beta(3) contains a cell surface receptor site for thyroid hormone that is linked to activation of mitogen-activated protein kinase and induction of angiogenesis. Endocrinology 146:2864-2871, 2005.
121. Baumann CT, Maruvada P, Hager GL, Yen PM: Nuclear cytoplasmic shuttling by thyroid hormone receptors. Multiple protein interactions are required for nuclear retention. J Biol Chem 276:11237-11245, 2001.
122. Storey NM, Gentile S, Ullah H, et al: Rapid signaling at the plasma membrane by a nuclear receptor for thyroid hormone. Proc Natl Acad Sci USA 103:5197-201, 2006.
123. Cao X, Kambe F, Moeller LC, et al: Thyroid hormone induces rapid activation of Akt/protein kinase B-mammalian target of rapamycin-p70S6K cascade through phosphatidylinositol 3-kinase in human fibroblasts. Mol Endocrinol 19:102-112, 2005.
124. Hiroi Y, Kim HH, Ying H, et al: Rapid nongenomic actions of thyroid hormone. Proc Natl Acad Sci U S A 103:14104-14109, 2006.
125. Klein I, Ojamaa K: Thyroid hormone and the cardiovascular system. N Engl J Med 344:501-509, 2001.
126. Moeller C, Dumitrescu AM, Refetoff S: Cytosolic action of thyroid hormone leads to induction of hypoxia-inducible factor-1alpha and glycolytic genes. Mol Endocrinol 19:2955-2963, 2005.
127. Wrutniak-Cabello C, Casas F, Cabello G: Thyroid hormone action in mitochondria. J Mol Endocrinol 26:67-77, 2001.
128. Casas F, Daury L, Grandemange S, et al: Endocrine regulation of mitochondrial activity: Involvement of truncated RXRalpha and c-Erb Aalpha1 proteins. FASEB J 17:426-436, 2003.
129. Davis PJ, Davis FB, Cody V: Membrane receptors mediating thyroid hormone action. Trends Endocrinol Metab 16:429-435, 2005.
130. Zhu XG, Hanover JA, Hager GL, Cheng SY: Hormone-induced translocation of thyroid hormone receptors in living cells visualized using a receptor green fluorescent protein chimera. J Biol Chem 273:27058-27063, 1998.
131. Shih A, Lin HY, Davis FB, Davis PJ: Thyroid hormone promotes serine phosphorylation of p53 by mitogen-activated protein kinase. Biochemistry 40:2870-2878, 2001.
132. Siegrist-Kaiser CA, Juge-Aubry C, Tranter MP, et al: Thyroxine-dependent modulation of actin polymerization in cultured astrocytes: A novel extranuclear action of thyroid hormone. J Biol Chem 265:5296-5302, 1990.
133. Davis PJ, Leonard JL, Davis FB: Mechanisms of nongenomic actions of thyroid hormone. Front Neuroendocrinol 29:211-218, 2008.
134. Farwell AP, DiBenedetto DJ, Leonard JL: Thyroxine targets different pathways of internalization of type II iodothyronine 5′-deiodinase in astrocytes. J Biol Chem 268:5055, 1993.
135. Farwell AP, Safran M, Dubord S, Leonard JL: Degradation and recycling of the substrate-binding subunit of type II iodothyronine 5′-deiodonase in astrocytes. J Biol Chem 271:16369-16374, 1996.
136. Cheng SY, Gong QH, Parkison C, et al: The nucleotide sequence of a human cellular thyroid hormone binding protein present in endoplasmic reticulum. J Biol Chem 262:11221-11227, 1987.
137. Kato H, Fukuda T, Parkinson C, et al: Cytoplasmic thyroid hormone-binding protein is a monomer of pyruvate kinase. Proc Natl Acad Sci U S A 86:7681-7685, 1990.
138. Ashizawa K, McPhie P, Lin KH, Cheng SY: An in vitro novel mechanism of regulating the activity of pyruvate kinase M2 by thyroid hormone and fructose 1,6-bisphosphate. Biochemistry 30:7105-7111, 1991.
139. Brenta G, Danzi S, Klein I: Potential therapeutic applications of thyroid hormone analogs. Nat Clin Pract Endocrinol Metab 3:632-640, 2007.
140. Grover GJ, Mellström K, Ye L, et al: Selective thyroid hormone receptor-beta activation: A strategy for reduction of weight, cholesterol, and lipoprotein (a) with reduced cardiovascular liability. Proc Natl Acad Sci U S A 100:10067-10072, 2003.
141. Berkenstam A, Kristensen J, Mellström K, et al: The thyroid hormone mimetic compound KB2115 lowers plasma LDL cholesterol and stimulates bile acid synthesis without cardiac effects in humans. Proc Natl Acad Sci U S A 105:663-667, 2008.
142. Mousa SA, O'Connor L, Davis FB, Davis PJ: Proangiogenesis action of the thyroid hormone analog 3,5-diiodothyropropionic acid (DITPA) is initiated at the cell surface and is integrin mediated. Endocrinology 147:1602-1607, 2006.
143. Morkin E, Pennock G, Spooner PH, et al: Pilot studies on the use of 3,5-diiodothyropropionic acid, a thyroid hormone analog, in the treatment of congestive heart failure. Cardiology 97:218-225, 2002.
144. Scanlan TS, Suchland KL, Hart ME, et al: 3-Iodothyronamine is an endogenous and rapid-acting derivative of thyroid hormone. Nat Med 10:638-642, 2004.
145. Doyle KP, Suchland KL, Ciesielski TM, et al: Novel thyroxine derivatives, thyronamine and 3-iodothyronamine, induce transient hypothermia and marked neuroprotection against stroke injury. Stroke 38:2569-2576, 2007.

Chapter 5

Thyroid Hormone Metabolism

Antonio C. Bianco and Brian W. Kim

Key Points

- The three deiodinases are selenoenzymes containing the rare amino acid selenocysteine.
- The deiodinases are coordinately regulated to promote thyroid hormone homeostasis.
- Primary changes in D2 or D3 expression and activity provide a mechanism for local control of thyroid hormone signaling.
- Novel roles for the deiodinases have emerged in development and metabolic control, based on linkage to hedgehog and bile acid signaling pathways.

The three deiodinases, enzymes that activate thyroxine (T_4) and inactivate both T_4 and triiodothyronine (T_3), are present in all vertebrates. Their relevance derives from the fact that T_3 is a long-lived prohormone molecule (half-life [$t_{1/2}$] is approximately 7 days in humans) that must be activated by deiodination to the short-lived biologically active form T_3 ($t_{1/2}$ is approximately 1 day) to initiate thyroid hormone action. T_3 modulates gene expression in almost every vertebrate tissue through ligand-dependent transcription factors, the thyroid hormone receptors. The deiodination of T_4 to T_3 occurs in the phenolic outer or 5′ ring of the T_4 molecule and is catalyzed by type 1 and type 2 iodothyronine deiodinase, D1 and D2 (Fig. 5-1). T_4 activation can be prevented and T_3 can be irreversibly inactivated by deiodination of the tyrosyl (inner or 5′) ring, a reaction catalyzed by the type 3 deiodinase (D3) and by D1.[1]

The coordinated changes in the expression and activity of these enzymes ensures thyroid hormone homeostasis and the constancy of T_3 production, constituting a major mechanism for adaptation to changes in the ingestion of iodine, starvation, and changes in environmental temperature. The study of animals with targeted disruption[2] or deficiency of D1 (C3H mouse),[3] targeted disruption of D2 ($Dio2^{-/-}$)[4,5] or D3 ($D3^{-/-}$),[6] and combinations[7] has not only confirmed this homeostatic role but revealed surprising new connections. Heightened interest in the field has been generated following the discovery that D2 can be an important component in the hedgehog signaling pathway and metabolically important G protein–coupled bile acid receptor 1 (GPBAR1)–mediated signaling cascade. The discovery of these new roles for the deiodinases indicates that tissue-specific deiodination plays a much broader role than once thought, extending into the realms of developmental biology and metabolism.[8]

DEIODINASES: THIOREDOXIN FOLD–CONTAINING PROTEINS

The three deiodinase proteins (D1, D2, and D3) show considerable similarity (approximately 50% sequence identity). All are integral membrane 29- to 33-kD proteins and have regions of high homology in the area surrounding the active center.[9-11] Structural analyses of these proteins have been hindered by their integral membrane nature and the inefficient eukaryotic-specific pathway for selenoprotein synthesis. Nevertheless, insights into their structures have been obtained through silicoprotein modeling (Fig. 5-2). Based on hydrophobic cluster analysis, it has become clear that the three deiodinases share a common general structure composed of a single transmembrane segment, which is present in the N termini of D1, D2, and D3, and several clusters, typical of alpha helices or beta strands, corresponding to core secondary structures of the deiodinase globular domains.[12] A striking common feature is the presence of the thioredoxin (TRX) fold, defined by βαβ and ββα motifs. It is interesting that within the canonical TRX fold, the relationship between the βαβ and ββα motifs is locally interrupted by interfering elements. These sequences correspond to distinct secondary structure elements added to the canonical TRX fold core, a feature also observed in other proteins of the TRX fold family.[13]

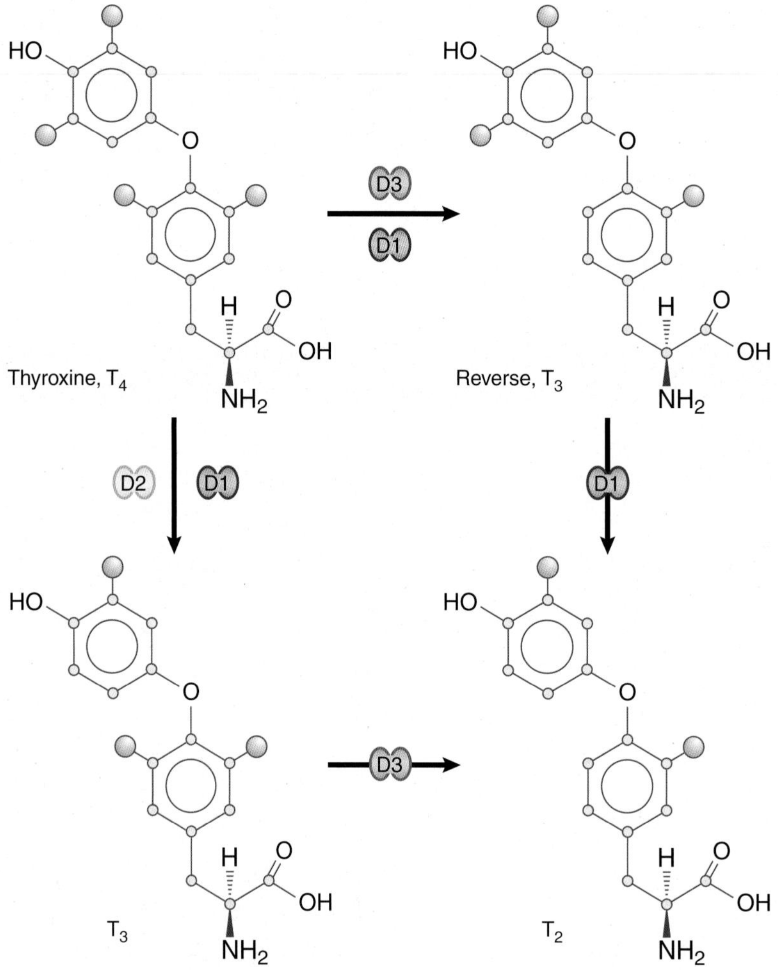

Figure 5–1 Basic deiodinase reactions. The reactions catalyzed by the deiodinases remove iodine moieties (blue spheres) from the phenolic (outer) or tyrosil (inner) ring of the iodothyronines. These pathways can activate thyroxine (T_4) by transforming it into triiodothyronine (T_3) via D1 or D2 or prevent it from being activated by conversion to the metabolically inactive form, reverse T_3 (via D1 or D3). T_2 is an inactive product common to both pathways that is rapidly metabolized by further deiodination.

The three-dimensional general model of the deiodinases predicts that the active center is a pocket defined by the β1-α1-β2 motifs of the TRX fold and one of the interfering elements. The critical element in the active center pocket is the rare amino acid selenocysteine (Sec), which catalyzes the deiodination reactions of all three deiodinases. Sec is encoded by UGA, which is recognized in the vast majority of mRNAs as a STOP codon.[9] However, a specific RNA stem loop immediately downstream of the UGA codon allows for the Sec incorporation in the STOP codon. This structure is termed the **S***ec* **I***nsertion* **S***equence*, or SECIS element, which is present in the deiodinases and all other selenoproteins.[14]

Distinct Subcellular Localizations of Deiodinases

D1 and D3 are located in the plasma membrane, whereas D2 is an endoplasmic reticulum (ER) resident protein.[15-17] The presence of D1 in the plasma membrane explains previous findings of rapid equilibration of plasma T_3 with T_3 generated via D1, as seen in liver and kidney, and the poor contribution of locally generated T_3 to the overall thyroid receptor (TR) occupancy in such tissues. In contrast, the action of D2 at the cytoplasmic face of the ER[16,18,19] generates T_3 in the perinuclear cytosol, which may facilitate access to its nuclear receptors.

D3 colocalizes with Na^+,K^+-ATPase alpha, with the early endosomal markers EEA-1 and clathrin but not with two ER-resident proteins.[15] There is constant internalization of D3 that is blocked by sucrose or methyl-β-cyclodextrin–containing medium. Exposing cells to a weak base such as primaquine increases the pool of internalized D3, suggesting that D3 is recycled between plasma membrane and early endosomes. Such recycling could account for the much longer half-life of D3 (12 hours) than D1 (8 hours) or D2 (~40 minutes). Although these studies also indicated that the D3 catalytic globular

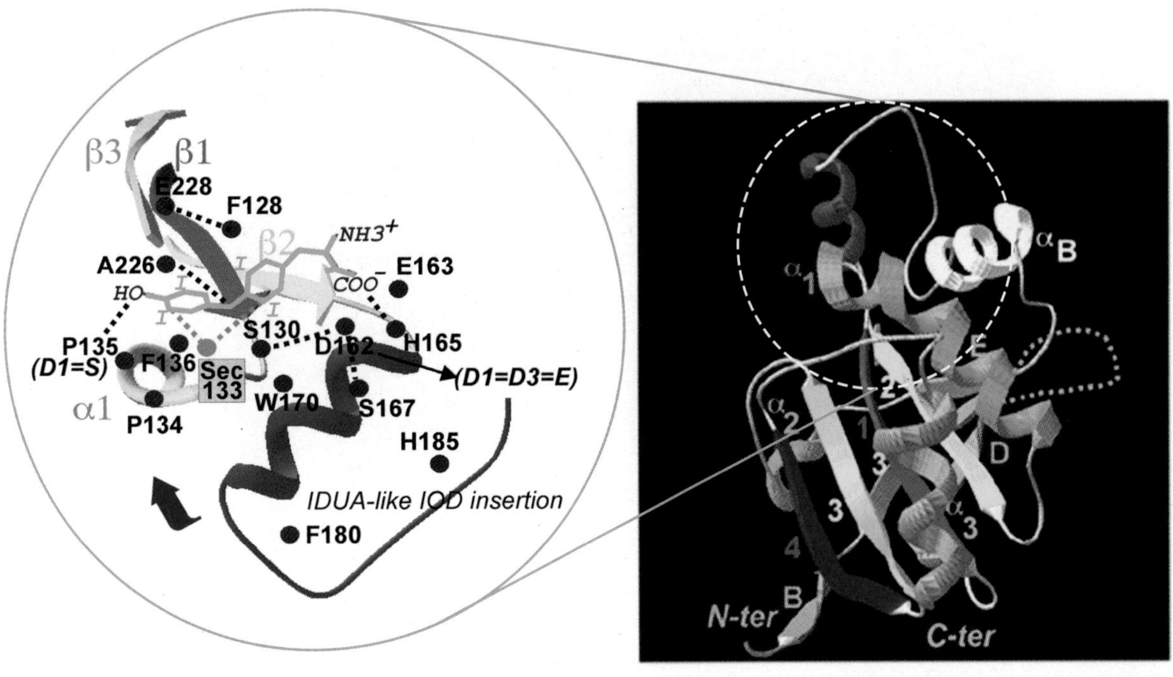

Figure 5–2 Structure of the deiodinases. Although the deiodinases have not yet been crystallized, protein modeling indicates that they share a common general structure composed of a single amino terminal anchoring segment, a short hinge region, and a thioredoxin fold–containing globular domain. A three-dimensional (3D) model of the D2 globular domain is shown on the right. Letters and numbers shown indicate different β sheets and α-helices. The orange dotted loop indicates the D2-specific segment that mediates interaction with the E3-ubiquitin ligase, WSB-1. **Inset,** The active center contains the rare amino acid selenocysteine (Sec), which is critical for nucleophilic attack during the deiodination reaction. The residues that putatively interact with the T_4 molecule (green) are also shown. Position 135, which in D2 and D3 is occupied by proline, is critical for enzyme kinetics. D2 and D3 have high affinity for their substrates and are not sensitive to inhibition by propylthiouracil (PTU). Replacement with serine, which is naturally found in D1, turns both D2 and D3 into low-affinity and PTU-sensitive enzymes.[12] C-ter, C terminus; N-ter, N terminus. *(Adapted from Callebaut I, Curcio-Morelli C, Mornon JP, et al: The iodothyronine selenodeiodinases are thioredoxin-fold family proteins containing a glycoside hydrolase-clan GH-A-like structure. J Biol Chem 278:36887-36896, 2003; and Dentice M, Bandyopadhyay A, Gereben B, et al: The Hedgehog-inducible ubiquitin ligase subunit WSB-1 modulates thyroid hormone activation and PTHrP secretion in the developing growth plate. Nat Cell Biol 7:698-705, 2005.)*

domain is located in the extracellular compartment, other studies have indicated that cellular entry of thyroid hormone via plasma membrane transporters is critical for D3-catalyzed deiodination, suggesting that the D3 active center is inside the cell.[20] More studies in this area are necessary to establish the determinants of D3 topology.

Inactivation of D2 by Ubiquitination Pathway

D2 is considered the critical homeostatic T_3-generating deiodinase because of its substantial physiologic plasticity.[1] A number of transcriptional and post-translational mechanisms have evolved to ensure limited expression and tight control of D2 levels, which is inherent to its homeostatic function.[21] D2 activity-to-mRNA ratios are variable, indicating that there is significant post-translational regulation of D2 expression.[22,23] The decisive biochemical property that characterizes D2's homeostatic behavior is its short half-life (approximately 40 minutes),[24] which can be further reduced by physiologic concentrations of its substrate, T_4, and in experimental situations by reverse T_3 or even high concentrations of T_3.[24-28] This downregulation of D2 by its substrate constitutes a rapid, potent generalized regulatory feedback loop that efficiently controls T_3 production and intracellular T_3 concentration based on how much T_4 is available.

The mechanism that underlies the feedback regulation of D2 by its substrate is ubiquitination. Important metabolic pathways often contain key rate-limiting enzymes whose half-lives can be modified by selective ubiquitination, a modification that targets proteins for destruction in the proteasomes.[29,30] The first evidence that D2 is regulated in this manner was obtained in GH4C1 cells, in which the half-life of endogenous D2 was noted to be stabilized by MG132, a proteasome inhibitor.[31] Substrate-induced loss of D2 activity was also inhibited by MG132 in these cells, indicating that both pathways affecting loss of D2 activity are mediated by the proteasomes.

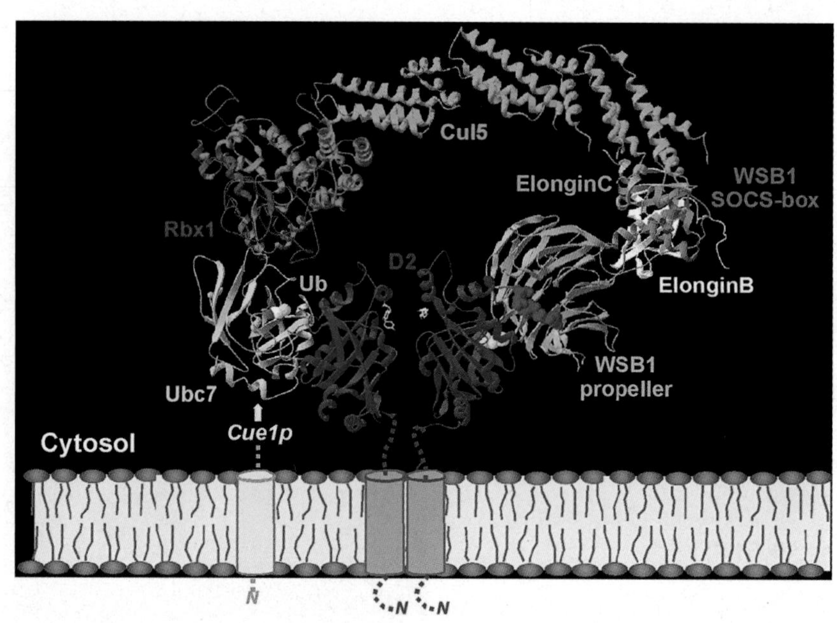

Figure 5–3 Ubiquitinating complex for D2. The hedgehog-inducible WSB-1 is an E3-ubiquitin ligase for D2. The WD40 propeller of WSB-1 recognizes an 18–amino acid loop in D2 that confers metabolic instability, whereas the SOCS-box domain mediates its interaction with ubiquitinating catalytic core complex, ECS^{WSB-1}, modeled as Elongin B-Cul5-Rbx1. *(Adapted from Dentice M, Bandyopadhyay A, Gereben B, et al: The Hedgehog-inducible ubiquitin ligase subunit WSB-1 modulates thyroid hormone activation and PTHrP secretion in the developing growth plate. Nat Cell Biol 7:698-705, 2005.)*

This implies that the loss of D2 activity is, at least partially, caused by proteolysis, a premise that was confirmed after the levels of immunoprecipitable labeled D2 were shown to parallel D2 activity, both under basal conditions and after exposure to substrate.[32]

A number of elements in the cellular ubiquitinating machinery have been identified as being important for D2 (Fig. 5-3).[33,34] In particular, the ubiquitin ligase responsible for the recognition of D2 by the ubiquitinating machinery has been identified as being WSB-1, a SOCS box–containing WD-40 protein of previously unknown function that is induced by hedgehog signaling in embryonic structures as shown in chicken development.[35,36] The WD-40 propeller of WSB-1 recognizes an 18–amino acid loop in D2 that confers metabolic instability, whereas the SOCS box domain mediates its interaction with an ubiquitinating catalytic core complex, modeled as Elongin BC-Cul5-Rbx1 (ECS^{WSB-1}). In the developing tibial growth plate, hedgehog-stimulated D2 ubiquitination via ECS^{WSB-1} induces parathyroid hormone–related peptide (PTHrP), thereby regulating chondrocyte differentiation. Thus, ECS^{WSB-1} mediates a novel mechanism whereby "locally generated" thyroid hormone can affect local control of the hedgehog-PTHrP negative feedback loop and thus skeletogenesis.[36]

The removal of the six amino terminal residues of the 18–amino acid D2 instability loop interferes with WSB-1–mediated ubiquitination so that D2 activity is not increased during WSB-1 knockdown.[19] However, this truncation does not eliminate the susceptibility to exposure to T_4 or prevent proteasomal degradation, suggesting that another E3 ligase could mediate the ubiquitination of D2. This is supported by a recent report in which yeast-expressed D2 is targeted by Doa10, a ubiquitin ligase known to ubiquitinate other ER resident proteins[37]; however, it is presently unknown whether TEB4, its likely human orthologue,[38] mediates D2 degradation in vertebrates.

Ubiquitinated D2 is not automatically degraded, but instead can be reactivated via the actions of the deubiquitinases VDU1 and VDU2.[39] The finding that VDU1 and VDU2 are coexpressed with D2 in many human tissues, including brain, heart, and skeletal muscle,[39-41] indicates that the importance of this mechanism may extend well beyond thermal homeostasis to include brain development, cardiac performance, glucose uptake, and energy expenditure.

Role of Deiodinases in Thyroid Hormone Homeostasis

Serum T_3 is relatively constant in healthy subjects, a finding that is not surprising considering that T_3 is a pleiotropic molecule. The deiodinases play an important role in the maintenance of thyroid hormone homeostasis, with deiodinase-mediated peripheral T_4 to T_3 conversion being the major source of plasma T_3 in humans, and with D2 being critical for feedback regulation of T_4 on thyroid-stimulating hormone (TSH) secretion.

The thyroid gland secretes T_4 and T_3 in a proportion determined by the T_4/T_3 ratio in thyroglobulin (15:1 in humans), modified to an unknown extent by intrathyroidal conversion of T_4 to T_3. Thus, the prohormone T_4 is the major secreted iodothyronine in healthy iodine-sufficient subjects. A number of lines of evidence have suggested that D2, rather than D1, is the pathway whereby most plasma T_3 is produced in euthyroid individuals. For example, in patients with primary hypothyroidism receiving fixed doses of exogenous T_4, propylthiouracil (PTU) treatment even at very high doses (1000 mg/day) only leads to a decrease of 25% in serum T_3.[42-46] More recent in vitro modeling estimates comparing T_3 production in cultured cells by the D1 or D2 pathway across a range of substrate concentrations have also favored the D2 pathway under euthyroid conditions, but also suggest that D1 becomes predominant as serum T_3 levels increase, as in thyrotoxic patients.[47]

The actions of the deiodinases are integrated, thus promoting the maintenance of serum T_3 concentrations. Fluctuations in serum T_4 and T_3 concentrations lead to homeostatic reciprocal changes in the activity of D2 and D3.[1] As serum T_3 concentrations increase, the D3 gene is upregulated, increasing T_3 clearance, whereas the D2 gene is modestly downregulated, decreasing T_3 production. The overall fractional conversion of T_4 to T_3 is increased in the hypothyroid patient, approximately 50% versus 25% in the euthyroid state.[48] This suggests that D2-catalyzed T_4 to T_3 conversion is an important mechanism to preserve T_3 production in primary hypothyroidism.[11,49,50] The increase in D2 seen in this setting has been particularly well documented for the brain, in which D2 activity and mRNA distribution are specifically concentrated in the hypothalamic tanycytes and the arcuate nucleus/median eminence region.[51-57] Brown adipose tissue (BAT) shows similar adaptation mechanisms. Because of the negative regulation of *Dio2* gene transcription by thyroid hormone,[23] D2 mRNA increases in iodine-deficient animals, especially within those subregions of the brain expressing high D2 activity. Not surprisingly, however, the increases in D2 activity are much greater than those in D2 mRNA.[22] This is explained by the hypothyroxinemia of iodine deficiency, accelerating D2 ubiquitination and degradation per se.

The clearance of T_3 from the brain is reduced during hypothyroidism, possibly as a result of a decrease in central nervous system (CNS) D3 activity. This decrease can be explained by the T_3 dependence of the *Dio3* gene—that is, the D3 message will be lower in hypothyroidism. Both total fetal and adult rat brain respond to iodine deficiency by decreasing D3 activity, although only modest (twofold) reductions have been observed.[10,55,58-60] As with D2, the distribution of D3 in the CNS is heterogeneous, with high focal expression in the hippocampus and cerebral cortex.[60,61] However, by focusing on specific brain subregions, it was found that D3 activity is decreased by 80% to 90% in the cerebral cortex, hippocampus, and cerebellum, changes of a much higher magnitude than those that occur in the brain in general.[55]

The increased fractional production of T_3 from T_4 by D2, combined with the prolonged residence time of T_3 (a result of low D3 activity), would be expected to mitigate the effects of severe iodine deficiency. This has been demonstrated in mild to moderate hypothyroidism by tracer studies in rodents[62] and confirmed directly by Campos-Barros and colleagues,[56] who measured thyroid hormone concentrations in various regions of the CNS in iodine-deficient rats. As expected, tissue T_4 was markedly decreased, whereas tissue T_3 concentrations were reduced by only 50%. This illustrates the effectiveness of these compensatory mechanisms.

D2 plays a key role in the feedback regulation of T_4 on TSH secretion (Fig. 5-4). This was first recognized following the observation that T_4 rapidly reduces TSH release in the hypothyroid rat in a PTU-insensitive manner.[63-66] Given that D1, but not D2, is inhibited by PTU, subsequent work was directed toward understanding the significance of D2 in the pituitary. Recently, it has been found that D2 and TSH are coexpressed in rat pituitary thyrotrophs and that hypothyroidism increases D2 expression in these cells.[66] Studies using two murine-derived thyrotroph cells, TtT-97 and TαT1, have demonstrated high expression of D2 in thyrotrophs and confirm its sensitivity to negative regulation by T_4-induced proteasomal degradation of this enzyme. Despite this, expression of the *Dio2* gene in TαT1 cells is higher than their T_4-induced D2 ubiquitinating capacity. As a result, D2 activity and net T_3 production in these cells are sustained, even at free T_4 concentrations that are several-fold above the physiologic range.

The presence of D2 in thyrotrophs can account for the requirement for physiologic levels of both T_4 and T_3 for normalization of TSH. It can also account for the increase in TSH at the early stages of iodine deficiency, when only T_4 is decreased.[67] D2 in the brain itself may also be important for TSH regulation, given evidence showing that the normalization of both circulating T_3 and T_4 are required to suppress TRH mRNA in the paraventricular nucleus

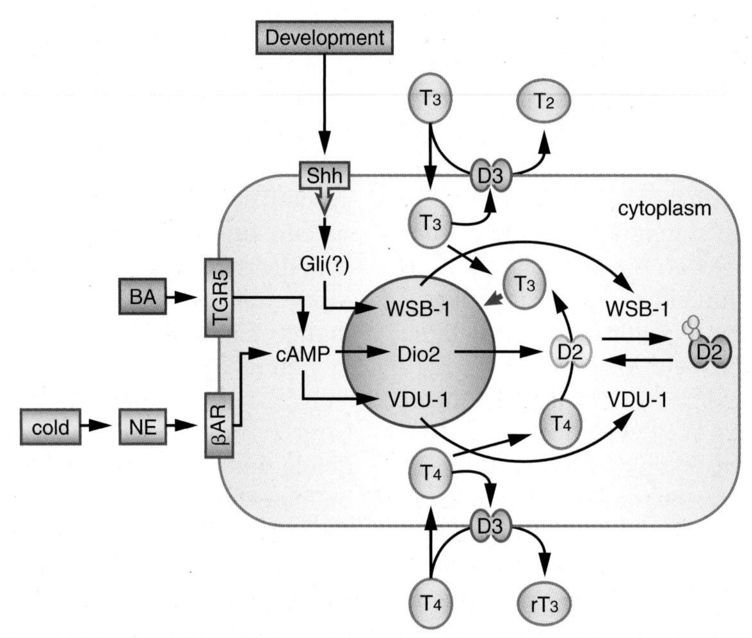

Figure 5–4 Pathways regulating D2 expression and thyroid hormone signaling. In D2-expressing cells such as brown adipocytes, stimulation of D2 expression increases local triiodothyronine (T_3) production, resulting in increased saturation of T_3 receptors. This increase can be mediated by norepinephrine (NE) stimulation of β-adrenergic receptors (βAR), such as during cold stimulation, or by bile acid (BA) stimulation of TGR5. Both these pathways activate cyclic AMP (cAMP) production and stimulate *Dio2* transcription (nucleus is a blue circle). In the brown fat, cAMP also promotes VDU-1 expression, amplifying the D2 induction via deubiquitination. Other signaling pathways can decrease D2 activity, resulting in relative local hypothyroidism. For example, the hedgehog cascade decreases D2 activity by promoting *WSB-1* expression and thus D2 ubquitination, presumably via the Gli cascade. *Shh*, sonic hedgehog.

of the hypothalamus. Surprisingly, D2 activity is not present in this portion of the hypothalamus but rather it is concentrated in the arcuate nucleus and median eminence, specifically in glial cells and tanycytes.[51-53,68,69] These specialized cells have their cell bodies in the inferior portion of the third ventricle, raising the possibility that a signal from T_4 in the central system fluid could be transduced to the thyrotrophs via T_3 released from the tanycyte processes into the pituitary portal plexus.

Tissue-Specific Control of Thyroid Hormone Signaling

At the cellular level, thyroid hormone action is initiated through the binding of T_3 to nuclear thyroid hormone receptors (TRs), high-affinity nuclear T_3 binding proteins that regulate the transcription of T_3-dependent genes. The extent of thyroid hormone signaling in a given cell ultimately depends on TR occupancy, which is determined by the affinity of the receptor for T_3 and the T_3 concentration in the nucleus. These values are such that at normal serum T_3 concentrations, the contribution from serum T_3 alone results in an approximately 50% saturation of thyroid hormone receptors in most tissues.

Although plasma thyroid hormones may provide a uniform signal to all tissues of the body, their biologic impact is not homogeneous. Tissues expressing D2 have an additional intracellular source of T_3; the nuclear T_3 concentration depends both on T_3 from the plasma and T_4 from the plasma that has been converted to T_3 by D2 (see Fig. 5-4).[70,71] The magnitude of the importance of D2 for nuclear T_3 levels is considerable: in liver and kidney, the saturation of the TRs is normally approximately 50% whereas in the CNS, where D2 is expressed, it is close to 95%. Furthermore, in brown adipose tissue the levels of D2 activity and TR occupancy are dynamic and change according to the metabolic requirements of the tissue (discussed later), increasing from a TR occupancy of approximately 70% at room temperature to approximately 100% during cold exposure.[54,72]

The importance of primary changes in deiodinase activity in determining local T_3-dependent effects has been clearly illustrated in studies of BAT in rodents. This tissue is the major site of adaptive thermogenesis in rodents, with heat being generated as a result of the actions of uncoupling protein 1 (UCP-1).[73] Cold-induced thermogenesis in BAT has been shown to depend on the cyclic adenosine monophosphate (cAMP)–mediated acceleration of D2-catalyzed T_3 production,[74] which in turn leads to the induction of T_3-responsive thermogenic genes including

UCP-1. In D2 knockout mice, survival in the cold is only possible because the mice begin shivering, a behavior not normally seen in small mammals.[5,75] An additional role played by D2 and thyroid hormones in brown adipose tissue (BAT) is to mediate a three- to fourfold increase in the activity of lipogenic proteins—malic enzyme (ME), glucose 6-phosphate dehydrogenase (G6PD), and Spot14—observed in this tissue during cold exposure, a response that is blunted in hypothyroid rats.[34,42-44] It is important to note that in spite of the large D2-mediated increase in BAT nuclear T_3 seen in cold-exposed animals, serum T_3 concentrations do not change, demonstrating that that D2 can have tissue-specific metabolic effects.

Novel Role for D2 in Metabolic Control

Given the generalized metabolic sensitivity to thyroid hormone documented in human subjects during hypo- and hyperthyroidism, one would anticipate a major physiologic role of this hormone in energy homeostasis. However, the relative constancy of serum T_3 concentration seemed to preclude a major role of T_3 in the basal metabolic rate (BMR) variations observed after a meal or during sleep. With the realization that deiodinases, in particular D2, could alter local intracellular thyroid status without necessarily altering serum T_3 concentrations, this presumption has been deservedly challenged.

Evidence for a role for D2 in the control of metabolic pathways beyond cold-induced thermogenesis was recently provided by the discovery that bile acids can confer resistance to diet-induced obesity in mice via upregulation of D2 expression in brown adipose tissue.[76] In this tissue, binding of bile acids to the plasma membrane G protein–coupled receptor TGR5 triggers an increase in cAMP formation and subsequently D2 expression. In normal mice fed a high-fat diet supplemented with bile acids, oxygen consumption increases and the mice did not gain weight or become as insulin-resistant as mice only fed the high fat diet. However, this effect is lost in D2 knockout mice. The importance of this mechanism in rodents fed a normal diet remains to be determined and D2-independent bile acid activated pathways may play a role. It is nonetheless noteworthy that D2 is overexpressed in two other rodent models of resistance to diet-induced obesity: UCP-1 knockout mice are paradoxically lean[77] and have ectopic expression of D2 in their white fat, whereas the double–liver X receptor (LXR) knockout mice express D2 ectopically in the liver.[78] If the ectopic expression of D2 in these animals results in tissue-specific thyrotoxicosis, as is suggested by gene expression profiling in the case of the double-LXR knockout mice, this would certainly support the concept that the D2 pathway increases energy expenditure.

Human newborns grow less dependent on BAT thermogenesis with maturity, and adult humans, unlike small mammals, do not have substantial amounts of BAT.[79] The mass of brown adipose tissue in humans peaks at the time of birth, when brown adipocytes comprise almost 1% of body weight.[80-82] It could thus be assumed that the D2 pathway is most important for thermogenesis in infants and less important in adults, except in those in whom brown adipose tissue mass is increased, such as patients with pheochromocytoma.[83] However, the amount of brown adipose tissue in adults may be greater than once thought, because studies using fluorodeoxyglucose (FDG) positron emission tomography (PET) or computed tomography (CT) imaging have identified focal deposits in the mediastinum and in extramediastinal areas.[84,85] More importantly, given the finding of D2 activity in human skeletal myocytes, a larger metabolic role for D2 in humans may be anticipated, because skeletal muscle is the predominant site of thermogenesis and insulin-induced glucose disposal in adult humans.[11,49]

Various studies have supported a previously unrecognized role of D2 in influencing the thyroid status and metabolic rate in humans. Earlier studies consistently found that diet-induced changes in serum thyroid hormones could be explained by changes in D2 activity. For example, the increase in BMR observed in subjects fed a high-carbohydrate diet is typically associated with an increase in the serum T_3/T_4 ratio,[86] a condition that is also observed in adult subjects chronically treated with terbutaline, a β-adrenergic receptor (β-AR) stimulator.[87] A connection with D2 can be easily imagined, given that it is the only cAMP-dependent deiodinase.[88] Furthermore, studies of patients receiving T_4 replacement at various dosages have shown a direct correlation of the BMR with free T_4 and inversely with serum TSH, but not with serum T_3.[89] Together, these data could indicate that D2-produced T_3 might be a significant physiologic determinant of energy expenditure in humans.

Thyroid hormone is one of the few truly potent stimulators of the metabolic rate, such that energy expenditure is several-fold higher in hyperthyroid as compared with hypothyroid patients.[90] However, little is known about how D2-generated T_3, or T_3 from plasma, accelerates energy expenditure. Although many T_3-responsive candidate genes have been identified, their exact contribution remains to be established. Increased mitochondrial uncoupling has been proposed as one mechanism, and this effect has been demonstrated in the skeletal muscle of mildly thyrotoxic human volunteers.[91] Similar results were reported in hepatocytes of thyrotoxic rats,[92] but it is not clear whether this effect is mediated by uncoupling proteins. Another general mechanism whereby T_3 may increase energy expenditure would be to accelerate the turnover of enzymes that use ATP. Several T_3-responsive genes have been implicated, such as the Na^+/K^+-ATPase[93,94] and the sarcoplasmic endoplasmic reticulum Ca^{2+}-ATPase (SERCA) gene[95,96] among others.[97-99] Which, if any, of these genes is most responsible for the observed increase in energy expenditure driven by T_3 remains to be determined, and it is possible that an as yet unidentified mechanism could play a major role.

DEIODINASES IN ILLNESS

Hyperthyroidism

Whereas D2 is thought to be the major T_3-producing deiodinase in euthyroid individuals, D1 becomes predominant during thyrotoxicosis. It has been established that the production rate of T_3 and its circulating concentration is about twofold higher relative to that of T_4 in hyperthyroid patients.[100] This is reflected in the markedly greater elevation in free T_3 than in free T_4 in such patients. Because the human *Dio1* promoter is T_3-responsive, one would anticipate that D1 activity or mRNA would be significantly increased in hyperthyroid patients; this has been demonstrated in Graves' thyroid tissue and in mononuclear leukocytes of patients with Graves' disease.[101-103]

Given that PTU blocks D1 activity, it is not surprising that its administration has a greater effect on thyrotoxic than on euthyroid subjects. This has been shown in a study in which the effects of PTU versus methimazole on serum T_3 production were examined in euthyroid and thyrotoxic patients.[100] These data, indicating a predominance of D1 in thyrotoxic subjects and inhibition of D1 by PTU, have led to the recommendation that large doses of PTU, or other agents that block T_4 to T_3 conversion, such as iopanoic or ipodipic acid, be used in the acute treatment of the severely hyperthyroid individual.[104-106]

AMIODARONE

Amiodarone is a potent iodine-containing cardiac antiarrhythmic that shares some structural homology with thyroid hormones. Thyroid function test results may be abnormal during its administration as a result of alterations in the metabolism of thyroid hormones,[107,108] with rapid development of increased plasma T_4 (approximately 40%) and reverse T_3 (170%) concentrations, along with decreases of T_3 by 10% to 25%. Similar changes occur in free T_3 and T_4.[109,110] These effects stem mainly from the fact that the drug is 37% iodine by weight, but there are also effects on deiodinases.

The T_4 to T_3 conversion rate may fall from 26% to 43% (range) to 10% to 17% during amiodarone therapy, but because T_4 production is increased, net T_3 production and plasma-free T_3 concentrations normalize.[111-113] Animal studies have suggested some primary effects of amiodarone on deiodinase activities. For example, in rats given amiodarone, D1 mRNA levels are normal,[114] but the enzyme activity is inhibited in homogenates of liver, heart, and kidney in a dose-dependent fashion.[115-119] The same is observed in hepatocytes exposed to amiodarone.[120] The mechanism of inhibition of D1 in amiodarone-treated animals is likely to be competitive inhibition with substrate by the drug per se or one of its metabolites.[121]

Deiodinases in Nonthyroidal Illness

Any critical illness, life-threatening trauma, or major surgery can trigger a stereotypic pattern of changes in pituitary-thyroid function sometimes referred to as the low T_3 syndrome or euthyroid sick syndrome. These patients exhibit low serum T_3 concentrations, with the decrease being inversely related to the severity of illness. The concentrations of T_4 and TSH may also decrease and an increase in total reverse T_3 may also be seen.[122-124]

Understanding the pathogenesis of the low T_3 syndrome has proven difficult, not only because of the protean nature of the underlying diseases but also because of interspecies variations in the response of the thyroid axis to illness. Nevertheless, changes in peripheral T_3 generation via the deiodinases and/or clearance of T_3 must certainly play a role. Serum TSH is not suppressed unless illness is extreme, suggesting that the severely reduced T_3 seen in ill patients does not stem from a lack of central T_3 production, but rather from decreased peripheral T_4 deiodination and/or increased clearance of T_3. This conclusion is further supported by the observation that serum T_3 and T_4 concentrations decrease during illness in patients with hypothyroidism who are given L-thyroxine every day during their illness.[125]

Recent data from critically ill patients have substantiated a previously unsuspected role for D3 in the pathogenesis of the low T_3 syndrome. D3 is normally expressed in multiple fetal structures, but the endometrium and the placenta are the only normal tissues known to express high levels of D3 activity in the mature human. The main previously recognized role for D3 had been in the regulation of maternal-fetal thyroid hormone transfer in the uteroplacental unit.[126] However, in a study that determined serum thyroid hormone levels and the expression of D1, D2, and D3 in liver and skeletal muscle from deceased intensive care patients, liver D1 was downregulated and D3 was induced ectopically in liver and skeletal muscle.[127] D1 and D3 mRNA levels corresponded with enzyme activities, suggesting regulation of the expression of both deiodinases at the pretranslational level. These observations may indicate tissue-specific mechanisms for the reduction of thyroid hormone bioactivity during illness.[127,128] Furthermore, an increase in D3 activity could contribute to the observed increase in reverse T_3 seen in the syndrome, along with decreased reverse T_3 clearance via D1.[129] Whether ectopic D3 occurs or is important in milder illness is not yet known.

The seemingly coordinated changes in the expression of the three deiodinases seen in ill patients could be taken as circumstantial evidence for the hypothesis that the nonthyroidal illness syndrome is in fact a physiologic response to illness, rather than a pathologic mechanism. In any case, although changes in peripheral deiodination may be necessary for the pathogenesis of the syndrome, they are probably not sufficient to cause it. Given the remarkable capacity of the hypothalamic-pituitary-thyroid axis to compensate for decreases in T_3 production in peripheral tissues, as demonstrated in the deiodinase-deficient mice, central hypothyroidism must also be part of the syndrome.[130] TSH secretion is decreased in critically ill subjects, and continuous infusion of TRH has been shown to increase serum T_4 and T_3 concentrations strikingly.[131] The molecular determinants of central hypothyroidism in these patients are not well characterized. Whereas dopamine and glucocorticoids play a suppressive role with respect to TSH,[132] leptin administration leads to increases in serum TSH, T_4, and T_3 concentrations in fasting rats[133] and humans.[135] Another pathway that could be involved is the nuclear factor κB (NF-κB) cascade, which upregulates D2 in the medial basal hypothalamus of rats following lipopolysaccharide injection,[135,136] although it remains speculative whether this induction of D2 leads to local thyrotoxicosis.

D3 in Hemangiomas

D3 expression has been found in human brain tumors, certain malignant cell lines, and vascular anomalies. D3 expression occurs at high levels in rare infantile hemangiomas.[137] If these tumors are sufficiently large, the rate of thyroid hormone inactivation can exceed the maximal rate of thyroid hormone synthesis. The first patient documented with this condition was 3 months old, presenting with severe hypothyroidism with an elevation in serum TSH, undetectable serum T_4 and T_3 concentrations, and high reverse T_3 and thyroglobulin levels. The relationship between infantile hemangiomas and D3 expression is notable because it identifies a previously unrecognized cause of hypothyroidism, which usually occurs at a critical age for neurologic development. Although extensive hepatic hemangiomas can be fatal, a significant fraction of these infants survive as a result of therapy and the natural tendency of these tumors is to regress. Accordingly, these patients may require replacement with large quantities of thyroid hormone in addition to therapy directed at their hemangiomas. Thyroid hormone treatment is also imperative to prevent the complication of irreversible mental retardation later in life.

Conclusions

From a broad perspective, deiodination of iodothyronines can be seen as an example of a paradigm in which hormones are activated or inactivated in a controlled fashion in specific extraglandular tissues. The deiodinases can be seen as playing an analogous role to that of 5α-reductase and cytochrome P-450 aromatase in sex steroid metabolism and to 11β-hydroxysteroid dehydrogenase in glucocorticoid metabolism. The three deiodinases constitute a major regulatory mechanism for thyroid hormone action, perhaps the most important peripheral regulatory mechanism at the prereceptor level. Their well-characterized homeostatic roles in the defense against hypothyroidism and the generation of thyrotoxicosis have obvious implications for the clinician. However, the breadth of actions of these enzymes is only now being recognized. If the role of deiodinases, particularly D2, in metabolic control is proven to be relevant for human subjects, then understanding these pathways may become of great importance for the treatment of diabetes, obesity, and the metabolic syndrome.

References

1. Bianco AC, Salvatore D, Gereben B, et al: Biochemistry, cellular and molecular biology and physiological roles of the iodothyronine selenodeiodinases. Endocrine Rev 23:38-89, 2002.
2. Schneider MJ, Fiering SN, Thai B: Targeted disruption of the type 1 selenodeiodinase gene (dio1) results in marked changes in thyroid hormone economy in mice. Endocrinology 147:580-589, 2006.

3. Berry MJ, Grieco D, Taylor BA, et al: Physiological and genetic analyses of inbred mouse strains with a type I iodothyronine 5′ deiodinase deficiency. J Clin Invest 92:1517-1528, 1993.
4. Schneider MJ, Fiering SN, Pallud SE, et al: Targeted disruption of the type 2 selenodeiodinase gene (Dio2) results in a phenotype of pituitary resistance to T4. Mol Endocrinol 15:2137-2148, 2001.
5. de Jesus LA, Carvalho SD, Ribeiro MO, et al: The type 2 iodothyronine deiodinase is essential for adaptive thermogenesis in brown adipose tissue. J Clin Invest 108:1379-1385, 2001.
6. Hernandez A, Martinez ME, Fiering S, et al: Type 3 deiodinase is critical for the maturation and function of the thyroid axis. J Clin Invest 116:476-484, 2006.
7. Christoffolete MA, Arrojo EDR, Gazoni F, et al: Mice with impaired extrathyroidal thyroxine to 3,5,3′-triiodothyronine (T_3) conversion maintain normal serum T_3 concentrations. Endocrinology, 148:954-960, 2006.
8. Bianco AC, Kim BW: Deiodinases: Implications of the local control of thyroid hormone action. J Clin Invest 116:2571-2579, 2006.
9. Berry MJ, Banu L, Larsen PR: Type I iodothyronine deiodinase is a selenocysteine-containing enzyme. Nature 349:438-440, 1991.
10. St. Germain DL, Schwartzman RA, Croteau W, et al: A thyroid hormone–regulated gene in Xenopus laevis encodes a type III iodothyronine 5-deiodinase. Proc Natl Acad Sci U S A 91:7767-7771, 1994.
11. Croteau W, Davey JC, Galton VA, St. Germain DL: Cloning of the mammalian type II iodothyronine deiodinase. A selenoprotein differentially expressed and regulated in human and rat brain and other tissues. J Clin Invest 98:405-417, 1996.
12. Callebaut I, Curcio-Morelli C, Mornon JP, et al: The iodothyronine selenodeiodinases are thioredoxin-fold family proteins containing a glycoside hydrolase-clan GH-A-like structure. J Biol Chem 278:36887-36896, 2003.
13. Martin JL: Thioredoxin—a fold for all reasons. Structure 3:245-250, 1995.
14. Berry MJ, Banu L, Chen YY, et al: Recognition of UGA as a selenocysteine codon in type I deiodinase requires sequences in the 3′ untranslated region. Nature 353:273-276, 1991.
15. Baqui MM, Botero D, Gereben B, et al: Human type 3 iodothyronine selenodeiodinase is located in the plasma membrane and undergoes rapid internalization to endosomes. J Biol Chem 278:1206-1211, 2003.
16. Baqui MM, Gereben B, Harney JW, et al: Distinct subcellular localization of transiently expressed types 1 and 2 iodothyronine deiodinases as determined by immunofluorescence confocal microscopy. Endocrinology 141:4309-4312, 2000.
17. Prabakaran D, Ahima RS, Harney JW, et al: Polarized targeting of epithelial cell proteins in thyrocytes and MDCK cells. J Cell Sci 112:1247-1256, 1999.
18. Curcio C, Baqui MM, Salvatore D, et al: The human type 2 iodothyronine deiodinase is a selenoprotein highly expressed in a mesothelioma cell line. J Biol Chem 276:30183-30187, 2001.
19. Zeold A, Pormuller L, Dentice M, et al: Metabolic instability of type 2 deiodinase is transferable to stable proteins independently of subcellular localization. J Biol Chem 281:31538-31543, 2006.
20. Friesema EC, Kuiper GG, Jansen J, et al: Thyroid hormone transport by the human monocarboxylate transporter 8 and its rate-limiting role in intracellular metabolism. Mol Endocrinol 20:2761-2772, 2006.
21. Gereben B, Kollar A, Harney JW, Larsen PR: The mRNA structure has potent regulatory effects on type 2 iodothyronine deiodinase expression. Mol Endocrinol 16:1667-1679, 2002.
22. Burmeister LA, Pachucki J, St. Germain DL: Thyroid hormones inhibit type 2 iodothyronine deiodinase in the rat cerebral cortex by both pre- and posttranslational mechanisms. Endocrinology 138:5231-5237, 1997.
23. Kim SW, Harney JW, Larsen PR: Studies of the hormonal regulation of type 2 5′-iodothyronine deiodinase messenger ribonucleic acid in pituitary tumor cells using semiquantitative reverse transcription-polymerase chain reaction. Endocrinology 139:4895-4905, 1998.
24. St. Germain DL: The effects and interactions of substrates, inhibitors, and the cellular thiol-disulfide balance on the regulation of type II iodothyronine 5′-deiodinase. Endocrinology 122: 1860-1868, 1988.
25. Leonard JL, Kaplan MM, Visser TJ, et al: Cerebral cortex responds rapidly to thyroid hormones. Science 214:571-573, 1981.
26. Koenig RJ, Leonard JL, Senator D, et al: 1984. Regulation of thyroxine 5′-deiodinase activity by T_3 in cultured rat anterior pituitary cells. Endocrinology 115:324-329, 1984.
27. Silva JE, Leonard JL: Regulation of rat cerebrocortical and adenohypophyseal type II 5′-deiodinase by thyroxine, triiodothyronine, and reverse triiodothyronine. Endocrinology 116:1627-1635, 1985.
28. Obregon MJ, Larsen PR, Silva JE: The role of 3,3′,5′-triiodothyronine in the regulation of type II iodothyronine 5′-deiodinase in the rat cerebral cortex. Endocrinology 119:2186-2192, 1986.
29. Pines J, Lindon C: Proteolysis: Anytime, any place, anywhere? Nat Cell Biol 7:731-735, 2005.
30. Ciechanover A: Proteolysis: From the lysosome to ubiquitin and the proteasome. Nat Rev Mol Cell Biol 6:79-87, 2005.
31. Steinsapir J, Harney J, Larsen PR: Type 2 iodothyronine deiodinase in rat pituitary tumor cells is inactivated in proteasomes. J Clin Invest 102:1895-1899, 1998.

32. Steinsapir J, Bianco AC, Buettner C, et al: Substrate-induced down-regulation of human type 2 deiodinase (hD2) is mediated through proteasomal degradation and requires interaction with the enzyme's active center. Endocrinology 141:1127-1135, 2000.
33. Botero D, Gereben B, Goncalves C, et al: Ubc6p and Ubc7p are required for normal and substrate-induced endoplasmic reticulum–associated degradation of the human selenoprotein type 2 iodothyronine monodeiodinase. Mol Endocrinol 16:1999-2007, 2002.
34. Kim BW, Zavacki AM, Harney JW, et al: The human type 2 iodothyronine selenodeiodinase (D2) is ubiquitinated via interaction with the mammalian ubiquitin conjugases MmUBC7 and MmUBC6. Presented at the 74th Meeting of the American Thyroid Association, Los Angeles, October 2002.
35. Hershko A, Ciechanover A: The ubiquitin system. Annu Rev Biochem 67:425-479, 1998.
36. Dentice M, Bandyopadhyay A, Gereben B, et al: The Hedgehog-inducible ubiquitin ligase subunit WSB-1 modulates thyroid hormone activation and PTHrP secretion in the developing growth plate. Nat Cell Biol 7:698-705, 2005.
37. Ravid T, Kreft SG, Hochstrasser M: Membrane and soluble substrates of the Doa10 ubiquitin ligase are degraded by distinct pathways. EMBO J 25:533-543, 2006.
38. Kreft SG, Wang L, Hochstrasser M: Membrane topology of the yeast endoplasmic reticulum-localized ubiquitin ligase Doa10 and comparison with its human ortholog TEB4 (MARCH-VI). J Biol Chem 281:4646-4653, 2006.
39. Curcio-Morelli C, Zavacki AM, Christofollete M, et al: Deubiquitination of type 2 iodothyronine deiodinase by pVHL-interacting deubiquitinating enzymes regulates thyroid hormone activation. J Clin Invest 112:189-196, 2003.
40. Li Z, Na X, Wang D, et al: Ubiquitination of a novel deubiquitinating enzyme requires direct binding to von Hippel-Lindau tumor suppressor protein. J Biol Chem 277:4656-4662, 2002.
41. Li Z, Wang D, Na X, et al: Identification of a deubiquitinating enzyme subfamily as substrates of the von Hippel-Lindau tumor suppressor. Biochem Biophys Res Commun 294:700-709, 2002.
42. Geffner DL, Azukizawa M, Hershman JM: Propylthiouracil blocks extrathyroidal conversion of thyroxine to triiodothyronine and augments thyrotropin secretion in man. J Clin Invest 55:224-229, 1975.
43. Saberi M, Sterling FH, Utiger RD: Reduction in extrathyroidal triiodothyronine production by propylthiouracil in man. J Clin Invest 55:218-223, 1975.
44. LoPresti JS, Eigen A, Kaptein E, et al: Alterations in 3,3′5′-triiodothyronine metabolism in response to propylthiouracil, dexamethasone, and thyroxine administration in man. J Clin Invest 84:1650-1656, 1989.
45. Lum SM, Nicoloff JT, Spencer CA, Kaptein EM: Peripheral tissue mechanism for maintenance of serum triiodothyronine values in a thyroxine-deficient state in man. J Clin Invest 73:570-575, 1984.
46. Nicoloff JT, Lum SM, Spencer CA, Morris R: Peripheral autoregulation of thyroxine to triiodothyronine conversion in man. Horm Metab Res Suppl 14:74-79, 1984.
47. Maia AL, Kim BW, Huang SA, et al: Type 2 iodothyronine deiodinase is the major source of plasma T_3 in euthyroid humans. J Clin Invest 115:2524-2533, 2005.
48. Inada M, Kasagi K, Kurata S, et al: Estimation of thyroxine and triiodothyronine distribution and of the conversion rate of thyroxine to triiodothyronine in man. J Clin Invest 55:1337-1348, 1975.
49. Salvatore D, Bartha T, Harney JW, Larsen PR: Molecular biological and biochemical characterization of the human type 2 selenodeiodinase. Endocrinology 137:3308-3315, 1996.
50. Hosoi Y, Murakami M, Mizuma H, et al: Expression and regulation of type II iodothyronine deiodinase in cultured human skeletal muscle cells. J Clin Endocrinol Metab 84:3293-3300, 1999.
51. Riskind PN, Kolodny JM, Larsen PR: The regional hypothalamic distribution of type II 5′-monodeiodinase in euthyroid and hypothyroid rats. Brain Res 420:194-198, 1987.
52. Tu HM, Kim SW, Salvatore D, et al: Regional distribution of type 2 thyroxine deiodinase messenger ribonucleic acid in rat hypothalamus and pituitary and its regulation by thyroid hormone. Endocrinology 138:3359-3368, 1997.
53. Guadano-Ferraz A, Obregon MJ, St. Germain DL, Bernal J: The type 2 iodothyronine deiodinase is expressed primarily in glial cells in the neonatal rat brain. Proc Natl Acad Sci U S A 94:10391-10396, 1997.
54. Larsen PR, Silva JE, Kaplan MM: Relationships between circulating and intracellular thyroid hormones: Physiological and clinical implications. Endocr Rev 2:87-102, 1981.
55. Meinhold H, Campos-Barros A, Behne D: Effects of selenium and iodine deficiency on iodothyronine deiodinases in brain, thyroid and peripheral tissue. Acta Med Austriaca 19:8-12, 1992.
56. Campos-Barros A, Meinhold H, Walzog B, Behne D: Effects of selenium and iodine deficiency on thyroid hormone concentrations in the central nervous system of the rat. Eur J Endocrinol 136:316-323, 1997.
57. Guadano-Ferraz A, Escamez MJ, Rausell E, Bernal J: Expression of type 2 iodothyronine deiodinase in hypothyroid rat brain indicates an important role of thyroid hormone in the development of specific primary sensory systems. J Neurosci 19:3430-3439, 1999.
58. Kaplan MM, Yaskoski KA: Phenolic and tyrosyl ring deiodination of iodothyronines in rat brain homogenates. J Clin Invest 66:551-552, 1980.

59. Schroder-van der Elst JP, van der Heide D, Morreale de Escoba G, Obregon MJ: Iodothyronine deiodinase activities in fetal rat tissues at several levels of iodine deficiency: A role for the skin in 3,5,3′-triiodothyronine economy? Endocrinology 139:2229-2234, 1998.
60. Tu HM, Legradi G, Bartha T, et al: Regional expression of the type 3 iodothyronine deiodinase messenger ribonucleic acid in the rat central nervous system and its regulation by thyroid hormone. Endocrinology 140:784-790, 1999.
61. Escamez MJ, Guadano-Ferraz A, Cuadrado A, Bernal J: Type 3 iodothyronine deiodinase is selectively expressed in areas related to sexual differentiation in the newborn rat brain. Endocrinology 140:5443-5446, 1999.
62. Silva JE, Larsen PR: Comparison of iodothyronine 5′-deiodinase and other thyroid-hormone-dependent enzyme activities in the cerebral cortex of hypothyroid neonatal rat. Evidence for adaptation to hypothyroidism. J Clin Invest 70:1110-1123, 1982.
63. Frumess RD, Larsen PR: Correlation of serum triiodothyronine (T_3) and thyroxine (T_4) with biologic effects of thyroid hormone replacement in propylthiouracil-treated rats. Metabolism 24:547-554, 975.
64. Larsen PR, Frumess RD: Comparison of the biological effects of thyroxine and triiodothyronine in the rat. Endocrinology 100:980-988, 1977.
65. Silva JE, Larsen PR: Peripheral metabolism of homologous thyrotropin in euthyroid and hypothyroid rats: Acute effects of thyrotropin-releasing hormone, triiodothyronine, and thyroxine. Endocrinology 102:1783-1796, 1978.
66. Christoffolete MA, Ribeiro R, Singru P, et al: Atypical expression of type 2 iodothyronine deiodinase in thyrotrophs explains the thyroxine-mediated pituitary TSH feedback mechanism. Endocrinology 147:1735-1743, 2006.
67. Riesco G, Taurog A, Larsen R, Krulich L: Acute and chronic responses to iodine deficiency in rats. Endocrinology 100:303-313, 1977.
68. Kakucska I, Rand W, Lechan RM: Thyrotropin-releasing hormone (TRH) gene expression in the hypothalamic paraventricular nucleus is dependent upon feedback regulation by both triiodothyronine and thyroxine. Endocrinology 130: 2845-2850, 1992.
69. Fekete C, Mihaly E, Herscovici S, et al: DARPP-32 and CREB are present in type 2 iodothyronine deiodinase producing tanycytes: Implications for the regulation of type 2 deiodinase activity. Brain Res 862:154-161, 2000.
70. Silva JE, Larsen PR: Pituitary nuclear 3,5,3′-triiodothyronine and thyrotropin secretion: An explanation for the effect of thyroxine. Science 198: 617-620, 1977.
71. Silva JE, Leonard JL, Crantz FR, Larsen PR: Evidence for two tissue-specific pathways for in vivo thyroxine 5′-deiodination in the rat. J Clin Invest 69:1176-1184, 1982.
72. Larsen PR: Regulation of thyrotropin secretion by 3,5,3′-triiodothyronine and thyroxine. Prog Clin Biol Res 74:81-93, 1981.
73. Lowell BB, Spiegelman BM: Towards a molecular understanding of adaptive thermogenesis. Nature 404:652-660, 2000.
74. Bianco AC, Silva JE: Intracellular conversion of thyroxine to triiodothyronine is required for the optimal thermogenic function of brown adipose tissue. J Clin Invest 79:295-300, 1987.
75. Christoffolete MA, Linardi CCG, de Jesus LA, et al: Mice with targeted disruption of the Dio2 gene have cold-induced overexpression of uncoupling protein 1 gene but fail to increase brown adipose tissue lipogenesis and adaptive thermogenesis. Diabetes 53:577-584, 2004.
76. Watanabe M, Houten SM, Mataki C, et al: Bile acids induce energy expenditure by promoting intracellular thyroid hormone activation. Nature 439:484-489, 2006.
77. Liu X, Rossmeisl M, McClaine J, et al: Paradoxical resistance to diet-induced obesity in UCP1-deficient mice. J Clin Invest 111:399-407, 2003.
78. Kalaany NY, Gauthier KC, Zavacki AM, et al: LXRx regulate the balance between fat storage and oxidation. Cell Metabolism 1:231-244, 2005.
79. Bruck K: Neonatal thermal regulation. In Polin RA, Fox WW (eds): Fetal and Neonatal Physiology. Philadelphia, WB Saunders, 1998, pp 676-702.
80. Hull D: Brown adipose tissue and the newborn infant's response to cold. In Philipp EE, Barnes J, Newton M (eds): Scientific Foundation of Obstetrics and Gynaecology. London, William Heinemann, 1977, pp 545-550.
81. Houstek J, Vizek K, Pavelka S, et al: Type II iodothyronine 5′-deiodinase and uncoupling protein in brown adipose tissue of human newborns. J Clin Endocrinol Metab 77:382-387, 1993.
82. Heaton JM: The distribution of brown adipose tissue in the human. J Anat 112:35-39, 1972.
83. Ricquier D, Nechad M, Mory G: Ultrastructural and biochemical characterization of human brown adipose tissue in pheochromocytoma. J Clin Endocrinol Metab 54:803-807, 1982.
84. Cohade C, Mourtzikos KA,Wahl RL: "USA-Fat": Prevalence is related to ambient outdoor temperature-evaluation with ^{18}F-FDG PET/CT. J Nucl Med 44:1267-1270, 2003.
85. Hany TF, Gharehpapagh E, Kamel EM, et al: Brown adipose tissue: A factor to consider in symmetrical tracer uptake in the neck and upper chest region. Eur J Nucl Med Mol Imaging 29:1393-1398, 2002.
86. Danforth E Jr, Horton ES, O'Connell M, et al: Dietary-induced alterations in thyroid hormone metabolism during overnutrition. J Clin Invest 64:1336-1347, 1979.
87. Scheidegger K, O'Connell M, Robbins DC, Danforth E Jr: Effects of chronic beta-receptor stimulation on sympathetic nervous system activity, energy expenditure, and thyroid hormones. J Clin Endocrinol Metab 58:895-903, 1984.

88. Bartha T, Kim SW, Salvatore D, et al: Characterization of the 5′-flanking and 5′-untranslated regions of the cyclic adenosine 3′,5′-monophosphate-responsive human type 2 iodothyronine deiodinase gene. Endocrinology 141:229-237, 2000.
89. al-Adsani H, Hoffe LJ, Silva JE: Resting energy expenditure is sensitive to small dose changes in patients on chronic thyroid hormone replacement. J Clin Endocrinol Metab 82:1118-1125, 1997.
90. Silva JE: Thyroid hormone and the energetic cost of keeping body temperature. Biosci Rep 25:129-148, 2005.
91. Lebon V, Dufour S, Petersen KF, et al: Effect of triiodothyronine on mitochondrial energy coupling in human skeletal muscle. J Clin Invest 108:733-737, 2001.
92. Harper ME, Brand MD: The quantitative contributions of mitochondrial proton leak and ATP turnover reactions to the changed respiration rates of hepatocytes from rats of different thyroid status. J Biol Chem 268:14850-14860, 1993.
93. Desai-Yajnik V, Zeng J, Omori K, et al: The effect of thyroid hormone treatment on the gene expression and enzyme activity of rat liver sodium-potassium dependent adenosine triphosphatase. Endocrinology 136:629-639, 1995.
94. Folke M, Sestoft L: Thyroid calorigenesis in isolated, perfused rat liver: Minor role of active sodium-potassium transport. J Physiol 269:407-419, 1977.
95. de Meis L: Role of the sarcoplasmic reticulum Ca^{2+}-ATPase on heat production and thermogenesis. Biosci Rep 21:113-137, 2001.
96. Reis M, Farage M, de Meis L: Thermogenesis and energy expenditure: Control of heat production by the Ca(2+)-ATPase of fast and slow muscle. Mol Membr Biol 19:301-310, 2002.
97. Izumo S, Nadal-Ginard B, Mahdavi V: All members of the MHC multigene family respond to thyroid hormone in a highly tissue-specific manner. Science 231:597-600, 1986.
98. Simonides WS, Thelen MH, van der Linden CG, et al: Mechanism of thyroid-hormone regulated expression of the SERCA genes in skeletal muscle: Implications for thermogenesis. Biosci Rep 21:139-154, 2001.
99. Oppenheimer JH, Schwartz HL, Lane JT, Thompson MP: Functional relationship of thyroid hormone-induced lipogenesis, lipolysis, and thermogenesis. J Clin Invest 87:125-132, 1991.
100. Abuid J, Larsen PR: Triiodothyronine and thyroxine in hyperthyroidism. Comparison of the acute changes during therapy with antithyroid agents. J Clin Invest 54:201-208, 1974.
101. Ishii H, Inada M, Tanaka K, et al: Triiodothyronine generation from thyroxine in human thyroid: Enhanced conversion in Graves' thyroid tissue. J Clin Endocrinol Metab 52:1211-1217, 1981.
102. Sugawara M, Lau R, Wasse HL, et al: Thyroid T_4 5′-deiodinase activity in normal and abnormal human thyroid glands. Metabolism 33:332-336, 1984.
103. Nishikawa M, Toyoda N, Yonemoto T, et al: Quantitative measurements for type 1 deiodinase messenger ribonucleic acid in human peripheral blood mononuclear cells: Mechanism of the preferential increase of T_3 in hyperthyroid Graves' disease. Biochem Biophys Res Commun 250:642-646, 1998.
104. Wu SY, Shyh TP, Chopra I: Comparison of sodium ipodate (Orografin) and propylthiouracil in early treatment of hyperthyroidism. J Clin Endocrinol Metab 54:630-634, 1982.
105. Burgi H, Wimpfheimer C, Burger A, et al: Changes of circulating thyroxine, triiodothyronine and reverse triiodothyronine after radiographic contrast agents. J Clin Endocrinol Metab 43:1203-1210, 1976.
106. Croxson MS, Hall TD, Nicoloff JT: Combination drug therapy for treatment of hyperthyroid Graves' disease. J Clin Endocrinol Metab 45:623-630, 1977.
107. Burger A, Dinchert D, Nirod P, et al: Effect of amiodarone on serum triiodothyronine, reverse triiodothyronine, thyroxine, and thyrotropin. J Clin Invest 58:255-259, 1976.
108. Melmed S, Nademanee K, Reed AW, et al: Hyperthyroxinemia with bradycardia and normal thyrotropin secretion after chronic amiodarone administration. J Clin Endocrinol Metab 53:997-1001, 1981.
109. Wiersinga WM, Trip MD: Amiodarone and thyroid hormone metabolism. Postgrad Med J 62:909-914, 1986.
110. Harjai KJ, Licata AA: Effects of amiodarone on thyroid function. Ann Intern Med 126:63-73, 1997.
111. Lambert MJ, Burger AG, Galeazzi RL, Engler D: Are selective increases in serum thyroxine (T_4) due to iodinated inhibitors of T_4 monodeiodination indicative of hyperthyroidism? J Clin Endocrinol Metab 55:1058-1065, 1982.
112. Borowski GD, Garofano CD, Rose LI, et al: Effect of long-term amiodarone therapy on thyroid hormone levels and thyroid function. Am J Med 78:443-450, 1985.
113. Hershman JM, Nademanee K, Sugawara M, et al: Thyroxine and triiodothyronine kinetics in cardiac patients taking amiodarone. Acta Endocrinol (Copenh) 111:193-199, 1986.
114. Hudig F, Bakker O, Wiersinga WM: Amiodarone-induced hypercholesterolemia is associated with a decrease in liver LDL receptor mRNA. FEBS Lett 341:86-90, 1994.
115. Balsam A, Ingbar SH: The influence of fasting, diabetes and several pharmacological agents of the pathways of thyroxine metabolism in rat liver. J Clin Invest 62:415-424, 1978.
116. Sogol PB, Hershman JM, Reed AW, Dillmann WH: The effects of amiodarone on serum thyroid hormones and hepatic thyroxine 5′-monodeiodination in rats. Endocrinology 113:1464-1469, 1983.

116. Pekary AE, Hershman JM, Reed AW, et al: Amiodarone inhibits T_4 to T_3 conversion and alpha-glycerophosphate dehydrogenase and malic enzyme levels in rat liver. Horm Metab Res 18:114-118, 1986.
118. Ceppi JA, Zaninovich AA: Effects of amiodarone on 5′-deiodination of thyroxine to tri-iodothyronine in rat myocardium. J Endocrinol 121:431-434, 1989.
119. Gotzsche LS, Boye N, Laurberg P, Andreasen F: Rat heart thyroxine 5′-deiodinase is sensitively depressed by amiodarone. J Cardiovasc Pharmacol 14:836-841, 1989.
129. Aanderud S, Sundsfjord J, Aarbakke J: Amiodarone inhibits the conversion of thyroxine to triiodothyronine in isolated rat hepatocytes. Endocrinology 115:1605-1608, 1984.
121. Ha HR, Stieger B, Grassi G, et al: Structure-effect relationships of amiodarone analogues on the inhibition of thyroxine deiodination. Eur J Clin Pharmacol 55:807-814, 2000.
122. Faber J, Siersbaek-Nielsen K: Serum free 3,5,3′-triiodothyronine (T3) in non-thyroidal somatic illness, as measured by ultrafiltration and immunoextraction. Clin Chim Acta 256:115-123, 1996.
123. Chopra IJ: Simultaneous measurement of free thyroxine and free 3,5,3′-triiodothyronine in undiluted serum by direct equilibrium dialysis/radioimmunoassay: Evidence that free triiodothyronine and free thyroxine are normal in many patients with the low triiodothyronine syndrome. Thyroid 8:249-257, 1998.
124. Kaplan MM, Larsen PR, Crantz FR, et al: Prevalence of abnormal thyroid function test results in patients with acute medical illnesses. Am J Med 72:9-16, 1982.
125. Wadwekar D, Kabadi UM: Thyroid hormone indices during illness in six hypothyroid subjects rendered euthyroid with levothyroxine therapy. Exp Clin Endocrinol Diabetes 112:373-377, 2004.
126. Huang SA: Physiology and pathophysiology of type 3 deiodinase in humans. Thyroid 15:875-881, 2005.
127. Peeters RP, Wouters PJ, Kaptein E, et al: Reduced activation and increased inactivation of thyroid hormone in tissues of critically ill patients. J Clin Endocrinol Metab 88:3202-3211, 2003.
128. Abe T, Kakyo M, Tokui T, et al: Identification of a novel gene family encoding human liver–specific organic anion transporter LST-1. J Biol Chem 274:17159-17163, 1999.
129. Docter R, Krenning EP, DeJong M, Hennemann G: The sick euthyroid syndrome: Changes in thyroid hormone serum parameters and hormone metabolism. Clin Endocrinol 39:499-518, 1993.
130. De Groot LJ: Non-thyroidal illness syndrome is a manifestation of hypothalamic-pituitary dysfunction, and in view of current evidence, should be treated with appropriate replacement therapies. Crit Care Clin 22:57-86, 2006.
131. Van den Berghe G, de Zeghe F, Baxter RC, et al: Neuroendocrinology of prolonged critical illness: Effects of exogenous thyrotropin-releasing hormone and its combination with growth hormone secretagogues. J Clin Endocrinol Metab 83:309-319, 1998.
132. Cavalieri RR: The effects of nonthyroid disease and drugs on thyroid function tests. Med Clin North Am 75:27-39, 1991.
133. Legradi G, Emerson CH, Ahima RS, et al: Leptin prevents fasting-induced suppression of prothyrotropin-releasing hormone messenger ribonucleic acid in neurons of the hypothalamic paraventricular nucleus. Endocrinology 138:2569-2576, 1997.
134. Chan JL, Heist K, DePaoli AM, et al: The role of falling leptin levels in the neuroendocrine and metabolic adaptation to short-term starvation in healthy men. J Clin Invest 111:1409-1421, 2003.
135. Fekete C, Gereben B, Doleschall M, et al: Lipopolysaccharide induces type 2 iodothyronine deiodinase in the mediobasal hypothalamus: Implications for the nonthyroidal illness syndrome. Endocrinology 145:1649-1655, 2004.
136. Zeold A, Doleschal M, Haffner MP, et al: Characterization of the NF-kappa B responsiveness of the human dio2 gene. Endocrinology 147:4419-4429, 2006.
137. Huang SA, Tu HM, Harney JW, et al: Severe hypothyroidism caused by type 3 iodothyronine deiodinase in infantile hemangiomas. N Engl J Med 343:185-189, 2000.

Section C

THYROID AXIS

Role of Thyrotropin-Releasing Hormone in the Regulation of the Thyroid Axis

Chapter 6

Anthony N. Hollenberg

Key Points

- Thyrotropin-releasing hormone (TRH) synthesis and secretion from the hypothalamus is required for normal thyroid function.
- TRH is primarily regulated by thyroid hormone levels.
- TRH and thyroid hormone levels may be influenced by nutritional status.
- TRH is regulated by critical illness; helps explain changes in thyroid function seen during such states.

The regulation of circulating thyroid hormone levels is critical for normal human physiologic function as thyroid hormone (TH) remains one of the principal regulators of human metabolism. To accomplish this, thyroid hormone levels must be set at the appropriate level for each individual. This is accomplished by a feedback system in which thyroid hormone targets its regulators to prevent over- or underproduction. Among the most important regulators of TH levels are a group of neurons in the hypothalamus that produce thyrotropin-releasing hormone (TRH). Genetic experiments in mice and human studies have demonstrated that the production and action of TRH are required for the synthesis and secretion of thyroid-stimulating hormone (TSH) from the pituitary and for normal TH levels.[1,2] In addition to allowing for the normal production of TSH and thyroid hormone, TRH neurons in the hypothalamus can be dynamically regulated by TH levels so that they can sense their deficiency and excess and respond to this feedback in an attempt to reset the thyroid axis. Furthermore, TRH neurons in the hypothalamus can sense states in which TH production may need to be curtailed, such as severe illness or nutritional deprivation, and downregulate the thyroid axis to limit metabolism.[3,4] Thus, an understanding of the regulation of TRH production in the hypothalamus is critical to understanding the regulation of the thyroid axis in health and disease.

THYROTROPIN-RELEASING HORMONE: STRUCTURE AND FUNCTION

Mature TRH is a tripeptide (pyroGlu-His-ProNH_2) produced from a larger prohormone (proTRH) by the enzymes proconvertase 1, proconvertase 2 (PC1 and PC2), and carboxypeptidase E. Genetic deficiency of these enzymes can disrupt the thyroid axis, presumably by impairing the production of mature TRH.[5-7] The gene encoding TRH in multiple species also allows for the production of other peptides that may play a role in physiology. However, these peptides appear to vary from species to species, making any judgment about their conserved role difficult.[5,8] Although the synthesis and release of TRH in the paraventricular nucleus of the hypothalamus (PVH; see later) is essential for normal regulation of the thyroid axis, TRH is also synthesized in other regions of the hypothalamus, brain, and peripheral organs, such as the pancreas and heart. Its function in these other areas is not clear, although mice lacking TRH develop glucose intolerance, suggesting that pancreatic TRH may play a role in glucose homeostasis.[2]

TRH signals through a single G protein–coupled receptor in humans, whereas other species appear to express a second TRH receptor whose function is unknown.[9] The principal action of TRH, once it is secreted into the portal system and reaches the pituitary, is to stimulate the production of TSH via its receptor on thyrotrophs. TRH receptors are also present on prolactin-secreting cells in the pituitary (lactotrophs) and, in hypothyroidism, when TRH levels are high, prolactin levels can also be high.[3] The TRH receptor is also expressed widely in the brain, supporting the notion that TRH may have other actions in addition to its central role in the regulation of the thyroid axis.[9]

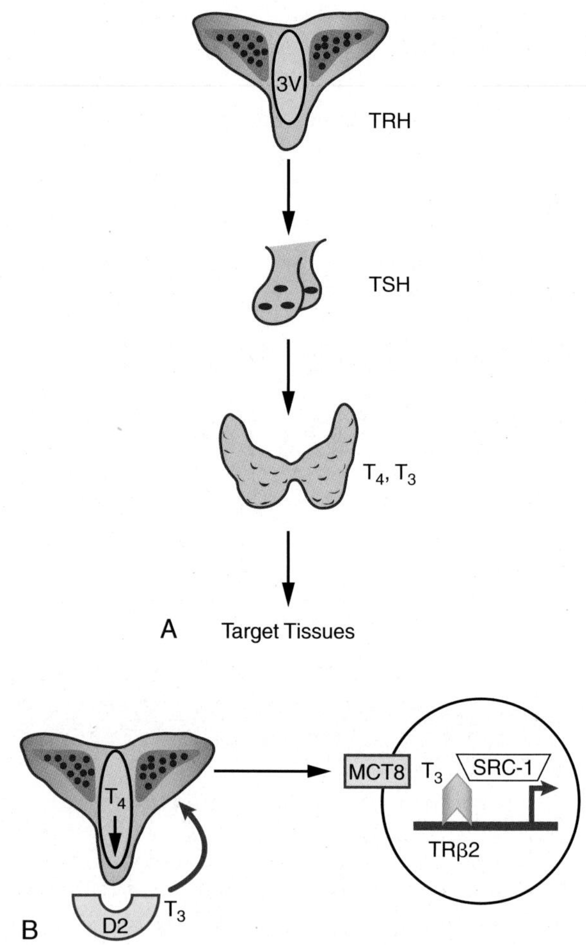

Figure 6–1 The hypothalamic-pituitary-thyroid axis. **A,** Hypophysiotropic thyrotropin-releasing hormone (TRH) neurons are present in the paraventricular nucleus of the hypothalamus that surrounds the third ventricle. The neurons project to the median eminence and release TRH into the portal system, which in turn reaches the pituitary and regulates thyroid-stimulating hormone (TSH) synthesis and secretion. TSH then acts on the thyroid to control thyroid hormone production. **B,** Triiodothyronine (T_3) feeds back at the level of the paraventricular nucleus of the hypothalamus (PVH) to regulate TRH synthesis. A model is shown in which local T_3 produced by type 2 deiodinase accesses TRH neurons in the PVH via the monocarboxylate 8 transporter (MCT8). T_4, thyroxine. *(Adapted from Hollenberg AN: The role of the thyrotropin-releasing hormone [TRH] neuron as a metabolic sensor. Thyroid 18:131, 2008.)*

Anatomy of Thyrotropin-Releasing Hormone Neurons

TRH is synthesized in multiple regions of the hypothalamus in addition to the paraventricular nucleus, including the ventromedial, dorsomedial, and lateral hypothalamus.[3,4,10] However, the function of TRH in these regions is not clear. The PVH is present on both sides of the third ventricle and is triangular in structure. Mature TRH that is synthesized in the PVH is transported to the median eminence, where it is released into the portal circulation and can regulate TSH subunit synthesis and secretion in the pituitary (Fig. 6-1A).[11] These TRH neurons are thus referred to as hypophysiotropic, given their key role in the regulation of pituitary TSH. The PVH also contains distinct neuronal populations that synthesize corticotropin-releasing hormone, oxytocin, and vasopressin.

To play a key role in the regulation of the thyroid axis, these hypophysiotropic neurons must be able to sense TH levels, interpret energy stores, and sense severe illness. It is likely that their discrete location in the PVH has developed to allow them to integrate all these inputs.

REGULATION OF THYROTROPIN-RELEASING HORMONE

Regulation by Thyroid Hormone

Critical to the role of TRH in maintaining the thyroid axis is its ability to sense circulating levels of TH, and in particular triiodothyronine (T_3). Seminal experiments performed 20 years ago demonstrated that T_3 specifically regulates TRH in the PVH so that TRH mRNA rises in the hypothyroid state and falls in the setting of hyperthyroidism. Remarkably, TRH mRNA is regulated by T_3 only in the PVH and not in other regions of the hypothalamus.[12,13] Thus, the hypophysiotropic TRH neurons have acquired the ability to mediate T_3 regulation of TRH through a unique ability to sense T_3 or the acquisition of a key molecular switch in the neuron that allows T_3 to act. Although it remains unclear which of these mechanisms is operative, it is important to understand how T_3 reaches the

PVH and how it acts at the molecular level to mediate regulation of TRH.

Most T_3 that acts on the TRH neurons in the PVH in the euthyroid or hypothyroid state is thought to be produced centrally from circulating thyroxine (T_4) by type 2 deiodinase (D2). D2 is present in tanycytes, a cell type that lines the third ventricle (see Fig. 6-1B).[14,15] The role of D2 in the central regulation of the thyroid axis is supported by the fact that D2 knockout mice have TSH levels that are inappropriately elevated in the setting of higher than normal TH levels presumably because central levels of T_3 are inadequate.[16] D2 plays a role in the local production of T_3 in the hypothalamus, but it is not clear that D2 activity is required at all sites in the brain for this purpose.[17] In addition, in the hyperthyroid state, when T_3 levels are high, as in the setting of Graves' disease or exogenous T_3 administration, T_3 can directly gain access to TRH neurons in the PVH without having to be produced locally. A role for the type 3 deiodinase D3, which normally inactivates T_3 in the hypothalamus, is suggested by the fact that D3 knockout mice have central hypothyroidism. This is the result of prolonged neonatal hyperthyroidism, which causes permanent suppression of the thyroid axis.[18]

Thus, a model can be proposed in which systemic T_4 is taken up by tanycytes and converted to T_3 by D2. The locally produced T_3 is then presented to the TRH neurons in the PVH. It is tempting to speculate that T_3 cannot be presented to other hypothalamic nuclei, which would explain the selective nature of regulation in the PVH. However, recent studies have shown that T_3 produced in the hypothalamus acts in the arcuate nucleus, making it unlikely that access to T_3 leads to cell-specific regulation, although it is possible that other hypothalamic areas that express TRH do not sense T_3.[19]

Once T_3 reaches the PVH, it is now clear that it must be actively transported into TRH neurons. The likely transporter is the monocarboxylate 8 transporter (MCT8), which was first identified as a T_3 transporter in 2003.[20] MCT8 was identified as the mutant gene present in the Allan-Herndon-Dudley syndrome, an X-linked disorder resulting in an early presentation of psychomotor retardation in affected males, with elevated T_3 levels in the setting of normal TSH and low T_4 levels.[21,22] MCT8 has been subsequently shown to be expressed in the brain, specifically on TRH neurons.[22] Two groups have recently disrupted the MCT8 gene in mice and, although there appears to be no gross neurologic phenotype in the knockout (KO) mice, the thyroid function test abnormalities are recapitulated.[23,24] These mice have hepatic hyperthyroidism, suggesting that T_3 does not require MCT8 to gain access to hepatocytes. In contrast, these animals have elevated TRH mRNA expression in the PVH, consistent with the requirement for MCT8 to transport T_3 into TRH neurons actively. When given large doses of T_4 or T_3, TRH can be partially suppressed in MCT8 knockout animals, suggesting that other mechanisms for T_3 access exist.[24] Thus, it can be hypothesized that delivery and transport of T_3 to and within TRH neurons in the PVH are required for its regulation. It is likely that this sensitive system plays a role in the unique ability of hypophysiotropic neurons to respond to T_3, although it still remains possible that the molecular mechanisms governing regulation of TRH mRNA and peptide production are specific to hypophysiotropic neurons.

It is now apparent that once T_3 gains access to TRH neurons, the regulation of TRH production within the PVH is at two levels:

1. TRH mRNA levels are directly regulated by T_3.
2. Processing of proTRH by PC1 and PC2 is regulated by T_3 via the direct regulation of PC1 and PC2 mRNAs.[25]

Thus, an understanding of the mechanisms underlying negative regulation by T_3 are key to understanding the regulation of TRH production in the PVH. Like positive regulation, negative regulation requires thyroid hormone receptor (TR) isoforms and a host of coregulatory proteins. These allow the TR to modify the local chromatin environment surrounding the TRH or PC1 and PC2 genes and allow for regulation by T_3. In the case of the TRH gene, much is known about how T_3 acts to mediate its regulation, which likely occurs at the level of transcription.

Whereas all TR isoforms have the ability to mediate negative regulation, elegant mouse genetic studies have demonstrated the requirement of the TRβ2 isoform for negative regulation of the TRH gene.[26] Mice that lack this isoform are unable to downregulate TRH mRNA in response to T_3. Furthermore, TRβ2 likely mediates its action via DNA binding, because mice expressing a mutant TRβ2 that is unable to bind DNA cannot mediate negative regulation in the hypothalamus and pituitary.[27] The role of DNA binding in the TRβ2 isoform regulation of the TRH gene is supported by earlier studies that demonstrated the presence of a unique negative thyroid hormone response element (nTRE) in the proximal promoter of the TRH promoter that is conserved across species. This nTRE, termed *site 4*, binds TRβ2 and mediates downregulation of the TRH promoter in cell culture experiments. Its role in vivo remains to be determined.[28,29]

TRβ2 likely binds to the TRH promoter to mediate negative regulation, but the role of coregulators in the actions of TRβ2 remain unclear. On a classic positive TRE, TR isoforms recruit the nuclear corepressors NCoR and SMRT in the absence of T_3, which in turn serve as a platform for a multiprotein complex that mediates transcriptional repression via histone deacetylation.[30-33] In the presence of T_3, the TR undergoes conformational changes, releases the corepressor complex, and recruits a multiprotein coactivator complex that mediates transcriptional activation via a variety of histone modifications, including acetylation and methylation.[34-37] Clearly, this paradigm cannot apply to negative regulation of TRH because TRH mRNA is upregulated in the absence of T_3 and downregulated in the presence of T_3. Surprisingly, mice that lack the coactivator steroid receptor coactivator 1 (SRC-1) have defective negative regulation of the thyroid-stimulating hormone (TSH)–beta gene, suggesting that coactivators may be paradoxically critical for negative regulation of TRH.[38,39] The in vivo role of NCoR and SMRT in the regulation of TRH has not been tested in genetic models.[40] A similar model for the regulation of PC1 and PC2 can likely be proposed because nTREs have been identified in the promoters of these genes.[41,42] However, like TRH, more work is necessary to understand negative regulation of these genes by T_3 completely.

Although the classic negative feedback of T_3 on TRH production in the hypothalamus predicts a rapid response, there are clearly cases in which long-term suppression of the thyroid axis occurs in the setting of persistently high T_3 levels. This suggests that there may be long-term actions of T_3 on TRH neurons in the PVH or on thyrotrophs in the pituitary. In patients with long-standing hyperthyroidism, treatment-induced low TH levels can still be associated with inappropriately low TSH levels for weeks following treatment.[43] Similarly, newborns of mothers with poorly controlled Graves' disease can present with central hypothyroidism requiring treatment.[44] Both these groups of patients appear refractory to TRH administration, which suggests that the defect is at the level of the pituitary, although permanent suppression of TRH synthesis in the PVH cannot be excluded. As noted, a similar situation is seen in D3 knockout mice, in which exposure to very high levels of T_3 during development leads to long-term suppression of TSH secretion and potentially TRH secretion.[18] It is likely that the molecular mechanism underlying this long-term suppression is separate and distinct from classic negative regulation.

Regulation of Synthesis by Nutritional Status

Although the regulation of TRH production in the PVH is controlled most dramatically by TH levels, it is also clear that other signaling pathways affect these neurons and possibly TH regulation. In the last 10 years, it has become clear that circulating leptin produced in adipocytes can regulate TRH mRNA expression and production in hypophysiotropic TRH neurons.[45] Given that leptin levels are reliable indicators of nutritional status, this is entirely consistent with the long-held view that fasting, which can dramatically reduce leptin levels, can regulate the thyroid axis in rodents and humans. Long-term fasting in humans causes a decrease in TSH and T_3 levels, whereas T_4 levels remain constant or may fall.[46,47] In contrast, fasting in rodents also causes a fall in T_4 levels; this was shown many years ago to be secondary to a dramatic decrease in TRH expression in the PVH.[48] Remarkably, in rodents, the administration of leptin prevents the fasting-induced suppression of the thyroid axis by rescuing TRH expression in the PVH.[49,50] The relevance of this axis in humans has been demonstrated by studies showing that the daily pulsations of TSH secretion, which are diminished by a 24-hour fast, can be rescued by physiologic leptin administration.[51] Furthermore, controlled weight loss experiments in human volunteers that cause a decrease in leptin levels have also demonstrated a decrease in thyroid hormone levels, without an increase in TSH levels. T_4 and T_3 levels can be restored by the administration of replacement doses of leptin.[52,53] Taken together, these data demonstrate that leptin regulates the thyroid axis via its ability to target the TRH neuron in the PVH. An understanding of the pathways involved is important, given the intersection of T_3 and leptin signaling in TRH neurons.

Leptin exerts its effects in the hypothalamus by engaging its cognate receptor, the leptin receptor, on target neurons in a number of separate nuclei (Fig. 6-2).[54] The arcuate nucleus of the hypothalamus is one of the most important nuclei in body weight regulation. The leptin receptor is expressed at high levels on two neuronal subpopulations in the arcuate nucleus that play a key role in body weight regulation and also project to the TRH neurons in the PVH.[55] In addition, leptin receptors are found on TRH neurons in the PVH.[56,57] Thus, leptin has the potential ability to target TRH production directly and indirectly via the arcuate nucleus. Importantly, the pathways that leptin engages play a central role in body weight regulation, which implies that regulation

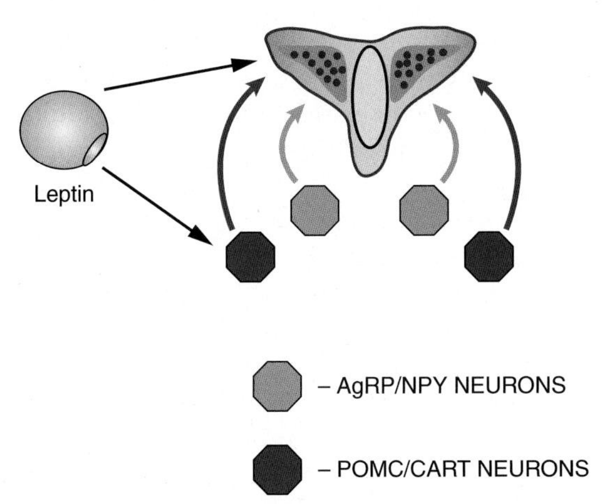

Figure 6–2 Thyrotropin-releasing hormone (TRH) neurons are regulated by leptin signaling. Leptin is produced peripherally by adipocytes and regulates TRH production via direct and indirect pathways. Leptin crosses the blood-brain barrier and activates proopiomelanocortin (POMC) and cocaine and amphetamine-related transcript (CART) neurons, which in turn project to the paraventricular nucleus of the hypothalamus (PVH) and stimulate TRH production in the PVH. In contrast, leptin inhibits agouti-related peptide (AgRP) and neuropeptide Y (NPY) neurons, which also project to the PVH and function to inhibit TRH production. Alternatively, leptin can signal directly to the PVH via its receptor and activate TRH production.

of the thyroid axis is an important arbiter of leptin action. The importance of leptin in the regulation of the thyroid axis is further supported by the fact that mouse models with defective leptin receptor function appear to have central hypothyroidism.[58] Interestingly, an initial report also suggested that the same was true in humans, but a more recent larger study has shown that humans with leptin receptor mutations have normal TH levels.[59,60]

As noted, leptin receptors in the arcuate nucleus are present on two groups of target neurons. The first group synthesizes the neuropeptides proopiomelanocortin (POMC) and cocaine and amphetamine-related transcript (CART) and are thus referred to as POMC/CART neurons.[61-63] The major product of POMC/CART neurons, α-melanocyte–stimulating hormone (α-MSH), is derived from the processing of POMC and is a potent anorexigenic hormone.[55] The second group synthesize agouti-related peptide (AgRP) and neuropeptide Y (NPY) and are referred to as AgRP/NPY neurons. Both AgRP and NPY are orexigenic and decrease energy expenditure. Although leptin receptors are present on both groups of neurons, leptin activates POMC/CART neurons while inhibiting AgRP/NPY neurons. Thus, in the presence of leptin, the production of α-MSH is increased and NPY and AgRP expression is decreased. In contrast, during a fast, when leptin levels are low, levels of α-MSH fall but AgRP and NPY levels are increased.[64-67] Many rodent models of diet-induced obesity manifest low levels of α-MSH and high levels of AgRP and NPY.

These critical neuropeptides regulate body weight based on their ability to project to second-order neurons, including those located in the PVH. Both α-MSH and AgRP signal principally through neurons in the PVH that express the melanocortin-4 receptor (MC4-R).[56] Whereas α-MSH is an agonist of the MC4-R, AgRP is an antagonist or inverse agonist, which explains their contrasting physiologic roles.[68] The importance of this system is supported by the fact that mutations in the MC4-R cause severe obesity in humans.[69,70] NPY signals through a variety of NPY receptor (NPY-R) isoforms; in particular, NPY-1R and NPY-5R are expressed in the PVH.[71,72] Moreover, both POMC/CART and ARP/NPY neurons synapse on hypophysiotropic TRH neurons and are thus poised to regulate TRH synthesis.[73] TRH neurons in the PVH coexpress the MC4-R and NPY-R isoforms, allowing the TRH neuron to sense arcuate nucleus output directly.[56,71] Both MC4-R and NPY-R isoforms engage the cyclic adenosine monophosphate (cAMP) signaling pathway and modulate the activity of the transcription factor cAMP response element–binding protein (CREB) through phosphorylation. Indeed, α-MSH activates CREB via the MC4-R and CREB, in turn, can bind to the TRH promoter to mediate activation of TRH expression. In contrast, AgRP and NPY prevent activation of CREB and inhibit TRH expression.[74-77] Thus, TRH gene expression can be driven by leptin's actions on the arcuate nucleus. However, both humans and mice with defective MC4-R signaling have normal TH levels, suggesting that other pathways must also affect TRH neurons.[69]

As noted, a portion of hypophysiotropic TRH neurons also express the leptin receptor; leptin-mediated activation of the transcription factor signal transducer and activator of transcription 3 (STAT3), a key mediator of the genomic actions of leptin signaling, can be seen in TRH neurons.[57] In addition, regulatory elements in the TRH promoter can respond to and bind STAT3.[78] Taken together, these results suggest that leptin can directly reach the PVH and regulate TRH without the need for arcuate nucleus input. Interestingly, there appear to be two groups of TRH neurons in the PVH that respond to leptin or α-MSH, with the predominant control of the thyroid axis emanating from those that respond to α-MSH.[79] Given the importance of the thyroid axis, it is likely that the direct and indirect pathways provide a redundant system to ensure that TH levels remain normal.

Although most evidence supports the notion that the leptin axis regulates TRH, it is also clear that D2 is upregulated by fasting, raising the possibility that local production of T_3 could be altered by fasting. This suggests that increased T_3 could be delivered to the PVH, leading to suppression of TRH expression.[80] Alternatively, increased local T_3 may act via a separate neuronal population that then projects to TRH neurons to suppress TRH expression. It has recently been shown that T_3 enhances the firing of AgRP/NPY neurons, which could potentially then mediate suppression of TRH expression in the PVH.[19] Although increased local T_3 could play a role in fasting-induced suppression of TRH expression, it is unlikely for two reasons: (1) when hypothyroid animals are fasted, TRH levels still fall when systemic TH levels are low, suggesting that even if D2 is increased there would be little T_4 available to produce T_3; and (2) in TRβ2 knockout mice, TRH mRNA is still actively suppressed during fasting, implying that T_3 action is not required.[26,81]

Regulation of TRH in the Euthyroid Sick Syndrome (Nonthyroidal Illness)

The euthyroid sick syndrome is viewed by most as an adaptive process that allows for a slowing of metabolism during acute or chronic illness. In humans, the euthyroid sick syndrome is heralded by a decrease in T_3 levels, with an increase in reverse T_3 (rT_3). This is likely secondary to the decreased production and action of D1 in the liver.[82,83] After this initial phase, in severe cases, there is often a decrease in T_4 and TSH, which is often associated with a higher mortality. This decrease in TSH is likely secondary to a decrease in TRH production in TRH neurons in the PVH. Elegant studies in humans have demonstrated that intensive care unit (ICU) patients who have died secondary to severe disease with low T_3 levels have suppressed expression of TRH in the PVH. In contrast, in patients who have succumbed acutely because of cardiac factors, without low T_3 levels, TRH expression is not suppressed. Furthermore, TRH mRNA expression in this first group of patients was directly proportional to serum TSH levels, supporting the concept that low TSH secretion in euthyroid sick syndrome is secondary to suppression of TRH secretion from hypophysiotropic neurons.[84] Similarly, inappropriate suppression of TRH in the PVH is seen in rodent models of euthyroid sick syndrome, consistent with the central origin of this portion of the disorder.

A number of different hypotheses have been proposed to explain the resistance of TRH neurons to the initial decrease in T_3 levels and then to the suppression of TRH mRNA production. Although glucocorticoid levels increase in inflammatory states and can suppress TRH production, their role in vivo remains uncertain because lipopolysaccharide (LPS) administration to rats, a model for nonthyroidal illness, can still suppress TRH expression in the absence of changes in glucocorticoids.[85] Certainly, a number of cytokines are predicted to play a role in severe illness, including interleukin 1(IL-1), IL-1β, and IL-6. Each of these could play a role in central suppression of the thyroid axis but definitive proof is lacking.[82,86]

More recently, it has become clear that D2 mRNA in tanycytes can also be upregulated by LPS administration to rodents, suggesting again that increased local production of T_3 could be responsible for the suppression of TRH mRNA expression in the PVH seen in euthyroid sick syndrome.[87,88] Furthermore, the human D2 promoter binds to and can be activated by nuclear factor-kappa B (NF-κB), a transcription factor complex that is activated by LPS administration and by other cytokines, thus linking D2 activity to cytokine activity.[89] However, the formal role of this pathway in euthyroid sick syndrome needs to be tested in D2 knockout mice.

Finally, it is tempting to speculate that the leptin axis somehow plays a role in the euthyroid sick syndrome. However, in patients with sepsis and low T_3 and TSH levels, it has been found that leptin levels are high rather than low, as would be expected if leptin signaling was playing a role in suppression of TRH production.[90] Moreover, the weight loss seen in mouse models of cachexia induced by LPS, tumor growth, or renal failure can be reversed by the use of an MC4-R antagonist, implying that the cachexia is induced by increases in α-MSH action.[91,92] Although the thyroid axis was not studied in these same experiments, such illness could be expected to induce the euthyroid sick syndrome. However, increased α-MSH action would be predicted to lead to an increase in TRH production. Further study of the role of other neuropeptides secreted by the arcuate nucleus is required to rule out a role for this axis in this disorder.

The exact cause of central hypothyroidism present in the euthyroid sick syndrome has not been determined, but it is becoming increasingly clear that those with central hypothyroidism do worse than those with just low T_3 syndromes. Thus, a better understanding of the pathways involved could lead to further insights for treating the underlying process.

CONCLUSIONS

The production of TRH in the PVH (hypophysiotropic TRH neurons) is absolutely required for the normal function of the thyroid axis. TRH production is not static, but is greatly influenced by TH levels, as well as by nutritional status and degree of illness. The TRH neuron in the PVH appears to carry the precise anatomic location and molecular networks so to receive feedback from the periphery and respond to it in an integrated fashion to regulate the thyroid axis. Undoubtedly, this regulation allows for appropriate adaptation in periods of excess or lack of TH, periods of malnutrition, and severe illness.

References

1. Collu R, Tang J, Castagne J, et al: A novel mechanism for isolated central hypothyroidism: Inactivating mutations in the thyrotropin-releasing hormone receptor gene. J Clin Endocrinol Metab 82:1561-1565, 1997.
2. Yamada M, Saga Y, Shibusawa N, et al: Tertiary hypothyroidism and hyperglycemia in mice with targeted disruption of the thyrotropin-releasing hormone gene. Proc Natl Acad Sci U S A 94:10862-10867, 1997.
3. Hollenberg AN: Regulation of thyrotropin secretion. In Braverman LE, Utiger RD (eds): Werner and Ingbar's The Thyroid: A Fundamental and Clinical Text, 9th ed. Philadelphia, Lippincott Williams & Wilkins, 2005, pp 197-214.
4. Lechan RM, Hollenberg AN: Thyrotropin-releasing hormone (TRH). In Henry HL, Norman AW (eds): Encyclopedia of Hormones. Philadelphia, Elsevier Science, 2003, pp 510-524.
5. Nillni EA, Sevarino KA: The biology of pro-thyrotropin-releasing hormone-derived peptides. Endocr Rev 20:599-648, 1999.
6. Nillni EA, Xie W, Mulcahy L, et al: Deficiencies in pro-thyrotropin-releasing hormone processing and abnormalities in thermoregulation in Cpefat/fat mice. J Biol Chem 277:48587-48595, 2002.
7. Schaner P, Todd RB, Seidah NG, Nillni EA: Processing of prothyrotropin-releasing hormone by the family of prohormone convertases. J Biol Chem 272:19958-19968, 1997.
8. Mori M, Yamada M, Satoh T, et al: Different post-translational processing of human preprothyrotropin-releasing hormone in the human placenta and hypothalamus. J Clin Endocrinol Metab 75:1535-1539, 1992.
9. Sun Y, Lu X, Gershengorn MC: Thyrotropin-releasing hormone receptors—similarities and differences. J Mol Endocrinol 30:87-97, 2003.
10. Lechan RM, Segerson TP: Pro-TRH gene expression and precursor peptides in rat brain. Observations by hybridization analysis and immunocytochemistry. Ann N Y Acad Sci 553:29-59, 1989.
11. Ishikawa K, Taniguchi Y, Inoue K, et al: Immunocytochemical delineation of thyrotrophic area: Origin of thyrotropin-releasing hormone in the median eminence. Neuroendocrinology 47:384-388, 1988.
12. Dyess EM, Segerson TP, Liposits Z, et al: Triiodothyronine exerts direct cell-specific regulation of thyrotropin-releasing hormone gene expression in the hypothalamic paraventricular nucleus. Endocrinology 123:2291-2297, 1988.
13. Segerson TP, Kauer J, Wolfe HC, et al: Thyroid hormone regulates TRH biosynthesis in the paraventricular nucleus of the rat hypothalamus. Science 238:78-80, 1987.
14. Kakucska I, Rand W, Lechan RM: Thyrotropin-releasing hormone gene expression in the hypothalamic paraventricular nucleus is dependent upon feedback regulation by both triiodothyronine and thyroxine. Endocrinology 130:2845-2850, 1992.
15. Tu HM, Kim SW, Salvatore D, et al: Regional distribution of type 2 thyroxine deiodinase messenger ribonucleic acid in rat hypothalamus and pituitary and its regulation by thyroid hormone. Endocrinology 138:3359-3368, 1997.
16. Schneider MJ, Fiering SN, Pallud SE, et al: Targeted disruption of the type 2 selenodeiodinase gene (DIO2) results in a phenotype of pituitary resistance to T4. Mol Endocrinol 15:2137-2148, 2001.
17. Galton VA, Wood ET, St. Germain EA, et al: Thyroid hormone homeostasis and action in the type 2 deiodinase-deficient rodent brain during development. Endocrinology 148:3080-3088, 2007.
18. Hernandez A, Martinez ME, Fiering S, et al: Type 3 deiodinase is critical for the maturation and function of the thyroid axis. J Clin Invest 116:476-484, 2006.
19. Coppola A, Liu ZW, Andrews ZB, et al: Central thermogenic-like mechanism in feeding regulation: An interplay between arcuate nucleus T3 and UCP2. Cell Metab 5:21-33, 2007.
20. Friesema EC, Ganguly S, Abdalla A, et al: Identification of monocarboxylate transporter 8 as a specific thyroid hormone transporter. J Biol Chem 278:40128-40135, 2003.
21. Dumitrescu AM, Liao XH, Best TB, et al: A novel syndrome combining thyroid and neurological abnormalities is associated with mutations in a monocarboxylate transporter gene. Am J Hum Genet 74:168-175, 2004.
22. Heuer H, Maier MK, Iden S, et al: The monocarboxylate transporter 8 linked to human psychomotor retardation is highly expressed in thyroid hormone-sensitive neuron populations. Endocrinology 146:1701-1706, 2005.
23. Dumitrescu AM, Liao XH, Weiss RE, et al: Tissue-specific thyroid hormone deprivation and excess in monocarboxylate transporter (mct) 8-deficient mice. Endocrinology 147:4036-4043, 2006.
24. Trajkovic M, Visser TJ, Mittag J, et al: Abnormal thyroid hormone metabolism in mice lacking the monocarboxylate transporter 8. J Clin Invest 117:627-635, 2007.
25. Perello M, Friedman T, Paez-Espinosa V, et al: Thyroid hormones selectively regulate the posttranslational processing of prothyrotropin-releasing hormone in the paraventricular nucleus of the hypothalamus. Endocrinology 147:2705-2716, 2006.

26. Abel ED, Ahima RS, Boers ME, et al: Critical role for thyroid hormone receptor beta2 in the regulation of paraventricular thyrotropin-releasing hormone neurons. J Clin Invest 107:1017-1023, 2001.
27. Shibusawa N, Hashimoto K, Nikrodhanond AA, et al: Thyroid hormone action in the absence of thyroid hormone receptor DNA-binding in vivo. J Clin Invest 112:588-597, 2003.
28. Hollenberg AN, Monden T, Flynn TR, et al: The human thyrotropin-releasing hormone gene is regulated by thyroid hormone through two distinct classes of negative thyroid hormone response elements. Mol Endocrinol 9:540-550, 1995.
29. Satoh T, Yamada M, Iwasaki T, Mori M: Negative regulation of the gene for the preprothyrotropin-releasing hormone from the mouse by thyroid hormone requires additional factors in conjunction with thyroid hormone receptors. J Biol Chem 271:27919-27926, 1996.
30. Guenther MG, Lane WS, Fischle W, et al: A core SMRT corepressor complex containing HDAC3 and TBL1, a WD40-repeat protein linked to deafness. Genes Dev 14:1048-1057, 2000.
31. Guenther MG, Yu J, Kao GD, et al: Assembly of the SMRT-histone deacetylase 3 repression complex requires the TCP-1 ring complex. Genes Dev 16:3130-3135, 2002.
32. Heinzel T, Lavinsky RM, Mullen TM, et al: A complex containing N-CoR, mSin3 and histone deacetylase mediates transcriptional repression. Nature 387:43-48, 1997.
33. Nagy L, Kao HY, Chakravarti D, et al: Nuclear receptor repression mediated by a complex containing SMRT, mSin3A, and histone deacetylase. Cell 89:373-380, 1997.
34. Fondell JD, Ge H, Roeder RG: Ligand induction of a transcriptionally active thyroid hormone receptor coactivator complex. Proc Natl Acad Sci U S A 93:8329-8333, 1996.
35. Glass CK, Rosenfeld MG: The coregulator exchange in transcriptional functions of nuclear receptors. Genes Dev 14:121-141, 2000.
36. Hollenberg AN, Jameson JL: Mechanisms of thyroid hormone action. In DeGroot L, Jameson JL (eds): Endocrinology, 5th ed. Philadelphia, WB Saunders, 2006, pp 1873-1899.
37. Onate SA, Tsai SY, Tsai MJ, O'Malley BW: Sequence and characterization of a coactivator for the steroid hormone receptor superfamily. Science 270:1354-1357, 1995.
38. Weiss RE, Gehin M, Xu J, et al: Thyroid function in mice with compound heterozygous and homozygous disruptions of SRC-1 and TIF-2 coactivators: Evidence for haploinsufficiency. Endocrinology 143:1554-1557, 2002.
39. Weiss RE, Xu J, Ning G, et al: Mice deficient in the steroid receptor co-activator 1 (SRC-1) are resistant to thyroid hormone. EMBO J 18:1900-1904, 1999.
40. Becker N, Seugnet I, Guissouma H, et al: Nuclear corepressor and silencing mediator of retinoic and thyroid hormone receptors corepressor expression is incompatible with T(3)-dependent TRH regulation. Endocrinology 142:5321-5331, 2001.
41. Shen X, Li QL, Brent GA, Friedman TC: Thyroid hormone regulation of prohormone convertase 1 (PC1): Regional expression in rat brain and in vitro characterization of negative thyroid hormone response elements. J Mol Endocrinol 33:21-33, 2004.
42. Shen X, Li QL, Brent GA, Friedman TC: Regulation of regional expression in rat brain PC2 by thyroid hormone/characterization of novel negative thyroid hormone response elements in the PC2 promoter. Am J Physiol Endocrinol Metab 288:E236-E245, 2005.
43. Uy HL, Reasner CA, Samuels MH: Pattern of recovery of the hypothalamic-pituitary-thyroid axis following radioactive iodine therapy in patients with Graves' disease. Am J Med 99:173-179, 1995.
44. Kempers MJ, van Tijn DA, van Trotsenburg AS, et al: Central congenital hypothyroidism due to gestational hyperthyroidism: Detection where prevention failed. J Clin Endocrinol Metab 88:5851-5857, 2003.
45. Hollenberg AN: The role of the thyrotropin-releasing hormone (TRH) neuron as a metabolic sensor. Thyroid 18:131-139, 2008.
46. Borst GC, Osburne RC, O'Brian JT, et al: Fasting decreases thyrotropin responsiveness to thyrotropin-releasing hormone: A potential cause of misinterpretation of thyroid function tests in the critically ill. J Clin Endocrinol Metab 57:380-383, 1983.
47. Komaki G, Tamai H, Kiyohara K, et al: Changes in the hypothalamic-pituitary-thyroid axis during acute starvation in non-obese patients. Endocrinol Jpn 33:303-308, 1986.
48. Blake NG, Eckland DJ, Foster OJ, Lightman SL: Inhibition of hypothalamic thyrotropin-releasing hormone messenger ribonucleic acid during food deprivation. Endocrinology 129:2714-2718, 1991.
49. Ahima RS, Prabakaran D, Mantzoros C, et al: Role of leptin in the neuroendocrine response to fasting. Nature 382:250-252, 1996.
50. Legradi G, Emerson CH, Ahima RS, et al: Leptin prevents fasting-induced suppression of prothyrotropin-releasing hormone messenger ribonucleic acid in neurons of the hypothalamic paraventricular nucleus. Endocrinology 138:2569-2576, 1997.
51. Chan JL, Heist K, DePaoli AM, et al: The role of falling leptin levels in the neuroendocrine and metabolic adaptation to short-term starvation in healthy men. J Clin Invest 111:1409-1421, 2003.
52. Rosenbaum M, Goldsmith R, Bloomfield D, et al: Low-dose leptin reverses skeletal muscle, autonomic, and neuroendocrine adaptations to maintenance of reduced weight. J Clin Invest 115:3579-3586, 2005.
53. Rosenbaum M, Murphy EM, Heymsfield SB, et al: Low-dose leptin administration reverses effects of sustained weight-reduction on energy expenditure and circulating concentrations of thyroid hormones. J Clin Endocrinol Metab 87:2391-2394, 2002.

54. Tartaglia LA, Dembski M, Weng X, et al: Identification and expression cloning of a leptin receptor, OB-R. Cell 83:1263-1271, 1995.
55. Bjorbaek C, Hollenberg AN: Leptin and melanocortin signaling in the hypothalamus. Vitam Horm 65:281-311, 2002.
56. Harris M, Aschkenasi C, Elias CF, et al: Transcriptional regulation of the thyrotropin-releasing hormone gene by leptin and melanocortin signaling. J Clin Invest 107:1-11, 2001.
57. Huo L, Munzberg H, Nillni EA, Bjorbaek C: Role of signal transducer and activator of transcription 3 in regulation of hypothalamic trh gene expression by leptin. Endocrinology 145:2516-2523, 2004.
58. Bates SH, Dundon TA, Seifert M, et al: LRb-STAT3 signaling is required for the neuroendocrine regulation of energy expenditure by leptin. Diabetes 53:3067-3073, 2004.
59. Clement K, Vaisse C, Lahlou N, et al: A mutation in the human leptin receptor gene causes obesity and pituitary dysfunction. Nature 392:398-401, 1998.
60. Farooqi IS, Wangensteen T, Collins S, et al: Clinical and molecular genetic spectrum of congenital deficiency of the leptin receptor. N Engl J Med 356:237-247, 2007.
61. Cheung CC, Clifton DK, Steiner RA: Proopiomelanocortin neurons are direct targets for leptin in the hypothalamus. Endocrinology 138:4489-4492, 1997.
62. Schwartz MW, Seeley RJ, Campfield LA, et al: Identification of targets of leptin action in rat hypothalamus. J Clin Invest 98:1101-1106, 1996.
63. Schwartz MW, Seeley RJ, Woods SC, et al: Leptin increases hypothalamic pro-opiomelanocortin mRNA expression in the rostral arcuate nucleus. Diabetes 46:2119-2123, 1997.
64. Mizuno TM, Kleopoulos SP, Bergen HT, et al: Hypothalamic pro-opiomelanocortin mRNA is reduced by fasting and [corrected] in ob/ob and db/db mice, but is stimulated by leptin. Diabetes 47:294-297, 1998.
65. Mizuno TM, Mobbs CV: Hypothalamic agouti-related protein messenger ribonucleic acid is inhibited by leptin and stimulated by fasting. Endocrinology 140:814-817, 1999.
66. Schwartz MW, Baskin DG, Bukowski TR, et al: Specificity of leptin action on elevated blood glucose levels and hypothalamic neuropeptide Y gene expression in ob/ob mice. Diabetes 45:531-535, 1996.
67. Stephens TW, Basinski M, Bristow PK, et al: The role of neuropeptide Y in the antiobesity action of the obese gene product. Nature 377:530-532, 1995.
68. Adan RA, Cone RD, Burbach JP, Gispen WH: Differential effects of melanocortin peptides on neural melanocortin receptors. Mol Pharmacol 46:1182-1190, 1994.
69. Farooqi IS, Keogh JM, Yeo GS, et al: Clinical spectrum of obesity and mutations in the melanocortin 4 receptor gene. N Engl J Med 348:1085-1095, 2003.
70. Huszar D, Lynch CA, Fairchild-Huntress V, et al: Targeted disruption of the melanocortin-4 receptor results in obesity in mice. Cell 88:131-141, 1997.
71. Fekete C, Sarkar S, Rand WM, et al: Neuropeptide Y1 and Y5 receptors mediate the effects of neuropeptide Y on the hypothalamic-pituitary-thyroid axis. Endocrinology 143:4513-4519, 2002.
72. Kishi T, Aschkenasi CJ, Choi BJ, et al: Neuropeptide Y Y1 receptor mRNA in rodent brain: Distribution and colocalization with melanocortin-4 receptor. J Comp Neurol 482:217-243, 2005.
73. Fekete C, Legradi G, Mihaly E, et al: (alpha)-Melanocyte-stimulating-hormone is contained in nerve terminals innervating thyrotropin-releasing hormone synthesizing neurons in the hypothalamic paraventricular nucleus and prevents fasting induced suppression of prothyrotropin-releasing hormone gene expression. J Neurosci 20:1550-1558, 2000.
74. Nijenhuis WA, Oosterom J, Adan RA: AgRP(83-132) acts as an inverse agonist on the human-melanocortin-4 receptor. Mol Endocrinol 15:164-171, 2001.
75. Ollmann MM, Wilson BD, Yang YK, et al: Antagonism of central melanocortin receptors in vitro and in vivo by agouti-related protein Science 278:135-138, 1998.
76. Sarkar S, Lechan RM: Central administration of neuropeptide Y reduces alpha-melanocyte-stimulating hormone-induced cyclic adenosine 5′-monophosphate response element binding protein (CREB) phosphorylation in pro-thyrotropin-releasing hormone neurons and increases CREB phosphorylation in corticotropin-releasing hormone neurons in the hypothalamic paraventricular nucleus. Endocrinology 144:281-291, 2003.
77. Sarkar S, Legradi G, Lechan RM: Intracerebroventricular administration of alpha-melanocyte stimulating hormone increases phosphorylation of CREB in TRH- and CRH-producing neurons of the hypothalamic paraventricular nucleus. Brain Res 945:50-59, 2002.
78. Guo F, Bakal K, Minokoshi Y, Hollenberg AN: Leptin signaling targets the thyrotropin-releasing hormone gene promoter in vivo. Endocrinology 145:2221-2227, 2004.
79. Perello M, Stuart RC, Nillni EA: The role of intracerebroventricular administration of leptin in the stimulation of prothyrotropin releasing hormone (proTRH) neurons in the hypothalamic paraventricular nucleus. Endocrinology 147:3296-3306, 2006.
80. Diano S, Naftolin F, Goglia F, Horvath TL: Fasting-induced increase in type II iodothyronine deiodinase activity and messenger ribonucleic acid levels is not reversed by thyroxine in the rat hypothalamus. Endocrinology 139:2879-2884, 1998.
81. Blake NG, Johnson MR, Eckland DJ, et al: Effect of food deprivation and altered thyroid status on the hypothalamic-pituitary-thyroid axis in the rat. J Endocrinol 133:183-188, 1992.

82. De Groot LJ: Dangerous dogmas in medicine: The nonthyroidal illness syndrome. J Clin Endocrinol Metab 84:151-164, 1999.
83. McIver B, Gorman CA: Euthyroid sick syndrome: An overview. Thyroid 7:125-132, 1997.
84. Fliers E, Guldenaar SE, Wiersinga WM, Swaab DF: Decreased hypothalamic thyrotropin-releasing hormone gene expression in patients with nonthyroidal illness. J Clin Endocrinol Metab 82:4032-4036, 1997.
85. Kondo K, Harbuz MS, Levy A, Lightman SL: Inhibition of the hypothalamic-pituitary-thyroid axis in response to lipopolysaccharide is independent of changes in circulating corticosteroids. Neuroimmunomodulation 4:188-194, 1997.
86. Kakucska I, Romero LI, Clark BD, et al: Suppression of thyrotropin-releasing hormone gene expression by interleukin-1-beta in the rat: Implications for nonthyroidal illness. Neuroendocrinology 59:129-137, 1994.
87. Fekete C, Lechan RM: Negative feedback regulation of hypophysiotropic thyrotropin-releasing hormone (TRH) synthesizing neurons: Role of neuronal afferents and type 2 deiodinase. Front Neuroendocrinol 28:97-114, 2007.
88. Fekete C, Sarkar S, Christoffolete MA, et al: Bacterial lipopolysaccharide (LPS)-induced type 2 iodothyronine deiodinase (D2) activation in the mediobasal hypothalamus (MBH) is independent of the LPS-induced fall in serum thyroid hormone levels. Brain Res 1056:97-99, 2005.
89. Zeold A, Doleschall M, Haffner MC, et al: Characterization of the nuclear factor-kappa B responsiveness of the human dio2 gene. Endocrinology 147:4419-4429, 2006.
90. Bornstein SR, Torpy DJ, Chrousos GP, et al: Leptin levels are elevated despite low thyroid hormone levels in the "euthyroid sick" syndrome. J Clin Endocrinol Metab 82:4278-4279, 1997.
91. Cheung W, Yu PX, Little BM, et al: Role of leptin and melanocortin signaling in uremia-associated cachexia. J Clin Invest 115:1659-1665, 2005.
92. Marks DL, Butler AA, Turner R, et al: Differential role of melanocortin receptor subtypes in cachexia. Endocrinology 144:1513-1523, 2003.

Chapter 7

Thyroid-Stimulating Hormone and Thyroid-Stimulating Hormone Receptor

Stéphanie Gaillard and Fredric E. Wondisford

Key Points

- Thyrotropin (thyroid-stimulating hormone, TSH), through its interaction with the TSH receptor (TSH-R), is the main regulator of thyroid hormone biosynthesis and secretion.
- Alterations in the regulation of TSH synthesis and mutations in the TSH beta subunit result in pathologic conditions, such as central hypothyroidism.
- Thyrotropin resistance syndrome is primarily caused by loss-of-function mutations in TSH-R, while gain of function mutations have been implicated in hyperfunctioning thyroid adenomas, toxic multinodular goiters, and congenital nonautoimmune hyperthyroidism.
- Stimulating autoantibodies to the TSH-R, as in Graves' disease, result in hyperproduction of thyroid hormone and thyrotoxicosis. TSH-R blocking antibodies inhibit receptor function resulting in chronic autoimmune hypothyroidism and thyroid atrophy.

Thyroid hormone synthesis involves the coordinated regulation of signals from the hypothalamus, pituitary, and thyroid. Thyrotropin (TSH) is the main stimulator of thyroid hormone production and its secretion is under the control of thyrotropin-releasing hormone (TRH) secreted by the hypothalamus (Fig. 7-1A). Negative feedback through inhibition of TSH and TRH production is effected by thyroxine (T_4) and triiodothyronine (T_3) activity on both the pituitary and hypothalamus. Thyrotropin primarily exerts its effects by binding to the thyrotropin receptor (TSH-R) on the basal surface of the follicular cells within the thyroid. Activation of the receptor results in activation of the cyclic adenosine monophosphate (cAMP) and phosphatidylinositol regulatory cascades that ultimately results in thyroid hormone synthesis and the modulation of thyroid hormone–responsive genes (see Fig. 7-1B).

THYROTROPIN

TSH is a member of the endocrine glycoprotein hormone family, which includes luteinizing hormone (LH), follicle-stimulating hormone (FSH), and chorionic gonadotropin (CG). These hormones are synthesized in the anterior lobe of the pituitary and in the placenta during pregnancy. Structurally, the hormones are noncovalently linked heterodimers composed of a common alpha subunit and a beta subunit unique to each hormone.[1] The beta subunit carries the biologic specificity of the hormone controlling receptor-specific binding and hormonal activity.

Structure

The human alpha subunit common to the four glycoprotein hormones consists of 92 amino acid residues encoded by a single gene located on chromosome 6. The gene is 9.4 kb long and is comprised of four exon regions separated by three introns.[2] The gene for the human thyrotropin beta subunit is located on chromosome 1, is 4.9 kb long, and is comprised of three exons and two introns.[3-5] The gene predicts a 118–amino acid coding region, but only a 112–amino acid protein is derived by purification of beta subunits in human pituitary preparations. There is no difference in the bioactivity of the two proteins and it has been speculated that the difference may reflect

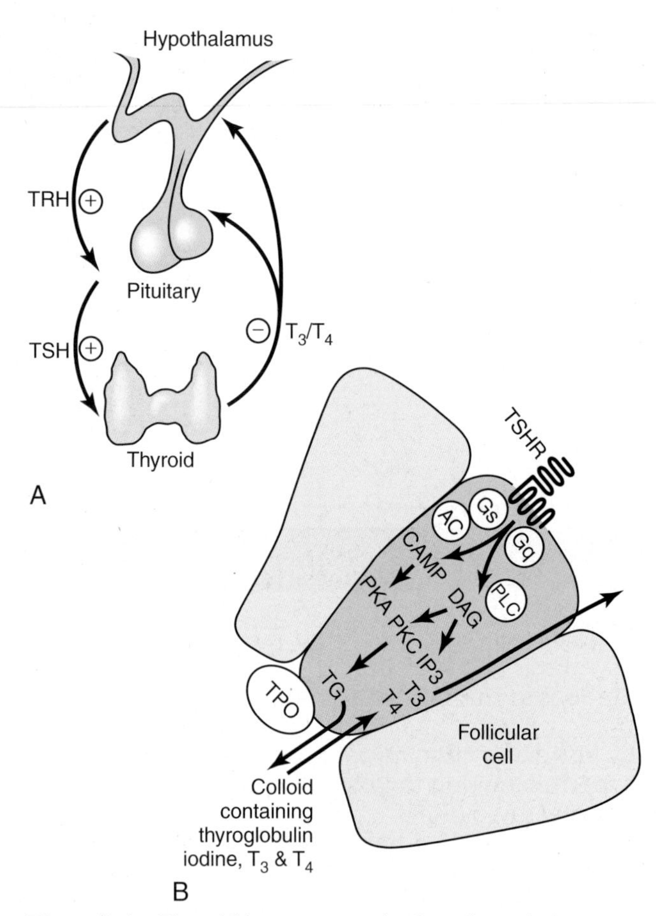

Figure 7–1 Thyroid hormone synthesis and regulation. **A,** The hypothalamus secretes thyrotropin-releasing hormone (TRH), stimulating the release of thyrotropin (TSH) from the anterior pituitary gland. TSH stimulates the follicular cells to synthesize and secrete thyroid hormones. **B,** The thyroid hormones, thyroxine (T_4) and triiodothyronine (T_3), in turn exhibit negative feedback to inhibit the hypothalamic production of TRH and pituitary production of TSH. *(Adapted from Kondo T, Ezzat S, Asa SL: Pathogenetic mechanisms in thyroid follicular-cell neoplasia. Nat Rev Cancer 6:292-306, 2006; and Braverman LE, Utiger RD: Werner and Ingbar's The Thyroid: A Fundamental and Clinical Text, 9th ed. Philadelphia, Lippincott, Williams & Wilkins, 2005.)*

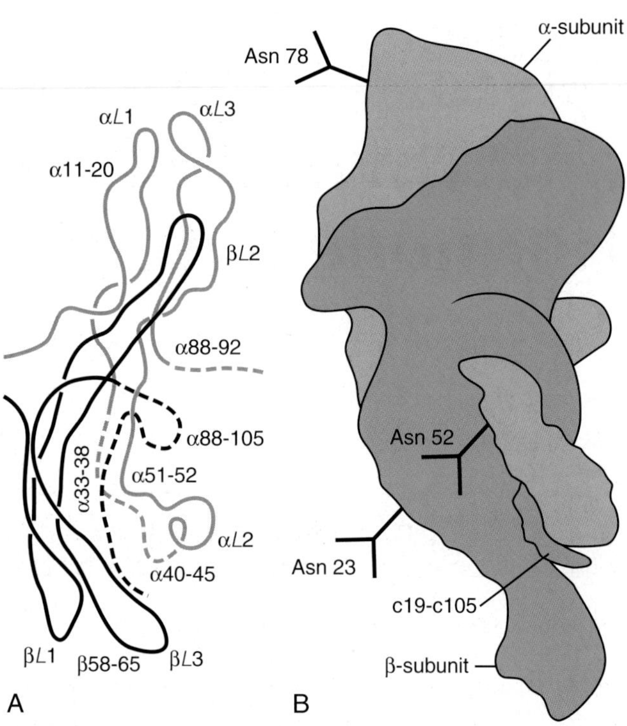

Figure 7–2 Diagram of the structure of human thyrotropin (TSH) based on human chorionic gonadotropin crystallography and TSH structure-function studies. The seat belt region is where the beta subunit wraps around loop 2 of the alpha subunit (αL2) and stabilizes the TSH heterodimer. **A,** In the ribbon model, the alpha subunit is represented by a gray line and the beta subunit is represented by a black line. **B,** The beta subunit (blue) wraps around loop 2 of the alpha subunit (violet), forming a seat belt. The c19-c105 cystine bond acts as the "buckle," securing the subunit in place. The sites of asparagine *N*-linked oligosaccharides are shown (Asn 23, Asn 52, Asn 78). αL, α-subunit loop; βL, β-subunit loop. ***(A** adapted from Szkudlinski MW, Fremont V, Ronin C, Weintraub BD: Thyroid-stimulating hormone and thyroid-stimulating hormone receptor structure-function relationships. Physiol Rev 82:473-502, 2002; **B** adapted from Medeiros-Neto G, Herodotou DT, Rajan S, et al: A circulating biologically inactive thyrotropin caused by a mutation in the beta subunit gene. J Clin Invest 97:1250-1256, 1996.)*

proteolytic cleavage during purification.[6,7] The three-dimensional structure of human CG (hCG) has been elucidated by x-ray crystallography, and homology models have confirmed expected structural similarities among the other glycoprotein hormones.[8,9] The alpha subunit contains 10 half-cystine residues, which form five intramolecular disulfide linkages that fold into a cystine knot motif; this is also found in some growth factors, such as transforming growth factor-β2 (TGF-β2) and platelet-derived growth factor.[10-12] Although there is no significant sequence similarity between the subunits, structurally the beta subunits of each glycoprotein hormone also fold into a cystine knot motif. The cystine knot of each subunit is flanked by two beta hairpin loops (L1 and L3) on the N-terminal side of the cystine knot, with a long loop (L2) of a double-stranded beta sheet–like structure on the C-terminal side (Fig. 7-2). A loop of the beta subunit wraps over the alpha subunit, giving the appearance of a seat belt holding the alpha subunit in place.[8] There is evidence that the seat belt region can confer glycoprotein hormone specificity.

The generation of chimeric hormone by replacing the seat belt region of TSH with the corresponding sequence of CG has resulted in binding of the chimeric protein to, and full activation of, the CG receptor. However, similar experiments replacing the seat belt region of TSH with that of FSH did not result in activation of the FSH receptor, indicating that other

Table 7–1 Natural Human Thyrotropin Beta Subunit Mutations

Type of Mutation	Amino Acid Change	Resultant Structural Change	Population
Missense	G29R	Arginine introduced into the cystine knot region prevents heterodimer formation	Japanese[15,16]
Missense	C85R	Disruption of disulfide bond C31-C85	Greek[17]
Nonsense	E12X	Truncated 11–amino acid N-terminal protein	Greek[18]
Nonsense	Q49X	Truncated 48–amino acid N-terminal protein	Greek,[17] Egyptian,[19] Turkish[20]
Frameshift and stop at codon 62	F57Sfs62X	Missense mutation amino acids 57-61, with truncation of amino acids 62-118	Not specified[21]
Frameshift and stop at codon 114	C105Vfs114X	Disrupts disulfide bond C19-C105 in the seat belt region	Brazilian,[22] German,[23-25] Belgian,[26,27] Swiss,[28] Argentinian[28,29]
Substitution	IVS2 + 5 G → A	G → A transition at +5 of donor splice site of intron 2; results in exon skipping and translation of an out of frame 25aa transcript	Not specified[31]

regions of the hormone are likely important in determining receptor specificity.[13] Mutagenesis studies of the alpha 33-38 domain have shown that mutation of alpha-alanine 36 to glutamic acid results in normal interactions with the hTSH beta subunit, leading to a bioactive heterodimer, but this does not form a dimer with the hCG beta subunit.[14] Other mutations in this region (alpha-phenylalanine 33 and alpha-arginine 35) are critical for hCG but not hTSH receptor binding. In similar experiments, mutagenesis of residues 11-20 of the alpha subunit increased receptor binding affinity and bioactivity.[9] Therefore the amino terminal portion of the alpha subunit is important for heterodimerization, receptor binding, and hormone activity.

Naturally Occurring Thyrotropin Mutations

Seven thyrotropin mutations have been identified that result in central hypothyroidism (Table 7-1).[15-31] Interestingly, no mutations in the gene for the common alpha subunit have been identified. Six of the mutations are located in the coding region for the beta subunit of TSH, whereas the seventh affects the donor splice site of intron 2. The mutations elucidate residues important for the proper synthesis of functional thyrotropin hormone. For example, in several families, conversion of the beta-glycine 29 to arginine in the CAGY region resulted in undetectable levels of TSH.[15,16] The CAGY region is conserved among all the glycoprotein hormone beta subunits and, in studies on hCG, was found to be essential for heterodimerization. This suggests that conservation of the glycine is essential to maintain proper subunit heterodimerization.[32] The most common mutation appears to be a frameshift mutation that substitutes a valine for the cysteine 105 residue on the beta subunit, which results in diminished beta subunit synthesis and impaired heterodimerization. This cysteine is critical for a disulfide linkage in the seat belt region of the beta subunit thought to lay across the alpha subunit with the C19-C105 cystine bond acting as the "buckle," securing the subunit in place (see Fig. 7-2).[8,22] TSH levels were typically diminished in patient with this mutation, but some TSH was detectable. Disruption of another disulfide bond (C31-C85) by substitution of arginine for cysteine at codon 85 (part of the cystine knot structural motif) likely results in conformational changes, decreased subunit stability, and impaired heterodimerization.[17] The Q49X, E12X, and F57Sfs62X mutations appear to result in severely truncated TSH beta subunits lacking the cystine knot, loops, or seat belt region. Mutation of the consensus region at the donor splicing site (IVS 2 + 5 G → A) results in exon skipping. The RNA transcript for the beta subunit does not have exon 2, along with its translational start site. It is possible that a mutant protein may be translated from the first ATG in exon 3, but this would result in a nonsense sequence of amino acids with no biologic activity.[31] Interestingly, all the mutations are inherited in an autosomal recessive fashion and most are the result of homozygous

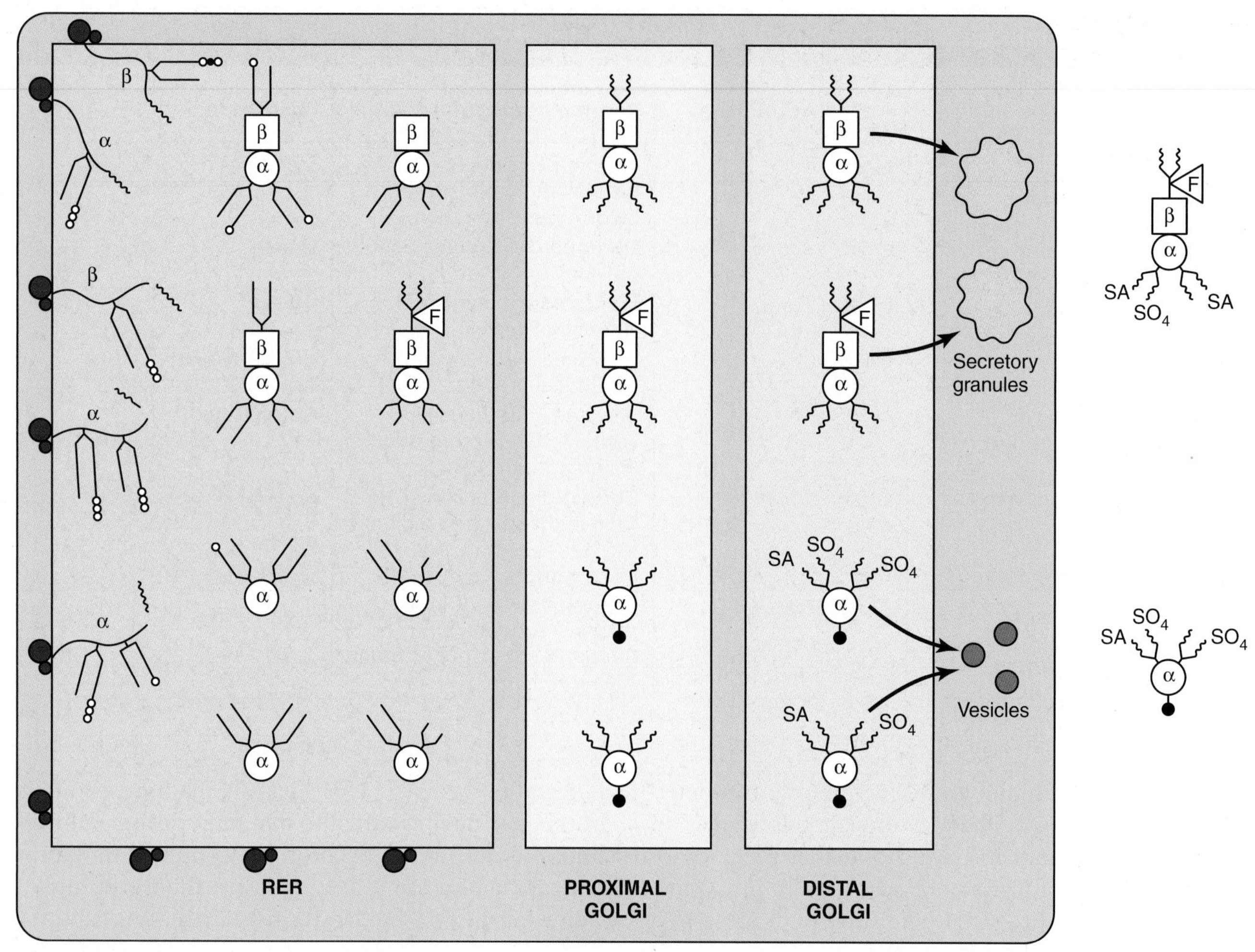

Figure 7–3 Model of thyrotropin (TSH) biosynthesis depicting transit through the rough endoplasmic reticulum (RER), proximal Golgi, distal Golgi, secretory vesicles, and granules toward secretion at the membrane of the thyrotroph cell. Circles and squares represent alpha and beta subunits of TSH, respectively. Cleavage of signal peptides (wavy lines) and glycosylation of asparagine residues occur in the RER. Two high-mannose carbohydrate units (Y) are added to the alpha subunit, whereas one is added to the beta subunit. Oligosaccharides added en bloc generally contain three glucose residues (small circles), two of which are rapidly removed, followed by removal of the final glucose residue. Combination of alpha and beta subunits begins in the RER while subunits still contain high-mannose oligosaccharides. In the Golgi complex, oligosaccharides are generated by the addition of *N*-acetylglucosamine, *N*-galactosamine, galactose, and fucose (F in triangle). Excess alpha subunits exist in the RER and also undergo glycosylation, particularly *O*-glycosylation (solid circle). Sulfate (SO_4) and/or sialic acid (SA) residues are added in the distal Golgi. TSH heterodimers enter a regulated pathway of secretory granules, and excess alpha subunits enter a more constitutive pathway of secretory vesicles. *(Adapted from Braverman LE, Utiger RD: Werner and Ingbar's The Thyroid: A Fundamental and Clinical Text, 8th ed. Philadelphia, Lippincott, Williams & Wilkins, 2000.)*

mutation. One example exists of congenital hypothyroidism resulting from compound heterozygous mutation, in which one allele encoded for the Q49X truncation and the other encoded for the disrupted seat belt disulfide bond (C105Vfs114X).[33]

Carbohydrate Modification of Thyrotropin

Synthesis and Secretion of Thyrotropin

The alpha and beta subunits of TSH, like those of the other glycoprotein hormones, are covalently linked to carbohydrate chains. The alpha subunit contains two asparagine *N*-linked oligosaccharide sites (N52 and N78) but the beta subunit only contains one (N23) (see Fig. 7-2). Glycosylation of the alpha and beta subunits occurs cotranslationally in the endoplasmic reticulum. The carbohydrate chains are formed from combinations of mannose, *N*-acetylglucosamine, *N*-acetylgalactosamine, fucose, galactose, and sialic acid. The cotranslational attachment of oligosaccharides protects against intracellular degradation and is essential for proper folding, heterodimer formation, and secretion of TSH (Fig. 7-3). In the endoplasmic reticulum, thyrotropin subunits are glycosylated with high-mannose precursors, oligosaccharides containing three glucose and nine mannose residues. A dolichol phosphate carrier is preassembled in the rough endoplasmic reticulum with the oligosaccharide, (glucose)3, and (mannose)9 (*N*-acetylglucosamine)2. The high-mannose precursors are transferred en bloc onto the asparagine residues of nascent peptides presenting the sequence asparagine-X-serine or asparagine-X-threonine (where X is any amino acid). The resultant glycoprotein is further processed by glucosidases and mannosidases to leave a three-unit core.[34,35] Post-translational processing continues as the glycoprotein is transported through the endoplasmic reticulum to the Golgi apparatus and complex oligosaccharides are generated by the addition of *N*-acetylglucosamine, *N*-galactosamine, galactose, and fucose. In addition, sulfate and sialic acid may be incorporated onto the terminal oligosaccharides.[36,37] Inhibition of proper oligosaccharide attachment during translation results in aggregation and intracellular degradation of TSH.[34,35,38] As a result of the multistep maturation process, secreted TSH molecules contain complex biantennary and triantennary carbohydrate structures terminating in a sulfate or sialic acid cap.

Biologic Activity and Metabolic Clearance of Thyrotropin

The role of oligosaccharides is not limited to the synthesis, transport, and secretion of thyrotropin. The biologic activity of TSH is also dependent on carbohydrate composition. Enzymatically deglycosylated TSH binds to its receptor, but its activity is markedly reduced.[39,40] The oligosaccharides located on the alpha subunit were shown to be necessary for full in vitro activity of the hormone, whereas sialylation was shown to attenuate the activity of the hormone.[41-43] More important than their effect on in vitro biologic activity, oligosaccharides also regulate metabolic clearance of the hormone, modulating circulating hormone levels and potency in vivo. At times, the results of in vitro and in vivo studies can appear to be at odds with each other. Although an enzymatically desialylated hormone was more biologically active, sialylated hormones in vivo displayed higher bioactivity largely because of a lower rate of metabolic clearance.[43-45] This emphasizes that effects on metabolic clearance can supersede effects on in vitro activity. Sulfated oligosaccharides are recognized by *N*-acetylgalactosamine (GalNAc) sulfate receptors located in the liver, shifting the proportion metabolized by the liver as compared with the kidney.[45] Liver metabolism of TSH is slower than in the kidney; thus the sialylation-to-sulfation ratio determines metabolic clearance and as a consequence, bioactivity. Location within the protein sequence of the subunit, in addition to type of carbohydrate structure, influences metabolic clearance. Glycosylation of the single carbohydrate chain of the beta subunit preferentially affects metabolic clearance of the hormone versus alpha subunit glycosylation, whereas glycosylation of N52 appears to be more important than that of N78 in the alpha subunit.[43,46] These studies emphasize the importance of post-translational modifications for proper heterodimer formation, transport, and secretion, as well as bioactivity and metabolic clearance.

Alteration of Carbohydrate Structures in Thyroid Function and Dysfunction

Thyrotropin is not secreted as one distinct hormone, but rather as a group of isohormones with different oligosaccharide composition, resulting in physiologic microheterogeneity. The functional effect of changes in the carbohydrate structure of TSH has not been completely elucidated, but alterations in carbohydrate structure are apparent in different thyroid states. In patients with primary hypothyroidism, there is an increase in the proportion of sialylated TSH secreted, which decreases in the setting of levothyroxine replacement therapy.[47-49] One mechanism of regulating sialylation is suggested by the finding that the level of mRNA of sialyltransferases in thyrotropes of the pituitary is increased in hypothyroid mice.[50,51] TRH stimulation also modulates microheterogeneity by varying sulfate and sialic acid content.[52,53] These findings likely reflect another element of the classic hypothalamic-pituitary-thyroid negative feedback loop, ensuring that the regulation of thyroid hormone production is tightly regulated in response to small variations in physiologic states. In addition to their presence in hypothyroid states, variable carbohydrate structures have also been identified in patients with central hypothyroidism, resistance to thyroid hormone (RTH), TSH-secreting pituitary adenomas, and in nonthyroidal illness such as chronic uremia and sick euthyroid illness.[47,54] Studies in patients with TSH-secreting pituitary adenomas have shown that heterogeneous isoforms of thyrotropin are secreted and octreotide treatment alters glycosylation patterns.[55-57] Different patterns of carbohydrate structures were also identified during the development and maturation of the rodent hypothalamus-pituitary-thyroid axis. Mature animals secreted a larger percentage of thyrotropin with complex oligosaccharides (multiantennary and complex biantennary

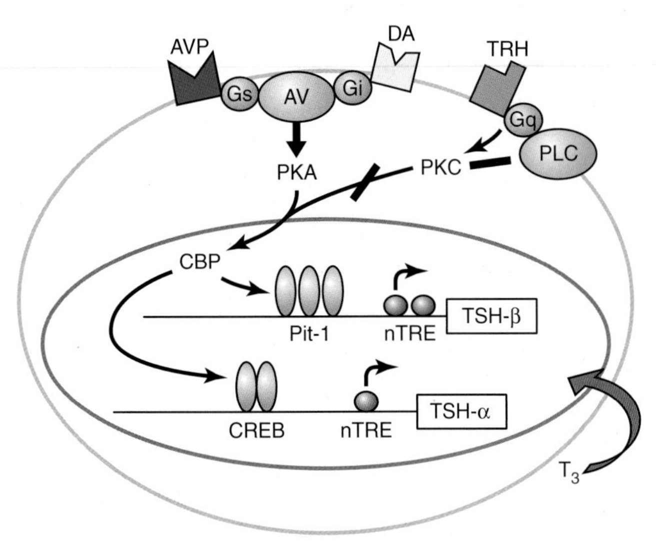

Figure 7–4 Overview of regulation of thyrotropin (TSH) subunit gene expression (see text for details). AC, adenylyl cyclase; AVP, arginine vasopressin; CBP, CREB-binding protein; CREB, cyclic adenosine monophosphate response element-binding protein; DA, dopamine; Gi, inhibitory guanine–nucleotide-binding protein; Gs, stimulatory guanine nucleotide-binding protein; nTRE, negative thyroid hormone response element; PKA, protein kinase A; PKC, protein kinase C; PLC, phospholipase C; TR, thyroid hormone receptor; TRH, thyrotropin-releasing hormone. *(Adapted from Braverman LE, Utiger RD: Werner and Ingbar's The Thyroid: A Fundamental and Clinical Text, 9th ed. Philadelphia, Lippincott, Williams & Wilkins, 2005.)*

structures) than prenatal or perinatal animals. In addition, the ratio of sialylated versus sulfated forms increased during development.[58] Higher sialylation 1was noted in normal patients during the nocturnal TSH surge as compared with the daytime circulating TSH in the same subject.[59] Thus, changes in the distribution of TSH isoforms occur as a result of diurnal variations, normal development and maturation, and pathologic states.

It is not yet clear, however, whether or how microheterogeneity and the relative balance of oligosaccharide composition result in the generation of different downstream signals. One possibility is that the oligosaccharide composition of TSH influences binding to TSH-R, resulting in different downstream effects (see later). This possibility is suggested by experiments in which pituitary TSH preparations, fractionated to isolate glycosylation variants, were shown to activate intracellular signal transduction pathways selectively.[60] Specifically, high-mannose variants were more potent stimulators of cAMP activity than biantennary variants, but stimulated inositol phosphate (IP) production to a similar degree. On the other hand, only fucosylated variants could stimulate IP production but unfucosylated forms did not, with no effect on the cAMP cascade.

Regulation of Thyrotropin Subunit Gene Expression

Physiologic stimuli regulate TSH subunit gene expression through the coordinated control of positive and negative regulatory pathways (Fig. 7-4). The hypothalamic hormone TRH is the predominant positive regulator of TSH subunit gene expression. In addition to the regulation of post-translational modifications described earlier, TRH acts through its receptor, TRH-R, a member of the seven-transmembrane G protein–coupled receptor superfamily. TRH binding results in the activation of both the inositol phospholipid-calcium-protein kinase C and cAMP-protein kinase A transduction pathways.[61-65] The transcriptional response to TRH stimulation by the TSH alpha and beta subunits is not identical, suggesting that different pathways downstream of TRH are involved in activating transcription.[66] Pit-1, a pituitary-specific transcription factor that is implicated in pituitary development and, when mutated, results in combined pituitary hormone deficiency and central hypothyroidism, is essential for the increase in transcription of the TSH beta subunit in response to TRH stimulation through three Pit-1 DNA-binding sites in the TSH beta subunit gene promoter.[67] Pit-1–mediated TSH beta subunit transcription is enhanced through interactions with the cAMP response element-binding (CREB) protein (CBP), a protein that integrates a number of signal transduction pathways and enhances transcription by recruiting transcriptional coactivators. The TSH alpha subunit promoter, on the other hand, does not contain any Pit-1 DNA-binding sites, but instead contains two cAMP response elements (CREs) that bind CREB. TRH stimulation results in phosphorylation of CREB, enhanced CBP binding, and enhanced gene transcription. CBP binding to another transcription factor, P-Lim (Lhx3), in a TRH-dependent manner contributes to alpha subunit transcription. Therefore, the transcription of TSH subunit genes is enhanced by TRH stimulation through increased CBP binding of different DNA-binding transcription factors.[65] Further studies have shown that TRH-directed stimulation of the TSH subunits is mediated through a complex array of other transcription factors, including GATA-2 and two members of the LIM family of homeobox genes, Lhx2 and Lhx3.[65,68-70]

Pit-1 and Lhx3 are two of several transcription factors that, when mutated, are implicated in the development of combined pituitary hormone deficiency (CPHD), a syndrome associated with abnormal hypothalamic-pituitary development that causes

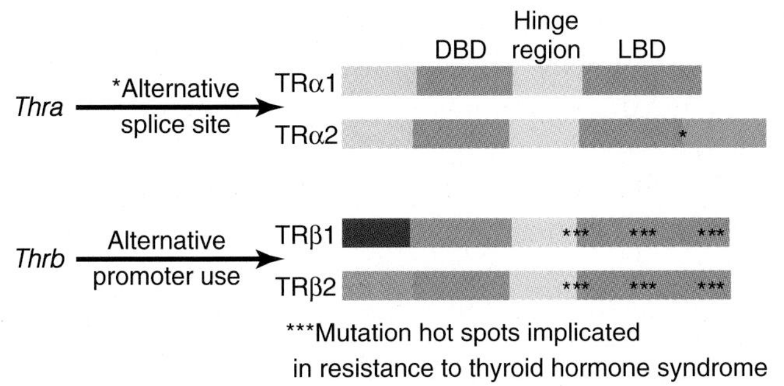

Figure 7–5 Schematic of thyroid hormone receptors. DBD, DNA-binding domain; LBD, ligand-binding domain; *Thra*, *Thrb*, genes encoding for thyroid receptor α (TRα) and TRβ, respectively.

deficiency of growth hormone, prolactin, and/or thyrotropin.[71] A common mutation of Pit-1 (R271W) occurs in the POU homeodomain of the Pit-1 protein, a region responsible for DNA binding.[72] This mutation leads to the production of a mutant Pit-1 that binds DNA but does not transactivate properly. Patients develop hypothyroidism but have inappropriately normal levels of TSH and do not respond to TRH stimulation, emphasizing the importance of Pit-1 in TRH-mediated transcription of TSH beta.

Interestingly, TRH is not required for the transcription of TSH. Knockout mice that lack the gene for TRH express slightly higher than normal levels of TSH, but the TSH expressed shows reduced biologic activity, resulting in central hypothyroidism.[73] Similarly, some patients with TRH-R mutations also have central hypothyroidism.[74,75] This suggests that the TRH-mediated regulation of TSH glycosylation is an important contributor to TSH activity. More recent studies have suggested that although TRH is not absolutely required for TSH synthesis, TRH deficiency results in decreased bioactivity.[76] However, this study also showed that TRH is absolutely required for TSH upregulation in the setting of hypothyroidism, suggesting crosstalk between the TRH and thyroid hormone signaling pathways in hypothyroidism.

Thyroid hormone is the predominant negative regulator of TSH subunit gene expression through regulation of TSH at the level of the pituitary and indirectly by reducing TRH production.[77-80] Thyroid hormone administration to mice results in a 75% decrease in TSH alpha subunit mRNA synthesis and a more than 95% decrease in TSH beta subunit mRNA.[77,78] Negative regulation of TSH subunit and TRH genes requires binding of the negative regulatory units in the subunit gene promoters by the thyroid hormone receptor (TR), a member of the nuclear hormone receptor superfamily (Fig. 7-5).[81,82] Like other nuclear hormone receptors, TRs consist of a DNA-binding domain that allows for binding to specific DNA elements (TREs in the case of TRs) and a ligand-binding domain that determines ligand-binding specificity. TRs can homodimerize or heterodimerize with the retinoid X receptor (RXR). In the absence of hormone, TRs bind constitutively to corepressors, a class of proteins that either have histone deacetylase activity or recruit proteins that have this activity. Histone deacetylation results in increased chromatin packing and decreased gene transcription. Once T_3 binds to the dimerized TR, the nuclear corepressors are released and coactivators are recruited that enhance transcriptional activity.

Two separate gene loci, *Thra* and *Thrb*, encode for the TRs, designated as TR alpha and TR beta. The TR alpha gene generates two isoforms, TR alpha 1 and alpha 2 (also designated c-erbAa-2), through alternative splicing. The alternative splicing of the C terminus of alpha 2 disrupts the ligand-binding domain and generates a non–T_3-binding isoform. The TR beta gene generates two isoforms through differential promoter usage, resulting in two beta receptors, each with a different amino terminus. The TR isoforms are variably expressed in mammalian tissues.[81] TR alpha 1 and TR beta 1 are expressed in most tissues; TR alpha 1 mRNA is more highly expressed in skeletal muscle and brown fat, whereas there is higher expression of TR beta 1 mRNA in the brain, liver, and kidney. TR beta 2 is almost exclusively expressed in the hypothalamus, pituitary, auditory system, and retina.[83,84] Knockout experiments in mice in which one or more of the TR isoforms were deleted have shown that the TR beta isoforms are the most potent regulators of thyroid-stimulating hormone.[85-87] TR beta 2 is the dominant mediator of the negative feedback regulation, particularly in the hypothalamus, because it appears to be the only isoform responsible for the negative regulation of the TRH gene.[88] Although TR beta 2 also appears to be the most important isoform for negative feedback in the pituitary, TR alpha 1 and TR beta 1 can also play a role.[89] TR-mediated inhibition of the hypothalamic-pituitary-thyroid axis is dependent on the DNA-binding activity of the receptor, as shown in mice with a knock-in mutation in the DNA binding domain of TR beta.[90,91] These mice displayed elevated serum levels of thyroid hormones and a hyperplastic thyroid gland caused by inappropriate secretion of TSH from the anterior pituitary. The thyroid hormone responsive regions of the TRH and TSH subunits have been localized to the proximal promoter regions.[92,93]

Resistance to Thyroid Hormone Syndromes

Mutations in the TR beta gene have been implicated as one cause of RTH syndrome, a rare syndrome in which there is decreased responsiveness of target tissues to thyroid hormone.[94,95] The syndrome is characterized by elevated levels of circulating thyroid hormone (both T_3 and T_4), with inappropriately normal or even slightly elevated levels of thyrotropin. Patients typically exhibit evidence of goiter, with mild to no evidence of thyrotoxicosis. RTH has clinically been shown to be caused by three molecular defects in the thyroid hormone signaling pathway: (1) impaired binding of T_3 to TR beta secondary to mutations within the TR beta hinge and ligand-binding domain; (2) defective transport of the receptor into cells caused by mutation of a thyroid hormone transporter, monocarboxylate transporter 8 (MCT8); and (3) impaired deiodinase activity as a result of mutation in SECISBP2, a protein involved in selenium incorporation and production of functional enzyme.[95] Mutations in TR beta are responsible for most cases of RTH syndrome and 122 mutations in the TR beta gene have been associated with this syndrome. The mutations cluster into three distinct hot spots, one within the hinge region and two within the ligand-binding domain (see Fig. 7-5). Mutant receptors retain the ability to dimerize and bind DNA-binding elements but have a reduced binding affinity for T_3. Mutant TR beta inhibits the function of TR alpha and nonmutant TR beta through heterodimerization, resulting in dominant negative inhibition. This phenomenon explains the autosomal dominant pattern of inheritance seen in all but one family in which RTH was caused by TR beta gene defects.

Regulation of Thyroid-Stimulating Hormone Secretion by Other Circulating Hormones

Thyrotropin secretion has been shown to be regulated by other hormones, including glucocorticoids, estrogens, androgens, vasopressin, somatostatin, and dopamine. Although their importance as regulatory hormones is likely less than that of TRH and thyroid hormone, they may play a role in some pathologic conditions or during exogenous hormone or drug administration. Studies in which subjects received exogenous dexamethasone or cortisol showed suppression of TSH secretion and lower circulating free T_3 levels as a result of glucocorticoid administration.[96,97] A similar effect was shown in a patient with Cushing's syndrome secondary to an adrenal adenoma; TSH and free T_4 suppression was reversed after surgical removal of the tumor.[98]

Two other steroid hormones, estradiol and dihydrotestosterone, were shown to enhance thyroid hormone suppression of TSH mRNA production in hypothyroid rats.[99,100] There was no effect on basal TSH concentrations and no effect was seen in euthyroid animals; however, increased suppression occurred in hypothyroid animals treated with T_3, as well as an increase in pituitary TR, suggesting that the sex hormones may influence TR synthesis.[101]

The neurotransmitter dopamine rapidly decreases TSH subunit secretion, possibly as a result of stimulation of dopamine receptors present on the surface of anterior pituitary cells.[102,103] Dopamine agonists (L-dopa and bromocriptine) and dobutamine, a beta1 agonist structurally similar to dopamine, have also been shown to decrease thyrotropin secretion.[104-106] Administration of a single therapeutic dose of a dopamine antagonist, metoclopramide, enhanced TSH secretion.[107] The physiologic role of dopamine regulation of TSH has not yet been elucidated, but these studies reflect the many factors that affect circulating TSH levels.

Recombinant Human Thyroid-Stimulating Hormone

The molecular cloning of the TSH subunits and an improved understanding of the importance of glycosylation in TSH activity have allowed for large-scale production of the hormone.[108-110] Recombinant human TSH (rhTSH) is produced for clinical use by a Chinese hamster ovary (CHO) cell line stably transfected with cDNAs for the alpha and beta subunits. CHO cells do not express the pituitary-specific *N*-acetylgalactosamine transferase (GalNAc-transferase) and GalNAc-sulfotransferase necessary to add the GalNAc and a terminal sulfate to TSH. Therefore, it is composed of oligosaccharide chains terminating sialic acid in a pattern that is more similar to the sialylated TSH that circulates in patients with primary hypothyroidism. As a result, the rhTSH is metabolically cleared more slowly and is slightly less potent compared with pituitary TSH from euthyroid patients.[111] However, the maximum stimulatory effect of rhTSH is similar to that of pituitary TSH in in vitro bio-and immunoassays.[110,112] Because of this, rhTSH has become an alternative to withdrawal of thyroid hormone for use in the detection of recurrence or metastases in well-differentiated thyroid carcinoma and is being evaluated for other uses, such as radioablation in nodular goiter.[113]

THYROTROPIN RECEPTOR

The thyrotropin receptor (TSH-R) is a member of the glycoprotein hormone receptor family, part of the larger superfamily of G protein–coupled receptors

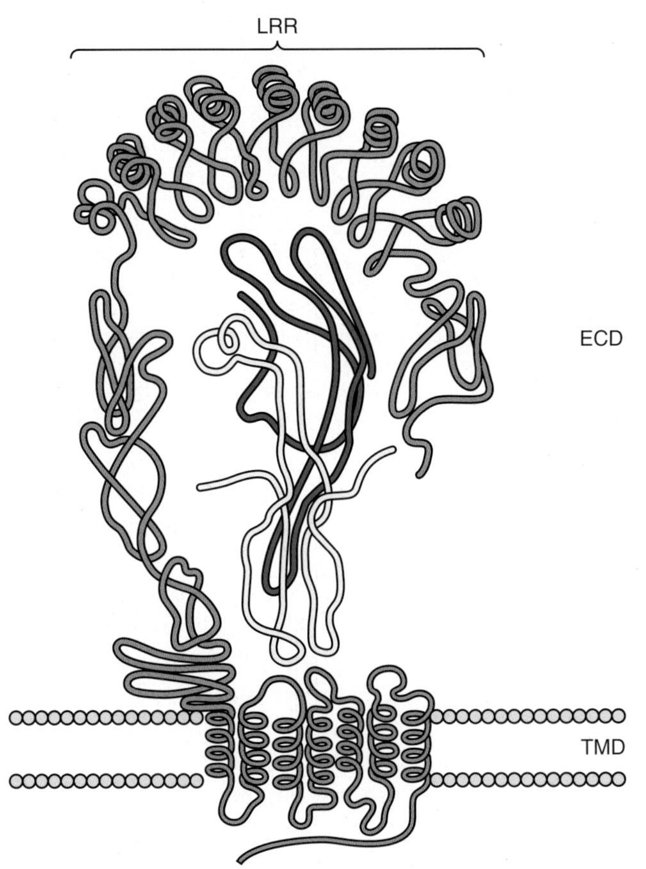

Figure 7–6 Schematic representation of thyrotropin (TSH) receptor in complex with thyroid-stimulating hormone (TSH). ECD, extracellular domain; LRR, leucine-rich repeats; TMD, transmembrane domain. *(Adapted from Szkudlinski MW, Fremont V, Ronin C, Weintraub BD: Thyroid-stimulating hormone and thyroid-stimulating hormone receptor structure-function relationships. Physiol Rev 82:473-502, 2002.)*

(GPCRs). The glycoprotein hormone receptors consist of a large extracellular ectodomain, a seven-transmembrane serpentine portion with many of the features typical of GPCRs, and a short C-terminal cytoplasmic arm (Fig. 7-6). The amino terminal ectodomain confers ligand-binding specificity to the receptor, and the transmembrane and cytoplasmic portions of the receptor interact with G proteins, dictating the activity of the receptor.

The gene encoding human TSH-R has been localized to chromosome 14q31[114] and encodes for a 764–amino acid protein, consisting of a 21–amino acid signal peptide that is cleaved prior to incorporation into the extracellular membrane, a 397–amino acid ectodomain, and a 346–amino acid transmembrane domain and cytoplasmic arm.[115-118] The gene is more than 60 kb long and is divided into 10 exons. The ectodomain is encoded by the first nine exons and part of the last exon, whereas the remainder of the last exon encodes for the entire transmembrane and cytoplasmic domains.[119] This is consistent with many genes for GPCRs that do not contain introns, and has led to the hypothesis that the glycoprotein hormone receptors evolved through the incorporation of an extracellular domain, conferring greater ligand specificity to a traditional GPCR.[120]

The thyrotropin receptor is primarily expressed on the basolateral surface of thyroid follicular cells. However, TSH-R mRNA transcripts and/or protein have been identified in adipocytes, orbital connective tissue, bone, leukocytes, skin, neurons, and astrocytes.[121-127] The role of TSH-R in nonthyroid tissue has not yet been clarified, although there appears to be evidence for a role in bone remodeling, in the dermatologic manifestations of thyroid disorders, and in the ophthalmopathic manifestations of Graves' disease. Studies of the TSH-R promoter have determined that it is primarily activated by thyroid transcription factor 1 (TTF-1), a transcription factor responsible for thyroid-specific gene expression, in cooperation with CREB.[128,129,130] The ability of TTF-1 to activate TSH-R transcription is enhanced when it is phosphorylated as a result of TSH activation of the protein kinase A (PKA) cascade.[131] Contrary to this, TSH has also been shown to regulate TSH-R expression negatively through at least two mechanisms: (1) TSH results in decreased TTF-1 mRNA production and in turn decreased TSHR expression; and (2) TSH can increase expression of TR alpha 1, which then downregulates TSH-R promoter activity in a T_3-dependent manner.[131,132] Thus, TSH can positively and negatively regulate the expression of its cognate receptor; however, the major effect of TSH appears to be downregulation of TSH-R expression. The promoter for the TSH-R in rats also appears to be positively regulated by insulin through an insulin-responsive element, but it is not known which transcription factors are involved in mediating this process.[133]

Structure of Thyrotropin Receptor

Extracellular Ectodomain (A or Alpha Subunit)

There is significant homology of the transmembrane domains among the glycoprotein receptors (approximately 70%), but homology among the ectodomains is significantly lower (35% to 45%), reflecting the specificity of each receptor while maintaining the similar nature of their signaling pathways.[134,135] Exchanging the ectodomains of the receptors changes the hormone binding specificity but does not impair activation of the downstream signaling cascades. The large extracellular domain of the TSHR accounts for approximately half of the receptor and is composed of two cysteine clusters flanking a central portion made of nine leucine-rich repeats (LRRs).[136] LRRs

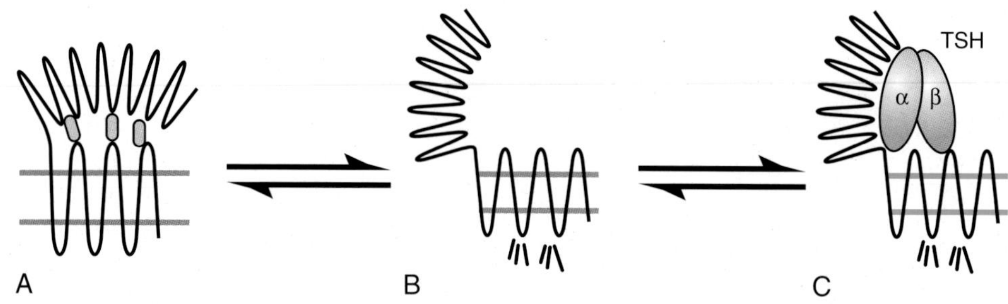

Figure 7–7 Model for thyroid-stimulating hormone receptor (TSH-R) activation. In this model, it is hypothesized that the TSH-R exists in two forms, the inactive or closed form **(A)** or the active or open form **(B)**. Binding of TSH to the receptor results in stabilization of the active conformation **(C)**, whereas the open form in the absence of ligand **(B)** results in constitutive activation of the receptor. *(Adapted from Duprez L, Parma J, Costagliola S, et al: Constitutive activation of the TSH receptor by spontaneous mutations affecting the N-terminal extracellular domain. FEBS Lett 409:469-474, 1997.)*

are found in a variety of proteins and are composed of a highly conserved consensus sequence that folds to form a beta sheet followed by an alpha helix. Modeling of the TSH-R based on the crystal structure of ribonuclease inhibitor, another LRR-containing protein, suggests that the LRRs together form a horseshoe-like structure and that TSH binds the concave surface of the ectodomain (see Fig. 7-6). The ectodomain alone is sufficient to interact with TSH with a similar affinity as the whole receptor, indicating that the transmembrane portion of the receptor does not play a significant role in hormone recognition.[137,138] The inner surface of the horseshoe, formed by the beta sheets, has been shown by mutagenesis studies to be responsible for hormone specificity.[139] Exchanging residues found on the inner surface of the receptor for those found on the inner surface of the LH receptor has resulted in a receptor with increased sensitivity to LH. In particular, three free acidic residues were shown to be important in the formation of an acidic groove in the center of the LRR domain. These three residues (positions X3 and X5 of LRR5 and X7 of LRR7) confer hormone-binding activity and specificity to the ectodomain. In addition, sulfation of a tyrosine residue (Y385) is essential for TSH binding and activation of the receptor.[140]

Transmembrane Serpentine Domain (B or Beta Subunit)

The B subunit of the receptor consists of seven hydrophobic transmembrane domains and an intracellular tail. Experiments in which most of the extracellular domain is removed have revealed that the transmembrane domain exhibits constitutive activity and does not require ligand binding for activation.[141] Spontaneous activating mutations within the extracellular domain of the receptor have been identified that abrogate an inhibitory interaction between the extracellular and transmembrane domains, resulting in increased constitutive activity.[142] These data have led to the hypothesis that in the unliganded state the ectodomain acts as an inverse agonist, inhibiting the constitutive activity of the receptor. In this model, TSH binding leads to stabilization of the full agonist conformation of the receptor (Fig. 7-7).[141-143]

Ligand-bound TSH-R results in the stimulation of adenylyl cyclase and phospholipase C cascades by interacting with Gs and Gq/11, although activation of the phospholipase C pathway requires higher concentrations of thyrotropin.[144,145] The two pathways are thought to regulate different downstream pathways; specifically, the cAMP cascade controls proliferation and differentiation of thyroid cells, whereas the inositol phosphate pathway regulates iodination and thyroid hormone synthesis. Studies of two mutations in the receptor, one in a family with resistance to TSH (see later) have shown that the two pathways are dissociable. Mutation of a tyrosine (TSH-R Y601H) in the fifth transmembrane domain has resulted in the inability of TSH to activate the phospholipase C–inositol phosphate signaling cascade, but adenylyl cyclase was only mildly reduced.[146] In addition, TSH-R Y601H was no longer constitutively active. A mutation of a distinct region of the B subunit, the third extracellular loop (TSH-R L653V), also resulted in reduced inositol phosphate signaling and reduced thyroid hormone synthesis.[147] These studies have indicated that the TSH-R may have several active conformations that allow for differential affinity to couple to Gs or Gq. Importantly, this may allow for the development of TSH analogues that preferentially activate a desired pathway.

Post-translational Modifications

Similar to thyrotropin, post-translational modifications are important in the synthesis, transport, and proper functioning of the TSH-R. Almost 40% of the mass of the extracellular domain is made of complex carbohydrates.[148] Glycosylation and the addition of complex carbohydrates can occur on six asparagine residues of the extracellular domain.[149] Although all six appear to be glycosylated in wild-type receptors, expression of a fully functional receptor is dependent on the glycosylation of at least four of the sites. Inhibition of glycosylation has resulted in improper protein folding, impaired intracellular trafficking, and reduced incorporation of the receptor into the extracellular membrane.[150]

Compared with the LH and FSH receptors, the TSH-R contains an additional 50 residues in the C-terminal portion of the ectodomain. This region is cleaved in the post-translational processing of the receptor, a process unique to the TSH-R among the glycoprotein receptors. There appear to be two intramolecular cleavage sites, resulting in the removal of a segment termed the *C peptide* (analogous to the C peptide produced in the processing of proinsulin).[151,152] However, no TSH-R C peptide has ever been isolated from cells or media expressing TSH-R, and it is likely that the resultant fragment is removed through sequential cleavage.[153] The two subunits are bound by disulfide bonds formed between the C-terminal region of the ectodomain and N-terminal portion of the transmembrane domains. The human TSH-R contains 11 cysteine residues, 8 of which are conserved in the other glycoprotein receptors.[154] Cysteine in position 41 has been identified as required for proper folding and multimerization of the receptor, suggesting that a disulfide bond at this position is a critical post-translational step in protein synthesis.[155]

There appear to be two populations of receptors on the surface of thyroid cells: cleaved, two-subunit receptors and uncleaved holoreceptors.[156] The relative proportions of cleaved and uncleaved receptors has been widely debated, with reports variously stating that the cleaved form of the receptor is either the minor or major form.[157-159] The physiologic significance of the two forms has yet to be defined, but each appears to interact with TSH with similar affinity and is activated to the same degree.[156,157,160] A protease involved in the proteolytic cleavage of the receptor was recently identified. ADAM10, a member of the disintegrin and metalloprotease (ADAM) family of metalloproteases specifically expressed in the thyroid, was shown to cleave the ectodomain.[161] The sequence recognized by ADAM10 is not the active proteolytic site, consistent with earlier studies which suggested that cleavage does not depend on a specific amino acid motif but rather a molecular ruler, in which the protein is cleaved at a fixed distance from a protease attachment site.[162] The activity of ADAM10 was increased in the presence of TSH, consistent with several reports showing that TSH enhances cleavage of the receptor.[161,163] After cleavage, a large portion of receptors lose the A subunit, termed *ectodomain shedding*, leaving behind the B subunit. This process requires receptor cleavage as well as reduction of the disulfide bridges by a protein disulfide isomerase.[164] The shed A subunit is considered to be the antigenic stimulus for the formation of the antithyrotropin receptor antibodies in Graves' disease (see later). It has been shown that there is proportionally two to three times more B subunits than A subunits on the surface of human thyroid cells.[165] This suggests that the A subunits may be lost into the bloodstream, where they may become the stimulus for autoimmune thyroid diseases.

TSH-R has been shown to form multimeric complexes on the surface of thyroid cells, a process that also occurs in other GPCRs.[166] In GPCRs, the formation of complexes is thought to regulate several processes, including protein trafficking, internalization, and signaling.[167,168] The transmembrane domain is sufficient for oligomerization. Although the ectodomain is not required, it may enhance complex formation.[169] There are conflicting results on the functional significance of TSH-R oligomerization. Recent studies have suggested that the TSH-R exists in oligomers in the inactivated state and that TSH induces dissociation of the receptors to monomers, promoting activation.[170] However, other reports have suggested that TSH-Rs are present as dimers in the inactive and active states.[169] In the latter, it was found that there is crosstalk between the monomers of the dimer. Cells were transfected with two different loss-of-function mutants; one is unable to bind TSH and the other can bind the hormone but cannot activate G protein signaling in response to binding. When the two were present together in the cells, they were able to restore the TSH signaling pathway, suggesting that they were functionally acting as a dimer. Whether TSH binding to one monomer of a pair of TSH-Rs leads to amplification of the signaling pathway is not yet known.

Thyroid Diseases Related to Inappropriate Function of the Thyrotropin Receptor

Several mechanisms of abrogating the appropriate function of the TSH-R have been identified. These include loss-of-function and gain-of-function mutations and thyroid-stimulating and thyroid-blocking antibodies. More than 50 different naturally occurring mutations have been indentified in the TSH-R (Fig. 7-8). In other glycoprotein hormone receptors, naturally occurring mutations, particularly activating mutations, are relatively rare.[171,172] These mutations have provided a unique opportunity to understand the molecular mechanisms regulating TSH-R action. Similarly, naturally occurring autoantibodies have not been identified to the LH-CG receptor and only rarely to the FSH receptor, in which they are thought to

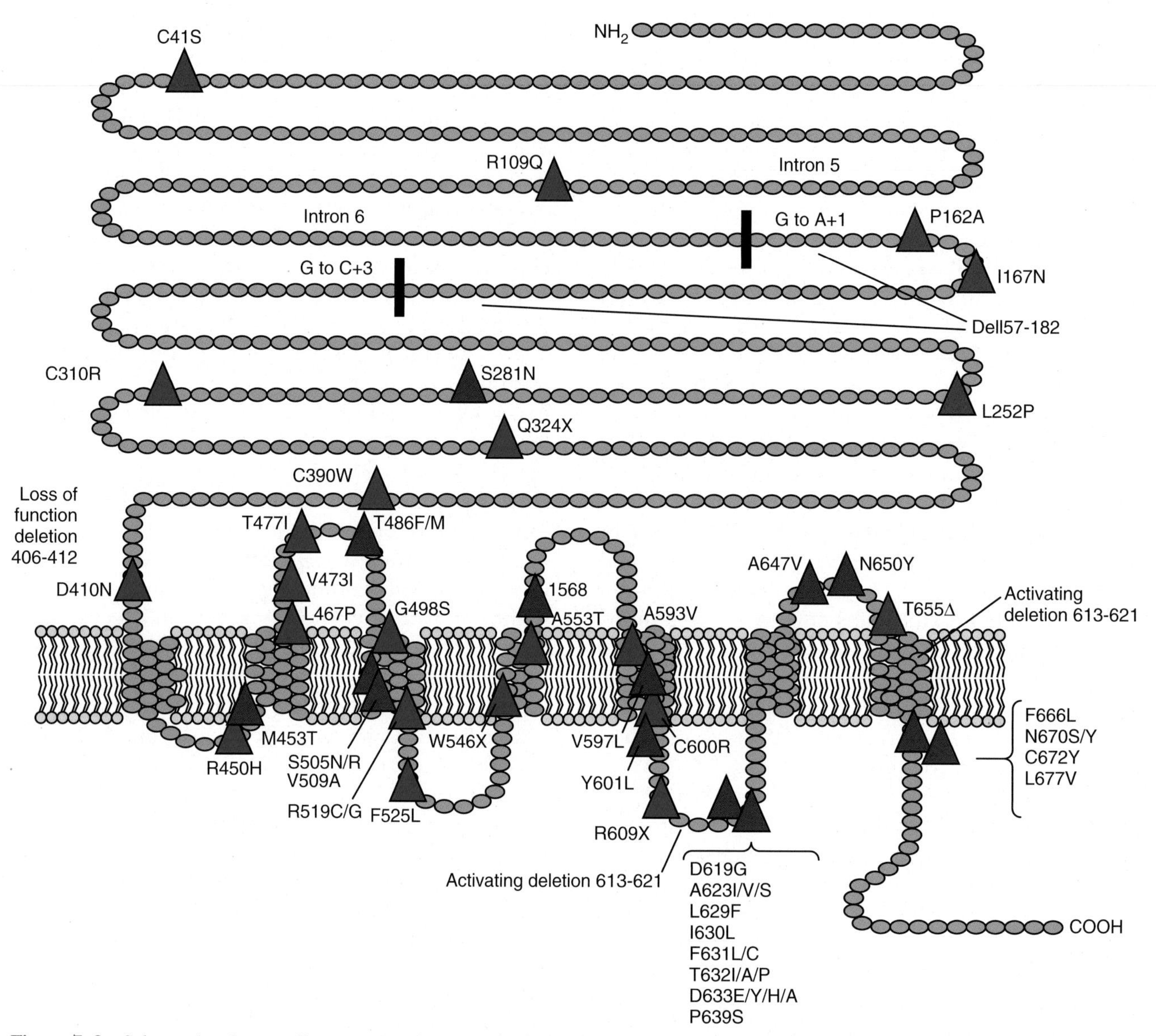

Figure 7–8 Schematic of naturally occurring thyroid-stimulating hormone receptor (TSH-R) mutations. Blue triangles identify loss-of-function exonic point mutations, red triangles identify gain-of-function mutations, and vertical bars illustrate intronic loss-of-function mutations. Positions of activating and loss-of-function deletions are also indicated by arrows. Loss-of-function mutations are widely distributed throughout the extracellular and intracellular domains, whereas gain-of-function mutations are concentrated in the intracellular domain with the exception of S281N. *(Adapted from Beck-Peccoz P, Persani L, Calebiro D, et al: Syndromes of hormone resistance in the hypothalamic-pituitary-thyroid axis. Best Pract Res Clin Endocrinol Metab 20:529-546, 2006.)*

cause premature ovarian failure. Thus, the common antigenic stimulation of the thyrotropin receptor seems to be a relatively unique feature.

Resistance to Thyrotropin

Thyrotropin resistance syndrome is primarily caused by loss-of-function mutations in the TSH-R, impairing the ability of the receptor to signal in response to TSH binding.[95] More than 30 different mutations have been identified; they reside both within the extracellular domain and the transmembrane domain and do not appear to concentrate in any particular location (see Fig. 7-8). The mutations result in a variety of receptor defects, including improper synthesis, targeting of the receptor, impaired TSH binding, and defective signaling through loss of appropriate crosstalk with downstream G proteins. The type of mutation dictates the mode of transmission (recessive versus dominant inheritance pattern), the level of receptor impairment, which can range from partial to complete resistance, and subsequently the phenotype of the disorder, ranging from mild to profound hypothyroidism.[173,174] Patients with thyrotropin resistance generally exhibit elevated TSH levels, low to normal levels of thyroid hormone, and a normal to hypoplastic thyroid gland. In profound TSH resistance, the condition is often recognized early in life because of the growth and developmental delays associated with congenital hypothyroidism. However, in patients with partial resistance, it may not be identified until later or may be found incidentally. Recently, it has been shown that some mutations can dissociate the two G protein signaling pathways (Gs from Gq/11), resulting in partial TSH resistance and isolated defects in one arm of the TSH signaling axis.[147]

Gain-of-Function Somatic Mutations

Constitutive activation of the TSH-R or the Gs secondary messenger leads to constitutive activation of adenylyl cyclase and has the potential to drive the formation of hyperfunctioning thyroid adenomas. Gain-of-function mutations of the TSH-R that constitutively activate the receptor and abrogate the need for binding to TSH have been implicated in hyperfunctioning thyroid adenomas, toxic multinodular goiters, and congenital nonautoimmune hyperthyroidism.[175,180] To date, the mutations are primarily concentrated in the transmembrane domain, particularly in the second extracellular loop, third intracellular loop, and sixth transmembrane segment (see Fig. 7-8), whereas only one activating mutation was found in the extracellular loop (Ser281Asn).[181] The third intracellular loop lies adjacent to the sixth transmembrane segment and the clustering of activating mutations in these regions suggests that they are important in maintaining the receptor in an inactive conformation. There is a direct interaction between Asp633 in the sixth transmembrane segment and Asn674 in the seventh transmembrane segment.[182] Mutations of either of these residues results in inappropriate constitutive activity. Polymorphisms have also been detected within the TSH-R gene, two in the extracellular domain (D36H and P52T) and one in the intracellular tail of the receptor (D727E).[183] The D727E polymorphism has been associated with increased cAMP activity in response to TSH stimulation and has been implicated in the pathogenesis of toxic multinodular goiter.[184] However, another study in 128 European patients failed to find an association between differences in codon 727 polymorphisms and toxic nonautoimmune thyroid disease.[185] Whether polymorphisms contribute to thyroid disease is still unclear. Activating mutations have also been identified in differentiated thyroid cancer, but whether the mutations result in malignant transformation has yet to be determined.[186,187] Therefore, at this time, the relationship between activating mutations and thyroid carcinoma is unproven, although transformation to malignancy rarely occurs in thyrotoxic adenomas.

Activation of the Thyroid-Stimulating Hormone Receptor by Chorionic Gonadotropin

The structural homology between TSH and hCG, and between their receptors, allows for the binding of hCG to the TSH-R when present in high concentrations. In high hCG states, such as during a brief period of the first trimester of pregnancy, this results in the promiscuous activation of TSH-R, thought to be a normal physiologic process of pregnancy.[188] However, prolonged expression of elevated hCG levels associated with molar pregnancy, choriocarcinoma, and hCG-secreting tumors results in thyrotoxicity. The thyrotoxic symptoms resolve after surgical removal of the pregnancy or tumor. A TSH-R mutation in the extracellular domain (K183R) has been associated with familial gestational hyperthyroidism, a condition in which women have recurrent thyrotoxic symptoms during pregnancy.[189] In these patients, the mutant receptor is more sensitive to hCG, resulting in activation of the receptor and hyperthyroidism despite normal hCG levels.

Thyrotropin Receptor–Stimulating Antibodies

In Graves' disease, autoantibodies directly bind TSHR inappropriately, activating adenylyl cyclase and inducing increased thyroid hormone secretion and thyroid proliferation.[190] Although Graves' disease patients have antibodies against several thyroid antigens, including thyroglobulin and thyroid peroxidase, it is the antibodies against TSH-R that are most critical in causing hyperproduction of thyroid hormone and thyrotoxicosis. When mice were immunized with either an adenovirus expressing the extracellular domain alone or an adenovirus expressing a holoreceptor unable to be cleaved, hyperthyroidism was more efficiently induced by the free subunit alone.[191] This supported the hypothesis that the free A subunit was the antigenic stimulus for autoantibody formation in Graves' disease patients. Further support for this hypothesis stems from studies that have shown that the epitope for the thyroid-stimulating antibodies is partially hidden in the holoreceptor but the epitope is exposed in the free A subunit.[192] Most epitopes for thyroid-stimulating hormones are located in the N-terminal region of the extracellular domain and compete with TSH for binding to the extracellular domain, but there is some heterogeneity among the antibody-binding sites and sites in the C-terminal region have been identified.[193-195] Although it is thought that TSH-R extracellular domains are shed as a result of normal processing of the receptor, thyroid-stimulating antibodies are not universally present. Therefore, there must be other factors that contribute to antibody formation and the progression to Graves' disease. Mouse studies have shown that aberrant MHC class I and class II expression, along with changes in the thyrocyte allowing it to become an antigen-presenting cell, all likely contribute to the pathogenesis of Graves' disease.[196,197]

Thyrotropin Receptor–Blocking Antibodies

TSH-R blocking antibodies bind to the receptor and prevent activation by TSH, inhibiting the receptor and resulting in chronic autoimmune hypothyroidism and, in some patients, thyroid atrophy.[198,199] These antibodies have been identified as the causative agents in some cases of Hashimoto's thyroiditis and idiopathic myxedema. In contrast to the TSH-R–stimulating antibodies, the epitope for the blocking antibodies is primarily located on the C-terminal portion of the extracellular domain.[200] TSH-R blocking antibodies have also been identified in patients with Graves' disease, in whom relative concentrations of the antibodies determine whether the patient experiences hyper- or hypothyroidism. Similarly, blocking TSHR antibodies that develop in patients with Graves' disease during pregnancy may cause fetal hypothyroidism.[201]

References

1. Pierce JG, Parsons TF: Glycoprotein hormones: Structure and function. Annu Rev Biochem 50:465-495, 1981.
2. Fiddes JC, Goodman HM: The gene encoding the common alpha subunit of the four human glycoprotein hormones. J Mol Appl Genet 1:3-18, 1981.
3. Wondisford FE, Radovick S, Moates JM, et al: Isolation and characterization of the human thyrotropin beta subunit gene. Differences in gene structure and promoter function from murine species. J Biol Chem 263:12538-12542, 1988.
4. Tatsumi K, Hayashizaki Y, Hiraoka Y, et al: The structure of the human thyrotropin beta subunit gene. Gene 73:489-497, 1988.
5. Dracopoli NC, Stanger BZ, Ito CY, et al: A genetic linkage map of 27 loci from PND to FY on the short arm of human chromosome I. Am J Hum Genet 43:462-470, 1988.
6. Takata K, Watanabe S, Hirono M, et al: The role of the carboxyl-terminal 6 amino acid extension of human TSH beta subunit. Biochem Biophys Res Commun 165:1035-1042, 1989.
7. Szkudlinski MW, Fremont V, Ronin C, Weintraub BD: Thyroid-stimulating hormone and thyroid-stimulating hormone receptor structure-function relationships. Physiol Rev 82:473-502, 2002.
8. Lapthorn AJ, Harris DC, Littlejohn A, et al: Crystal structure of human chorionic gonadotropin. Nature 369:455-461, 1994.
9. Szkudlinski MW, Te NG, Grossmann M, et al: Engineering human glycoprotein hormone superactive analogues. Nat Biotechnol 14:1257-1263, 1996.
10. Sun PD, Davies DR: The cystine-knot growth-factor superfamily. Annu Rev Biophys Biomol Struct 24:269-291, 1995.
11. Oefner C, D'Arcy A, Winkler FK, et al: Crystal structure of human platelet-derived growth factor BB. EMBO J 11:3921-3926, 1992.
12. Schlunegger MP, Grutter MG: Refined crystal structure of human transforming growth factor beta 2 at 1.95 A resolution. J Mol Biol 231:445-458, 1993.
13. Grossmann M, Szkudlinski MW, Wong R, et al: Substitution of the seat-belt region of the thyroid-stimulating hormone TSH beta subunit with the corresponding regions of choriogonadotropin or follitropin confers luteotropic but not follitropic activity to chimeric TSH. J Biol Chem 272:15532-15540, 1997.
14. Grossmann M, Szkudlinski MW, Dias JA, et al: D. Site-directed mutagenesis of amino acids 33-44 of the common alpha-subunit reveals different structural requirements for heterodimer expression among the glycoprotein hormones and suggests that cyclic adenosine 3′,5′-monophosphate production and growth promotion are potentially dissociable functions of human thyrotropin. Mol Endocrinol 10:769-779, 1996.
15. Hayashizaki Y, Hiraoka Y, Endo, et al: Thyroid-stimulating hormone TSH deficiency caused by a single base substitution in the CAGYC region of the beta-subunit. EMBO J 8:2291-2296, 1989.
16. Hayashizaki Y, Hiraoka Y, Tatsumi K, et al: Deoxyribonucleic acid analyses of five families with familial inherited thyroid stimulating hormone deficiency. J Clin Endocrinol Metab 71:792-796, 1990.
17. Sertedaki A, Papadimitriou A, Voutetakis A, et al: Low TSH congenital hypothyroidism: Identification of a novel mutation of the TSH beta subunit gene in one sporadic case C85R and of mutation Q49stop in two siblings with congenital hypothyroidism. Pediatr Res 52:935-941, 2002.
18. Dacou-Voutetakis C, Feltquate DM, Drakopoulou M, et al: Familial hypothyroidism caused by a nonsense mutation in the thyroid-stimulating hormone beta subunit gene. Am J Hum Genet 46:988-993, 1990.
19. Bonomi M, Proverbio MC, Weber G, et al: Hyperplastic pituitary gland, high serum glycoprotein hormone alpha-subunit, and variable circulating thyrotropin TSH levels as hallmark of central hypothyroidism due to mutations of the TSH beta gene. J Clin Endocrinol Metab 86:1600-1604, 2001.
20. Vuissoz JM, Deladoey J, Buyukgebiz A, et al: New autosomal recessive mutation of the TSH-beta subunit gene causing central isolated hypothyroidism. J Clin Endocrinol Metab 86:4468-4471, 2001.

21. Morales AE, Shi JD, Wang CY, et al: Novel TSH beta subunit gene mutation causing congenital central hypothyroidism in a newborn male. J Pediatr Endocrinol Metab 17:355-359, 2004.
22. Medeiros-Neto G, Herodotou DT, Rajan S, et al: A circulating biologically inactive thyrotropin caused by a mutation in the beta subunit gene. J Clin Invest 97:1250-1256, 1996.
23. Doeker BM, Pfaffle RW, Pohlenz J, Andler W: Congenital central hypothyroidism due to a homozygous mutation in the thyrotropin beta subunit gene follows an autosomal recessive inheritance. J Clin Endocrinol Metab 83:1762-1765, 1998.
24. Partsch CJ, Riepe FG, Krone N, et al: Initially elevated TSH and congenital central hypothyroidism due to a homozygous mutation of the TSH beta subunit gene: Case report and review of the literature. Exp Clin Endocrinol Diabetes 114:227-234, 2006.
25. Brumm H, Pfeufer A, Biebermann H, et al: Congenital central hypothyroidism due to homozygous thyrotropin beta 313 delta T mutation is caused by a founder effect. J Clin Endocrinol Metab 87:4811-4816, 2002.
26. Biebermann H, Liesenkotter KP, Emeis M, et al: Severe congenital hypothyroidism due to a homozygous mutation of the betaTSH gene. Pediatr Res 46:170-173, 1999.
27. Heinrichs C, Parma J, Scherberg NH, et al: Congenital central isolated hypothyroidism caused by a homozygous mutation in the TSH-beta subunit gene. Thyroid 10:387-391, 2000.
28. Deladoey J, Vuissoz JM, Domene HM, et al: Congenital secondary hypothyroidism due to a mutation C105Vfs114X thyrotropin-beta mutation: Genetic study of five unrelated families from Switzerland and Argentina. Thyroid 13:553-559, 2003.
29. Domene HM, Gruneiro-Papendieck L, Chiesa A, et al: The C105fs114X is the prevalent thyrotropin beta subunit gene mutation in Argentinean patients with congenital central hypothyroidism. Horm Res 61:41-46, 2004.
30. McDermott MT, Haugen BR, Black JN, et al: Congenital isolated central hypothyroidism caused by a "hot spot" mutation in the thyrotropin-beta gene. Thyroid 12:1141-1146, 2002.
31. Pohlenz J, Dumitrescu A, Aumann U, et al: Congenital secondary hypothyroidism caused by exon skipping due to a homozygous donor splice site mutation in the TSH beta subunit gene. J Clin Endocrinol Metab 87:336-339, 2002.
32. Suganuma N, Matzuk MM, Boime I: Elimination of disulfide bonds affects assembly and secretion of the human chorionic gonadotropin beta subunit. J Biol Chem 264:19302-19307, 1989.
33. Karges B, LeHeup B, Schoenle E, et al: Compound heterozygous and homozygous mutations of the TSHbeta gene as a cause of congenital central hypothyroidism in Europe. Horm Res 62:149-155, 2004.
34. Stannard BS, Gesundheit N, Ronin C, et al: Differential carbohydrate processing and secretion of thyrotropin and free alpha subunit. Effects of 1-deoxynojirimycin. J Biol Chem 263:8309-8317, 1988.
35. Stannard BS, Gesundheit N, Thotakura NR, et al: Differential effect of inhibitors of oligosaccharide processing on the secretion of thyrotropin from dispersed rodent pituitary cells. Biochem Biophys Res Commun 165:788-794, 1989.
36. Green ED, Baenziger JU: Asparagine-linked oligosaccharides on lutropin, follitropin, and thyrotropin. II. Distributions of sulfated and sialylated oligosaccharides on bovine, ovine, and human pituitary glycoprotein hormones. J Biol Chem 263:36-44, 1988.
37. Green ED, Baenziger JU: Asparagine-linked oligosaccharides on lutropin, follitropin, and thyrotropin. I. Structural elucidation of the sulfated and sialylated oligosaccharides on bovine, ovine, and human pituitary glycoprotein hormones. J Biol Chem 263:25-35, 1988.
38. Weintraub BD, Stannard BS, Meyers L: Glycosylation of thyroid-stimulating hormone in pituitary tumor cells: Influence of high mannose oligosaccharide units on subunit aggregation, combination, and intracellular degradation. Endocrinology 112:1331-1345,1983.
39. Berman MI, Thomas CG Jr, Manjunath P, et al: The role of the carbohydrate moiety in thyrotropin action. Biochem Biophys Res Commun 133:680-687, 1985.
40. Thotakura NR, LiCalz L, Weintraub BD: The role of carbohydrate in thyrotropin action assessed by a novel approach using enzymatic deglycosylation. J Biol Chem 265:11527-11534, 1990.
41. Sairam MR, Bhargavi GN: A role for glycosylation of the alpha subunit in transduction of biological signal in glycoprotein hormones. Science 229: 65-67, 1985.
42. Papandreou MJ, Sergi I, Medri G, et al: Differential effect of glycosylation on the expression of antigenic and bioactive domains in human thyrotropin. Mol Cell Endocrinol 78:137-150, 1991.
43. Szkudlinski MW, Thotakura NR, Weintraub BD: Subunit-specific functions of N-linked oligosaccharides in human thyrotropin: Role of terminal residues of alpha- and beta subunit oligosaccharides in metabolic clearance and bioactivity. Proc Natl Acad Sci U S A 92:9062-9066, 1995.
44. Joshi L, Murata Y, Wondisford FE, et al: Recombinant thyrotropin containing a beta subunit chimera with the human chorionic gonadotropin-beta carboxy-terminus is biologically active, with a prolonged plasma half-life: Role of carbohydrate in bioactivity and metabolic clearance. Endocrinology 136:3839-3848, 1995.
45. Szkudlinski MW, Thotakura NR, Tropea JE, et al: Asparagine-linked oligosaccharide structures determine clearance and organ distribution of pituitary and recombinant thyrotropin. Endocrinology 136:3325-3330, 1995.

46. Grossmann M, Szkudlinski MW, Tropea JE, et al: Expression of human thyrotropin in cell lines with different glycosylation patterns combined with mutagenesis of specific glycosylation sites. Characterization of a novel role for the oligosaccharides in the in vitro and in vivo bioactivity. J Biol Chem 270:29378-29385, 1995.
47. Papandreou MJ, Persani L, Asteria C, et al: Variable carbohydrate structures of circulating thyrotropin as studied by lectin affinity chromatography in different clinical conditions. J Clin Endocrinol Metab 77:393-398, 1993.
48. Oliveira JH, Barbosa ER, Kasamatsu T, Abucham J: Evidence for thyroid hormone as a positive regulator of serum thyrotropin bioactivity. J Clin Endocrinol Metab 92:3108-3113, 2007.
49. Gyves PW, Gesundheit N, Thotakura NR, et al: Changes in the sialylation and sulfation of secreted thyrotropin in congenital hypothyroidism. Proc Natl Acad Sci U S A 87:3792-3796, 1990.
50. Helton TE, Magner JA: Sialyltransferase messenger ribonucleic acid increases in thyrotrophs of hypothyroid mice: An in situ hybridization study. Endocrinology 134:2347-2353, 1994.
51. Helton TE, Magner JA: Beta-galactoside alpha-2,3-sialyltransferase messenger RNA increases in thyrotrophs of hypothyroid mice. Thyroid 5:315-317, 1995.
52. Gesundheit N, Magner JA, Chen T, Weintraub BD: Differential sulfation and sialylation of secreted mouse thyrotropin TSH subunits: Regulation by TSH-releasing hormone. Endocrinology 119:455-463, 1986.
53. Weintraub BD, Gesundheit N, Taylor T, Gyves PW: Effect of TRH on TSH glycosylation and biological action. Ann N Y Acad Sci 553:205-213, 1989.
54. Lee HY, Suhl J, Pekary AE, Hershman JM: Secretion of thyrotropin with reduced concanavalin A-binding activity in patients with severe nonthyroid illness. J Clin Endocrinol Metab 65:942-945, 1987.
55. Magner J, Klibanski A, Fein H, et al: Ricin and lentil lectin-affinity chromatography reveals oligosaccharide heterogeneity of thyrotropin secreted by 12 human pituitary tumors. Metabolism 41:1009-1015, 1992.
56. Francis TB, Smallridge RC, Kane J, Magner JA: Octreotide changes serum thyrotropin TSH glycoisomer distribution as assessed by lectin chromatography in a TSH macroadenoma patient. J Clin Endocrinol Metab 77:183-187, 1993.
57. Sergi I, Medri G, Papandreou MJ, et al: Polymorphism of thyrotropin and alpha subunit in human pituitary adenomas. J Endocrinol Invest 16:45-55, 1993.
58. Gyves PW, Gesundheit N, Stannard BS, et al: Alterations in the glycosylation of secreted thyrotropin during ontogenesis. Analysis of sialylated and sulfated oligosaccharides. J Biol Chem 264:6104-6110, 1989.
59. Persani L, Borgato S, Romoli R, et al: Changes in the degree of sialylation of carbohydrate chains modify the biological properties of circulating thyrotropin isoforms in various physiological and pathological states. J Clin Endocrinol Metab 83:2486-2489, 1998.
60. Schaaf L, Leiprecht A, Saji M, et al: Glycosylation variants of human TSH selectively activate signal transduction pathways. Mol Cell Endocrinol 132:185-194, 1997.
61. Carr FE, Fisher CU, Fein HG, Smallridge RC: Thyrotropin-releasing hormone stimulates c-jun and c-fos messenger ribonucleic acid levels: Implications for calcium mobilization and protein kinase-C activation. Endocrinology 133:1700-1707, 1993.
62. Carr FE, Galloway RJ, Reid AH, et al: Thyrotropin-releasing hormone regulation of thyrotropin beta subunit gene expression involves intracellular calcium and protein kinase C. Biochemistry 30:3721-3728, 1991.
63. Carr FE, Shupnik MA, Burnside J, Chin WW: Thyrotropin-releasing hormone stimulates the activity of the rat thyrotropin beta subunit gene promoter transfected into pituitary cells. Mol Endocrinol 3:717-724, 1989.
64. Gershengorn MC: Mechanism of signal transduction by TRH. Ann N Y Acad Sci 553:191-196, 1989.
65. Hashimoto K, Zanger K, Hollenberg AN, et al: cAMP response element-binding protein-binding protein mediates thyrotropin-releasing hormone signaling on thyrotropin subunit genes. J Biol Chem 275:33365-33372, 2000.
66. Shupnik MA, Greenspan SL, Ridgway EC: Transcriptional regulation of thyrotropin subunit genes by thyrotropin-releasing hormone and dopamine in pituitary cell culture. J Biol Chem 261:12675-12679, 1986.
67. Steinfelder HJ, Radovick S, Wondisford FE: Hormonal regulation of the thyrotropin beta subunit gene by phosphorylation of the pituitary-specific transcription factor Pit-1. Proc Natl Acad Sci U S A 89:5942-5945, 1992.
68. Gordon DF, Lewis SR, Haugen BR, et al: Pit-1 and GATA-2 interact and functionally cooperate to activate the thyrotropin beta subunit promoter. J Biol Chem 272:24339-24347, 1997.
69. Kim KK, Song SB, Kang KI, et al: Activation of the thyroid-stimulating hormone beta subunit gene by LIM homeodomain transcription factor Lhx2. Endocrinology 148:3468-34676, 2007.
70. Bach I, Rhodes SJ, Pearse RV 2nd, et al: P-Lim, a LIM homeodomain factor, is expressed during pituitary organ and cell commitment and synergizes with Pit-1. Proc Natl Acad Sci U S A 92: 2720-2724, 1995.
71. Kelberman D, Dattani MT: The role of transcription factors implicated in anterior pituitary development in the aetiology of congenital hypopituitarism. Ann Med 38:560-577, 2006.

72. Cohen LE, Wondisford FE, Salvatoni A, et al: A "hot spot" in the Pit-1 gene responsible for combined pituitary hormone deficiency: Clinical and molecular correlates. J Clin Endocrinol Metab 80:679-684, 1995.
73. Yamada M, Saga Y, Shibusawa N, et al: Tertiary hypothyroidism and hyperglycemia in mice with targeted disruption of the thyrotropin-releasing hormone gene. Proc Natl Acad Sci U S A 94:10862-10867, 1997.
74. Collu R: Genetic aspects of central hypothyroidism. J Endocrinol Invest 23:125-134, 2000.
75. Collu R, Tang J, Castagne J, et al: A novel mechanism for isolated central hypothyroidism: Inactivating mutations in the thyrotropin-releasing hormone receptor gene. J Clin Endocrinol Metab 82:1561-1565, 1997.
76. Nikrodhanond AA, Ortiga-Carvalho TM, Shibusawa N, et al: Dominant role of thyrotropin-releasing hormone in the hypothalamic-pituitary-thyroid axis. J Biol Chem 281:5000-5007, 2006.
77. Shupnik MA, Chi WW, Habener JF, Ridgway EC: Transcriptional regulation of the thyrotropin subunit genes by thyroid hormone. J Biol Chem 260:2900-2903, 1985.
78. Gurr JA, Kourides IA: Thyroid hormone regulation of thyrotropin alpha- and beta subunit gene transcription. DNA 4:301-307, 1985.
79. Segerson TP, Kauer J, Wolfe HC, et al: Thyroid hormone regulates TRH biosynthesis in the paraventricular nucleus of the rat hypothalamus. Science 238:78-80, 1987.
80. Taylor T, Wondisford FE, Blaine T, Weintraub BD: The paraventricular nucleus of the hypothalamus has a major role in thyroid hormone feedback regulation of thyrotropin synthesis and secretion. Endocrinology 126:317-324, 1990.
81. Lazar MA: Thyroid hormone receptors: Multiple forms, multiple possibilities. Endocr Rev 14:184-193, 1993.
82. Oetting A, Yen PM: New insights into thyroid hormone action. Best Pract Res Clin Endocrinol Metab 21:193-208, 2007.
83. Bradley DJ, Towle HC, Young WS 3rd: Alpha and beta thyroid hormone receptor TR gene expression during auditory neurogenesis: Evidence for TR isoform-specific transcriptional regulation in vivo. Proc Natl Acad Sci U S A 91:439-443, 1994.
84. Jones I, Ng L, Liu H, Forrest D: An intron control region differentially regulates expression of thyroid hormone receptor beta2 in the cochlea, pituitary, and cone photoreceptors. Mol Endocrinol 21:1108-1119, 2007.
85. Gauthier K, Chassande O, Plateroti M, et al: Different functions for the thyroid hormone receptors TR alpha and TR beta in the control of thyroid hormone production and post-natal development. EMBO J 18:623-631, 1999.
86. Abel ED, Boers ME, Pazos-Moura C, et al: Divergent roles for thyroid hormone receptor beta isoforms in the endocrine axis and auditory system. J Clin Invest 104:291-300, 1999.
87. Abel ED, Kaulbach HC, Campos-Barros A, et al: Novel insight from transgenic mice into thyroid hormone resistance and the regulation of thyrotropin. J Clin Invest 103:271-279, 1999.
88. Abel ED, Ahima RS, Boers ME, et al: Critical role for thyroid hormone receptor $beta_2$ in the regulation of paraventricular thyrotropin-releasing hormone neurons. J Clin Invest 107:1017-1023, 2001.
89. Abel ED, Moura EG, Ahima RS, et al: Dominant inhibition of thyroid hormone action selectively in the pituitary of thyroid hormone receptor-beta null mice abolishes the regulation of thyrotropin by thyroid hormone. Mol Endocrinol 17:1767-1776, 2003.
90. Shibusawa N, Hollenberg AN, Wondisford FE: Thyroid hormone receptor DNA binding is required for both positive and negative gene regulation. J Biol Chem 278:732-738, 2003.
91. Shibusawa N, Hashimoto K, Nikrodhanond A, et al: Thyroid hormone action in the absence of thyroid hormone receptor DNA-binding in vivo. J Clin Invest 112:588-597, 2003.
92. Bodenner DL, Mroczynski MA, Weintraub BD, et al: A detailed functional and structural analysis of a major thyroid hormone inhibitory element in the human thyrotropin beta subunit gene. J Biol Chem 266:21666-21673, 1991.
93. Hollenberg AN, Monden T, Flynn TR, et al: The human thyrotropin-releasing hormone gene is regulated by thyroid hormone through two distinct classes of negative thyroid hormone response elements. Mol Endocrinol 9:540-550, 1995.
94. Olateju TO, Vanderpump MP: Thyroid hormone resistance. Ann Clin Biochem 43:431-440, 2006.
95. Beck-Peccoz P, Persani L, Calebiro D, et al: Syndromes of hormone resistance in the hypothalamic-pituitary-thyroid axis. Best Pract Res Clin Endocrinol Metab 20:529-546, 2006.
96. Wilber JF, Utiger RD: The effect of glucocorticoids on thyrotropin secretion. J Clin Invest 48:2096-2103, 1969.
97. Re RN, Kourides IA, Ridgway EC, et al: The effect of glucocorticoid administration on human pituitary secretion of thyrotropin and prolactin. J Clin Endocrinol Metab 43:338-346, 1976.
98. Inagaki K, Otsuka F, Miyoshi T, et al: Reversible pituitary dysfunction in a patient with Cushing's syndrome discovered as adrenal incidentaloma. Endocr J 51:201-206, 2004.
99. Ahlquist JA, Franklyn JA, Ramsden DB, Sheppard MC: Regulation of alpha and thyrotropin-beta subunit mRNA levels by androgens in the female rat. J Mol Endocrinol 5:1-6, 1990.

100. Ahlquist JA, Franklyn JA, Wood DF, et al: Hormonal regulation of thyrotropin synthesis and secretion. Horm Metab Res Suppl 17:86-89, 1987.
101. Franklyn JA, Wood DF, Balfour NJ, et al: Modulation by oestrogen of thyroid hormone effects on thyrotropin gene expression. J Endocrinol 115: 53-59, 1987.
102. Cooper DS, Klibanski A, Ridgway EC: Dopaminergic modulation of TSH and its subunits: In vivo and in vitro studies. Clin Endocrinol Oxf 18:265-275, 1983.
103. Foord SM, Peters JR, Dieguez C, et al: Hypothyroid pituitary cells in culture: An analysis of thyrotropin and prolactin responses to dopamine DA and DA receptor binding. Endocrinology 115: 407-415, 1984.
104. Refetoff S, Fang VS, Rapoport B, Friesen HG: Interrelationships in the regulation of TSH and prolactin secretion in man: Effects of L-dopa, TRH and thyroid hormone in various combinations. J Clin Endocrinol Metab 38:450-457, 1974.
105. Felt V, Nedvdkova J: Effect of bromocryptine on the secretion of thyrotropic hormone TSH, prolactin Pr, human growth hormone HGH, thyroxine T_4 and triiodothyroxine T_3 in hypothyroidism. Horm Metab Res 9:274-277, 1977.
106. Lee E, Chen P, Rao H, et al: Effect of acute high dose dobutamine administration on serum thyrotrophin TSH. Clin Endocrinol Oxf 50:487-492, 1999.
107. Scanlon MF, Weightman DR, Shale DJ, et al: Dopamine is a physiological regulator of thyrotrophin TSH secretion in normal man. Clin Endocrinol Oxf 10:7-15, 1979.
108. Wondisford FE, Usala SJ, DeCherney GS, et al: Cloning of the human thyrotropin beta subunit gene and transient expression of biologically active human thyrotropin after gene transfection. Mol Endocrinol 2:32-39, 1988.
109. Watanabe S, Hayashizaki Y, Endo Y, et al: Production of human thyroid-stimulating hormone in Chinese hamster ovary cells. Biochem Biophys Res Commun 149:1149-1155, 1987.
110. Thotakura NR, Desai RK, Bates LG, et al: Biological activity and metabolic clearance of a recombinant human thyrotropin produced in Chinese hamster ovary cells. Endocrinology 128: 341-348, 1991.
111. Szkudlinski MW, Thotakura NR, Bucci I, et al: Purification and characterization of recombinant human thyrotropin TSH isoforms produced by Chinese hamster ovary cells: The role of sialylation and sulfation in TSH bioactivity. Endocrinology 133:1490-1503, 1993.
112. Ribela MT, Bianco AC, Bartolini P: The use of recombinant human thyrotropin produced by Chinese hamster ovary cells for the preparation of immunoassay reagents. J Clin Endocrinol Metab 81:249-256, 1996.
113. Duntas LH, Cooper DS: Review on the occasion of a decade of recombinant human TSH: Prospects and novel uses. Thyroid 18:509-516, 2008.
114. Rousseau-Merck MF, Misrahi M, Loosfelt H, et al: Assignment of the human thyroid stimulating hormone receptor TSHR gene to chromosome 14q31. Genomics 8:233-236, 1990.
115. Frazier AL, Robbins LS, Stork PJ, et al: Isolation of TSH and LH/CG receptor cDNAs from human thyroid: Regulation by tissue specific splicing. Mol Endocrinol 4:1264-1276, 1990.
116. Parmentier M, Libert F, Maenhaut C, et al: Molecular cloning of the thyrotropin receptor. Science 246:1620-1622, 1989.
117. Misrahi M, Loosfelt H, Atger M, et al: Cloning, sequencing and expression of human TSH receptor. Biochem Biophys Res Commun 166:394-403, 1990.
118. Nagayama Y, Kaufman KD, Seto P, Rapoport B: Molecular cloning, sequence and functional expression of the cDNA for the human thyrotropin receptor. Biochem Biophys Res Commun 165:1184-1190, 1989.
119. Gross B, Misrahi M, Sar S, Milgrom E: Composite structure of the human thyrotropin receptor gene. Biochem Biophys Res Commun 177: 679-687, 1991.
120. Farid NR, Szkudlinski MW: Minireview: Structural and functional evolution of the thyrotropin receptor. Endocrinology 145:4048-4057, 2004.
121. Crisp MS, Lane C, Halliwell M, et al: Thyrotropin receptor transcripts in human adipose tissue. J Clin Endocrinol Metab 82:2003-2005, 1997.
122. Bahn RS: Thyrotropin receptor expression in orbital adipose/connective tissues from patients with thyroid-associated ophthalmopathy. Thyroid 12:193-195, 2002.
123. Sorisky A, Bell A, Gagnon A: TSH receptor in adipose cells. Horm Metab Res 32:468-474, 2000.
124. Klein JR: Physiological relevance of thyroid stimulating hormone and thyroid stimulating hormone receptor in tissues other than the thyroid. Autoimmunity 36:417-421, 2003.
125. Abe E, Marians RC, Yu W, et al: TSH is a negative regulator of skeletal remodeling. Cell 115:151-162, 2003.
126. Crisanti P, Omri B, Hughes E, et al: The expression of thyrotropin receptor in the brain. Endocrinology 142:812-822, 2001.
127. Slominski A, Wortsman J, Kohn L, et al: Expression of hypothalamic-pituitary-thyroid axis related genes in the human skin. J Invest Dermatol 119:1449-1455, 2002.
128. Ohmori M, Shimura H, Shimura Y, et al: Characterization of an upstream thyroid transcription factor-1-binding site in the thyrotropin receptor promoter. Endocrinology 136:269-282, 1995.
129. Civitareale D, Castelli MP, Falasca P, Saiardi A: Thyroid transcription factor 1 activates the promoter of the thyrotropin receptor gene. Mol Endocrinol 7:1589-1595, 1993.
130. Saiardi A, Falasca P, Civitareale D: Synergistic transcriptional activation of the thyrotropin receptor promoter by cyclic AMP-responsive-element-binding protein and thyroid transcription factor 1. Biochem J 310(Pt 2):491-496, 1995.

131. Shimura H, Okajima F, Ikuyama S, et al: Thyroid-specific expression and cyclic adenosine 3′,5′-monophosphate autoregulation of the thyrotropin receptor gene involves thyroid transcription factor-1. Mol Endocrinol 8:1049-1069, 1994.
132. Saiardi A, Falasca P, Civitareale D: The thyroid hormone inhibits the thyrotropin receptor promoter activity: Evidence for a short loop regulation. Biochem Biophys Res Commun 205:230-237, 1994.
133. Shimura Y, Shimura H, Ohmori M, et al: Identification of a novel insulin-responsive element in the rat thyrotropin receptor promoter. J Biol Chem 269:31908-31914, 1994.
134. Braun T, Schofield PR, Sprengel R: Amino-terminal leucine-rich repeats in gonadotropin receptors determine hormone selectivity. EMBO J 10:1885-1890, 1991.
135. Rapoport B, Chazenbalk GD, Jaume JC, McLachlan SM: The thyrotropin TSH receptor: Interaction with TSH and autoantibodies. Endocr Rev 19:673-716, 1998.
136. Kajava AV, Vassart G, Wodak SJ: Modeling of the three-dimensional structure of proteins with the typical leucine-rich repeats. Structure 3:867-877, 1995.
137. Da Costa CR, Johnstone AP: Production of the thyrotrophin receptor extracellular domain as a glycosylphosphatidylinositol-anchored membrane protein and its interaction with thyrotropin and autoantibodies. J Biol Chem 273:11874-11880, 1998.
138. Seetharamaiah GS, Kurosky A, Desai RK, et al: A recombinant extracellular domain of the thyrotropin TSH receptor binds TSH in the absence of membranes. Endocrinology 134:549-554, 1994.
139. Smits G, Campillo M, Govaerts C, et al: Glycoprotein hormone receptors: Determinants in leucine-rich repeats responsible for ligand specificity. EMBO J 22:2692-2703, 2003.
140. Costagliola S, Panneels V, Bonomi M, et al: Tyrosine sulfation is required for agonist recognition by glycoprotein hormone receptors. EMBO J 21:504-513, 2002.
141. Zhang M, Tong KP, Fremont V, et al: The extracellular domain suppresses constitutive activity of the transmembrane domain of the human TSH receptor: Implications for hormone-receptor interaction and antagonist design. Endocrinology 141:3514-3517, 2000.
142. Duprez L, Parma J, Costagliola S, et al: Constitutive activation of the TSH receptor by spontaneous mutations affecting the N-terminal extracellular domain. FEBS Lett 409:469-474, 1997.
143. Vlaeminck-Guillem V, Ho SC, Rodien P, et al: Activation of the cAMP pathway by the TSH receptor involves switching of the ectodomain from a tethered inverse agonist to an agonist. Mol Endocrinol 16:736-746, 2002.
144. Laurent E, Mockel J, Van Sande J: Dual activation by thyrotropin of the phospholipase C and cyclic AMP cascades in human thyroid. Mol Cell Endocrinol 52:273-278, 1987.
145. Allgeier A, Offermanns S, Van Sande J, et al: The human thyrotropin receptor activates G-proteins Gs and Gq/11. J Biol Chem 269:13733-13735, 1994.
146. Biebermann H, Schoneberg T, Schulz A, et al: A conserved tyrosine residue Y601 in transmembrane domain 5 of the human thyrotropin receptor serves as a molecular switch to determine G-protein coupling. FASEB J 12:1461-1471, 1998.
147. Grasberger H, Van Sande J, Hag-Dahood Mahameed A, Tenenbaum-Rakover Y: A familial thyrotropin TSH receptor mutation provides in vivo evidence that the inositol phosphates/Ca^{2+} cascade mediates TSH action on thyroid hormone synthesis. J Clin Endocrinol Metab 92:2816-2820, 2007.
148. Rapoport B, McLachlan SM, Kakinuma A, Chazenbalk GD: Critical relationship between autoantibody recognition and thyrotropin receptor maturation as reflected in the acquisition of complex carbohydrate. J Clin Endocrinol Metab 81:2525-2533, 1996.
149. Nagayama Y, Nishihara E, Namba H, et al: Identification of the sites of asparagine-linked glycosylation on the human thyrotropin receptor and studies on their role in receptor function and expression. J Pharmacol Exp Ther 295:404-409, 2000.
150. Nagayama Y, Namba H, Yokoyama N, et al: Role of asparagine-linked oligosaccharides in protein folding, membrane targeting, and thyrotropin and autoantibody binding of the human thyrotropin receptor. J Biol Chem 273:33423-33428, 1998.
151. Chazenbalk GD, Tanaka K, Nagayama Y, et al: Evidence that the thyrotropin receptor ectodomain contains not one, but two, cleavage sites. Endocrinology 138:2893-2899, 1997.
152. Tanaka K, Chazenbalk GD, McLachlan SM, Rapoport B: Thyrotropin receptor cleavage at site 1 does not involve a specific amino acid motif but instead depends on the presence of the unique, 50 amino acid insertion. J Biol Chem 273:1959-1963, 1998.
153. de Bernard S, Misrahi M, Huet JC, et al: Sequential cleavage and excision of a segment of the thyrotropin receptor ectodomain. J Biol Chem 274:101-107, 1999.
154. Kursawe R, Paschke R: Modulation of TSHR signaling by posttranslational modifications. Trends Endocrinol Metab 18:199-207, 2007.
155. Graves PN, Vlase H, Davies TF: Folding of the recombinant human thyrotropin TSH receptor extracellular domain: Identification of folded monomeric and tetrameric complexes that bind TSH receptor autoantibodies. Endocrinology 136:521-527, 1995.
156. Furmaniak J, Hashim FA, Buckland PR, et al: Photoaffinity labelling of the TSH receptor on FRTL5 cells. FEBS Lett 215:316-322, 1987.
157. Russo D, Chazenbalk GD, Nagayama Y, et al: A new structural model for the thyrotropin TSH receptor, as determined by covalent cross-linking of TSH to the recombinant receptor in intact cells: Evidence for a single polypeptide chain. Mol Endocrinol 5:1607-1612, 1987.

158. Chen CR, Chazenbalk GD, Wawrowsky KA, et al: Evidence that human thyroid cells express uncleaved, single-chain thyrotropin receptors on their surface. Endocrinology 147:3107-3113, 2006.
159. Misrahi M, Ghine N, Sar S, et al: Processing of the precursors of the human thyroid-stimulating hormone receptor in various eukaryotic cells (human thyrocytes, transfected L cells and baculovirus-infected insect cells). Eur J Biochem 222:711-719, 1994.
160. Vassart G, Costagliola S: A physiological role for the posttranslational cleavage of the thyrotropin receptor? Endocrinology 145:1-3, 2004.
161. Kaczur V, Puskas LG, Nagy ZU, et al: Cleavage of the human thyrotropin receptor by ADAM10 is regulated by thyrotropin. J Mol Recognit 20:392-404, 2007.
162. Tanaka K, Chazenbalk GD, McLachlan SM, Rapoport B: Evidence that cleavage of the thyrotropin receptor involves a "molecular ruler" mechanism: Deletion of amino acid residues 305-320 causes a spatial shift in cleavage site 1 independent of amino acid motif. Endocrinology 141:3573-3577, 2000.
163. Latif R, Ando T, Davies TF: Monomerization as a prerequisite for intramolecular cleavage and shedding of the thyrotropin receptor. Endocrinology 145:5580-5588, 2004.
164. Couet J, de Bernard S, Loosfelt H, et al: Cell surface protein disulfide-isomerase is involved in the shedding of human thyrotropin receptor ectodomain. Biochemistry 35:14800-14805, 1996.
165. Loosfelt H, Pichon C, Jolivet A, et al: Two-subunit structure of the human thyrotropin receptor. Proc Natl Acad Sci U S A. 89:3765-3769, 1992.
166. Graves PN, Vlase H, Bobovnikova Y, Davies TF: Multimeric complex formation by the thyrotropin receptor in solubilized thyroid membranes. Endocrinology 137:3915-3920, 1996.
167. Gomes I, Jordan BA, Gupta A, et al: G protein coupled receptor dimerization: Implications in modulating receptor function. J Mol Med 79:226-242, 2001.
168. Rios CD, Jordan BA, Gomes I, Devi LA: G-protein-coupled receptor dimerization: Modulation of receptor function. Pharmacol Ther 92:71-87, 2001.
169. Urizar E, Montanelli L, Loy T, et al: Glycoprotein hormone receptors: Link between receptor homodimerization and negative cooperativity. EMBO J 24:1954-1964, 2005.
170. Latif R, Graves P, Davies TF: Ligand-dependent inhibition of oligomerization at the human thyrotropin receptor. J Biol Chem 277:45059-45067, 2002.
171. Themmen APN, Huhtaniemi IT: Mutations of gonadotropins and gonadotropin receptors: Elucidating the physiology and pathophysiology of pituitary-gonadal function. Endocr Rev 21: 551-583, 2000.
172. Kudo M, Osuga Y, Kobilka BK, Hsueh AJ: Transmembrane regions V and VI of the human luteinizing hormone receptor are required for constitutive activation by a mutation in the third intracellular loop. J Biol Chem 271:22470-22478, 1996.
173. Sunthornthepvarakui T, Gottschalk ME, Hayashi Y, Refetoff S: Brief report: Resistance to thyrotropin caused by mutations in the thyrotropin-receptor gene. N Engl J Med 332:155-160, 1995.
174. Abramowicz MJ, Duprez L, Parma J, et al: Familial congenital hypothyroidism due to inactivating mutation of the thyrotropin receptor causing profound hypoplasia of the thyroid gland. J Clin Invest 99:3018-3024, 1997.
175. Yen PM: Thyrotropin receptor mutations in thyroid diseases. Rev Endocr Metab Disord 1:123-129, 2000.
176. Corvilain B, Van Sande J, Dumont JE, Vassart G: Somatic and germline mutations of the TSH receptor and thyroid diseases. Clin Endocrinol Oxf 55:143-158, 2001.
177. Parma J, Duprez L, Van Sande J: Somatic mutations in the thyrotropin receptor gene cause hyperfunctioning thyroid adenomas. Nature 365:649-651, 1993.
178. Duprez L, Parma J, Van Sande J, et al: Germline mutations in the thyrotropin receptor gene cause non-autoimmune autosomal dominant hyperthyroidism. Nat Genet 7:396-401,1994.
179. Kopp P, van Sande J, Parma J, et al: Brief report: Congenital hyperthyroidism caused by a mutation in the thyrotropin-receptor gene. N Engl J Med 332:150-154, 1995.
180. Tonacchera M, Agretti P, Chiovato L, et al: Activating thyrotropin receptor mutations are present in nonadenomatous hyperfunctioning nodules of toxic or autonomous multinodular goiter. J Clin Endocrinol Metab 85:2270-2274, 2000.
181. Fuhrer D, Holzapfel HP, Wonerow P, et al: Somatic mutations in the thyrotropin receptor gene and not in the Gs alpha protein gene in 31 toxic thyroid nodules. J Clin Endocrinol Metab 82:3885-3891, 1997.
182. Govaerts C, Lefort A, Costagliola S, et al: A conserved Asn in transmembrane helix 7 is an on/off switch in the activation of the thyrotropin receptor. J Biol Chem 276:22991-22999, 2001.
183. Tonacchera M, Pinchera A: Thyrotropin receptor polymorphisms and thyroid diseases. J Clin Endocrinol Metab 85:2637-2639, 2000.
184. Gabriel EM, Bergert ER, Grant CS, et al: Germline polymorphism of codon 727 of human thyroid-stimulating hormone receptor is associated with toxic multinodular goiter. J Clin Endocrinol Metab 84:3328-3335, 1999.
185. Muhlberg T, Herrmann K, Joba W, et al: Lack of association of nonautoimmune hyperfunctioning thyroid disorders and a germline polymorphism of codon 727 of the human thyrotropin receptor in a European Caucasian population. J Clin Endocrinol Metab 85:2640-2643, 2000.
186. Russo D, Arturi F, Schlumberger M, et al: Activating mutations of the TSH receptor in differentiated thyroid carcinomas. Oncogene 11:1907-1911, 1995.

187. Spambalg D, Sharifi N, Elisei R, et al: Structural studies of the thyrotropin receptor and Gs alpha in human thyroid cancers: Low prevalence of mutations predicts infrequent involvement in malignant transformation. J Clin Endocrinol Metab 81:3898-3901, 1996.
188. Glinoer D: The regulation of thyroid function in pregnancy: Pathways of endocrine adaptation from physiology to pathology. Endocr Rev 18:404-433, 1997.
189. Rodien P, Bremont C, Sanson ML, et al: Familial gestational hyperthyroidism caused by a mutant thyrotropin receptor hypersensitive to human chorionic gonadotropin. N Engl J Med 339:1823-1826, 1998.
190. Rapoport B, McLachlan SM: The thyrotropin receptor in Graves' disease. Thyroid 17:911-922, 2007.
191. Nagayama Y, Kita-Furuyama M, Ando T, et al: A novel murine model of Graves' hyperthyroidism with intramuscular injecton of adenovirus expressing the thyrotropin receptor. J Immunol 168:2789-2794, 2002.
192. Chazenbalk GD, Pichurin P, Chen CR, et al: Thyroid-stimulating autoantibodies in Graves' disease preferentially recognize the free A subunit, not the thyrotropin holoreceptor. J Clin Invest 110:209-217, 2002.
193. Tahara K, Ishikawa N, Yamamoto K, et al: Epitopes for thyroid stimulating and blocking autoantibodies on the extracellular domain of the human thyrotropin receptor. Thyroid 7:867-877, 1997.
194. Kikuoka S, Shimojo N, Yamaguchi KI, et al: The formation of thyrotropin receptor TSHR antibodies in a Graves' animal model requires the N-terminal segment of the TSHR extracellular domain. Endocrinology 139:1891-1898, 1998.
195. Morgenthaler NG, Minich WB, Willnich M, et al: Affinity purification and diagnostic use of TSH receptor autoantibodies from human serum. Mol Cell Endocrinol 212:73-79, 2003.
196. Kohn LD, Napolitano G, Singer DS, et al: Graves' disease: A host defense mechanism gone awry. Int Rev Immunol 19:633-664, 2000.
197. Shimojo N, Arima T, Yamaguchi K, et al: A novel mouse model of Graves' disease: Implications for a role of aberrant MHC class II expression in its pathogenesis. Int Rev Immunol 19:619-631, 2000.
198. Tokuda Y, Kasagi K, Iida Y, et al: Inhibition of thyrotropin-stimulated iodide uptake in FRTL-5 thyroid cells by crude immunoglobulin fractions from patients with goitrous and atrophic autoimmune thyroiditis. J Clin Endocrinol Metab 67: 251-258, 1988.
199. Kohn LD, Harii N: Thyrotropin receptor autoantibodies TSHRAbs: Epitopes, origins and clinical significance. Autoimmunity 36:331-337, 2003.
200. Kosugi S, Ban T, Akamizu T, Kohn LD: Identification of separate determinants on the thyrotropin receptor reactive with Graves' thyroid-stimulating antibodies and with thyroid-stimulating blocking antibodies in idiopathic myxedema: These determinants have no homologous sequence on gonadotropin receptors. Mol Endocrinol 6:168-180, 1992.
201. Kung AW, Lau KS, Kohn LD: Epitope mapping of tsh receptor-blocking antibodies in Graves' disease that appear during pregnancy. J Clin Endocrinol Metab 86:3647-3653, 2001.

PART II

Pediatric Thyroid Disease

Chapter 8

Screening for Congenital Disease

Annette Grueters-Kieslich

Since the introduction of newborn screening programs, the management of the newborn and infant with congenital hypothyroidism (CH) has undergone significant changes. Screening strategies have changed and new technologies, including molecular genetic studies, were made available in the procedures of the conformational diagnosis. The replacement therapy with thyroid hormones has been adjusted to the results of outcome studies. Special aspects of the management of patients with congenital hypothyroidism are related to newborns with persistent, mildly elevated thyroid-stimulating hormone (TSH) levels and normal peripheral thyroid hormone concentrations, and to those newborns with severe CH in whom TSH levels remain elevated despite an adequate dosage of thyroid hormone replacement therapy and compliance to treatment.

SCREENING STRATEGIES

Newborn screening for CH has been introduced more than 30 years ago and now is routine in most industrialized countries.[1] Screening for CH is usually performed in dried blood spot samples, which are collected for a variety of newborn screening tests including amino acid disorders, disorders of fatty acid oxidation, congenital adrenal hyperplasia, and galactosemia. Although screening program protocols vary, most current programs screen for elevated serum TSH concentrations as the most reliable marker of primary hypothyroidism. The average threshold value for a significant TSH elevation is 15 to 25 mU/L and the common time for sampling is 48 to 72 hours after birth. However, some mothers are discharged from the hospital as early as within 24 hours after birth. Early measurement of TSH increases the prevalence of infants demonstrating elevation of TSH concentration caused by a physiologic neonatal TSH surge, which varies considerably from individual to individual. Thus, early screening for CH increases the frequency of false-positive results, depending on the threshold value established for a significant TSH elevation for infants discharged within 24 hours of birth.

It has been shown that as many as 5% of CH infants are missed in newborn screening programs.[2] Most of these relate to errors in specimen handling, testing, data analysis, or communication of the results. In rare cases, the increase in serum TSH concentration in the affected infant is delayed for several days or weeks after delivery. The reasons are unclear, and immaturity of the hypothalamic-pituitary axis has been suggested as a possible cause.[3] The prevalence of the confirmed cases of CH detected by newborn screening programs is 1 in 3500 to 4000 births. Causes include thyroid dysgenesis (e.g., aplasia, hypoplasia, ectopy, hemithyroidea), defects of thyroid hormone biosynthesis, central hypothyroidism (only in programs measuring TSH and thyroxine [T_4]), and transient forms of hypothyroidism. The most common forms are thyroid dysgenesis (75% to 80%) and defects of thyroid hormone biosynthesis (10% to 15%; Table 8-1). Modifications of CH screening programs have been introduced to improve the detection of infants with delayed increase in serum TSH concentration and those with central hypothyroidism.[4] Repeated testing at 2 to 6 weeks of age has detected an additional 10% of infants with CH[5] and addition of a T_4 or T_4 plus thyroxine-binding globulin (TBG) has been shown to detect newborns with central hypothyroidism. Most of these newborns have multiple pituitary hormones deficiencies and isolated TSH deficiency, most commonly caused by mutations of the TSH-beta gene, is rare.[6]

In a recent consensus paper of the American Academy of Pediatrics, the simultaneous measurement of T_4 and TSH was considered as the "ideal screening approach" and, depending on the varying screening strategies, different approaches for the confirmational diagnosis have been recommended.[7]

Table 8–1 Thyroid Disorders Detected in Newborn Screening Programs

Disorder	Examples
Thyroid dysgenesis (70%-80%)	Agenesis, hypoplasia, ectopy, hemithyroidea
Defects of thyroid hormone biosynthesis (10%-15%)	Defects in sodium-iodide symporter, TPO,THOX2, thyroglobulin, dehalogenase
Central hypothyroidism (only detectable in programs combining TSH and T_4-FT_4)	Developmental defects of the hypothalamus or pituitary, isolated TSH deficiency
Transient hypothyroidism, hyperthyrotropinemia	Iodine contamination, antithyroid drugs, maternal antibodies, TSH receptor defect

FT_4, free thyroxine; T_4, thyroxine; THOX2, thyroid oxidase 2; TPO, thyroid peroxidase; TSH, thyroid-stimulating hormone.

CONFIRMATIONAL DIAGNOSIS

A positive screening report for CH in a newborn demands the prompt evaluation of the newborn so as not to delay the onset of treatment. The goals of the diagnostic procedures in a newborn with a screening result suggesting CH are the confirmation of hypothyroidism and the attempt to specify the cause of CH. To confirm or rule out CH, a determination of serum TSH and T_4 or free T_4 (FT_4) concentration is performed. It is crucial that the results are interpreted according to age and method-related reference data because TSH and T_4 levels in the first weeks of life are significantly different from those in later life. Hypothyroidism is confirmed when TSH levels are higher than the age-related reference range and T_4 (FT_4) levels are below the age-related reference range. In infants with proven CH, 90% have TSH levels above 50 mU/L and 75% have T_4 concentrations below 84 nmol/L (6.5 µg/dL). If only the TSH level is elevated, the correct definition would be hyperthyrotropinemia and other differential diagnoses, such as hypothalamic dysfunction, specific genetic syndromes (e.g., Down syndrome, Williams-Beuren syndrome, or loss-of-function mutations of the TSH receptor have to be considered as possible causes). Hypothalamic-pituitary hypothyroidism is more difficult to diagnose. Most of these infants are missed in screening programs unless a simultaneous T_4 (FT_4)-TSH or TSH-T_4-TBG measurement is performed.[6] To investigate the cause of congenital hypothyroidism, imaging studies are initially performed to distinguish between the different forms of thyroid dysgenesis and defects of thyroid hormone biosynthesis with a normally developed or enlarged thyroid gland. Ultrasound studies have been accepted as the first-line investigation. If accompanied by the determination of the serum thyroglobulin concentration, it is even possible to distinguish between thyroid agenesis and ectopy without scintigraphy. This can be done because in newborns, in whom no thyroid tissue is detectable in the normal position but T_4 and thyroglobulin (Tg) are measurable, some functional thyroid tissue must be present in an ectopic position (Table 8-2). With new ultrasound techniques using Doppler sonography, the direct detection of small thyroid remnants in a typical and ectopic position has been described. This has also been elegantly shown with magnetic resonance imaging (MRI), but MRI studies are not recommended as a routine procedure, because anesthesia of the newborn or infant is necessary.[8]

If hypothyroidism is confirmed by the analysis of serum TSH and T_4, these investigations have to be performed immediately. It is not acceptable to delay the replacement therapy—for example, if imaging studies are not readily available. However, imaging studies and the measurement of Tg may avoid the interruption of replacement therapy, which should be performed at the age of 2 to 3 years if there is doubt that hypothyroidism is permanent. If there is no gland visible on ultrasound despite high TSH concentration, an interruption of replacement therapy is not necessary. The same is true for patients who have shown repeatedly elevated TSH levels during replacement therapy. Thus, an interruption of therapy can be restricted to infants with a normally developed or enlarged gland with constant normal or suppressed TSH levels during thyroid hormone replacement therapy.

Thyroid Dysgenesis

The term *thyroid dysgenesis* describes infants with developmental defects of the thyroid, including hemithyroidea and ectopic or hypoplastic thyroid glands as well as those with total thyroid agenesis. Thyroid dysgenesis usually is sporadic and the mechanism(s) for the defective organogenesis remain obscure in most affected infants. Dysgenesis is more prevalent in female than in male infants; the female-to-male ratio approximates 2 to 3:1. The disorder has been

Table 8–2 Diagnostic Approach for Newborns with Elevated Thyroid-Stimulating Hormone*

Screening Test	Findings		
Ultrasound	No gland	No gland	Eutopic gland
Serum T_4	Low/absent	Low/absent	Low
Serum Tg	Low/absent	Meas/normal	Meas/normal/ high
	↓	↓	↓
Diagnosis	Agenesis	Ectopy	Defect of biosynthesis

*Found by newborn screening.
Meas, measurable; T_4, thyroxine; Tg, thyroglobulin.

reported to be less prevalent in black (1:32,000) than in white infants and is more frequent (1:2,000) in Hispanic infants. Approximately 2% to 3% of thyroid dysgenesis cases are familial and can be attributed to mutations in genes encoding for transcription factors or the TSH receptor. An increased prevalence (8% to 10%) of other anomalies has been reported in infants with congenital hypothyroidism.[9] The most prevalent are cardiac but include anomalies of the nervous, musculoskeletal, digestive, and urologic systems and cleft palate and eye. First-degree relatives of children with thyroid dysgenesis have an increased prevalence of thyroglossal duct cysts, a pyramidal thyroid lobe, thyroid hemiagenesis, and ectopic thyroid.[10] These abnormalities are compatible with an autosomal dominant mode of inheritance with a low penetrance, supporting the hypothesis of a genetic predisposition.

Defects of Thyroid Hormone Biosynthesis

These disorders usually are transmitted as autosomal recessive traits. Except for the familial incidence and tendency of affected individuals to develop a goiter, the clinical manifestations of congenital hypothyroidism caused by a biochemical defect are similar to those in infants with thyroid dysgenesis. Thyroid enlargement may be manifest at birth but patients detected by newborn screening and treated early, with good long-term compliance, may never develop a goiter. These disorders are summarized in Table 8-3.

RESISTANCE TO THYROID-STIMULATING HORMONE

Newborns with defective TSH signaling are usually detected by newborn screening with low or normal serum T_4 and increased TSH concentrations. Thyroid radioiodine uptake is low or low-normal and unresponsive to TSH.

The thyroid follicular cell response to TSH involves a series of coordinated steps, including TSH binding to a receptor in the plasma membrane, activation of adenylyl cyclase, synthesis of cyclic adenosine monophosphate (cAMP), activation of protein kinase(s), phosphorylation of receptor protein(s), and stimulation of the several intracellular events of thyroid hormone synthesis and release. A defect at one of several sites could lead to an abnormality in thyroid responsiveness to TSH.

Germline mutations of the thyrotropin receptor gene have been described in association with congenital or acquired thyroid disease; both loss-of-function and gain-of-function phenotypes have been described.[11] Most of the loss-of-function defects lead to asymptomatic hyperthyrotropinemia and most patients described have been compound heterozygous, with normal heterozygous parents. A few cases of severe CH with absent iodine uptake and thyroid hypoplasia on ultrasound and apparent athyrosis on scintigraphy have been reported.[12]

Defects in Gs subunits have been reported in families with dominantly inherited pseudohypoparathyroidism and in patients with Albright's hereditary osteodystrophy. Affected subjects may have reduced TSH responsiveness and hyperthyrotropinemia or hypothyroidism.[13,14]

SODIUM-IODIDE SYMPORTER DEFECTS

Several reports have documented mutations in the Na^+-I^- symporter (NIS) gene in patients with congenital hypothyroidism.[15] These patients present with CH and the diagnosis is based on the presence of goiter, limited or absent radioiodine uptake, and an elevated serum TSH level. Heterozygous family members were not clinically affected.

ORGANIFICATION DEFECTS

Newborns with defective organification of iodide have been reported to present with increased TSH in newborn screening.[16] The defects include a complete deficiency of thyroid peroxidase (TPO); abnormal, functionally defective TPO; or a deficiency of hydrogen peroxide generation. The complete defect can be detected by a perchlorate discharge test, with a rapid and profound discharge of thyroidal radioiodine during a 1- to 2-hour period. Molecular genetic studies (sequencing of the TPO gene) are necessary for a definitive diagnosis. More than 20 different mutations have been described, including homozygous and compound

Table 8–3 Inborn Errors of Thyroid Hormone Metabolism*

Disorder	Inheritance	Goiter	Diagnostic Feature	Molecular Genetics
Familial TSH deficiency	AR	No	Absent TSH response to TRH	TSH-beta gene mutations
Developmental defect (hypopituitarism)	AD, AR	No	GH and other pituitary hormone deficiencies	Pit-1, Prop-1, Hesx-1, LHX3, and LHX4 gene mutations
TSH resistance	AR	No	Normal gland, hypoplasia or apparent athyrosis	Mutations of the TSH receptor gene
Iodide transport defect	AR	Yes	Salivary, gastric tissues also fail to concentrate iodide	Mutations of the Na^+-I^- symporter (NIS)
Organification defects	AR	Yes	Positive perchlorate discharge test	Thyroid peroxidase and THOX2 gene mutations
Thyroglobulin defects	AR	Yes	Usually low Tg, with no Tg response to TSH	Tg gene mutations
Iodotyronine deiodinase defect	AR	Yes	High serum MIT, DIT	DEHAL1 gene mutations

*Detectable by newborn screening.
AD, autosomal dominant; AR, autosomal recessive; DIT, diiodotyrosine; GH, growth hormone; MIT, monoiodotyrosine; Tg, thyroglobulin; TRH, thyrotropin-releasing hormone; TSH, thyroid-stimulating hormone.

heterozygous missense mutations, frame shift mutations, base pair duplications, and single-nucleotide substitutions.[16]

Recently, two genes encoding nicotinamide adenine dinucleotide phosphate (NADPH) oxidases have been cloned, referred to as thyroid oxidase 1 and 2 (THOX1, THOX2).[17] The proteins colocalize with TPO at the apical membrane of thyroid follicular cells. Inactivating mutations in THOX2 were originally described in four patients and inactivating mutations were seen in four other patients, associated with transient (heterozygous mutation) or severe (homozygous mutation) CH.[18]

Defects in Thyroglobulin Synthesis

Thyroglobulin synthesis defects occur in about 1 in 80,000 to 1 in 100,000 newborns.[19] A goiter frequently is already present at birth.

IODOTYROSINE DEIODINASE DEFECT

Failure to deiodinate thyroid monoiodotyrosine (MIT) and diiodotyrosine (DIT) as they are released from thyroglobulin leads to severe iodine wastage, because the nondeiodinated MIT and DIT leak out of the thyroid and are excreted in urine. The patients originally described were hypothyroid, with goiters presenting at birth or shortly thereafter. Recently, the gene encoding the iodothyronine dehalogenase (DEHAL1) has been cloned.[20] Mutations of the DEHAL1 gene have been identified in patients with congenital hypothyroidism from three different families. The phenotype is variable and includes goiter, mental retardation, or normal mental development despite delayed thyroid hormone substitution.[21]

Hypothalamic-Pituitary Hypothyroidism

Newborns with central hypothyroidism are relatively uncommon, with a prevalence in the range of 1 in 20,000 to 30,000 newborns. These infants are only detected in newborn thyroid screening programs using initial T_4 and/or T_4/TBG ratio measurements or simultaneous TSH and T_4 measurements to detect infants with central hypothyroidism.[6] Hypothalamic-pituitary or central hypothyroidism can result from hypothalamic and/or pituitary dysgenesis or isolated TSH deficiency. Various transcription factor gene defects have been described in association with hypothalamic-pituitary dysgenesis. GLi2, SHH, ZIC2, and SIX3 defects have been identified in patients with holoprosencephaly, HESX1 defects in association with septo-optic dysplasia, GLi3 mutation in the Pallister-Hall syndrome, and LHX3, LHX4, PROP1, and POUIFI defects in hypopituitarism.[22]

Familial isolated TSH deficiency is a rare disorder. Serum T_4 and TSH concentrations are low while other pituitary functions are intact. A number of homozygous mutations in the TSHβ subunit gene on chromosome 1 have been described.[23] The most prevalent mutation identified in different populations is derived from a common ancestor and results in severe congenital hypothyroidism.[24] It involves a 1 bp deletion from codon 105 of the βTSH-beta gene (C105V).

Therapy of hypothyroidism in these infants is similar to therapy for other CH states. In addition, replacement of other pituitary or end-organ hormone deficiencies is necessary.

Transient Congenital Hypothyroidism

Transient CH comprises 5% to 10% of infants detected in newborn thyroid screening programs. These infants manifest low or normal T_4 levels, with variably elevated serum TSH concentrations. The most common causes in North America are goitrogenic agents and transplacentally derived TSH receptor blocking maternal autoantibodies. Autoantibody-mediated CH accounts for 1% to 2% of cases.[25] In areas of endemic iodine deficiency, transient CH is more frequent and is caused by a relative iodine deficiency associated with increased thyroid hormone requirements in the neonatal period.[26] Maternal iodine or possibly antithyroid drug ingestion should be considered in all cases of CH. The thyroid scan result varies depending on the cause; iodine usually inhibits technetium or radioiodine uptake, whereas drug or dietary goitrogens typically increase uptake and produce a positive scan. Maternal TSH receptor blocking antibody-induced hypothyroidism should be suspected in any case in which the mother has a history of autoimmune thyroid disease.[27] The transient CH in these infants usually is of short duration (1 to 2 weeks) in the case of drugs or longer duration (1 to 4 months) if related to maternal blocking antibody. If biochemical hypothyroidism CH persists beyond 2 weeks, treatment should be instituted.

THYROID HORMONE REPLACEMENT THERAPY

The goal of newborn CH screening is the institution of early, adequate thyroid hormone replacement therapy. Because most of thyroid hormone in the CNS is derived from local T_4 to triiodothyronine (T_3) conversion,[28] the preferred thyroid hormone preparation for treatment of infants with CH is T_4.

The dosage of T_4 should normalize the serum T_4 level as quickly as possible.[29-32] Regarding the higher thyroid hormone concentrations in the first weeks of life and to guarantee adequate hormone to all infants, it is desirable to maintain the serum T_4 and FT_4 levels in the upper half of the normal age-related reference range during therapy. To normalize the serum T_4 concentration in the CH infant rapidly, an initial dose of levothyroxine (L-T_4) of 10 to 15 μg/kg/day is recommended.[29] For the average term infant weighing 3 to 4.5 kg, an initial dose of 50 μg daily is therefore recommended.

Physical growth and development of infants with CH usually are normalized by early and adequate therapy.[33] IQ scores and mental and motor development also are normalized in most infants with CH.[34] However, low-normal or occasionally low IQ values and motor impairments have been reported in treated children with severe CH as assessed by a very low serum T_4 level and delayed bone maturation at birth.[35-37] This outcome has been found in programs using a relatively low replacement dose of T_4 or in infants in whom treatment is delayed.[38] This deficit, although variable, amounts to several IQ points for every week of delayed early treatment. Early therapy with 10 to 15 μg/kg/day of levothyroxine reduces the serum TSH level more rapidly and minimizes the early IQ loss. More recent studies with a double-blind randomized approach have demonstrated that thyroid hormone replacement with an adequate dosage can completely restore normal mental development, even in patients with severe CH.[29]

In some patients with remaining deficits and neurologic problems, mutations in the transcription factor NKX2-1, which is expressed not only in the thyroid but also in the central nervous system during development, explain the unfavorable outcome.[39]

SPECIAL CONSIDERATIONS

Since the introduction of newborn screening programs, asymptomatic hyperthyrotropinemia has become a relatively common disorder and may be transient or permanent. The prevalence of transient hyperthyrotropinemia in Europe approximates 1 in 8000 births, with 50% caused by perinatal iodine exposure.[40] Other causes could include defects of the biologic activity of TSH or the TSH receptor, a mild thyroid hormone biosynthesis defect, subtle developmental defects such as a hemithyroid, or a disturbance of the TSH feedback control system. Germline mutations of the TSH receptor gene have been associated with a phenotype of asymptomatic hyperthyrotropinemia. Most were compound heterozygotes with normal heterozygous parents.[41,42]

Transient neonatal hyperthyrotropinemia is not as rare in Japan, where it is detected in about 1 in 18,000 newborns.[43] Elevated TSH values frequently normalize spontaneously within 6 months, excluding an abnormal TSH molecule or TSH receptor defect in these subjects. The mechanism in patients with persistent TSH elevations remains unclear. Partially inactivating mutations in the TSH receptor gene accounts for some of the familial cases.[44] Hyperthyrotropinemia in the newborn is usually treated but, in the presence of FT_4 levels in the upper half of the normal range, he or she could be managed expectantly.[45]

Serum TSH concentrations in some treated infants with proven CH may remain relatively elevated, despite normalized levels of T_4 or FT_4. The elevation of serum TSH is marked during the first 2 years of therapy but can persist to some degree in a minority of patients.[46] The elevated serum TSH concentration relative to T_4 concentration in CH infants presumably is caused by a difference in the feedback threshold for T_4 suppression of TSH release in CH. This difference exists perinatally, but the mechanism remains obscure. As long as there are no prospective randomized IQ outcome data for this particular group of children with hyperthyrotropinemia, the question of whether treatment to decrease TSH levels in these children is beneficial remains open.

Newborn screening for CH and early thyroid hormone replacement in affected newborns has effectively prevented symptoms of CH, especially mental retardation, in 1 of 3500 to 4000 newborns. Therefore, screening for CH can be considered as one of the major achievements of pediatrics in the last 3 decades.

References

1. Fisher DA: Screening for congenital hypothyroidism: Status report. Trends Endocrinol 2:129, 1991.
2. Fisher DA: Effectiveness of newborn screening programs for congenital hypothyroidism: Prevalence of missed cases. Pediatr Clin N Amer 34:881, 1987.
3. LaFranchi SH, Hanna CE, Krainz PL, et al: Screening for congenital hypothyroidism with specimen collection at two time periods. Results of the Northwest Regional screening program. Pediatrics 76:734, 1985.
4. Delange F: Neonatal screening for congenital hypothyroidism. Results and perspectives. Horm Res 48: 51, 1997.
5. Tylek-Lemanska D, Kumorowicz-Kopiec M, Starzyk J: Screening for congenital hypothyroidism: The value of retesting after four months in neonates with low or very low birth weight. J Med Screening 12:166, 2005.
6. van Tijn DA, de Vijlder JJM, Verbeeten B Jr, et al: Neonatal detection of congenital hypothyroidism of central origin. J Clin Endocrinol Metab 90:3350, 2005.
7. American Academy of Pediatrics, Rose SR; Section on Endocrinology and Committee on Genetics, American Thyroid Association, Brown RS; Public Health Committee, Lawson Wilkins Pediatric Endocrine Society, Foley T, et al: Update of newborn screening and therapy for congenital hypothyroidism. Pediatrics 117:2290, 2006.
8. Ohnishi H, Sato H, Noda H, et al: Color Doppler ultrasonography: Diagnosis of ectopic thyroid gland in patients with congenital hypothyroidism caused by thyroid dysgenesis. J Clin Endocrinol Metab 88:5145, 2003.
9. Olivieri A, Stazi MA, Mastroiacovo P, et al: A population-based study on the frequency of additional congenital malformatons in infants with congenital hypothyroidism: Data from the Italian Registry for Congenital Hypothyroidism (1991-1998). J Clin Endocrinol Metab 87:557, 2002.
10. Leger J, Marinovic D, Garel C, et al: Thyroid developmental anomalies in first-degree relatives of children with congenital hypothyroidism. J Clin Endocrinol Metab 87:575, 2002.
11. Corvillain B, Van Sande J, Dumont JE, Vassart G: Somatic and germline mutations of the TSH receptor and thyroid diseases. Clin Endocrinol 55:143, 2001.
12. Abramowicz MJ, Duprez L, Parma J, et al: Familial congenital hypothyroidism due to inactivating mutation of the thyrotropin receptor causing profound hypoplasia of the thyroid gland. J Clin Invest 99:3018, 1997.
13. Spiegel AM: The molecular basis of disorders caused by defects in G proteins. Horm Res 47:89, 1997.
14. Szinnai G, Kusugi S, Derriene, et al: Extending the clinical heterogeneity of iodide transport defect (ITD): A novel mutation R124H of the sodium/iodide symporter gene and review of genotype-phenotype correlations in ITD. J Clin Endocrinol Metab 91:1199, 2006.
15. Vulsma T, De Vijlder JJM: Genetic defects causing hypothyroidism. In Braverman LE, Utiger RD (eds): The Thyroid, 9th ed. Philadelphia, Lippincott, Williams & Wilkins, 2005, pp 714-730.
16. Vassart G, Dumont JE, Refetoff S: Thyroid disorders. In Beudet AL, Sly WS, Valle D (eds): The Metabolic and Molecular Bases of Inherited Disease, 7th ed. New York, McGraw Hill, 1995, pp 2883-2887.
17. DeDeken X, Wang D, Many MC, et al: Cloning of two human thyroid cDNAs encoding new members of the NADPH oxidase family. J Biol Chem 275:23227, 2000.
18. Moreno JC, Bikker H, Kempers MJE, et al: Inactivating mutations in the gene for thyroid oxidase 2 (THOX2) and congenital hypothyroidism. N Engl J Med 347:95, 2002.
19. Knobel M, Medeiros-Neto G: An outline of inherited disorders of the thyroid hormone generating system. Thyroid 13:771, 2003.
20. Gnidehou S, Caillou B, Talbot M, et al: Iodothyronine dehalogenase (DEHAL1) is a transmembrane protein involved in recycling of iodide close to the thyroglobulin iodination site. FASEB J 18:1574, 2004.
21. Moreno JC: European Society for Paediatric Endocrinology (ESPE) 45th Annual Meeting, Rotterdam, June-July 2006. Horm Res 65 (Suppl 4), 2006.
22. Tran PV, Savage JJ, Ingraham HA, Rhodes SJ: Molecular genetics of hypothalamic-pituitary development. In Pescovitz OH, Eugster EA (eds): Pediatric Endocrinology. Philadelphia, Lippincott, Williams & Wilkins, 2004, pp 63-79.

23. Medeiros-Neto GA, de Laserda L, Wondisford FE: Familial congenital hypothyroidism caused by abnormal and bioinactive TSH due to mutations in the β subunit gene. Trends Endocrinol 8:15, 1997.
24. Brumm J, Pfeufer A, Biebermann H, et al: Congenital central hypothyroidism due to a homozygous thyrotropin beta 313 delta T mutation is caused by a founder effect. J Clin Endocrinol Metab 87:4811, 2002.
25. Brown R, Bellisario R, Botero D, et al: Incidence of transient congenital hypothyroidism due to maternal thyrotropin receptor blocking antibodies in over one million babies. J Clin Endocrinol Metab 81:1147, 1996.
26. Glinoer D, Delange F, Laboureur I, et al: Maternal and neonatal thyroid function at birth in an area of marginally low iodine intake. J Clin Endocrinol Metab 75:800, 1992.
27. Iseki M, Shimizu M, Oikawa T, et al: Sequential serum measurements of thyrotropin binding inhibiting immunoglobulin G in transient neonatal hypothyroidism. J Clin Endocrinol Metab 57:384, 1983.
28. Calvo R, Obregon MJ, Ruiz de Ona C, et al: Congenital hypothyroidism as studied in rats: Crucial role of maternal thyroxine but not of 3,5,3′-triiodothyronine in the protection of the fetal brain. J Clin Invest 86:889, 1990.
29. Bongers-Schokking JJ, de Muinck Keizer-Schrama SM: Influence of timing and dose of thyroid hormone replacement on mental, psychomotor and behavioral development in children with congenital hypothyroidism. J Pediatr 147:768, 2005.
30. LaFranchi S: Congenital hypothyroidism, etiologies, diagnosis and management. Thyroid 9:735, 1999.
31. Selva K, Harper A, Downs A, et al: Neurodevelopmental outcomes in congenital hypothyroidism: Comparison of initial T_4 dose and time to reach target T_4 and TSH. J Pediatr 147:775, 2005.
32. Bakker B, Kempers MJE, DeVijlder JJM, et al: Dynamics of the plasma concentrations of TSH FT_4 and T_3 following thyroxine supplementation in congenital hypothyroidism. Clin Endocrinol 57:529, 2002.
33. Grant DB: Growth in early treated congenital hypothyroidism. Arch Dis Child 70:464, 1994.
34. Heyerdahl S, Kase BF, Lie SO: Intellectual development of children with congenital hypothyroidism in relation to recommended thyroxine treatment. J Pediatr 118:850, 1991.
35. Boileau P, Bain P, Rivas S, Toublanc JE: Earlier onset of treatment or increment in LT_4 dose in screened congenital hypothyroidism: Which was the more important factor for IQ at 7 years? Horm Res 61:228, 2004.
36. Simoneau-Roy J, Marti S, Deal C, et al: Cognition and behavior at school entry in children with congenital hypothyroidism treated early with high-dose levothyroxine. J Pediatr 144:747, 2004.
37. Rovet JF: Congenital hypothyroidism: Long-term outcome. Thyroid 9:741, 1999.
38. Dubuis JM, Glorieux J, Richer F, et al: Outcome of severe congenital hypothyroidism: Closing the developmental gap with early high dose levothyroxine treatment. J Clin Endocrinol Metab 81:222, 1996.
39. Krude H, Schuetz B, Biebermann H, et al: Choreoathetosis, hypothyroidism, and pulmonary alterations due to human NKX2-1 haploinsufficiency. J Clin Invest 109:475, 2002.
40. Kohler B, Schnabel D, Biebermann H, Grueters A: Transient congenital hypothyroidism and hyperthyrotropinemia: Normal thyroid function and physical development at the ages of 6-14 years. J Clin Endocrinol Metab 81:1563, 1996.
41. Duprez L, Parma J, Van Sande J, et al: TSH receptor mutations and thyroid disease. Trends Endocrinol 9:133, 1998.
42. Corvillain B, Van Sande J, Dumont JE, Vassart G: Somatic and germline mutations of the TSH receptor and thyroid diseases. Clin Endocrinol 55:143, 2001.
43. Miki J, Nose O, Miyai K, et al: Transient infantile hyperthyrotropinemia. Arch Dis Child 64:1177, 1989.
44. Matsuura N, Yamada Y, Nohara Y, et al: Familial, neonatal transient hypothyroidism due to maternal TSH-binding inhibitor immunoglobulins. N Engl J Med 303:738, 1980.
45. Fisher DA: Management of congenital hypothyroidism. J Clin Endocrinol Metab 72:523, 1991.
46. Fisher DA, Schoen EJ, LaFranchi S, et al: The hypothalamic-pituitary-thyroid negative feedback control axis in children with treated congenital hypothyroidism. J Clin Endocrinol Metab 85:2722, 2000.

Chapter 9

Genetics and Epigenetics of Congenital Hypothyroidism

Guy Van Vliet

Key Points

- Congenital hypothyroidism (CH) is the most common congenital endocrine disorder.
- CH most often results from defects in thyroid development (thyroid dysgenesis).
- Thyroid dysgenesis is predominantly non-Mendelian.
- Functional defects leading to CH (thyroid dyshormonogenesis) are inherited in autosomal recessive fashion.

Hypothyroidism, which affects one neonate in about 3000, is the most common congenital endocrine disorder.[1] As is true at other stages of life, the defect most commonly lies at the level of the thyroid gland itself and is of a permanent nature (permanent primary congenital hypothyroidism [PPCH]). PPCH is therefore reviewed first in this chapter. Recently, even some transient forms of primary CH have been shown to have a genetic basis. Finally, central hypothyroidism can also occur, either isolated or associated with other pituitary hormone deficiencies, and may have a genetic basis as well.

PERMANENT PRIMARY CONGENITAL HYPOTHYROIDISM

Nomenclature and Clinical Features

PPCH most often results from defects in the development of the gland during embryogenesis, which are collectively called thyroid dysgenesis. The development of the thyroid is reviewed elsewhere in this text (see Chapter 2). In humans, the most common developmental defect associated with PPCH is an arrest in the migration of the median thyroid anlage anywhere along its normal path of descent between the foramen cecum and the neck. This results in an ectopic mass of otherwise well-differentiated thyroid follicular cells, which is best evidenced by radionuclide scanning.[2] In addition to their abnormal location, ectopic thyroid glands have an abnormal shape, lacking the lateral lobes typical of the normal thyroid. Because ectopic thyroid cells are functional, it is unclear why patients whose only thyroid tissue is ectopic are generally hypothyroid, but this may simply reflect a smaller number of cells. The contribution of the lateral thyroid anlage to the pool of follicular cells is controversial, but this lateral anlage appears to be essential to the lobulation process and may play a role in the development of an appropriate vascular supply to the gland.[3]

The second most common defect underlying PPCH is thyroid aplasia or agenesis (athyreosis). It is important to realize that up to 50% of patients with no detectable uptake on radionuclide scan have detectable plasma thyroglobulin levels.[4] Whether the thyroglobulin-producing tissue is ectopic or orthotopic in these patients is unknown. We have used the term *apparent athyreosis* to describe the condition of these patients and *true athyreosis* when there is no detectable radionuclide uptake *and* an undetectable plasma thyroglobulin.[5] In the latter situation, it is unknown whether these are individuals in whom no follicular cell ever differentiated during organogenesis or if thyroid cells differentiated initially and then disappeared. It is noteworthy that in mice in whom thyroid transcription factor 1 (Ttf-1, Ttf-2), or Pax8 has been genetically ablated, the median thyroid bud always forms and disappears later. Apoptosis has specifically been demonstrated to be responsible for the disappearance of the thyroid in *Ttf-1 −/−* mice.[6]

The third gross developmental defect, the absence of one of the lobes—and, occasionally, of the isthmus as well—is only rarely encountered in patients with PPCH. Most subjects with thyroid hemiagenesis remain euthyroid. Systematic studies of schoolchildren by ultrasound have shown that this anatomic variant is encountered in about 1 in 500 individuals.[7] The mechanism underlying the hypothyroidism in the small fraction of patients with hemiagenesis who present with PPCH is unknown.

Finally, a small percentage of patients with PPCH have thyroid glands that are of normal shape and location but that are small (orthotopic hypoplasia). If PPCH is severe, these small orthotopic glands will not take up radionuclides but may be visualized on very careful ultrasonography. These patients have generally had detectable and even high, relative to the amount of thyroid tissue, plasma thyroglobulin (see earlier, apparent athyreosis).

Ironically, it is in patients with orthotopic hypoplasia, who account for less than 5% of cases of PPCH, that single-gene disorders have been identified. Thus, the molecular mechanisms underlying the vast majority of cases of thyroid dysgenesis remain unknown. Assessing progress in this area requires understanding that the phenotypic characterization of the specific defect in thyroid development is essential and that radionuclide scanning is the technique of choice for revealing ectopic thyroid tissue.[8] Whether all types of thyroid dysgenesis represent a spectrum with potentially common mechanisms or discrete entities with specific causes is controversial. In favor of athyreosis and ectopy being part of a spectrum is the observation that in the rare familial forms, athyreosis and ectopy have been reported in the same pedigree,[9] although one should realize that the quality of imaging may not have been the same in all cases from the same family, especially when they were from different generations. On the other hand, the different gender ratios in ectopy and in athyreosis (with female predominance more pronounced in the former) suggest that, if there is a common molecular cause to the two phenotypes, it is modulated by sexually dimorphic mechanisms.[10]

Possible Molecular Mechanisms

CH from thyroid dysgenesis was classically described as a sporadic entity until, in 2001, a nationwide survey in France revealed that the percentage of familial cases was 2%, a figure 15-fold higher than by chance alone.[9] At about the same time, a systematic survey of monozygotic twins revealed a discordance rate of 92%.[11] Deladoey and associates have[12] proposed a unifying model that would be compatible with the evidence of a genetic contribution and with the almost universal discordance of monozygotic twins. In this two-hit model, a germline mutation would be combined with a somatic mutation or epigenetic difference in genes involved in thyroid development. The putative germline mutation is unlikely to be in *PAX-8*, *TTF-1*, or *TTF-2*, because systematic screening of relatively large numbers of patients with CH from thyroid dysgenesis for mutations in these genes has yielded negative results.[13-16] Another sporadic congenital endocrine disorder that is much less common than thyroid dysgenesis, focal hyperinsulinism, has been shown to result from such a two-hit model.[17] In the pancreatic lesions found in these patients, a paternally inherited mutation in the *SUR1* or *KIR6.2* genes is found, together with loss of the maternal 11p15 allele (loss of heterozygosity). The loss of heterozygosity is a somatic event restricted to the pancreatic lesion, which explains why focal congenital hyperinsulinism is a sporadic disease. In contrast to thyroid dysgenesis, no familial case of focal hyperinsulinism has been observed (C. A. Stanley, personal communication, 2007), but this may reflect the extreme rarity of the latter condition. Whether the two-hit model is applicable to thyroid dysgenesis remains to be determined. Rather than speculating further, the rare single-gene disorders that have been shown to be associated with PPCH will be reviewed (Table 9-1). Although they account for a small proportion of PPCH, their study at the molecular level has yielded interesting insights about the genetic control of thyroid gland development and function.

Thyrotropin Resistance

During prenatal development, the thyroid-stimulating hormone (TSH) receptor (TSH-R) becomes expressed in the fetal thyroid well after it has completed its initial differentiation and migration.[18] Accordingly, inactivation of the TSH-R should not interfere with migration and, indeed, even patients bearing mutations that severely impair TSH-R function in the homozygous or compound heterozygous state have apparent athyreosis, as defined earlier, but not ectopy. This phenotype is transmitted in an autosomal recessive fashion. Milder TSH resistance can also be observed as part of pseudohypoparathyroidism[19] or with an autosomal dominant pattern of inheritance; this can be caused by heterozygosity for TSH-R–inactivating mutations[20] or by other still undefined mechanisms.[21]

PAX8 Mutations

Relatively speaking, heterozygous mutations in *PAX8* are the ones that have been most frequently encountered in patients with PPCH. However, the total number of mutations identified to date is still only about 10.

Table 9–1 Gene Disorders Shown to Be from Thyroid Dysgenesis Associated with Primary Congenital Hypothyroidism

Gene Name(s)	Transmission	Thyroid Morphology	Other Abnormalities
TTF-1 or *TITF-1* *T/EBP* *NKX2.1*	Dominant De novo	Normal Orthotopic hypoplasia Apparent athyreosis	Hypotonia Choreoathetosis Respiratory distress
TTF-2 or *TITF-2* *FKHL15* *FOXE1*	Recessive	True athyreosis	Cleft palate Kinky hair Bifid epiglottis
PAX 8	Dominant	Normal Orthotopic hypoplasia Apparent athyreosis	None
TSHR	Recessive	Normal Orthotopic hypoplasia Apparent athyreosis	None
GLIS3	Recessive	Apparent athyreosis	Neonatal diabetes Hepatic fibrosis Congenital glaucoma Polycystic kidneys

They were observed in either sporadic or familial cases with dominant transmission. The phenotype is very variable both between families and even within the same family. It has also recently been shown that *PAX8* mutations can lead to early onset rather than to congenital hypothyroidism.[22] The case initially reported as "hypoplasia and ectopy"[23] in fact never had a scintiscan and likely had orthotopic hypoplasia, as had all the others. The reason why heterozygous mutations in *PAX8* lead to a phenotype in humans and not in mice is unknown. Postulated mechanisms include monoallelic expression of the mutant allele in the thyroid.[24]

TTF-1 Mutations

The initial description of the TTF-1 deficiency syndrome in humans was based on an infant with a heterozygous chromosomal 14q13 deletion detected by fluorescence in situ hybridization.[25] The concept that haploinsufficiency for TTF-1 itself is responsible for the association of respiratory distress, primary thyroid failure, and neurologic symptoms has since been confirmed.[26,27] Mutations inactivating TTF-1 have now also been found in a condition that had been described as benign hereditary chorea.[28] Initially, most cases were sporadic, but autosomal dominant transmission of the full syndrome has now been reported.[29] The spectrum of severity of all three components of the syndrome has now been shown to be wide and includes lethal neonatal respiratory distress caused by the effect of TTF-1 on surfactant production.[30] Morphologically, the thyroid is normal or hypoplastic but is always in the normal position and has a normal shape.

TTF-2 Mutations

Consistent with the expression pattern of this transcription factor, germline mutations in *TTF-2* result in a phenotype that is not restricted to the thyroid. A complex syndrome of athyreosis, cleft palate, kinky hair, and bifid epiglottis, originally described by Bamforth and colleagues,[31] has now been shown to be caused by homozygous *TTF-2* mutations in the offspring of three marriages between first cousins.[32-34] However, most cases of CH with cleft palate do not have *TTF-2* mutations.[10,16] The length of the polyalanine tract in *TTF-2*, which is polymorphic, may play a role in the genetic predisposition to CH from thyroid dysgenesis,[35] but this remains controversial.[16,36]

NKX2.5 Mutations

Aside from the rare syndromes described earlier, CH from thyroid dysgenesis is typically isolated. However, several studies have found an increased incidence of mild congenital heart malformations, mostly septation defects.[9,10,37] Dominant transmission of heart conduction defects caused by mutations in *NKX2.5* had been described in 1998.[38] More recently, rare *NKX2.5* sequence variants were found in 4 of 241 patients with CH (the imaging modality used to establish cause was not specified), some of whom had cardiac anomalies. These sequence variants were transmitted by one of the parents, who did not have CH, and only one had a heart defect. The involvement of *NKX2.5* in CH in humans therefore remains to be confirmed.

GLIS3 Mutations

A recessively inherited syndrome of CH associated with neonatal diabetes, congenital glaucoma, hepatic fibrosis, and polycystic kidneys has been shown to be caused by mutations in *GLIS3*, encoding GLI similar 3, a recently identified transcription factor. The thyroid phenotype corresponds to that of apparent athyreosis, as defined earlier.[39]

Syndromes Associated with Permanent Primary Congenital Hypothyroidism

A great many dysmorphic syndromes are thought to be associated with hypothyroidism, but its precise nature has not always been well defined. Among the best studied and most common syndromes are trisomy 21 and DiGeorge and Williams syndrome. The studies of van Trotsenburg and associates have clearly shown that patients with trisomy 21 present a mild form of PPCH, with orthotopic thyroid hypoplasia.[40] In DiGeorge syndrome, which results from a deletion of chromosome region 22q11, PPCH has been reported but without scintigraphic diagnosis.[41] Our group has been following a 5-year-old girl with DiGeorge syndrome and PPCH with normal thyroid morphology on technetium scanning. In Williams syndrome, which is caused by a deletion of the elastin gene on 7q11.23, PPCH is usually mild and associated with orthotopic thyroid hypoplasia.[42] In DiGeorge syndrome, the candidate gene is *TBX1* and disruption in the development of the arterial supply, essential for stabilization and growth of the thyroid lobes, may be the link to PPCH,[43] but in trisomy 21 and Williams syndrome, the mechanisms underlying the link between the chromosomal lesion and PPCH are unknown.

PERMANENT PRIMARY CONGENITAL HYPOTHYROIDISM CAUSED BY THYROID DYSHORMONOGENESIS

Mutations inactivating any one of the steps involved in thyroid hormone synthesis (Table 9-2), from the uptake of iodine through the sodium-iodine symporter (NIS) to its recycling through dehalogenase (DEHAL), can cause CH and will lead to goiter formation. However, the goiter may not be present at birth and can develop over the lifespan. Moreover, goiters are difficult to detect with certainty in neonates, even when the neck is hyperextended and an experienced clinician is available. With very few exceptions, PPCH from thyroid dyshormonogenesis is an autosomal recessive disease. Trying to establish a specific diagnosis does not affect genetic counseling and should never delay treatment. If there is a goiter clinically and/or by ultrasound, but no uptake of radioisotope, a mutation in NIS is likely, but this appears to be rare. In centers using iodine rather than technetium (which is not organified) as the radiopharmaceutical for the diagnostic scintiscan, the perchlorate discharge test can be used to determine whether iodide organification is abnormal, in which case a mutation in thyroperoxidase (TPO) is the most likely. However, intermediate values may not be easy to interpret and perchlorate is not available in all centers. With the increased availability of sequencing techniques, a search for mutations in the genes involved in thyroid hormone synthesis can now be carried out whenever a specific molecular diagnosis is sought, even if a perchlorate discharge test is not available.[44]

TPO Mutations

Ever since their first description in 1992,[45] *TPO* mutations have been found to be the most common cause of goitrous PPCH, accounting for up to 46% of patients.[46] A goiter is almost invariably present and the plasma thyroglobulin (TG) level is high.[47] Although the transmission of TPO deficiency is typically autosomal recessive, apparently manifesting heterozygotes are common, suggesting promoter or intronic mutations or monoallelic expression.[48] Partial maternal isodisomy for chromosome 2p, to which the *TPO* gene maps, has also been described.[49] Finally, given that carriers of mutated *TPO* alleles are frequently found in the general population, pseudodominant transmission can be expected, even in nonconsanguineous families, and Deladoey and coworkers[44] have recently observed such a pedigree.

Thyroglobulin Mutations

The first description of a mutation in TG in humans was in a hypothyroid patient with a large goiter contrasting with a low plasma TG.[50] However, a linkage study of 23 families in Sweden with presumably autosomal recessive CH and no goiter has revealed linkage to the TG locus in 44.5%. Interestingly, in two families, the goiter was not only absent at birth but did not develop during childhood in spite of growth and

Table 9–2 Mutations Inactivating Steps Involved in Thyroid Hormone Synthesis

Gene Name(s)	Goiter	Hypothyroidism	Scintigraphy and PDT Findings
TPO	++	++	High uptake; PDT, abnormal
TG	May be absent	++	High uptake; PDT, usually normal
NIS	Depends on iodine intake		No uptake
PDS	Develops late		High uptake; PDT, normal or abnormal
DEHAL	++	May develop after birth	High uptake; PDT, normal

PDT, perchlorate discharge test.

mental retardation from late treatment of CH. The notion that *TG* mutations do not necessarily lead to goiter formation also stems from observations in the WIC-*rdw* rat, which bears the G2320R mutation in TG and does not develop a goiter, presumably because the *rdw* mutation is toxic to the host thyrocytes.[51]

NIS Mutations

Since the first description of a mutation in *NIS* in 1997,[52] only 30 more patients have been described.[53] A high iodine intake may prevent or delay the expression of the full phenotype of hypothyroidism and goiter.[54] The residual enzyme activity of the mutated gene products is correlated with the age at which the phenotype becomes apparent.

PDS Mutations

Pendred's syndrome, or the association of deaf mutism and goiter, is thought to account for 10% of congenital deafness. It is caused by mutations in *PDS*, a gene that encodes pendrin, a transmembrane protein involved in the transport of iodine across the apical membrane of the thyroid follicular cells. Pendrin is also expressed in the cochlea, where its role is thought to be through its chloride transport capacity.[55] The thyroid phenotype is variable and affected patients are only rarely identified by neonatal TSH screening.[56,57] More typically, hypothyroidism and goiter develop in late childhood and adulthood.

Dehalogenase Mutations

Mutations affecting dehalogenation, the enzymatic activity responsible for the recycling of iodine contained in iodotyrosines, have been postulated to explain an autosomal recessive form of goitrous CH with excessive loss of iodine, mimicking iodine deficiency, and whose expression strongly depends on iodine intake. Recently, mutations in *DEHAL1* have been described in four patients with this phenotype.[58] Importantly, the hypothyroidism may not be present at the time of neonatal screening but develop in infancy and still lead to mental deficiency.

TRANSIENT PRIMARY CONGENITAL HYPOTHYROIDISM: MUTATIONS IN DUOX2

Until 2002, all recognized causes of transient CH were not genetic, involving the transplacental transfer of anti–TSH-R antibodies, chronic iodine deficiency, and/or acute iodine overload. Screening patients with CH caused by a total iodide organification defect of unknown cause, Moreno and colleagues[59] have found one patient with PPCH who was homozygous for mutations in the gene encoding dual oxidase 2 (DUOX2), the enzyme responsible for the generation of H_2O_2 at the apical membrane of the thyroid follicular cells. However, contrasting with other forms of dyshormonogenesis, heterozygous subjects had transient CH. This first demonstration of a genetic origin for transient CH has been confirmed in nine other patients.[60] On the other hand, the expression of DUOX activity in vitro requires a maturation factor,[61] and mutations in the gene encoding this maturation factor have recently been identified in humans.[61a]

CENTRAL CONGENITAL HYPOTHYROIDISM

Central congenital hypothyroidism is approximately 10 times less common than PPCH.[62] It is generally caused by sporadic developmental defects of the hypothalamopituitary unit and is associated with deficiencies of other pituitary hormones. It is the clinical expression of the latter (e.g., hypoglycemia, microphallus) that leads to the diagnosis.[63] However, rare cases of isolated central hypothyroidism have also been reported.

Isolated Central Congenital Hypothyroidism

Mutations in the Thyrotropin-Releasing Hormone Receptor (TRHR)

So far, only one case of compound heterozygous mutations in the thyrotropin-releasing hormone receptor (TRH-R) has been reported. Although thyroxine was low at neonatal screening, TSH was not elevated, so the patient was not recalled. He presented with a relatively mild phenotype (slow growth, retarded bone maturation, and bradycardia) at the age of 9 years. Biochemically, neither TSH nor prolactin rose after exogenous TRH, which was the clue to the molecular diagnosis.[64]

Mutations in the Thyroid-Stimulating Hormone Beta Subunit Gene

In contrast to the single patient with a TRH-R mutation described earlier, all patients with mutations in the gene encoding the TSH beta subunit gene that have been reported since 1990[65,66] presented with a severe phenotype and were consequently at risk for mental retardation if not promptly recognized.[67] Biochemically, plasma TSH may be recognized in some immunoassays and the TSH value may be slightly elevated, but not as would be expected for the degree of hypothyroxinemia.[68] After TRH, TSH increases slightly, whereas the high basal prolactin level increases further. The most common mutation appears to be *C105Vfs114X*, but whether this represents a founder effect or a hot spot is controversial.[69,70]

Central Congenital Hypothyroidism Associated with Other Pituitary Hormone Deficiencies

In patients with mutations of *PIT-1*, central CH occurs in association with severe growth hormone and prolactin deficiency.[71] Patients with *PROP1* mutations present with the same combination of deficiencies but may develop partial deficiencies of gonadotropin and adrenocorticotropin over their lifespan. Central CH with various combinations of other anterior pituitary hormone deficiencies can also be observed in patients with mutations in the pituitary transcription factors LHX3, LHX4, and HESX1.[72]

References

1. Van Vliet G: Hypothyroidism in infants and children. In Braverman LE, Utiger RD (eds): Werner and Ingbar's The Thyroid: A Fundamental and Clinical Text, 9th ed. Philadelphia, Lippincott, Williams & Wilkins, 2005, pp 1029-1047.
2. Schoen EJ, Clapp W, To TT, Fireman BH: The key role of newborn thyroid scintigraphy with isotopic iodide (^{123}I) in defining and managing congenital hypothyroidism. Pediatrics 114:e683-e688, 2004.
3. Fagman H, Andersson L, Nilsson M: The developing mouse thyroid: Embryonic vessel contacts and parenchymal growth pattern during specification, budding, migration, and lobulation. Dev Dyn 235:444-455, 2006.
4. Djemli A, Fillion M, Belgoudi J, et al: Twenty years later: A reevaluation of the contribution of plasma thyroglobulin to the diagnosis of thyroid dysgenesis in infants with congenital hypothyroidism. Clin Biochem 37:818-822, 2004.
5. Gagne N, Parma J, Deal C, et al: Apparent congenital athyreosis contrasting with normal plasma thyroglobulin levels and associated with inactivating mutations in the thyrotropin receptor gene: Are athyreosis and ectopic thyroid distinct entities? J Clin Endocrinol Metab 83:1771-1775, 1998.
6. Kimura S, Ward JM, Minoo P: Thyroid-specific enhancer-binding protein/thyroid transcription factor 1 is not required for the initial specification of the thyroid and lung primordia. Biochimie 81: 321-327, 1999.
7. Shabana W, Delange F, Freson M, et al: Prevalence of thyroid hemiagenesis: Ultrasound screening in normal children. Eur J Pediatr 159:456-458, 2000.
8. Perry RJ, Maroo S, Maclennan AC, et al: Combined ultrasound and isotope scanning is more informative in the diagnosis of congenital hypothyroidism than single scanning. Arch Dis Child 24:972-976, 2006.
9. Castanet M, Polak M, Bonaiti-Pellie C, et al: Nineteen years of national screenbing for congenital hypothyroidism: Familial cases with thyroid dysgenesis suggest the involvement of genetic factors. J Clin Endocrinol Metab 86:2009-2014, 2001.
10. Devos H, Rodd C, Gagne N, et al: A search for the possible molecular mechanisms of thyroid dysgenesis: Sex ratios and associated malformations. J Clin Endocrinol Metab 84:2502-2506, 1999.
11. Perry R, Heinrichs C, Bourdoux P, et al: Discordance of monozygotic twins for thyroid dysgenesis: Implications for screening and for molecular pathophysiology. J Clin Endocrinol Metab 87: 4072-4077, 2002.
12. Deladoey J, Vassart G, Van Vliet G: Possible non-mendelian mechanisms of thyroid dysgenesis. Endocr Dev 10:29-42, 2007.
13. Lanzerath K, Bettendorf M, Haag C, et al: Screening for Pax8 mutations in patients with congenital hypothyroidism in South-West Germany. Horm Res 66:96-100, 2006.
14. Lapi P, Macchia PE, Chiovato L, et al: Mutations in the gene encoding thyroid transcription factor-1 (TTF-1) are not a frequent cause of congenital hypothyroidism (CH) with thyroid dysgenesis. Thyroid 7:383-387, 1997.

15. Perna MG, Civitareale D, De Filippis V, et al: Absence of mutations in the gene encoding thyroid transcription factor- 1 (TTF-1) in patients with thyroid dysgenesis. Thyroid 7:377-381, 1997.
16. Tonacchera M, Banco M, Lapi P, et al: Genetic analysis of TTF-2 gene in children with congenital hypothyroidism and cleft palate, congenital hypothyroidism, or isolated cleft palate. Thyroid 14:584-588, 2004.
17. Giurgea I, Bellanne-Chantelot C, Ribeiro M, et al: Molecular mechanisms of neonatal hyperinsulinism. Horm Res 66:289-296, 2006.
18. Trueba SS, Auge J, Mattei G, et al: PAX8, TITF1, and FOXE1 gene expression patterns during human development: New insights into human thyroid development and thyroid dysgenesis-associated malformations. J Clin Endocrinol Metab 90:455-462, 2005.
19. Yokoro S, Matsuo M, Ohtsuka T, Ohzeki T: Hyperthyrotropinemia in a neonate with normal thyroid hormone levels: The earliest diagnostic clue for pseudohypoparathyroidism. Biol Neonate 58: 69-72, 1990.
20. Alberti L, Proverbio MC, Costagliola S, et al: Germline mutations of TSH receptor gene as cause of nonautoimmune subclinical hypothyroidism. J Clin Endocrinol Metab 87:2549-2555, 2002.
21. Grasberger H, Mimouni-Bloch A, Vantyghem MC, et al: Autosomal dominant resistance to thyrotropin as a distinct entity in five multigenerational kindreds: Clinical characterization and exclusion of candidate loci. J Clin Endocrinol Metab 90:4025-4034, 2005.
22. Al Taji E, Biebermann H, Limanova Z, et al: Screening for mutations in transcription factors in a Czech cohort of 170 patients with congenital and early-onset hypothyroidism: Identification of a novel PAX8 mutation in dominantly inherited early-onset nonautoimmune hypothyroidism. Eur J Endocrinol 156:521-529, 2007.
23. Macchia PE, Lapi P, Krude H, et al: PAX8 mutations associated with congenital hypothyroidism caused by thyroid dysgenesis. Nat Genet 19:83-86, 1998.
24. Vilain C, Rydlewski C, Duprez L, et al: Autosomal dominant transmission of congenital thyroid hypoplasia due to loss-of-function mutation of PAX8. J Clin Endocrinol Metab 86:234-238, 2001.
25. Devriendt K, Vanhole C, Matthijs G, de Zegher F. Deletion of thyroid transcription factor-1 gene in an infant with neonatal thyroid dysfunction and respiratory failure. N Engl J Med 1998 Apr 30;338 (18):1317-8, 1998.
26. Pohlenz J, Dumitrescu A, Zundel D, et al: Partial deficiency of thyroid transcription factor 1 produces predominantly neurological defects in humans and mice. J Clin Invest 109:469-473, 2002.
27. Krude H, Schutz B, Biebermann H, et al: Choreoathetosis, hypothyroidism, and pulmonary alterations due to human NKX2-1 haploinsufficiency. J Clin Invest 109:475-480, 2002.
28. Breedveld GJ, van Dongen JW, Danesino C, et al: Mutations in TITF-1 are associated with benign hereditary chorea. Hum Mol Genet 11:971-979, 2002.
29. Doyle DA, Gonzalez I, Thomas B, Scavina M: Autosomal dominant transmission of congenital hypothyroidism, neonatal respiratory distress, and ataxia caused by a mutation of NKX2-1. J Pediatr 145: 190-193, 2004.
30. Maquet E, Costagliola S, Parma J, et al: Lethal respiratory failure and mild primary hypothyroidism in a term girl with a de novo heterozygous mutation in the TTF1 gene. J Clin Endocrinol Metab 94:197-203, 2008.
31. Bamforth JS, Hughes IA, Lazarus JH, et al: Congenital hypothyroidism, spiky hair, and cleft palate. J Med Genet 26:49-51, 1989.
32. Clifton-Bligh RJ, Wentworth JM, et al: Mutation of the gene encoding human TTF-2 associated with thyroid agenesis, cleft palate and choanal atresia. Nat Genet 19:399-401, 1998.
33. Castanet M, Park SM, Smith A, et al: A novel loss-of-function mutation in TTF-2 is associated with congenital hypothyroidism, thyroid agenesis and cleft palate. Hum Mol Genet 11:2051-2059, 2002.
34. Baris I, Arisoy AE, Smith A, et al: A novel missense mutation in human TTF-2 (FKHL15) gene associated with congenital hypothyroidism but not athyreosis. J Clin Endocrinol Metab 91:4183-4187, 2006.
35. Carré A, Castanet M, Sura-Trueba S, et al: Polymorphic length of FOXE1 alanine stretch: Evidence for genetic susceptibility to thyroid dysgenesis. Hum Genet 122:467-476, 2007.
36. Hishinuma A, Ohyama Y, Kuribayashi T, et al: Polymorphism of the polyalanine tract of thyroid transcription factor-2 gene in patients with thyroid dysgenesis. Eur J Endocrinol 145:385-389, 2001.
37. Olivieri A, Stazi MA, Mastroiacovo P, et al: A population-based study on the frequency of additional congenital malformations in infants with congenital hypothyroidism: Data from the Italian Registry for Congenital Hypothyroidism (1991-1998). Clin Endocrinol Metab 87:557-562, 2002.
38. Schott JJ, Benson DW, Basson CT, et al: Congenital heart disease caused by mutations in the transcription factor NKX2-5. Science 281:108-111, 1998.
39. Senee V, Chelala C, Duchatelet S, et al: Mutations in GLIS3 are responsible for a rare syndrome with neonatal diabetes mellitus and congenital hypothyroidism. Nat Genet 38:682-687, 2006.
40. van Trotsenburg AS, Kempers MJ, Endert E, et al: Trisomy 21 causes persistent congenital hypothyroidism presumably of thyroidal origin. Thyroid 16:671-680, 2006.
41. Scuccimarri R, Rodd C. Thyroid abnormalities as a feature of DiGeorge syndrome: A patient report and review of the literature. J Pediatr Endocrinol Metab 11:273-276, 1998.
42. Cambiaso P, Orazi C, Digilio MC, et al: Thyroid morphology and subclinical hypothyroidism in children and adolescents with Williams syndrome. J Pediatr 150:62-65, 2007.
43. Alt B, Elsalini OA, Schrumpf P, et al: Arteries define the position of the thyroid gland during its developmental relocalisation. Development 133:3797-3804, 2006.

44. Deladoey J, Pfarr N, Vuissoz JM, et al: Pseudodominant inheritance of goitrous congenital hypothyroidism caused by TPO mutations: Molecular and in silico studies. J Clin Endocrinol Metab 93:627-633, 2008.
45. Abramowicz MJ, Targovnik HM, Varela V, et al: Identification of a mutation in the coding sequence of the human thyroid peroxidase gene causing congenital goiter. J Clin Invest 90:1200-1204, 1992.
46. Avbelj M, Tahirovic H, Debeljak M, et al: High prevalence of thyroid peroxidase gene mutations in patients with thyroid dyshormonogenesis. Eur J Endocrinol 156:511-519, 2007.
47. Rodrigues C, Jorge P, Soares JP, et al: Mutation screening of the thyroid peroxidase gene in a cohort of 55 Portuguese patients with congenital hypothyroidism. Eur J Endocrinol 152:193-198, 2005.
48. Fugazzola L, Cerutti N, Mannavola D, et al: Monoallelic expression of mutant thyroid peroxidase allele causing total iodide organification defect. J Clin Endocrinol Metab 88:3264-3271, 2003.
49. Bakker B, Bikker H, Hennekam RC, et al: Maternal isodisomy for chromosome 2p causing severe congenital hypothyroidism. J Clin Endocrinol Metab 86:1164-1168, 2001.
50. Ieiri T, Cochaux P, Targovnik HM, et al: A 3′ splice site mutation in the thyroglobulin gene responsible for congenital goiter with hypothyroidism. J Clin Invest 88:1901-1905, 1991.
51. Kim PS, Ding M, Menon S, et al: A missense mutation G2320R in the thyroglobulin gene causes non-goitrous congenital primary hypothyroidism in the WIC-rdw rat. Mol Endocrinol 14:1944-1953, 2000.
52. Fujiwara H: Congenital hypothyroidism caused by a mutation in the Na^+/I^- symporter. Nat Genet 17:122, 1997.
53. Szinnai G, Kosugi S, Derrien C, et al: Extending the clinical heterogeneity of iodide transport defect (ITD): A novel mutation R124H of the sodium/iodide symporter (NIS) gene and review of genotype-phenotype correlations in ITD. J Clin Endocrinol Metab 91:1199-1204, 2006.
54. Kosugi S, Bhayana S, Dean HJ: A novel mutation in the sodium/iodide symporter gene in the largest family with iodide transport defect. J Clin Endocrinol Metab 84:3248-3253, 1999.
55. Everett LA, Glaser B, Beck JC, et al: Pendred syndrome is caused by mutations in a putative sulphate transporter gene (PDS). Nat Genet 17:411-422, 1997.
56. Gaudino R, Garel C, Czernichow P, Leger J: Proportion of various types of thyroid disorders among newborns with congenital hypothyroidism and normally located gland: A regional cohort study. Clin Endocrinol (Oxf) 62:444-448, 2005.
57. Banghova K, Al TE, Cinek O, et al: Pendred syndrome among patients with congenital hypothyroidism detected by neonatal screening: Identification of two novel PDS/SLC26A4 mutations. Eur J Pediatr 167:777-783, 2008.
58. Moreno JC, Klootwijk W, van TH, et al: Mutations in the iodotyrosine deiodinase gene and hypothyroidism. N Engl J Med 358:1811-188, 2008.
59. Moreno JC, Bikker H, Kempers MJ, et al: Inactivating mutations in the gene for thyroid oxidase 2 (THOX2) and congenital hypothyroidism. N Engl J Med 347:95-102, 2002.
60. Moreno JC, Visser TJ: New phenotypes in thyroid dyshormonogenesis: Hypothyroidism due to DUOX2 mutations. Endocr Dev 10:99-117, 2007.
61. Grasberger H, Refetoff S: Identification of the maturation factor for dual oxidase. Evolution of an eukaryotic operon equivalent. J Biol Chem 281: 18269-18272, 2006.
61a. Zamproni I, Grasberger H, Cortinovis F, et al: Biallelic inactivation of the dual oxidase maturation factor 2 (DUOXA2) gene as a novel cause of congenital hypothyroidism. J Clin Endocrinol Metab 93:605-610, 2008.
62. Kempers MJ, Lanting CI, van Heijst AF, et al: Neonatal screening for congenital hypothyroidism based on thyroxine, thyrotropin, and thyroxine-binding globulin measurement: Potentials and pitfalls. J Clin Endocrinol Metab 91:3370-3376, 2006.
63. Lovinger RD, Kaplan SL, Grumbach MM: Congenital hypopituitarism associated with neonatal hypoglycemia and microphallus: Four cases secondary to hypothalamic hormone deficiencies. J Pediatr 87(Pt 2):1171-1181, 1975.
64. Collu R, Tang J, Castagne J, et al: A novel mechanism for isolated central hypothyroidism: Inactivating mutations in the thyrotropin-releasing hormone receptor gene. J Clin Endocrinol Metab 82:1561-1565, 1997.
65. Hayashizaki Y, Hiraoka Y, Tatsumi K, et al: Deoxyribonucleic acid analyses of five families with familial inherited thyroid stimulating hormone deficiency. J Clin Endocrinol Metab 71:792-796, 1990.
66. Dacou-Voutetakis C, Feltquate DM, et al: Familial hypothyroidism caused by a nonsense mutation in the thyroid-stimulating hormone beta-subunit gene. Am J Hum Genet 46:988-993, 1990.
67. Partsch CJ, Riepe FG, Krone N, et al: Initially elevated TSH and congenital central hypothyroidism due to a homozygous mutation of the TSH beta subunit gene: Case report and review of the literature. Exp Clin Endocrinol Diabetes 114:227-234, 2006.
68. Heinrichs C, Parma J, Scherberg NH, et al: Congenital central isolated hypothyroidism caused by a homozygous mutation in the TSH-beta subunit gene. Thyroid 10:387-391, 2000.
69. Brumm H, Pfeufer A, Biebermann H, et al: Congenital central hypothyroidism due to homozygous thyrotropin beta 313 Delta T mutation is caused by a Founder effect. J Clin Endocrinol Metab 87: 4811-4816, 2002.
70. Deladoey J, Vuissoz JM, Domene HM, et al: Congenital secondary hypothyroidism due to a mutation C105Vfs114X thyrotropin-beta mutation: Genetic study of five unrelated families from Switzerland and Argentina. Thyroid 13:553-559, 2003.

71. Ward L, Chavez M, Huot C, et al: Severe congenital hypopituitarism with low prolactin levels and age-dependent anterior pituitary hypoplasia: A clue to a PIT-1 mutation. J Pediatr 132:1036-1038, 1998.

72. Kelberman D, Dattani MT: The role of transcription factors implicated in anterior pituitary development in the aetiology of congenital hypopituitarism. Ann Med 38:560-577, 2006.

Chapter 10

Hypothyroidism

Joanne F. Rovet, Thomas P. Foley, Jr., and Meranda Nakhla

Key Points

- Distinct challenges in managing hypothyroidism in the pediatric population
- Thyroid hormones' unique role in early brain development and subsequent brain function
- Congenital and acquired hypothyroidism—causes, clinical features, diagnosis, and treatment; common pitfalls in diagnosis or misdiagnosis, including consequences of late diagnosis
- Persisting subtle deficits in adequately treated congenital hypothyroidism and associated risk factors
- Outcome following therapy for acquired hypothyroidism and potential adverse effects of therapy

Hypothyroidism is caused by a deficiency in the secretion of thyroid hormones produced in the thyroid gland. Because thyroid hormone is essential for normal growth and development, adequate metabolism, and proper brain development, the consequences of hypothyroidism in childhood can be devastating, particularly in children with neonatal hypothyroidism. A delay of treatment in this group can result in permanent brain damage and mental retardation.

There are two major forms of hypothyroidism in the pediatric population: (1) congenital hypothyroidism (CH), which represents a group of diseases developing at conception or during gestation and are present at birth; and (2) acquired hypothyroidism (AH), which usually appears after 6 months of age and arises from autoimmune destruction of the thyroid. The management of hypothyroidism in an infant or young child poses challenges distinct from those of adult hypothyroidism because of the need to diagnose and treat affected children as quickly as possible. This is particularly vital for children younger than 3 years. Additionally, among older children presenting with severe AH, it is important to introduce replacement hormone slowly to prevent adverse reactions that may result from exposing the brain to high levels of exogenous hormone after having adjusted to its hypothyroid state over the long term.

Regarding the loss of thyroid hormone in infants and children, results of extensive animal studies have demonstrated that thyroid hormone is essential for early brain development and plays a key role in later brain functioning.[1] Thyroid hormone is involved in fundamental neurobiologic processes such as neurogenesis,[2] axon and dendrite formation,[3] neuronal migration,[4-6] myelination,[7] and synaptogenesis,[8] with the timing of need for thyroid hormone varying among different brain structures. In the brain, the need for thyroid hormone proceeds in a subcortical to cortical direction and, within the cortex, in a posterior to anterior direction, with the frontal lobes needing thyroid hormone last.[9] Structures showing the greatest need for thyroid hormone include the following: the thalamus, which is important for perception; the cerebellum, important for motor coordination; the caudate, important for attention; the hippocampus, important for memory; and the cortex, important for multiple aspects of cognitive functioning. In addition, thyroid hormone is also involved in cochlear[10] and retinal[11] development and, in the retina, rod versus cone distribution and the patterning of the cone subtypes underlying color vision.[12-14] In rodents, a lack of thyroid hormone during gestation and/or early life contributes to damage in the various thyroid hormone–dependent brain structures; although this can be reversed or minimized by the administration of exogenous hormone, it must be provided within a critical developmental window to have an effect.[15,16]

Thyroid hormone acts by regulating specific brain genes,[17,18] which underlie the basic processes of brain development described. Thyroid-specific gene regulation is accomplished via a set of distinct thyroid hormone receptors,[2,19,20] which along with specific coactivators and corepressors[21,22] activate or deactivate particular brain genes.[23] Receptor distribution varies ontologically and regionally,[24] with some brain structures showing a greater need for thyroid hormone than others.[25] This finding is significant for humans, in whom impairment from early thyroid hormone loss is more likely to result in specific rather than global deficits; the exact nature will depend on the precise timing of thyroid hormone insufficiency.

Thyroid hormone also plays an important role in neurotransmission.[26-30] During early life, thyroid hormone controls production of neurotransmitter systems[29] whereas in later life, thyroid hormone regulates catecholamine production and responsiveness.[31,32] Studies with transgenic hypothyroid mice show impaired GABAminergic (gamma-aminobutyric acid, GABA) circuit formation accompanied by reduced exploratory behavior and increased freezing in fear conditioning.[33] Thyroid hormone also modulates the production of tyrosine hydroxylase, the rate-limiting enzyme in dopamine and norepinephrine production,[34] and is thought to act as a cotransmitter,[35] traveling along central noradrenergic pathways.[36] In addition, thyroid hormone (1) activates neurons via astrocytes,[37] (2) affects synaptic transmission between neurons through the release of glutamate,[8] (3) upregulates a sodium-dependent neurotransmitter transporter gene[38] and other genes involved in neurotransmitter function,[39] and (4) controls GABA release and reuptake,[40] as well as GABA receptor function.[38] Furthermore, thyroid hormone effects on neurotransmitter function are different in the developing than in the adult brain[38] where, for example, thyroid hormone stimulates GABA function in early life and inhibits it later. Because these actions have functional implications for humans, they underscore the need to maintain proper levels of thyroid hormone beyond the period of early brain growth. Thus, a further purpose of this chapter will be to examine outcomes in children with CH and AH in relation to adequacy of therapy.

EPIDEMIOLOGY, RISK FACTORS, AND PATHOGENESIS

The epidemiology and associated risk factors for congenital and acquired hypothyroidism vary, depending on the cause. Table 10-1 compares some of the most common causes of the two conditions.

Congenital Hypothyroidism

In areas of iodine sufficiency, CH sporadically affects between 1 in 3000 to 4000 newborns. This incidence is higher in areas of iodine insufficiency. CH is more common in Hispanic than white infants and less common in blacks than in whites. CH is also comorbid with Down syndrome (DS) and may occur in as many as 1 in 128 DS cases.[41]

The two major CH subcategories are (1) primary hypothyroidism, resulting from a defect at the level of the thyroid gland and (2) central hypothyroidism, reflecting a defect in hypothalamic or pituitary regulation of thyroid hormone levels. At the thyroidal level, CH can result from thyroid dysgenesis caused by a missing, ectopic (lingual or sublingual), or hypoplastic gland or from thyroid dyshormonogenesis caused by a gene defect in one of the many stages of thyroid hormone synthesis and transport[42] (see Chapter 9). In thyroid dysgenesis, girls are twice as frequently affected as boys and, in most forms, this occurs sporadically.[43] Several genes found to be associated with thyroid dysgenesis include *TTF-1*, *TTF-2*, and *PAX8*; however, because defects in these genes have accounted only for about 10% of all cases with thyroid dysgenesis to date, the picture is far from complete. In thyroid dyshormonogenesis, males and females are equally affected and inheritance is autosomal recessive, often with multiple family members affected.

Additionally, 1 in 50,000 children may have thyroid hormone resistance caused by a mutation in the gene encoding the thyroid hormone receptor β (TRβ) receptors. Inheritance is autosomal dominant and the distribution of receptor mutations within an individual and family is generally heterogeneous. Thyroid hormone resistance is classically categorized as the following: (1) central, with receptors within the pituitary affected; (2) peripheral, with only receptors in the peripheral tissue affected; or (3) generalized, with receptors in both the central nervous system (CNS) and peripheral tissue affected. Clinically, patients may be hypothyroid (2, 3), euthyroid (1, 2, 3), or hyperthyroid (1), depending on the severity of the receptor mutation and tissue distribution of the mutant genes.

In a small proportion of children, CH may be transient because of intrauterine transmission of maternal antibodies, which block the developing fetal thyroid from functioning, or because of pre- and perinatal exposure to excess iodine from radiocontrast and antiseptic solutions.[44,45] Based on animal studies, it is also possible that some children can experience mild hypothyroidism from certain environmental chemicals,[46] such as flame retardants or polybrominated diphenyl ethers (PBDEs), mercury, lead, dioxins, and polychlorinated biphenyls (PCBs).[47] However, studies directly examining the impact of these chemicals on children's thyroid function have not been conducted.

Table 10–1 Causes of Hypothyroidism

Congenital Hypothyroidism	Acquired Hypothyroidism
Permanent Sporadic Hypothyroidism	Late-onset, mild congenital hypothyroidism
Thyroid dysgenesis	Ectopic thyroid dysgenesis
Athyrosis	Familial thyroid dyshormonogenesis
Ectopia	Peripheral resistance to thyroid hormone action
Hypoplasia, iatrogenic	Acquired primary hypothyroidism
Maternal exposure to ^{131}I-iodine—congenital defects in embryogenesis; PAX8, TTF1, TTF2	Chronic autoimmune thyroiditis
Idiopathic hyperthyrotropinemia (subclinical hypothyroidism of infancy)	Lymphocytic thyroiditis of childhood and adolescence with thyromegaly
Isolated	Hashimoto's thyroiditis with thyromegaly
Down syndrome	Chronic fibrous variant
Idiopathic primary hypothyroidism—PAX8, TTF1, TTF2	Acquired autoimmune-mediated infantile hypothyroidism
Permanent Familial Hypothyroidism	Drug-induced hypothyroidism
Dyshormonogenesis	Antithyroid drugs (propylthiouracil, methimazole, carbimazole)
TSH-beta loss-of-function mutations	Lithium (therapeutic doses to treat bipolar diseases)
TSH receptor loss-of-function mutations	Endemic goiter
Unresponsiveness with mild-to-severe hypothyroidism	Iodine deficiency with or without selenium deficiency
Iodide trapping defect (sodium iodide symporter mutations)	Environmental goitrogens
Iodide oxidation defects	Therapeutic radioiodine
Pendred's syndrome	Environmental exposure to thyroid disruptors (PCBs, PBDEs, lead, dioxins, perchlorate)
Thyroperoxidase mtuations	Surgical excision (cancer, hyperthyroidism)
Iodotyrosine deiodinase defect	Subacute thyroiditis: transient phase
Permanent hypothalamic-pituitary hypothyroidism	External irradiation of nonthyroid tumors
Multiple hypothalamic hormone deficiencies	Irradiation of thyroid by external irradiation, ingestion and inhalation from environmental sources (e.g., nuclear power plant accidents, atomic bomb detonations, terrorist attacks with dirty bombs)
Idiopathic	
Familial	
Associated with midline central nervous system anatomic defects	
Isolated TRH deficiency	
Isolated TSH deficiency	
Transient hypothyroidism	
Iodine deficiency	
Nutritional	
Congenital nephrosis, iatrogenic	
Maternal or neonatal exposure to iodine	
Maternal antithyroid drug therapy	
Maternal TSH receptor-blocking antibodies	
Maternal chronic autoimmune thyroiditis	
Transient dyshormonogenesis	
Oxidation defect	

PBDEs, polybrominated diphenyl ethers; PCBs, polychlorinated biphenyls; TRH, thyrotropin-releasing hormone; TSH, thyroid-stimulating hormone.

Acquired Hypothyroidism

AH can affect as many as 1% to 2% of adolescents. AH is more common in children older than 10 years, very rare in infants, and more frequent in females than males.

The most common cause of AH is Hashimoto's thyroiditis, an autoimmune disorder caused by abnormalities of the humoral and cellular immune systems. Although the specific genetically programmed immune-mediated mechanisms producing

AH are poorly understood, the primary effect appears to be an immune response against normal thyroid cells, which leads to inflammation, destruction, and death of thyroid follicular cells, destroying as much as 75% of the thyroid tissue. Hashimoto's thyroiditis is also often associated with other autoimmune diseases, such as type 1 diabetes mellitus, Addison's disease, and rheumatoid arthritis, and it is common in DS and Turner's syndrome.

In addition, AH may be induced by certain psychotropic medications, which can also alter thyroid function tests to yield false-positive data indicative of hypothyroidism. For example, lithium carbonate in high doses used to treat bipolar diseases, iodinated drugs such as amiodarone, and cytokines (e.g., interferon-gamma [IFN-γ], interleukin-6 [IL-6], granulocyte-monocyte colony stimulating-factor [GM-CSF]) all interfere with thyroid hormone synthesis and/or secretion to cause primary hypothyroidism. This effect usually occurs in biochemically and clinically euthyroid patients with little thyroid reserve caused by an existing thyroid disease, such as autoimmune thyroiditis. In similar patients, as well as those on a fixed dose of thyroxine, antiepileptics (e.g., phenobarbital, phenytoin, carbamazepine) and the antituberculosis drug rifampicin can stimulate cytochrome P450 inducers to accelerate the hepatic degradation of thyroxine, whereas other drugs such as propylthiouracil (PTU), beta blockers, dexamethasone, and other iodinated preparations inhibit 5′-deiodinase. Phenytoin and substances such as heparin, free fatty acids, and salicylates compete with thyroxine (T_4) for T_4-binding proteins to cause low T_4 values and even interfere with many of the free T_4 tests. Thus, when thyroid function test results do not make sense, the problem could be other medications that might be inducing hypothyroidism or interfere with the laboratory analysis.

CLINICAL FEATURES

The most common symptoms and signs of CH and AH are listed in Table 10-2. The appearance of a specific symptom or sign depends on the age at which the hypothyroidism develops, duration of the disease, and disease severity. Often, findings may not be obvious to parents or physicians until the child's growth velocity declines or hypothyroidism progresses to a moderate or severe stage.

Congenital Hypothyroidism

Today, almost all infants with CH born in the United States and Canada are identified through newborn screening programs, which assess for abnormal thyroid-stimulating hormone (TSH) and/or T_4 levels (see Chapter 8). Typically, diagnosis from newborn screening occurs before most physical signs and symptoms are evident. In neonates, the most common signs and symptoms of CH after birth are prolonged neonatal jaundice, hypothermia, large anterior and posterior fontanelles, an umbilical hernia, and a puffy face. An Australian study has reported that 62% of infants diagnosed with CH have jaundice, 54% have an umbilical hernia, 41% have edema, and 21% have a protruding tongue, whereas only 6% show an enlarged thyroid on palpation.[48] In addition, approximately 15% of CH children also show an increased incidence of major congenital malformations,[48] particularly cardiac (7%) and urogenital (3%) abnormalities.

Most neonates with CH are born full term, with a substantial number born past 42 weeks gestation and at birth weights more than 4 kg. With age, those infants not promptly treated show generalized myxedema, carotenemia of the skin, wiry and/or excessive dark hair, macroglossia, and increased floppiness and muscle weakness (Fig. 10-1) and may also develop strabismus and nystagmus. In addition, they display marked lethargy, little activity, decreased appetite, and severe constipation over time.

Rarely, but not uncommonly, some children with CH are missed by the newborn screening program. Lack of detection can arise from problems in submitting and shipping samples, errors in labeling, laboratory error, and problems with data entry. In a few cases, children may fail to receive the newborn screening test for reasons such as transfer to another hospital or home birth. In other cases, children may pass the screening test but show delayed presentation of CH, particularly if T4 screening is used; in still others, the particular condition may not be identified by the particular screening method (e.g., central hypothyroidism and the TSH test). Although some states provide a second screen between 2 and 4 weeks of age, which is capable of catching these delayed presentation cases, second screening is not universal and costly and it is not known to what degree these children still suffer residual damage during the period between the two screening tests. Although many parents of children missed by screening are usually very aware and concerned their infant was not developing normally, their physicians failed to make the proper diagnosis and did not conduct diagnostic tests despite seeking advice from geneticists, ophthalmologists, and gastroenterologists (who also failed to make the diagnosis). Thus it is critical that all physicians be cognizant of the possibility for a missed screening test and thus be prudent of the need to diagnose CH clinically,

Table 10–2 Common Symptoms and Signs of Hypothyroidism

Congenital Hypothyroidism	Acquired Hypothyroidism
Findings During the First 2 Postnatal Weeks	***Findings Between 6 Months and 3 Years of Age***
Prolonged neonatal jaundice	Deceleration of linear growth
Edema of the eyelids, hands, and feet	Coarse facial features
Gestation > 42 wk	Dry skin with carotenemia
Birth weight > 4 kg	Hoarse cry and large tongue
Poor feeding	Umbilical hernia
Hypothermia	Muscular pseudohypertrophy (enlargement of the arm and leg muscles)
Protuberant abdomen	***Findings During Childhood***
Large anterior and posterior fontanelles	Deceleration of linear growth with or without short stature
Findings Beyond Age 1 Month	Delay in eruption of teeth and in shedding of primary teeth
Darkened and mottled skin	Muscle weakness and pseudohypertrophy (enlargement of the arm and leg muscles)
Stressful, frequent, and labored breathing	Infrequent and hard stools
Failure to gain weight	Dry skin with carotenemia
Poor sucking ability	Generalized swelling or myxedema
Decreased stool frequency	Precocious sexual development—breast development without sexual hair in girls; enlarged testes without sexual hair in boys
Decreased activity and lethargy	***Findings During Adolescence***
Findings During the First 3 Months	Delayed onset of puberty
Umbilical hernia	Generalized swelling of myxedema
Infrequent and hard stools	Infrequent and hard stools
Dry skin with carotenemia	Cool, dry pale skin with carotenemia, sallow color, keratoderma
Macroglossia	Peripheral vasoconstriction and, rarely, ecchymoses
Generalized swelling or myxedema	Dry, coarse brittle hair with diffuse or partial alopecia
Hoarse cry	Madarosis or loss of the lateral third of eyebrow hair
	Thick, brittle, and slow-growing nails
	Galactorrhea (girls)

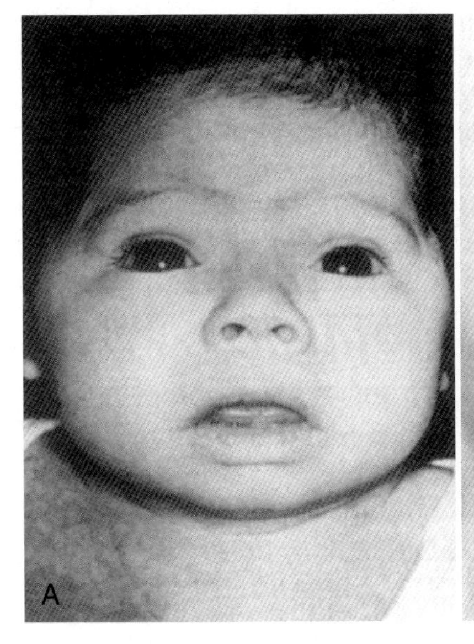

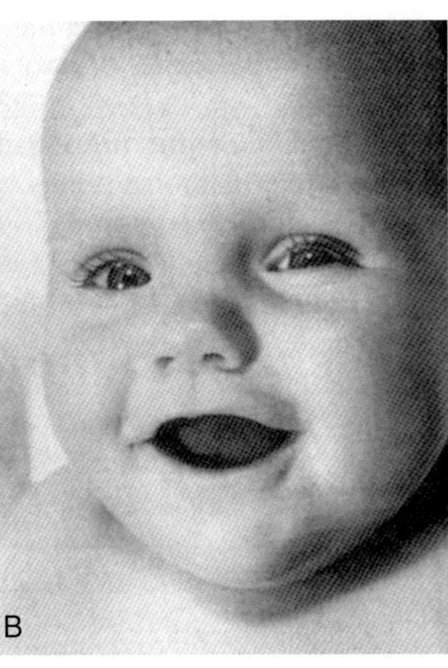

Figure 10–1 Children with congenital hypothyroidism prior to **(A)** and after **(B)** newborn screening.

particularly given the devastating consequences of delaying a diagnosis.

Acquired Hypothyroidism

In acquired hypothyroidism, the most common presenting feature is failure or deceleration of growth with delayed skeletal maturation. Although changes in body shape and a coarsening of facial features do become evident over time, the appearance of a child with AH is usually not as striking as a child with cretinism (Fig. 10-2). Children with AH may be slow in shedding their primary or developing teeth and also have constipation, myxedema, coldness, dry skin, and muscle weakness. They also present with delayed puberty or rarely isosexual precocious puberty.

Because the onset of AH is insidious, its diagnosis is often delayed for months after a prolonged period of abnormal linear growth. Moreover, because children with AH are generally well behaved and achieving satisfactorily at school in the hypothyroid state, concern may be minimal. However, in rare cases where the disorder does develop in infancy, these children often show many of the same features as late-treated CH including deceleration of growth, coarse facial features, dry skin, wiry hair, hoarse cry, large tongue, an umbilical hernia, delayed dentition, delayed closure of the fontanelles, and lethargy. Toddlers and preschoolers with AH may also show regression of intellectual and motor development following the onset of hypothyroidism as well as engage in severe temper tantrums and show increased irritability.[50] Because of the brain's high need for thyroid hormone up to 3 years of age, these children will likely be permanently affected and show neurodevelopmental delays.

DIAGNOSIS

Congenital Hypothyroidism

The diagnosis of CH should be made as soon as possible after the newborn screening results are available. Diagnostic tests should include a serum free T_4 (FT_4), serum thyroglobulin if the thyroid gland is not palpable, and thyroid ultrasonography or technetium scan to establish the cause of hypothyroidism. Table 10-3 summarizes the evaluation of thyroid function in different types of hypothyroidism. At 3 years of age, children should be taken off therapy for 1 month and thyroid function tests repeated to ascertain whether the hypothyroidism was transient.[51] In patients with central hypothyroidism, other pituitary and peripheral hormones should be measured, especially cortisol, before thyroxine therapy is started.

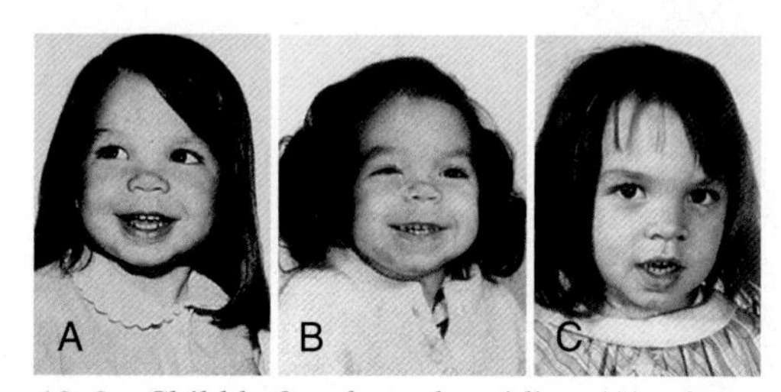

Figure 10–2 Child before hypothyroidism **(A)**, after onset of acquired hypothyroidism **(B)**, and after treatment **(C)**.

Acquired Hypothyroidism

The diagnostic procedures for AH should include thyroid function tests and measuring thyroid peroxidase and thyroglobulin antibodies to establish the diagnosis of autoimmune thyroiditis. FT_4 is preferred over total T_4 because the latter may yield misleading results from binding with thyroid-binding proteins. The investigation should also include examination of the neck for an enlarged thyroid, measurement of linear growth and growth velocity, assessment for signs and symptoms of hypothyroidism, and determining a family history of thyroid disease. Additionally, serum levels of gonadotropins, morning cortisol, and prolactin should be measured in patients with delayed puberty or concern of central hypothyroidism. Bone age, which is typically delayed, is often used as a marker of the onset of AH. Computed tomography and magnetic resonance imaging (MRI) of the brain may reveal an enlarged sella turcica caused by pituitary thyrotroph hypertrophy.[52] An empty sella and other CNS dysmorphic features, such as septo-optic dysplasia, may also be apparent.

TREATMENT

The treatment of hypothyroidism is relatively easy and inexpensive and the treatment of choice for infants and children is levothyroxine (L-T_4). Although the total dose increases about three- to fivefold from infancy to adult life, the daily dose per body weight steadily decreases to an adult dose in adolescence. Treatment must be individualized because thyroxine absorption and metabolism differ among individuals, making careful monitoring essential. Because certain foods (e.g., soy formulas, fiber-containing foods) can block intestinal absorption of L-T_4, these should be limited or closely monitored. Similarly, because medications containing iron or calcium can also block L-T_4 absorption, these should be given at different times of day than L-T_4.

There are no complications from L-T_4 therapy if the proper dose is taken and blood tests are monitored on a regular basis. Complications can be associated with unrecognized or inadequately treated hypothyroidism, the worst being delayed treatment in infancy. Premature craniosynostosis following a high dose level for many weeks in infancy is generally not seen, as long as thyroid hormone levels are closely monitored.

Table 10–3 Thyroid Function Test Results

Thyroid Function Test	Primary Hypothyroidism	Hypothalamic Hypothyroidism	Pituitary Hypothyroidism
TSH	Elevated	Normal or low	Low
Free T_4	Low	Low	Low
TSH response to TRH	Exaggerated	Normal or delayed and exaggerated	Absent

T_4, thyroxine; TRH, thyrotropin-releasing hormone; TSH, thyroid-stimulating hormone.
Adapted from Germak JA, Foley TP Jr: Longitudinal assessment of L-thyroxine therapy for congenital hypothyroidism. J Pediatr 117:211-219, 1990.

Congenital Hypothyroidism

The American Academy of Pediatrics recommends a starting dose of L-T_4 from 10 to 15 μg/kg/day taken at least 30 minutes before food intake. The goal of therapy is to normalize T_4 within 2 weeks and TSH within 1 month. Thus, infants with athyreosis who have very low or undetectable FT_4 and highly elevated TSH levels are prescribed to start with 13 to 15 mg/kg/day of L-T_4. For infants with a TSH higher than 20 mU/L and normal T_4 values, a starting L-T_4 dose of 37.5 mg/day should be sufficient if the birth weight is normal and the baby was born full term. Thereafter, it is important to maintain TSH between 0.5 and 2.0 mU/L and T_4 and/or FT_4 in the upper half of the reference range for the first 3 years of life.[43] In patients for whom compliance is suspected to be poor, and because of the major sequelae associated with poor compliance, initial and ongoing counseling of parents is recommended.

L-T_4 is available for infants in 25-, 50-, 75-μg, and higher tablets. During infancy, 25-μg tablets should be prescribed and children should be given, for example, one-and-a-half, two, or two-and-a-half tablets to get daily dosages of 37.5, 50, or 62.5 μg. Subtle dosage adjustments can also be achieved by the addition or omission of one tablet/wk or by 12.5-μg increments daily. The pill should be crushed in a suspension of formula, breast milk, or water. Care should be taken to avoid concomitant administration of soy, fiber, calcium, or iron and the dose should be adjusted according to the infant's clinical response and serum FT_4 and TSH concentrations.[43] The U.S. Food and Drug Administration (FDA) has deemed that several L-T_4 products are bioequivalent to some current brands. Any change in source of L-T_4, especially if not a standard brand, may require dose retitration.[43]

If a parent misses a dose or thinks the dose was missed, the dosage on the next day should be doubled. As a rule, starting dose levels of 10 to 15 μg/kg can allow for normalization of serum T_4 and TSH within 3 days and 2 weeks, respectively.[53] The exact duration of hypothyroid therapy usually reflects disease severity, age when treatment is initiated, and dosage of replacement hormone, although there is a small subset of children who are refractory to treatment[54] and may have a less sensitive than normal hypothalamic-pituitary-thyroid axis.[55] Breast feeding can mildly offset the thyroid insufficiency[56] because mother's milk contains small amounts of thyroxine.[57,58]

In managing a child with CH, the recommended protocol is to evaluate the children at 2 and 4 weeks after diagnosis, monthly to age 6 months, trimonthly or quarterly between 6 months and 3 years of age, and semiannually or annually from 3 years until growth has ceased.[52] Children showing serum TSH elevations should receive a dose increment; hypothyroidism with a particular cause may need more frequent adjustments than others.[59] In follow-up, a dose should be provided that maintains FT_4 levels in the upper end of the normal range for at least the first 3 years of life. Occasionally, TSH levels may be undetectable despite normal FT_4 levels. If this is associated with clinical thyrotoxicosis, the dose of L-T_4 should be reduced until the TSH is measurable and the clinical symptoms subside. However, if the child is clinically euthyroid, it is advisable to decrease the dose slightly by half to one tablet/wk to retain normal FT_4 with a measurable TSH.

Because children from rural communities or who live in small cities that lack academic health care facilities are typically treated by primary physicians who may not be cognizant of the American Academy of Pediatrics guidelines, it is important that information about treatment and management of CH be conveyed broadly. We are aware of a number of cases of children who received inadequate care for CH (e.g., no dose increments, overtreatment, or improper parental education) from uninformed primary health care physicians and their professional staff. It is therefore essential that there be strict adherence to the guidelines for clinical and thyroid function monitoring and at the prescribed intervals for infants and children with CH to avoid permanent detrimental consequences for the affected child.

It is also important to assess for the permanence of CH. Confirmation of the cause can be accomplished by thyroid imaging using ^{99m}Tc-technetium or ^{123}I-iodine scans and ultrasound using standard protocols for the evaluation of the permanent, sporadic, and familial causes of CH. If the initial scan shows an ectopic or absent gland, the CH is permanent. If the initial TSH level is lower than 50 mU/L and there is no increase in TSH after the newborn period, then a trial off therapy should be considered at age 3[51]; if the TSH level increases off therapy, the CH can be considered permanent and the individual will need to continue L-T_4 therapy throughout life.

Acquired Hypothyroidism

Treatment of AH involves oral L-T_4 taken in a single daily dose, determined by the child's size. The recommended daily dosage by age is 8 to 10 µg/kg at 3 to 6 months, 6 to 8 µg/kg from 6 to 12 months,[52] 6 µg/kg from 1 to 5 years, 4 µg/kg from 6 to 10 years, and 2 to 3 µg/kg from 11 to 20 years.[60,61] The optimal maintenance dosage should normalize levels of serum TSH and maintain serum FT_4 or total T_4 levels in the middle or upper range of normal for age. A prudent approach based on our earlier studies is to provide a low dosage initially and gradually titrate the dose upward until euthyroidism is achieved. This approach is optimal for children with severe and long-standing hypothyroidism. Excessive dosages should be avoided to prevent accelerated skeletal maturation and consequently compromised final adult height and hyperthyroidism as well. It is also important to note that the L-T_4 dose may need to be increased if an infant is on a soy-containing formula or a child is taking iron and calcium medications or high dietary fiber in food, because these can impair thyroxine absorption. Similarly, children with malabsorptive disorders (e.g., celiac disease, inflammatory bowel disease) may need an increase in their thyroxine dose to maintain euthyroidism.

If diagnosis is delayed or treatment is inadequate for several years in late childhood or early adolescence, the final adult height may be less than expected, despite appropriate treatment. Prolonged hypothyroidism is also associated with high levels of cholesterol, slowing of activity, episodic hip or knee pain caused by unilateral or bilateral slipped capital femoral epiphysis that often requires surgical intervention, and chronic constipation.[60] Except for attenuation in expected adult height, these abnormalities usually disappear with appropriate treatment. Although most children are well behaved and achieve satisfactorily at school, a few children show slowing of mental function and poor school performance in the hypothyroid state; however, this usually disappears following treatment in most, but not all, cases.[62]

A small proportion of children may also experience visual impairment with papilledema and pseudotumor cerebri, with severe headaches following initiation of replacement therapy.[63] Although these effects are especially evident in children between 8 and 13 years of age,[64,65] pseudotumor cerebri has also been reported in an infant with AH following treatment.[66] Treatment of the pseudotumor is usually based on expert opinion, with visual function as the key to severity, and on the need for invasive interventions that rarely are seen in patients on L-T_4 therapy for AH. Temporary reduction in dose should be helpful. The diagnostic lumbar puncture may cause improvement. The cornerstone of medical management is dosage of acetazolamide of 25 mg/kg/day in three divided doses, up to 250 mg three times daily. Serial objective measurements of vision determine treatment decisions. Cerebral venous sinus thrombosis should be excluded by MRI examination. In obese patients, weight loss is an important intervention.

PROGNOSIS

Congenital Hypothyroidism

Prior to the advent of newborn thyroid screening, most children diagnosed clinically with CH were at risk for mental retardation, with severity of the impairment reflecting the length of delay in treatment.[67-69] As a rule, treatment past 3 months of age was associated with frank and severe mental retardation, whereas treatment before this age was associated with a lesser degree of retardation. In addition to retardation, these children often showed significant neurobehavioral impairments, neuropsychological deficits, and neurologic abnormalities,[70-72] as well as ophthalmologic difficulties. Children missed by newborn screening and treated late often show the same characteristics as those prior to screening, with neurologic damage appearing to originate prenatally and more serious damage occurring if hypothyroidism was not treated until 3 months of age.[73]

Because newborn screening is almost universal in the developed world and is also seen in many developing nations (see Chapter 8), the prognosis for children with CH is far better than in the prescreening era and the risk of mental retardation is very low, particularly if thyroxine therapy is initiated promptly and subsequent treatment is adequate. Most children identified by screening show normal growth and development and attain IQs within the normal range.[74]

PHYSICAL DEVELOPMENT

Although children often fail to grow during the period of thyroid hormone insufficiency, physical recovery is generally good and stature usually normalizes unless treatment is excessively delayed. One longitudinal study followed a cohort of 74 children with congenital hypothyroidism until 3 years of age and measured linear growth and its association to the severity of CH.[75] The mean age at diagnosis and start of treatment was 16.9 ± 5.2 days with an initial starting dose of L-T_4 12.9 ± 2 μg/kg/day.[75] By the age of 3 years, children with CH had normal heights compared to Tanner and Whitehouse growth standards. Also, the severity of CH at diagnosis was not found to be an associated risk factor for linear growth.

In another retrospective cohort study, linear growth and head circumference were examined in 125 children with CH, from diagnosis until 3 years of age.[76] Subjects were categorized based on the cause of CH—athyreosis, ectopia, and dyshormonogenesis. Throughout the 3-year study period, the mean length standard deviation (SD) was within 1 SD of normal population standards and did not differ among the three groups. Also, no difference was found among the three variants as to length SD at diagnosis and 3 years of age and no differences were observed between boys and girls. However, children with athyreosis between 1 to 3 years of age showed significantly larger head circumferences compared with children with ectopia and dyshormonogenesis, and they had a significant increase in head circumference between diagnosis and 3 years of age.[76] The total T_4 at diagnosis was negatively correlated with head circumference SD at 3 years and significantly predicted height. It was postulated that the larger head circumference in children with the athyreotic variant might reflect a compensatory growth of the calvarium as a result of a shortened cranial base. Another theory is that there is an increase in neuronal mass following thyroxine replacement in those with thyroid athyreosis.[76]

A third prospective study from Australia has followed the physical development of a cohort of 152 children with CH to age 12 years.[77] As with the two previous studies, linear growth was normal in the children with CH and persisted throughout the follow-up period. Across both genders, median weights were found to be heavier when compared with U.S. standards. Consistent with other studies, head circumferences were larger in affected children at all ages compared with Australian reference data[77]; the median value in boys was 1.1 to 2.0 cm above reference values and, in girls, 0.6 to 1.4 cm above. Mean bone age lagged narrowly behind the chronologic age across all age groups,[77] and was most pronounced in the group with athyreosis, and was least pronounced in the ectopic group.

A retrospective study from Italy examining pubertal development and final height of patients with CH has reported that pubertal development occurs at normal ages in both genders. In boys, testicular volume of 4 mL was seen at 11.3 years.[78] In girls, breast development reached Tanner stage 2 at a mean age of 10.3 years, with the mean age of menarche occurring at 12.5 years. Final height, which was evaluated at a mean age of 16.5 ± 0.5 years in females and 17.5 ± 0.5 years in males, was normal when compared with British reference standards.[79] Further analyses revealed that onset of pubertal development and final heights are independent of cause and severity of CH at diagnosis.

Overall, the findings from these four studies indicate that timely identification and treatment of children with CH results in the attainment of normal final height and pubertal development.

PSYCHOLOGICAL DEVELOPMENT

The psychological follow-up studies of children with CH identified by screening can be categorized according to eras or generations, depending on the available guidelines for treatment at the time the children were diagnosed. First-generation studies, when children tended to be treated toward the end of the first month of life (e.g., 27 days in Quebec and 29 days in the Netherlands[78,80]) and with dosages of thyroxine from 5 to 10 mg/kg, reported mean IQ levels were significantly below expectation and below unaffected sibling controls,[81,82] although still in the normal range. A 1996 meta-analysis of seven studies from the first cohort reported a 6.3-point IQ differential from sibling or closely matched controls,[83,84] a difference maintained into adolescence[85] and adulthood.[80,86] As a rule, the lowest scores were attained by children with athyreosis or the lowest levels of thyroid hormone at diagnosis. In addition, low IQs were also associated with the length of time to achieve euthyroidism, which depended on several treatment factors (e.g., age at starting treatment, dosage). Other factors influencing intelligence scores included the child's thyroid hormone levels at time of testing,[87] country of residence, ethnic and socioeconomic background, age at assessment, and when the study was conducted in relation to the derivation of the test norms, given the upward drift in scores over time in a population.[88]

Children with CH from the second wave of follow-up studies appeared to achieve a smaller decline in IQ of approximately 4 points[74] compared with the first-generation cases. Nevertheless, those with more severe presentation at birth had reduced IQs, regardless of treatment age.[89,90] A surprising finding from the Netherlands comparing cohorts of CH children born a decade apart, with the later cohort receiving superior treatment, showed improved outcome only in the children with mild thyroid hormone insufficiency.[91] Because the cost of a 4- to 6-point loss in IQ in the general population is not insignificant,[92] efforts to improve treatment time should still continue.

Another major treatment variable is the starting dose level of L-T_4, given that time to achieve euthyroidism or duration of hypothyroidism is highly dependent on dosage.[93] At the beginning of the newborn screening era, when the starting dose level selected by some groups was relatively low (typically less than 8 μg/kg/day), the usual time to achieve euthyroidism often ranged from days to several months for T_4 and from weeks to months for TSH.[94] Comparisons of children stratified according to their starting dose levels revealed higher IQ levels in the higher dose subgroups,[95-97] and the difference was largest in children with the most severe hypothyroidism. In the mid-1990s, both the American Academy of Pediatrics[98,88] and the European Pediatric Society[47] raised the recommended starting dose levels to 10 to 15 μg/kg, with the normalization time defined as the time to achieve a 50% gain in T_4 or lowering of TSH level. These new standards decreased the time for achieving normal serum T_4 levels to 3 days and for normal TSH to 2 weeks.[53] The most recent guidelines of the American Academy of Pediatrics now recommend 10 to 15 μg/kg of L-T_4, taking into account the severity of the initial hypothyroidism.[43] Studies to identify third-generation cases treated more individually are now under way[91] and may signify further improvement in scores.

In addition to lower IQ scores, children with CH may experience a number of specific cognitive and neuromotor deficits. Across studies, findings have revealed the following: (1) delays in speech acquisition with catch-up and subsequently reduced verbal ability; (2) weak motor skills and general clumsiness; (3) visual, visuomotor, and visuospatial impairments; and (4) attention and memory problems.[99,100] Furthermore certain abilities within specific cognitive domains are affected to a greater degree than others and some may be totally spared. Among the various deficits seen in these children, deficits in the visual domain appear to be most apparent and evident very early in life. Table 10-4 lists some of the specific deficits that have been described in these children to date, along with the contributing disease and/or treatment factors.

Regarding language development, children with CH may show subtle speech and language deficits,[101] particularly if they have the athyreotic cause.[82] Delayed speech acquisition is often evident around 3 years of age[100]; however, most children show later catch-up. Language testing reveals weak expressive and receptive skills, particularly for word knowledge but not grammar,[102] a finding that continues into adulthood.[103]

Table 10–4 Specific Deficits in Congenital Hypothyroidism in Relation to Disease and Treatment Factors

Domain	Ability Affected	Contributing Factor	Nonaffected Ability
Language	Expressive speech	Athyreosis; time to normalization	Expressive grammar
	Word comprehension	Time to normalization	Understanding grammar
Visual	Contrast sensitivity	Disease severity	Visual acuity
	Blue-yellow color vision	Disease severity	Red-green color vision
Visuospatial	Object location and orientation	Initial disease severity	Object identification, face discrimination
Attention	Focus, sustain	Initial disease severity; levels at time of testing	Inhibit, shift, divide
Memory	Span size, associative learning, place learning, everyday memory	Time to achieve euthyroidism	Face recognition, working memory, story recall
Executive function		Delay in treatment and normalization	Working memory, decision making, controlled attention

Deficits are seen in multiple aspects of visual and visuospatial function, including contrast detection,[104] color vision,[105] and abilities in manipulating mental images, locating objects in space, forming block constructions, and solving puzzles.[80,82,103,106] These deficits are typically associated with initial disease severity factors, implicating a gestational need for thyroid hormone in the neural substrates supporting these abilities.

Attentional skills may also be problematic in children with CH who are identified and treated early in life. Particularly affected appear to be the abilities in focusing and sustaining attention in contrast to abilities involved in inhibiting, shifting, and dividing attention, which are unaffected.[107] In children with CH, their weak attentional skills reflect factors relating to both initial disease severity and abnormal thyroid hormone levels at the time of testing.[108-111]

Memory is a further area of vulnerability in children with CH who are treated early. Particularly affected are their digit span, memory for locations, and associative learning skills.[55,100,112] Deficits in these memory skills appear to reflect the delay in achieving euthyroidism. According to parents, difficulties in attention and everyday memory functioning seem to affect the child's daily functioning.[113] Executive function skills are generally unaffected, unless treatment is significantly delayed.[106]

Selective motor deficits are seen in children and adults with CH and reflect reduced strength and balance[80,114,115] and increased clumsiness.[101] On tests assessing specific aspects of cerebellar functioning (e.g., dysmetria, dysdiadochokinesia, motor timing), children with CH performed atypically relative to controls but showed no evidence of cerebellar involvement.[116] In addition, children with CH show fine motor deficits in visuomotor integration, manual dexterity, and ball throwing. A recent study has reported an association between postural control and time to TSH normalization.[117]

At school, children with CH identified by newborn screening generally perform satisfactorily, but their levels of achievement are lower than their siblings or classmates.[118] Moreover, children with CH are at greater risk of a learning disability in the nonverbal area, which affects primarily their arithmetic abilities.[112] Unless the children have an associated hearing deficit, which is seen in about 20% of cases, their reading abilities are usually normal.[119] Their learning profile continues into adulthood[86] and the CH group is also less likely to graduate from high school than siblings.[80] School success has also been correlated with initial L-T_4 dose.

Behavior problems reflect increased temperamental difficulty in infancy, due to elevated arousal levels and increased environmental sensitivity.[120] At an older age, difficulties with attention, introversion, and social maturity are frequent.[121,122] Because some of the behavior problems are positively correlated with starting dose level,[123] this suggests the need to monitor the children closely to prevent overtreatment.

Only a few studies have as yet examined neuroanatomy and neurologic function in children with CH. Autopsy findings reveal extensive neuropathology in children with late diagnosis or who died for other reasons. Although studies of small samples of late-treated cases reported atrophy in the frontal and parietal lobes, as well as delayed myelination,[124] comparable small-scale studies of infants detected by screening have shown no morphologic defects.[125,126] However, a study of 10- to 16-year olds with CH diagnosed via screening found an increased incidence of abnormal MRI scans in CH relative to controls[127] and abnormal spectroscopy results in the hippocampus.[128,129] Although preliminary hippocampal measurements revealed no difference in volume between CH and controls, hippocampal size did correlate with memory performance in the CH but not the control group.[127]

Children with a delayed diagnosis of CH typically attain IQs about 2 SDs below their parents and siblings and also show marked cognitive deficiencies, particularly in language, attention, memory, and executive function skills. In addition, they are at risk for severe behavioral problems, including attention-deficit hyperactivity disorder, pervasive developmental disorder, anxiety, depression, and social awkwardness. Moreover, their adaptive skills are weak and they are unable to function independently in adulthood. These children have a high need for professional services (e.g., speech therapy, physiotherapy, occupational therapy) and special class placements.

In summary, although CH children identified by newborn screening and treated in a timely manner show a relatively good outcome, they may still have a slight lowering of IQ and subtle neurocognitive and behavioral deficits. Factors contributing to the different specific deficits in CH include initial disease severity and the delay in achieving euthyroidism, reflecting when treatment was initiated and the starting dose levels. One variable that has received limited attention so far is the adequacy of the maintenance dose.[130] In addition, a small proportion of children may experience a delay in diagnosis of CH because of an error in screening or sampling. Because prolonged hypothyroidism is associated with permanent brain damage and poor psychological outcome, it is important that all physicians be aware of the possibility of missed detection and therefore may need to diagnose CH clinically.

Acquired Hypothyroidism

GROWTH

Children with prolonged and severe AH may fail to achieve their predicted final height. In a study of the long-term growth of children with severe primary hypothyroidism treated with L-T_4 for maintenance of normal thyroid function, findings revealed that skeletal maturation exceeds expectation for statural growth.[131] As a result, the children were approximately 2 SDs below the normal adult stature for gender as well as below their predicted midparental heights. Duration of hypothyroidism prior to the institution of treatment was significantly related to the decrease in adult stature.

NEUROPSYCHOLOGICAL DEVELOPMENT

The severe mental deficiency typically seen in late-treated CH is seldom, if ever, seen in AH. However, school achievement may be subnormal and intelligence lower than normal if AH develops at a relatively young age. In a study of very young AH patients, mild mental retardation or significant language delays were observed in three of four cases presenting with acquired primary hypothyroidism in infancy. The least affected child was a girl who acquired her hypothyroidism past 1 year of age and was treated shortly thereafter, whereas the other three children, all boys, either sustained a longer period of hypothyroidism or developed it earlier in infancy.[50] The two cases most severely affected experienced significant growth deceleration and a long delay before treatment was initiated. One of these patients also experienced a persistent neurosensory deficit.

Older children are frequently described as well behaved and high achievers at school when they are in the hypothyroid state, possibly because of their pliant behavior and reduced activity levels. Although behavior problems are rare before treatment, a teenager described in 1993 presented with psychosis (new-onset auditory hallucinations and severe obsessions), which subsequently abated following diagnosis and treatment of hypothyroidism.[132] A follow-up after discontinuation of psychotropic medication (but not L-T_4) and a psychotic relapse suggested that his hypothyroidism was probably an aggravating factor, rather than the primary cause of the psychosis originally, and that his AH and psychosis needed continuous and appropriate therapy.

In adults, behavioral problems are not uncommon after initiation of treatment for AH[133,134] and a case of a murder after T_4 treatment was ascribed to myxedema madness.[135] We described three adolescents with AH who demonstrated significant and marked behavior abnormalities following L-T_4 therapy.[136] One was a 13½-year-old girl who went from being an above-average student with superior mathematics ability and advanced artistic talents to a student whose work deteriorated significantly and was not able to concentrate, perform at school, or draw following the onset of L-T_4 therapy. She showed features of organic brain syndrome and an inability to concentrate and acquire new information. The second case involved a 12-year-old boy who was diagnosed with AH after a 2-year history of slow growth. He had been an honor student with no signs of hyperactivity or major behavior problems. Shortly after initiation of treatment, he developed an acute psychosis and petit mal seizures and subsequently sustained severe concentration, organization, and behavioral difficulties and was failing at school. The third case was a 16-year-old boy diagnosed with AH following a 3-year period of growth failure. After treatment, he sexually assaulted an older neighbor and subsequently suffered significant school and behavioral problems.

Our experience with these three adolescents prompted a prospective study in which 23 newly diagnosed children and adolescents with AH were evaluated with neuropsychological tests right after diagnosis and prior to onset of L-T_4 therapy as well at 6, 12, and 24 months postdiagnosis.[62] Results showed considerable variability in response, with 17% developing de novo behavior problems (temper tantrums, moodiness, aggression, irritability) and 17% developing attention problems; however, 22% showed improved behavior because of increased energy levels and a better attitude. Although no major changes were noted in overall intelligence, 26% showed a significant decline, whereas a further 26% showed significant improvement (Fig. 10-3). In the entire group, a significant overall decline in visuomotor integration ability was seen over the 2-year period. Although achievement testing revealed only a slight and nonsignificant decline in scores over the 2-year period, parents reported on questionnaires that their children showed significant declines in writing, arithmetic, and spelling abilities, as well as an increased incidence of academic problems. Only about one third of the children showed appropriate school-related gains, whereas one third showed no gain at 3 months but caught up after 1 year, and another third failed to make any gains in reading or arithmetic over the 2-year period. Children with the worst outcome were those with the more severe and long-standing hypothyroidism initially, who also achieved euthyroidism quickly and whose thyroid hormone levels were high. Nevertheless, none of

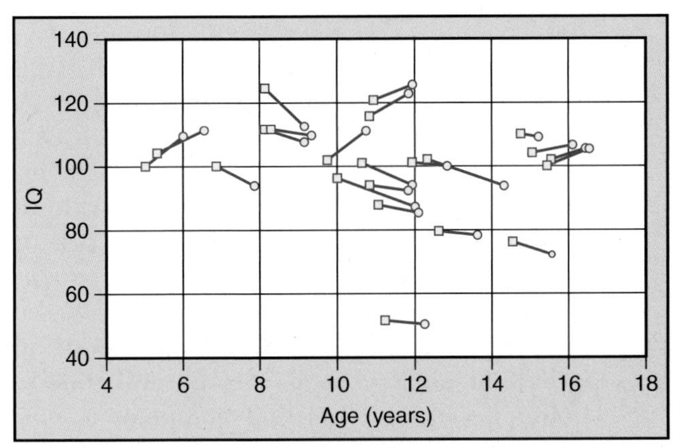

Figure 10–3 Individual pretreatment (square) and posttreatment (circle) IQ scores in sample of children with juvenile hypothyroidism.

these children showed behavioral problems as severe as the three patients described earlier.

In summary, children older than 3 years of age generally show few behavioral or learning problems in the hypothyroid state, whereas a small proportion of children will experience severe learning and memory deficits and behavior and attention problems following L-T_4 therapy, especially if the period of hypothyroidism was prolonged.

PREVENTION

Prevention of thyroid disease in children is essentially nonexistent. Possibilities in the future might involve gene therapy for the familial forms of dysgenesis. However, as long as the disease is diagnosed early and treatment (which is relatively inexpensive) is provided early, gene therapy may be unnecessary except for children with receptor and transporter defect disorders, who have more severe and debilitating phenotypes. Discontinuing the excessive use of iodine-containing drugs or cutaneous applications of iodine in infancy could help prevent iodine-induced transient hypothyroidism. Iodine supplementation during pregnancy and lactation is critical in iodine-deficient countries to prevent iodine deficiency–associated hypothyroidism in the fetus and infant. Similarly, in iodine-sufficient regions,[137] it is still necessary to supplement iodine intake during pregnancy and lactation. In addition, other trace metal deficiencies often coexist with iodine deficiency. Selenium, essential for normal activity of the monodeiodinase enzymes,[138,139] should be tested, especially if iodine levels are deficient, because the thyroidal response to iodine supplementation is attenuated in the presence of selenium and iron deficiencies.[140,141] At an environmental level, it is also important to reduce, if not eliminate, unnecessary exposure to the chemical compounds that may interfere with iodine synthesis and/or thyroid production and transport. Pediatric patients undergoing therapy for certain psychiatric illnesses, such as lithium therapy for bipolar disease, which is increasing in the pediatric population, should have their TSH levels monitored regularly during therapy to prevent iatrogenic hypothyroidism.

PITFALLS, COMPLICATIONS, AND CONTROVERSIES

Congenital Hypothyroidism

As noted, screening programs can, for various reasons, fail to diagnose a small subset of children. For example, children with a low total T_4 and normal TSH profile because of hypothalamic immaturity, prematurity, illness, or thyroxine-binding globulin (TBG) deficiency may be missed on TSH screening. In rare cases (1 in 100,000), some children with primary hypothyroidism have a delayed rise in TSH. Inhibition of TSH release can also result from constant infusions of dopamine or high-dose glucocorticoids. Similarly, although T_4 screening programs can diagnosis central hypothyroidism, these programs may miss children with milder forms of CH who, at the time of screening, are capable of producing low levels of thyroid hormone, which are sufficiently high to pass the neonatal screening program. Because many of the latter group of children would be compensating for their low (but recognizable) levels of T_4, they would have been identified on TSH screening. Although screening for both hormones is ideal and performed by a few programs (in the United States, only Alabama and Delaware), this approach adds significantly to the cost of the screening program. T_4 determination by tandem mass spectrometry will obviate the cost issue.[142,143]

In many preterm infants, transient hypothyroxinemia from immaturity of the hypothalamic-pituitary axis or nonthyroidal illness is not uncommon. Because of the delayed rise in TSH associated with extreme prematurity, cardiovascular abnormalities, and severe illness, some programs have chosen to repeat the neonatal screening in these infants at 2 and 6 weeks of age or at 36 weeks projected gestation to capture possible false-negative cases missed on the first screen. A major controversy surrounding transient hypothyroxinemia of prematurity is whether to treat these infants, given the findings that adverse effects of treatment were seen in selected gestational age subgroups, despite definite benefits in other gestational age subgroups.[144,145] Additional issues concerning hypothyroxinemia of prematurity include identifying the optimal dosage of treatment, dosing regimen, duration of therapy, and appropriate biochemical markers to use for monitoring of therapy.[146,147]

Transient hypothyroidism may also occur in healthy full-term infants as a result of intrauterine exposure to maternal antithyroid drugs, maternal TSH receptor antibodies, heterozygous thyroid oxidase 2 deficiency, germline mutations in the TSH receptor, iodine deficiency, or prenatal or postnatal exposure to excess iodides (e.g., povidone iodine, iodinated contrast materials). These causes should be evaluated by careful history taking and, because they cannot be distinguished clinically from true hypothyroidism, it is important to determine at a later age (usually about 3 years) whether the hypothyroidism is permanent by discontinuing the medication briefly and retesting the child.

Because of the possibility of a missed or false-negative screening test result, it is still necessary to know how to diagnose CH clinically. Because cretinism is now a rare phenomenon, it is essential that physicians remain prudent of the critical signs and symptoms to make a clinical diagnosis. Thus, appropriate education and training regarding the disorder should continue to be provided.

Another persisting and controversial issue concerns the benefit of thyroid imaging at diagnosis. Although a thyroid scan will help determine whether a condition is permanent, its severity (e.g., ectopic gland versus aplasia), and/or whether the condition is heritable and the risk for subsequent offspring, the tests may expose the child to ionizing radiation and some hospitals may not having scanning facilities available. Ultrasound is safe and provides a reasonable alternative; however, gray-scale ultrasonography is less sensitive than iodine 123 or technetium scanning and an ectopic thyroid gland, the most common form of CH, may be missed. Color Doppler ultrasonography may provide a suitable alternative. If a genetically mediated thyroid synthetic enzyme deficit is identified, it is important to arrange for genetic counseling for families planning to have more children.

Occasionally, some children with CH may encounter problems associated with treatment of hypothyroidism because of the following:

- Thyrotoxicosis from dose levels that are too high. This may require a dose reduction, particularly because prolonged hyperthyroidism can lead to premature craniosynostosis. Despite recent guidelines for relatively high starting doses of L-T_4, it is important to take into account the cause of the CH and disease severity when assigning the dose, which may be too high for children with partial thyroid function at diagnosis.
- Undetectable TSH levels with normal FT_4 because of inconsistent compliance with treatment and overdosing just prior to testing.
- Intermittent elevations of serum TSH levels associated with normal or high T_4 and FT_4 values from inconsistent compliance, with or without overdosing just prior to testing. In this case, it may be necessary to arrange for more frequent TSH and FT_4 tests, and possibly increase the dose despite episodes of thyrotoxicosis during periods of good compliance. Careful inquiry should be made regarding compliance, dosing, and mode of administration. If problems are suspected, education and counseling of the parents are necessary.
- Persistent elevations in serum TSH caused by problems in absorption or metabolism of L-T_4 (e.g., iron, calcium, certain foods). In this case, it may be necessary to increase the dose, despite episodes of thyrotoxicosis during periods of improved absorption, or eliminate the suspected compound, if possible.
- Intermittent elevations of serum TSH levels associated with variable potency of the medication. It may be necessary to change brands of levothyroxine and determine whether the medication is fresh by checking the date of production of the specific lot number.
- Elevated levels of TSH, FT_4, and T_3 caused by abnormal feedback control of pituitary TSH secretion. In these cases, it may be necessary to reduce the dose of L-T_4 until the child is clinically euthyroid and FT_4 and T_3 levels are normal, regardless of the serum TSH level.

Good continued management of children with CH is also critical. Because the vast majority of these children are not followed throughout childhood by pediatric endocrinologists, it is important for treating physicians to be fully informed of the condition and the child's special needs. Additional testing and dose changes may be necessary at times of increased growth, such as the pubertal growth spurt. Although it has been established that growth and pubertal onset are normal in this population and that some of these patients are now having children of their own, detailed studies of puberty and reproduction have not been conducted in the CH population.

Children and parents have frequent concerns about the disease and its impact on life, so support groups and informational meetings for parents and patients are often helpful. When transitioning to adult health facilities, including adult endocrinology clinics, it is important that all physicians be well informed about the special needs of these patients, including reproductive issues. For example, a dose increment of about 150% should be considered in women of reproductive age contemplating pregnancy and during the early months of pregnancy.[148]

Follow-up studies have shown that despite IQs in the normal range, a number of children with CH may evidence subtle to severe cognitive and school-related problems. In dealing with the commonly reported difficulties in focusing attention, physicians may consider psychostimulant medications; however, these should be administered under a controlled trial. Although associated learning disabilities will require special education or outside tutoring, these children may not qualify for traditional identification and remediation because they are caused by a preexisting illness, according to some criteria. Thus, it is important that the children be assessed at critical time points in their education, if needed, to ensure that proper interventions are provided. In addition, because some children with CH will be at risk for certain auditory and visual problems, their hearing and vision should be routinely tested. Similarly, some children with persisting clumsiness may need physiotherapy and/or occupational therapy.

Acquired Hypothyroidism

Controversies surrounding AH concern adequacy of treatment and titration of the dose, especially if children have the disorder for a long time. Children showing adverse reactions to therapy need the additional resources of psychologists and psychiatrists, and some children may also need psychostimulant medications. Because infants and very young children with AH would have passed the newborn screening test, it is important that physicians recognize the hallmarks of this disorder and be able to make a clinical diagnosis quickly to prevent any brain damage during critical windows of development. Provisions for special education and counseling should be made for children showing an adverse effect to AH treatment. Another pitfall is the failure to diagnose other problems or their causes seen in the newly diagnosed AH patient, such as family disturbance and stressful events.

In AH caused by an autoimmune process, other autoimmune diseases may be present or develop subsequently in a patient with autoimmune AH. Families and their physicians must be aware of the association of other autoimmune diseases, which occur more often in patients with autoimmune thyroiditis with hypothyroidism.

Because some acute psychiatric illnesses, particularly during adolescence, are caused by AH, it is important to evaluate thyroid status in these children, especially if no previous signs of mental illness or deviance were ever noted. On the other hand, some forms of AH may be caused by exposure to psychotropic medications; thus, it is important that a careful history be taken in the diagnostic process.

CONCLUSIONS

Congenital and acquired hypothyroidism represent distinct conditions from hypothyroidism in the adult, particularly with regard to diagnosis, treatment, and management. In CH, it is essential to diagnose and treat as soon as possible after the positive newborn screening levels have been determined. The dosage, in micrograms per unit of body weight, should be relatively high to achieve euthyroidism quickly and thus reduce the risk of brain damage. It is also important to manage these children appropriately throughout childhood and adolescence. Because a few children will be missed by each screening method or because of an error in the screening process, physicians must still be prudent about the need for the clinical diagnosis of CH and timely treatment. In AH, because severe problems following therapy may occur, it is important to titrate the dosage slowly to prevent adverse reactions, particularly if the hypothyroidism was long-standing. AH can also occur in infants who might have passed the newborn screening test but also could be vulnerable to brain damage associated with a lack of TH in infancy, so it is critical that the physician be aware of this possibility when seeing a child who fails to grow and/or shows an unexplained decline in neurodevelopment.

References

1. Bernal J, Nunez J: Thyroid hormones and brain development. Eur J Endocrinol 133:390-398, 1995.
2. Shapiro S: Metabolic and maturational effects of thyroxine in the infant rat. Endocrinology 78:527-532, 1966.
3. Legrand J: Effects of thyroid hormones on central nervous system development. In Yanat J (ed): Neurobehavioral Teratology. Amsterdam, Elsevier, 1984, pp 331-363.
4. Potter B, Mano M, Belling G, et al: Retarded fetal brain development resulting from severe dietary iodine deficiency in sheep. Neuropath Appl Neurobiol 8:303-313, 1982.
5. Lavado-Autric R, Ausó E, García-Velasco JV, et al: Early maternal hypothyroxinemia alters histogenesis and cerebral cortex cytoarchitecture of the progeny. J Clin Invest 111:1073-1082, 2003.
6. Ausó E, Cases O, Fouquet C, et al: Protracted expression of serotonin transporter and altered thalamocortical projections in the barrel field of hypothyroid rats. Eur J Neurosci 14:1968-1980, 2001.

7. Rosman N, Malone M, Helfenstein M, et al: The effect of thyroid deficiency on myelination of the brain. Neurology 22:99-106, 1972.
8. Vara H, Martinez B, Santos A, et al: Thyroid hormone regulates neurotransmitter release in neonatal rat hippocampus. Neuroscience 110:19-28, 2002.
9. Gould E, Butcher LL: Developing cholinergic basal forebrain neurons are sensitive to thyroid hormone. J Neurosci 9:3346-3358, 1989.
10. Rüsch A, Erway L, Oliver D, et al: Thyroid hormone receptor beta-dependent expression of a potassium conductance in inner hair cells at the onset of hearing. Proc Natl Acad Sci U S A 95:15758-15762, 1998.
11. Kelley MW, Turner JK, Reh TA: Regulation of proliferation and photoreceptor differentiation in fetal human retinal cell cultures. Invest Ophth Vis Sci 36:1280-1289, 1995.
12. Ng L, Hurley J, Dierks B, et al: A thyroid hormone receptor that is required for the development of green cone photoreceptors. Nat Genet 27:94-98, 2001.
13. Forrest D: The developing brain and maternal thyroid hormone: Finding the links. Endocrinology 145:4034-4036, 2004.
14. Roberts M, Srinivas M, Forrest D, et al: Making the gradient: Thyroid hormone regulates cone opsin expression in the developing mouse retina. Proc Natl Acad Sci U S A 103:6218-6223, 2006.
15. Zoeller RT, Rovet J: Timing of thyroid hormone action in the developing brain: Clinical observations and experimental findings. J Neuroendocrinol 16:809-818, 2004.
16. Morreale de Escobar G, Obregon MJ, Escobar del Rey F: Role of thyroid hormone in early brain development. Eur J Endocrinol 151(Suppl 3):U25-U37, 2004.
17. Bernal J: Action of thyroid hormone in brain. J Endocrinol Invest 25:268-288, 2002.
18. Nunez J, Celi FS, Ng L, Forrest D: Multigenic control of thyroid hormone functions in the nervous system. Mol Cell Endocinol 287:1-12, 2008.
19. Harbers M, Wahlstrom GM, Vennstrom B: Transactivation by the thyroid hormone receptor is dependent on the spacer sequence in hormone response elements containing directly repeated half-sites. Nucleic Acids Res 24:2252-2259, 1996.
20. Perlmann T, Umesono K, Rangarajan PN, et al: Two distinct dimerization interfaces differentially modulate target gene specificity of nuclear hormone receptors. Mol Endocrinol 10:958-966, 1996.
21. Anderson GW, Schoonover CM, Jones SA: Control of thyroid hormone action in the developing rat brain. Thyroid 13:1039-1056, 2003.
22. Thompson CC, Potter GB: Thyroid hormone action in neural development. Cereb Cortex 10:939-945, 2000.
23. Brent GA: The molecular basis of thyroid hormone action. N Engl J Med 221:847-853, 1994.
24. Bradley DJ, Towle HC, Young WSI: Spatial and temporal expression of α- and β-thyroid hormone receptor mRNAs, including the β2-subtype, in the developing mammalian nervous system. J Neurosci 12:2288-2302, 1992.
25. Iniguez MA, De Lecea L, Guadano-Ferraz A: Cell-specific effects of thyroid hormone on RC3/neurogranin expression in rat brain. Endocrinol 137:1032-1041, 1996.
26. Puymirat J, Luo M, Dussault JH: Immunocytochemical localization of thyroid hormone nuclear receptors in cultured hypothalamic dopaminergic neurons. Neuroscience 30:443-449, 1989.
27. Virgili M, Saverino O, Vaccari M, et al: Temporal, regional and cellular selectivity of neonatal alteration of the thyroid state on neurochemical maturation in the rat. Exp Brain Res 83:556-561, 1991.
28. Berbel P, Guadanao-Ferraz A, Angulo A, et al: Role of thyroid hormones in the maturation of interhemispheric connections in rats. Behav Brain Res 64:9-14, 1994.
29. Evans IM, Sinha AK, Pickard MR, et al: Maternal hypothyroxinemia disrupts neurotransmitter metabolic enzymes in developing brain. J Endocrinol 161:273-279, 1999.
30. Hashimoto Y, Furkawa S, Omae F, et al: Correlative regulation of nerve growth factor level and choline aceyltransferase activity by thyroxine in particular regions of infant rat brain. J Neurochem 63:326-332, 1994.
31. Savard P, Merand Y, Di Paolo T, et al: Effects of thyroid state on serotonin, 5-hydroxyindoleacetic acid and substance P contents in discrete brain nuclei of adult rats. Neuroscience 10:1399-1404, 1983.
32. Rastogi R, Singhal RL: Influence of neonatal and adult hyperthyroidism on behavior and biosynthetic capacity for neorepinephrine, dopamine, and 5-hydroxytryptamine in rat brain. J Pharmacol Exp Ther 198:609-618, 1976.
33. Guadano-Ferraz A, Escamez MJ, Rausell E, et al: Expression of type 2 iodothyronine deiodinase in the hypothyroid rat brain indicates an important role of thyroid hormone in the development of specific primary sensory systems. J Neurosci 19:3430-3439, 1999.
34. Claustre J, Balende C, Pujol JF: Influence of the thyroid hormone status on tyrosine hydroxylase in central and peripheral catecholaminergic structures. Neurochem Int 28:277-281, 1996.
35. Dratman MB, Gordon JT: Thyroid hormones as neurotransmitters. Thyroid 6:639-647, 1996.
36. Rozanov CB, Dratman MB: Immunohistochemical mapping of brain triiodothyronine reveals prominent localization in central noradrenergic systems. Neurosci 74:897-915, 1996.
37. Farwell AP, Dubord-Tomasetti SA, Pietrzykowski AZ, et al: Dynamic non-genomic actions of thyroid hormone in the developing rat brain. Endocrinology 147:2567-2574, 2006.

38. Wiens SC, Trudeau VL: Thyroid hormone and γ-aminobutyric acid (GABA) interactions in neuroendocrine systems. Comp Biochem Physiol 144:332-344, 2006.
39. Haas MJ, Mreyoud A, Fishman M, et al: Microarray analysis of thyroid hormone-induced changes in mRNA expression in the adult rat brain. Neurosci Lett 365:14-18, 2004.
40. Mason GA, Walker CH, Prange AJ, Bondy SC: GABA uptake is inhibited by thyroid hormones: Implications for depression. Psychoneuroendocrinology 12:284-289, 1987.
41. Fort P, Lifshitz F, Bellisario R, et al: Abnormalities of thyroid function in infants with Down syndrome. J Pediatr 104:545-549, 1984.
42. Moreno JC, de Vijlder JJM, Vulsma T, et al: Genetic basis of hypothyroidism: Recent advances, gaps and strategies for future research. Trends Endocrinol Metab 14:318-326, 2003.
43. American Academy of Pediatrics, Rose SR; Section on Endocrinology and Committee on Genetics, American Thyroid Association, Brown RS; Public Health Committee, Lawson Wilkins Pediatric Endocrine Society, Foley T, et al: Update of newborn screening and therapy for congenital hypothyroidism. Pediatrics 117:2290-2303, 2006.
44. Brown RS, Bloomfield S, Bednarek FJ, et al: Routine skin cleansing with povidone-iodine is not a common cause of transient neonatal hypothyroidism in North America: A prospective controlled study. Thyroid 7:395-400, 1997.
45. Weber G, Vigone MC, Rapa A, et al: Neonatal transient hypothyroidism: Aetiological study. Italian Collaborative Study on Transient Hypothyroidism. Arch Dis Child Fetal Neonatal Ed 79:F70-F72, 1998.
46. Howdeshell KL: A model of the development of the brain as a construct of the thyroid system. Envir Health Persp 110:337-348, 2002.
47. Gauger KJ, Kato Y, Haraguchi K, et al: Polychlorinated biphenyls (PCBs) exert thyroid hormone-like effects in the fetal rat brain but do not bind to thyroid hormone receptors. Envir Health Persp 112:516-523, 2004.
48. Connelly JF, Coakley JC, Gold H, et al: Newborn screening for congenital hypothyroidism, Victoria, Australia, 1977-1997. Part 1: The screening programme, demography, baseline perinatal data and diagnostic classification. J Pediatr Endocrinol Metab 14:1597-1610, 2001.
49. Stoll CG, Roth MP, Dott B, et al: Study of 290 cases of polyhydramnios and congenital malformations in a series of 225,669 consecutive births. Community Genet 2:36-42, 1999.
50. Foley TP, Abbassi V, Copeland KC, et al: Hypothyroidism caused by chronic autoimmune thyroiditis in very young infants. N Engl J Med 330:466-468, 1994.
51. Davy T, Daneman D, Walfish PG, et al: Congenital hypothyroidism. The effect of stopping treatment at 3 years of age. Am J Dis Child 139:1028-1030, 1985.
52. LaFranchi S: Thyroiditis and acquired hypothyroidism. Pediatr Ann 21:32-39, 1992.
53. Bakker B, Kempers MJ, de Vijlder JJM, et al: Dynamics of the plasma concentrations of TSH, FT_4 and T_3 following thyroxine supplementation in congenital hypothyroidism. Clin Endocrinol (Oxf) 57:529-537, 2002.
54. Fisher DA, Schoen EJ, La Franchi S, et al: The hypothalamic-pituitary-thyroid negative feedback control axis in children with treated congenital hypothyroidism. J Clin Endocrinol Metab 85:2722-2727, 2000.
55. Song S, Daneman D, Rovet J: The influence of etiology and treatment factors on intellectual outcome in congenital hypothyroidism. J Dev Behav Pediatr 22:376-384, 2001.
56. Rovet JF: Does breast feeding protect the hypothyroid infant diagnosed by newborn screening? Am J Dis Child 144:319-323, 1990.
57. Bode HH, Vanjonack WJ, Crawford JD: Mitigation of cretinism by breast-feeding. Pediatrics 62:13-16, 1978.
58. Hahn HB, Brown LO, Hillis A, et al: Breast feeding and neonatal screening for congenital hypothyroidism. Tex Med 82:46-47, 1986.
59. Hanukogulu A, Perlman K, Shamis I, et al: Relation of etiology to treatment in patients with congenital hypothyroidism. J Clin Endocrinol Metab 86:86-191, 2001.
60. Foley TP Jr: Hypothyroidism. Pediatr Rev 25:94-100, 2004.
61. Fisher DA: Acquired juvenile hypothyroidism. In Braverman LE, Utiger RD (eds): Werner and Ingbar's The Thyroid, 7th ed. Philadelphia, JB Lippincott, 1993, pp 1228-1236.
62. Rovet J, Daneman D: Behavioral and cognitive abnormalities associated with juvenile acquired hypothyroidism. In Hauser P, Rovet J (eds): Thyroid Disorders in Infancy and Childhood. Washington, DC, American Psychiatric Press, 1998, pp 163-185.
63. Cappell J, Patterson MC: Pseudotumor cerebri syndrome. In Burg FD, Ingelfinger JR, Polin RA, Gershon AA (eds): Current Pediatric Therapy. Philadelphia, Saunders Elsevier, 2006, pp 407-410.
64. McVie R: Abnormal TSH regulation, pseudotumor cerebri, and empty sella after replacement therapy in juvenile hypothyroidism. J Pediatr 105:768-770, 1984.
65. Van Dop C, Conte FA, Koch TK, et al: Pseudotumor cerebri associated with initiation of levothyroxine therapy for juvenile hypothyroidism. N Engl J Med 308:1076-1080, 1983.
66. Raghavan S, DiMartino-Nardi J, Saenger P, et al: Pseudotumor cerebri in an infant after L-thyroxine therapy for transient neonatal hypothyroidism. J Pediatr 130:478-480, 1997.
67. Maenpaa J: Congenital hypothyroidism. Aetiological and clinical aspects. Arch Dis Child 47:914-923, 1972.

68. Hulse A: Congenital hypothyroidism and neurological development. J Child Psychol Psychiatry 24:629-635, 1983.
69. Klein RZ: Neonatal screening for hypothyroidism. Adv Pediatr 26:417-440, 1979.
70. Macfaul R, Dorner S, Brett EM, et al: Neurological abnormalities in patients treated for hypothyroidism from early life. Arch Dis Child 53:611-619, 1978.
71. Wolter R, Noel P, De Cock P, et al: Neuropsychological study in treated thyroid dysgenesis. Acta Paediatr Scand Suppl 277:41-46, 1979.
72. Frost GL, Parkin JM: A comparison between the neurological and intellectual abnormalities in children and adults with congenital hypothyroidism. Eur J Pediatr 145:480-484, 1986.
73. Virtanen M, Maenpaa J, Santavuori P, et al: Congenital hypothyroidism: Age at start of treatment versus outcome. Acta Paediatr Scand 72:197-201, 1983.
74. Rovet J: Congenital hypothyroidism: Treatment and outcome. Curr Opin Endocrinol Diabetes Obes 12:42-52, 2005.
75. Morin A, Giumarey L, Apezteguia M, et al: Linear growth in children with congenital hypothyroidism detected by neonatal screening and treated early: A longitudinal study. J Pediatr Endocrinol Metab 15:973-977, 2002.
76. Ng SM, Wong SC, Didi M: Head circumference and linear growth during the first 3 years in treated congenital hypothyroidism in relation to aetiology and initial biochemical severity. Clin Endocrinol 61:155-159, 2004.
77. Connelly JF, Rickards AL, Coakley JC: Newborn screening for congenital hypothyroidism, Victoria, Australia, 1977-1997. Part 2: Treatment, progress and outcome. J Pediatr Endocrinol Metab 14:1611-1634, 2001.
78. Glorieux J, Dussault JH, Morissette J, et al: Follow-up at ages 5 and 7 years on mental development in children with hypothyroidism detected by Quebec Screening Program. J Pediatr 107:913-915, 1985.
79. Salerno M, Micillo M, Di Maio S, et al: Longitudinal growth, sexual maturation and final height in patients with congenital hypothyroidism detected by neonatal screening. Eur J Endocrinol 145: 377-383, 2001.
80. Kempers MJ, van der Sluijs Veer L, Nijhuis-van der Sanden MW, et al: Intellectual and motor development of young adults with congenital hypothyroidism diagnosed by neonatal screening. J Clin Endocrinol Metab 91:418-424, 2006.
81. Glorieux J, Dussault J, Van Vliet G: Intellectual development at age 12 years of children with congenital hypothyroidism diagnosed by neonatal screening. J Pediatr 121:581-584, 1992.
82. Rovet JF: Neurodevelopmental outcome in infants and preschool children following newborn screening for congenital hypothyroidism. J Pediatr Psychol 17:187-213, 1992.
83. Derksen-Lubsen G, Verkerk PH: Neuropsychologic development in early-treated congenital hypothyroidism: Analysis of literature data. Pediatr Res 39:561-566, 1996.
84. Heyerdahl S, Oerbeck B: Congenital hypothyroidism: Developmental outcome in relation to levothyroxine treatment variables. Thyroid 13:1029-1038, 2003.
85. Rovet J: Long-term neuropsychological sequelae of early-treated congenital hypothyroidism: Effects in adolescence. Acta Paediatr 432:88-95, 199.
86. Oerbeck B, Sundet K, Kase BF, et al: Congenital hypothyroidism: Influence of disease severity and L-thyroxine treatment on intellectual, motor, and school-associated outcomes in young adults. Pediatrics 112:923-930, 2003.
87. Rovet J: Long-term follow-up of children born with sporadic congenital hypothyroidism. Ann Endocrinol (Paris) 64:58-61, 2003.
88. Rovet J, Daneman D: Congenital hypothyroidism: A review of current diagnostic and treatment practices in relation to neuropsychologic outcome. Pediatr Drugs 5:141-149, 2003.
89. Labarta J, Mayayo E, Puga B: Psychomotor development in congenital hypothyroidism: Spanish experience. In Morreale de Escobar G, de Vijlder J, Butz S (eds): The Thyroid and Brain. Stuttgart, Germany, Schattauer, 2003, pp 259-272.
90. Bongers-Schokking JJ, de Muinck Keizer-Schrama SM: Influence of timing and dose of thyroid hormone replacement on mental, psychomotor, and behavioral development in children with congenital hypothyroidism. J Pediatr 147:768-774, 2005.
91. Kempers MJ, van der Sluijs Veer L, Nijhuis-van der Sanden RW, et al: Neonatal screening for congenital hypothyroidism in the Netherlands: Cognitive and motor outcome at 10 years of age. J Clin Endocrinol Metab 92:919-924, 2007.
92. Muir T, Zegarac M: Societal costs of exposure to toxic substances: Economic and health costs of four case studies that are candidates for environmental causation. Environ Health Perspect 109:885-903, 2001.
93. Selva KA, Harper A, Downs A, et al: Neurodevelopmental outcomes in congenital hypothyroidism: Comparison of initial T_4 dose and time to reach target T_4 and TSH. J Pediatr 147:775-780, 2005.
94. Germak JA, Foley TP Jr: Longitudinal assessment of L-thyroxine therapy for congenital hypothyroidism. J Pediatr 117:211-219, 1990.
95. Hrystiuk K, Gilbert R, Logan S, et al: Starting dose of levothyroxine for the treatment of congenital hypothyroidism: A systematic review. Arch Pediatr Adol Med 156:485-491, 2002.
96. Fisher DA: The importance of early management in optimizing IQ in infants with congenital hypothyroidism [editorial]. J Pediatr 136:273-274, 2000.
97. Touati G, Leger J, Toublanc JE, et al: An initial dosage of 8 μg/kg is appropriate for the vast majority of children with congenital hypothyroidism. In Farriaux JP, Dhondt JK (eds): New Horizons in Neonatal Screening. Amsterdam, Elsevier, 1994, pp 145-148.

98. American Academy of Pediatrics, Section on Endocrinology and Committee on Genetics, and American Thyroid Association Committee on Public Health: Newborn screening for congenital hypothyroidism: Recommended guidelines. Pediatrics 91:1203-1209, 1993.
99. Working Group on Congenital Hypothyroidism of the European Society for Paediatric Endocrinology: Guidelines for neonatal screening programmes for congenital hypothyroidism. Eur J Pediatr 152:974-975, 1993.
100. Rovet J: Congenital hypothyroidism: Persisting deficits and associated factors. Child Neuropsychol 8:150-162, 2003.
101. Gottschalk B, Richman R, Lewandowski L: Subtle speech and motor deficits of children with congenital hypothyroidism treated early. Dev Med Child Neurol 36:216-220, 1994.
102. Rovet J, Brown R: Congenital hypothyroidism: Genetic and biochemical influences on brain development and neuropsychological functioning. In Mazzocco M, Ross J (eds): Neurogenetic Developmental Disorders: Manifestation and Identification in Childhood. Boston, MIT Press, 2007, pp 266-295.
103. Oerbeck B, Sundet K, Kase BF, et al: Congenital hypothyroidism: No adverse effects of high-dose thyroxine treatment on adult memory, attention, and behaviour. Arch Dis Child 90:132-137, 2005.
104. Mirabella G, Westall C, Asztalos E, et al: The development of contrast sensitivity in infants with prenatal and neonatal thyroid hormone insufficiencies. Pediatr Res 57:902-907, 2005.
105. Borkowski S: The effects of an early life transient thyroid hormone deficiency on the subsequent colour vision capabilities of children. Master's thesis, Department of Psychology, University of Toronto, Toronto, 2005.
106. Rovet JF: Outcome in congenital hypothyroidism. Thyroid 9:741-748, 1999.
107. Rovet J, Hepworth S: Attention problems in adolescents with congenital hypothyroidism: A multicomponential analysis. J Int Neuropsychol Soc 7:734-744, 2001.
108. Rovet J, Alvarez M: Thyroid hormone and attention in congenital hypothyroidism. J Pediatr Endocrinol Metab 9:63-66, 1996.
109. Rovet J, Hepworth SL: Dissociating attention deficits in children with ADHD and congenital hypothyroidism using multiple CPTs. J Child Psychol Psychiatry 42:1049-1056, 2001.
110. Rovet JF, Hepworth S: Attention problems in adolescents with congenital hypothyroidism: A multicomponential analysis. J Int Neuropsychol Soc 7:734-744, 2001.
111. Kooistra L, van der Meere JJ, Vulsma T, et al: Sustained attention problems in children with early treated congenital hypothyroidism. Acta Paediatr Scand 85:425-429, 1996.
112. Rovet J: Congenital hypothyroidism and nonverbal learning disabilities. In Rourke B (ed): Syndrome of NLD: Manifestations in Neurological Disease, Disorder, and Dysfunction. New York, Guilford Press, 1995, pp 255-281.
113. Rovet J: Neuropsychological follow-up of early-treated congenital hypothyroidism following newborn screening. In Morreale de Escobar G, de Vijlder J, Butz S (eds): The Thyroid and Brain. Stuttgart, Germany, Schattauer, 2003, pp 242-258.
114. Rovet J: Neuromotor deficiencies in six-year-old hypothyroid children identified by newborn screening. In Pass K (ed): Proceedings of the Eighth National Neonatal Screening Symposium and XXI Birth Defects Symposium. Washington, DC, Association of State and Territorial Public Health Laboratory Directors, 1992, pp 378-381.
115. Weber G, Siragusa V, Rondanini GF, et al: Neurophysiologic studies and cognitive function in congenital hypothyroid children. Pediatr Res 37: 736-740, 1995.
116. Kooistra L, Laane C, Vulsma T, et al: Motor and cognitive development in children with congenital hypothyroidism: A long-term evaluation of the effects of neonatal treatment. J Pediatr 124: 903-909, 1994.
117. Gauchard GC, Deviterne D, Leheup B, et al: Effect of age at thyroid-stimulating hormone normalization on postural control in children with congenital hypothyroidism. Dev Med Child Neurol 146:107-113, 2006.
118. Rovet J, Ehrlich RM: The psychoeducational characteristics of children with early-treated congenital hypothyroidism. Pediatrics 105:515-522, 2000.
119. Rovet J, Walker W, Bliss B, et al: Long-term sequelae of hearing impairment in congenital hypothyroidism. J Pediatr 127:776-783, 1997.
120. Rovet J, Ehrlich R, Sorbara D: The effect of thyroid hormone on temperament in infants with congenital hypothyroidism detected by newborn screening. J Pediatr 114:63-69, 1989.
121. Rovet JF: Neurobehavioral consequences of congenital hypothyroidism identified by newborn screening. In Stabler B, Berscu B (eds): Therapeutic Outcome of Endocrine Disorders. Efficacy, Innovation, and Quality of Life. New York, Springer-Verlag, 2000, pp 235-254.
122. Kooistra L, Stemerdink N, van der Meere J, et al: Behavioural correlates of early-treated congenital hypothyroidism. Acta Paediatrica 90:1141-1146, 2001.
123. Rovet JF, Ehrlich RM: Long-term effects of L-thyroxine therapy for congenital hypothyroidism. J Pediatr 126:380-386, 1995.
124. Gupta RK, Bhatia V, Poptani H, et al: Brain metabolite changes on in vivo proton magnetic resonance spectroscopy in children with congenital hypothyroidism. J Pediatr 126:389-392, 1995.

125. Alves C, Eidson M, Engle H, et al: Changes in brain maturation detected by magnetic resonance imaging in congenital hypothyroidism. J Pediatr 115:600-603, 1989.
126. Siragusa V, Boffelli S, Weber G, et al: Brain magnetic resonance imaging in congenital hypothyroid infants at diagnosis. Thyroid 7:761-764, 1997.
127. Rovet J, Williamson M, Nash K, et al: Using magnetic resonance spectroscopy (MRS) to study thyroid hormone's role in hippocampal development. Thyroid 16:919-920, 2006.
128. Rovet JF, Desrocher M, Williamson M, et al: Abnormal MRS profiles in children with congenital hypothyroidism. Presented at the International Neuropsychological Society 34th Annual Meeting, Boston, February 2006.
129. Williamson M, Nash K, Sheard E, et al: Abnormal MRS profiles in children with congenital hypothyroidism. Presented at the Fifth Annual Imaging Network of Ontario Symposium. Toronto, Ontario, March 2007.
130. Rovet J, Daneman D: Congenital hypothyroidism: A review of current diagnostic and treatment practices in relation to neuropsychologic outcome. Pediatr Drugs 5:141-149, 2003.
131. Rivkees SA, Bode HH, Crawford JD: Long-term growth in juvenile acquired hypothyroidism: The failure to achieve normal adult stature. N Engl J Med 318:599-602, 1988.
132. Bhatara VS, McMillin J, Bandettini F: Behavioral manifestations of hypothyroidism versus thyroxine effects. J Pediatr 123:840-841, 1993.
133. Josephson AM, Mackenzie TB: Thyroid-induced mania in hypothyroid patients. Br J Psychiatry 137:222-228, 1980.
134. Heinrich TW, Grahm G: Hypothyroidism presenting as psychosis: Myxedema madness revisited. Prim Care Companion J Clin Psychiatry 5:260-266, 2003.
135. Easson WM: Myxedema psychosis—insanity defense in homicide. J Clin Psychiatry 41:316-318, 1980.
136. Rovet JF, Daneman D, Bailey J: Adverse psychological consequences of thyroxine therapy for juvenile acquired hypothyroidism. J Pediatr 122:543-549, 1993.
137. Public Health Committee of the American Thyroid Association, Becker DV, Braverman LE, Delange F, et al: Iodine supplementation for pregnancy and lactation—United States and Canada: Recommendations of the American Thyroid Association. Thyroid 16:949-951, 2006.
138. Bianco AC, Kim BW: Deiodinases: Implications of the local control of thyroid hormone action. J Clin Invest 116:2571-2579, 2006.
139. Bianco AC, Salvatore D, Gereben B, et al: Biochemistry, cellular and molecular biology, and physiological roles of the iodothyronine selenodeiodinases. Endocrinol Rev 23:38-89, 2002.
140. Zimmermann MB, Wegmueller R, Zeder C, et al: Triple fortification of salt with microcapsules of iodine, iron, and vitamin A. Am J Clin Nutr 80:1283-1290, 2004.
141. Vanderpas J: Nutritional epidemiology and thyroid hormone metabolism. Ann Rev Nutr 26:293-322, 2006.
142. Kelleher AS, Clark RN, Steinbach M, et al: The influence of amino-acid supplementation, gestational age and time on thyroxine levels in premature neonates. J Perinatol 28:270-274, 2008.
143. Chace DH: Mass spectrometry in newborn and metabolic screnning: Historical perspective and future directions. J Mass Spectrom. 44:163-170, 2009.
144. van Wassenaer AG, Kok JH, de Vijlder JJ, et al: Effects of thyroxine supplementation on neurologic development in infants born at less than 30 weeks' gestation. N Engl J Med 336:21-26, 1997.
145. van Wassenaer AG, Westera J, Houtzager BA, Kok JH: Ten-year follow-up of children born at <30 weeks' gestational age supplemented with thyroxine in the neonatal period in a randomized, controlled trial. Pediatrics 116:e613-e618, 2005.
146. La Gamma EF, van Wassenaer AG, Golombek SG, et al: Neonatal thyroxine supplementation for transient hypothyroxinemia of prematurity: Beneficial or detrimental? Treat Endocrinol 5:335-346, 2006.
147. Asztalos EV: Thyroid hormone supplementation in preterm infants. Master's of science thesis, Hamilton, Ontario, McMaster University, 2002.
148. Alexander EK, Maqusee E, Lawrence J, et al: Timing and magnitude of increases in levothyroxine requirements during pregnancy in women with hypothyroidism. N Engl J Med 351:241-249, 2004.

Chapter 11

Hyperthyroidism

Juliane Léger

Key Points

- Thyrotoxicosis is a rare disorder in childhood, occurring most frequently as a consequence of Graves' disease (GD).
- Antithyroid drug (ATD) is usually recommended as initial treatment for hyperthyroidism in children.
- Overall frequency of relapse is higher in children than in adults; about 30% of children achieve lasting remission after about 24 months of ATD.
- Indications for radical treatment (thyroidectomy or radioactive iodine) include relapse after appropriate course of ATD, lack of compliance, and antithyroid drug toxicity.
- Pregnant women with GD or euthyroid with a history of GD should undergo thyrotropin receptor antibody (TRAb) determinations at the beginning of pregnancy. If TRAbs are detected, the fetus should be considered at risk of developing thyrotoxicosis and monitored accordingly.

Thyrotoxicosis is a rare disorder in childhood,[1] occurring most frequently as a consequence of Graves' disease (GD), an autoimmune disorder resulting from thyrotropin (thyroid-stimulating hormone, TSH) receptor stimulation by autoantibodies. Acute or subacute thyroiditis, chronic lymphocytic thyroiditis, and acute or chronic administration of thyroid hormones and/or iodides may also result in transient thyrotoxicosis. McCune-Albright syndrome and germline and somatic gain-of-function mutations of the TSH receptor gene, which may be associated with the presence of diffuse hyperplasia and toxic nodules, are also rare causes of thyrotoxicosis, as are TSH-secreting pituitary tumors and thyroid hormone resistance (Table 11-1).

GRAVES' DISEASE

Pathogenesis

The cause of GD remains unclear, but is believed to result from a complex interaction among genetic background (heredity), environmental factors, and the immune system. For unknown reasons, the immune system produces an antibody (TSH receptor antibody) that stimulates the thyroid gland to produce excess thyroid hormone. Genetic susceptibility to the disease is thought to be polygenic. GD has been reported to be associated with the human leukocyte antigen (HLA) gene on chromosome 6p, the cytotoxic T-lymphocyte antigen-4 (CTLA-4) gene on chromosome 2q33, and the PTPN22 (lymphoid tyrosine phosphatase) gene on chromosome 1p13. Data from twin studies and the higher prevalence of Graves' disease in first-degree relatives of patients with this disease than in controls suggest that about 80% of the susceptibility to GD is determined by genetic factors.[2,3]

The thyroid-stimulating immunoglobulin (TSI) binds to and stimulates the TSH receptor on the thyroid cell membrane, resulting in follicular cell growth, an increase in vascularity, and the excessive synthesis and secretion of thyroid hormone. The thyroid gland typically displays lymphocytic infiltration, with T-lymphocyte abnormality and an absence of follicular destruction. T cells activate local inflammation and tissue remodeling by producing and releasing cytokines, leading to B-cell dysregulation and an increase in autoantibody production. An imbalance between pathogenic and regulatory T cells is thought to be involved in both the development of GD and its severity.[4]

Incidence

GD is a rare disease in children, accounting for 1% to 5% of all patients with GD. In adults, this disease affects approximately 2% of women and 0.2% of men, mostly in their teens and 20s.[5,6] In both adults and children, GD is much more frequent in female than in male subjects. It may occur at any age during childhood, but it increases in frequency with age, peaking during adolescence (Fig. 11-1). The incidence is thought to be rising and is about 0.1/100,000 person-years in young children to 3/100,000 person-years in adolescents.[1] A frequency of up to 14/100,000 patient-years has been reported in Hong-Kong, with no relationship to differences in iodine nutritional status.[7,8] GD is more frequent in children with other autoimmune conditions, and in children with a familial history of autoimmune thyroid disease.

Clinical Manifestations

Most patients present the classic symptoms and signs of hyperthyroidism. The early symptoms are subtle, with changes in behavior, irritability, emotional lability, fatigue, nervousness, palpitations, insomnia, excessive perspiration, an increase in appetite accompanied by no weight gain or even weight loss, and diarrhea. A decline in academic performance and deteriorations in attention are often associated.

The size of the thyroid gland is highly variable and the goiter may go unnoticed in patients with a slightly enlarged thyroid gland. The thyroid gland is usually symmetrically enlarged, firm, uniformly smooth, and not tender. A palpable thrill may be present, reflecting the increase in blood flow through the gland. Ophthalmic abnormalities are less severe in children than in adults, with staring eyes, retraction of the upper lid, and a wide palpebral aperture. True exophthalmos is rare in children. Other signs include tachycardia, an increase in blood pressure, precordial thrill, and an ejection murmur caused by functional insufficiency of the mitral valve. Increases in height velocity, with advanced bone age, are related to the duration of hyperthyroidism (Fig. 11-2). As in adults, children with GD may have a lower than normal bone mass.[9] Pretibial myxedema

Table 11–1 Causes of Thyrotoxicosis in Children

Causes
Graves' disease
Autoimmune neonatal hyperthyroidism (passage of maternal TRAbs across the placenta)
Thyroiditis
Subacute thyroiditis
Chronic lymphocytic thyroiditis (Hashimoto's disease)
Exogenous causes
Exogenous thyroid hormone (acute or chronic)
Iodine-induced hyperthyroidism—iodine, radiocontrast agents, amiodarone
Autonomous functioning nodules
Somatic activating mutation of *Gsα*—McCune-Albright syndrome
Somatic activating mutation of the TSH receptor gene
Toxic adenoma
Hyperfunctioning papillary or follicular carcinoma
Congenital activating mutations of the TSH receptor gene (hereditary or de novo)—congenital hyperthyroidism
Selective pituitary resistance to thyroid hormones
TSH-secreting pituitary tumors

TRAbs, thyrotropin receptor antibodies; TSH, thyroid-stimulating hormone.

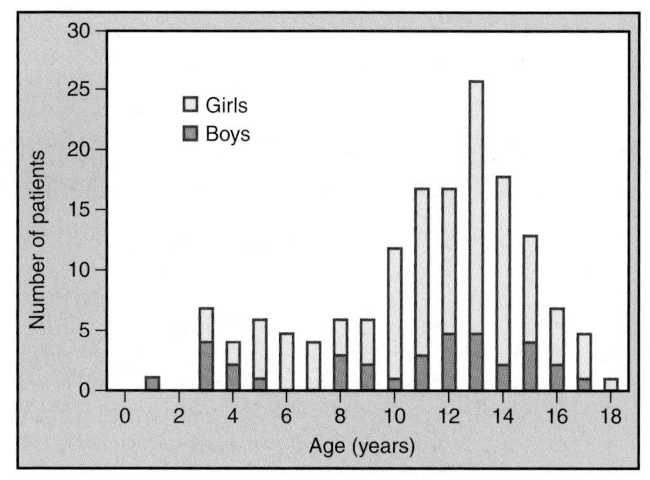

Figure 11–1 Distribution of age at diagnosis of thyrotoxicosis in childhood in 155 patients with Graves' disease. The frequency of this condition increases with age, peaking in adolescence. Girls are more frequently affected than boys.

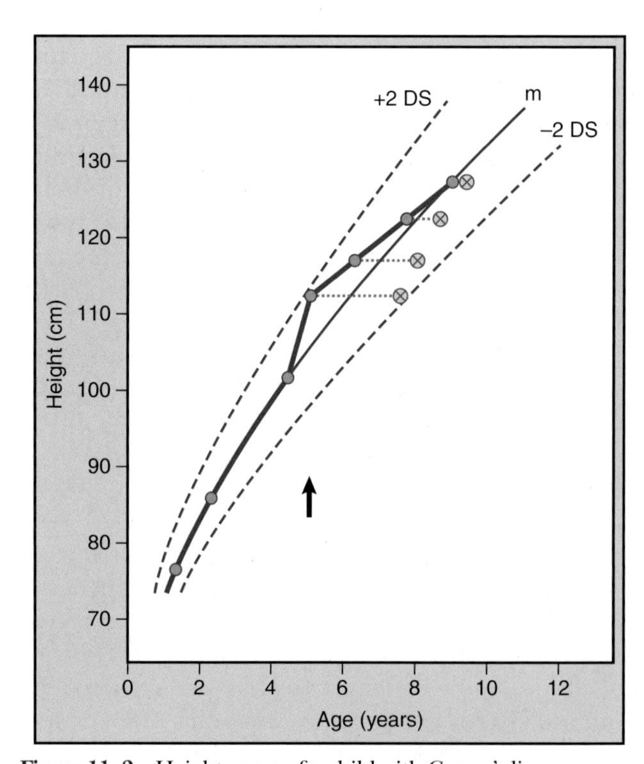

Figure 11–2 Height curve of a child with Graves' disease diagnosed at the age of 5 years, before and during the course of antithyroid drug (ATD) therapy. An increase in growth velocity with advanced bone age can clearly be seen. Hyperthyroidism went unrecognized for 1 year before the initiation of ATD treatment. Once euthyroidism had been established through ATD treatment, height velocity decreased and height normalized and followed its previous course. m, meters.

is rare. Various symptoms are observed, and children may initially be referred to cardiologists, ophthalmologists, psychiatrists, and/or gastroenterologists before being referred to an endocrinologist.[10]

Laboratory Diagnosis

The diagnosis is confirmed by thyroid hormone measurements. TSH is undetectable in the serum (less than 0.3 mU/L) in all patients. Most children with hyperthyroidism have high serum free thyroxine (FT_4) and free triiodothyronine (FT_3) concentrations. However, some patients may have normal FT_4 levels and high FT_3 levels — a condition termed *triiodothyronine toxicosis*, which may be observed at diagnosis or at times of relapse during the course of the disease. In some patients with mild hyperthyroidism and serum FT_4 and FT_3 levels close to the upper limit of normal values, a TRH test may be carried out. In this test, the inhibition of TSH release in response to TRH stimulation confirms the diagnosis of hyperthyroidism.

Thyrotropin receptor antibodies (TRAbs) are detected in most patients, with highly variable titers. Determinations of circulating thyroid peroxidase levels and, in some cases, tests for antibodies against thyroglobulin, may be useful for the confirmation of thyroid autoimmune disease.

Thyroid Imaging

Thyroid imaging with radioisotopes is not required for the diagnosis of GD and has been replaced by ultrasound scans. The thyroid gland is diffusely enlarged, and often homogenous. The gland may display normal echogenicity or may be hypoechogenic, as in thyroiditis. Diffuse parenchymal hypervascularity is observed. High-grade hypervascularization is not observed to the same extent in patients with chronic autoimmune thyroiditis. Goiter size is variable, and the goiter may be small, moderate, or large.[11] In rare cases, thyroid volume is normal.

Treatment

The optimal treatment of GD in childhood remains a matter of debate (Table 11-2),[12,13] and prospective randomized long-term clinical studies are required to compare treatment failure frequencies and the short- and long-term side effects of the different therapeutic options. Current treatment options include antithyroid drugs, subtotal or near-total thyroidectomy, and radioactive iodine (iodine 131). There is no specific cure for the disease and each therapeutic option has associated complications. Most patients are initially treated with antithyroid drugs (ATDs). However, it is difficult to achieve long-term compliance and the rate of relapse is high in children. Surgical removal of the thyroid gland or destruction of the gland by radioiodine treatment are therefore often used as alternatives. Indications for radical treatment in children include relapse after an appropriate course of drug treatment, a lack of compliance on the part of the patient or the parents, and ATD toxicity. As in many rare diseases, there is currently no evidence-based strategy for the management of this disease in children, in contrast to the situation in adults, in whom the disease is more frequent.[14,15] GD treatment policy varies considerably within and between countries and depends on local traditions and resources, the age and preference of the patient, the size of the goiter, and the severity of the disease.

Table 11–2 List of Controversies for Optimal Management of GD in Childhood

Duration of antithyroid drug therapy
Radical treatment options:
  near-total thyroidectomy *or*
  radioiodine therapy

Additional treatment with beta blockers (except in patients with asthma or cardiac failure) during the first 2 weeks of management may help to reduce the patient's symptoms. This treatment (propanolol) can be given orally twice daily, at a dosage of 2 mg/kg/day, and stopped when the patient becomes euthyroid.

ANTITHYROID DRUG THERAPY

Antithyroid drug treatment is usually recommended as the initial treatment for hyperthyroidism in children and adolescents. The most commonly used ATDs are carbimazole and its active metabolite, methimazole (MMI), and propylthiouracil (PTU). These drugs inhibit thyroid hormone synthesis by interfering with the thyroid peroxidase–mediated iodination of tyrosine residues in thyroglobulin. PTU can also block the conversion of T_4 to T_3, whereas MMI cannot. Both MMI and PTU are associated with minor reactions (rash, urticaria, arthralgia, gastrointestinal problems) in about 5% to 25% of cases. The frequency of agranulocytosis is between 0.2% and 0.5% for both drugs and other major, rare side effects include drug-induced hepatitis and the production of cytoplasmic antineutrophil antibodies. Antibody-positive vasculitis occurs only in exceptional cases. The frequency of side effects may be dose-related and is very small for severe side effects in patients receiving MMI at a dosage of less than 10 mg/day.[15] MMI is more effective in the short term than PTU.[16] MMI also presents a major advantage over PTU in terms of compliance, because MMI has a longer half-life and is effective when given as a single daily dose. The initial starting dose of PTU is 5 to 10 mg/kg/day, with a maximum of 300 mg/day in three equal doses, whereas that of MMI (or carbimazole) is 0.5 to 1 mg/kg/day, with a maximal dose of 30 mg/day. After 2 to 4 weeks, when thyroid hormone secretion is effectively blocked and thyroid hormone levels have normalized, the initial dose is gradually reduced by 30% to 50%. No additional benefit accrues from the maintenance of a high dose of ATD, administered with replacement doses of levothyroxine (L-T_4). Recent studies have even suggested that high-dose therapy may be harmful, because the frequency of side effects is dose-dependent. There is also currently no rationale for the use of L-T_4 in combination with ATDs to enhance remission rates.[15] GD remission on ATD therapy is linked to the restoration of euthyroidism rather than the immunosuppressive effects of the drugs. Hyperthyroidism itself has been shown to worsen the autoimmune aberration, and autoimmunity leads to the generation of more TSH receptor antibodies and a worsening of hyperthyroidism. Once this cycle is broken by ATD treatment rendering the patient euthyroid or by surgery, the patient may experience gradual remission of the disease.[17] More prolonged use of ATD (at least 2 years) in children than in adults may be required to achieve remission. Compliance is therefore an important issue in the management of these children and should be improved by educational strategies. However, the inhibition of autoantibodies obtained by treatment is difficult to predict, probably because the treatment does not target B cells or autoantibodies directly. B lymphocytes are important self-antigen–presenting cells and precursors of antibody-secreting plasma cells. Temporary B-lymphocyte depletion with the monoclonal antibody rituximab may therefore efficiently decrease or abolish the production of TRAbs. Large clinical trials of this treatment are currently required.[18,19]

Less than 30% of children achieve lasting remission after about 24 months of ATD.[11,20-23] For the remaining patients, near-total thyroidectomy or radioiodine therapy are the definitive therapeutic options, but both carry a high risk of permanent hypothyroidism. Unfortunately, prospective randomized trials are still lacking to evaluate the efficacy of short- and long-term ATD therapy to increase the remission rate in children, and further studies are required to increase our knowledge of ATD treatment in children.

SURGICAL TREATMENT

Total (or near-total) thyroidectomy is often currently preferred to subtotal (or partial) thyroidectomy to reduce the risk of recurrent hyperthyroidism.[13] The vascularity of the gland is decreased by adding iodine to ATD (5 to 10 drops of Lugol's solution) for 1 week before surgery.[24] L-T_4 replacement therapy should be initiated within days of surgery and the patient should undergo long-term follow-up. Complications such as hypoparathyroidism, vocal cord palsy, and keloid formation are rare for operations performed by a pediatric surgeon with extensive experience. For patients with recurrent hyperthyroidism after surgery, radioactive iodine (RAI) treatment is recommended because the risk of complications is higher for a second operation.[13]

This radical option is often recommended for patients with a large goiter or with ophthalmopathy. For other cases, there is still some debate about whether RAI treatment or surgical ablation should be preferred as the definitive treatment for pediatric GD.[12,13]

IODINE TREATMENT

RAI treatment is effective in children with hyperthyroidism caused by GD, and most patients can be successfully treated with a single oral dose. Larger doses (220 to 275 μCi/g, corresponding to about 250 Gy) should be preferred over smaller doses of ^{131}I.[25] Euthyroidism caused by the radioiodine-mediated destruction of the thyroid gland is different, because radioiodine therapy has a particular effect on thyroid autoimmunity. There is no evidence of reproductive dysfunction or higher frequencies of abnormalities in the offspring of treated patients.[26] RAI is absolutely contraindicated during pregnancy and breastfeeding. RAI should also be avoided in very young children because of an increased potential risk of neoplasia. Concerns about potential thyroid malignancy, hyperparathyroidism, and mortality rates have highlighted the need for a large, randomized control study with long-term follow-up to settle this issue definitively.[27] Hypothyroidism is likely to occur after treatment, and appropriate doses of L-T_4 must therefore be administered throughout the patient's life.

Long-term Outcome

Less than 30% of children treated with ATDs achieve remission lasting at least 2 years, whereas ATD treatment results in long-term remission in about 40% to 60% of adult patients.[11,20-23,28] Consequently, the overall frequency of relapse is higher in children than in adults, and may reach 70% to 80%. About 75% of patients relapse within 6 months of the end of drug treatment, whereas only 10% relapse after 18 months. Methods for identifying the patients who are unlikely to have remission after drug treatment would greatly improve patient management, because they would facilitate the identification of patients requiring long-term ATD or early radical treatment. Previous studies had their limitations but evaluated age, goiter size, decrease in body mass index, severity of biochemical hyperthyroidism at onset, TRAb levels at onset and end of treatment, and duration of medical treatment as predictive markers of GD relapse during childhood.[11,23,29-33] However, all these studies but one[33] were retrospective and none has led to widespread changes in clinical practice. A recent prospective study[34] has shown that the risk of relapse is increasing with nonwhite ethnicity, young age, and the severity of the disease at diagnosis, as demonstrated by high serum TRAb and FT_4 levels. Conversely, relapse risk decreased with duration of the first course of ATD; every additional year of treatment was associated with a decrease in relapse rate. These results highlight the positive impact of a long period of primary ATD treatment on outcome to minimize thyroid autoimmunity and recurrence of the disease. In this study, a prognostic score was constructed that allowed the identification of three different risk groups at diagnosis. This score would greatly improve patient counseling and appropriate therapeutic decisions. Other factors, such as genetic background, gender, iodine intake, and smoking, have been thought to modulate individual responsiveness in adults.[28,35-37] Large prospective randomized studies in children are therefore required to resolve these issues.

Negative consequences for health-related quality of life during and after treatment, even after 14 to 21 years, particularly in regard to mental performance and vitality, have been demonstrated in adult patients with GD. These problems do not seem to be accounted for by the patient's thyroid hormone status during follow-up. However, the mode of treatment, whether drug-based, surgical, or based on the use of radioiodine, has been shown to have little impact on health-related quality of life in the long term.[38] These considerations have not been studied in children, but it would seem prudent to monitor subjects with hyperthyroidism in childhood over the longer term for neuropsychological, emotional, and/or behavioural functioning.

NEONATAL HYPERTHYROIDISM

Pathogenesis

Autoimmune neonatal hyperthyroidism is commonly caused by the passage across the placenta of maternal stimulating antibodies directed against the TSH receptor (TRAbs), which stimulate the adenylate cyclase in fetal thyrocytes, leading to thyroid hormone hypersecretion. Hyperthyroidism in pregnancy has a prevalence of approximately 0.2% and mostly results from Graves' disease.[39] Graves' thyrotoxicosis generally improves in the second half of pregnancy, caused by decreases in serum TRAb concentration, but then worsens after delivery.[40] In maternal gestational autoimmune GD, the preservation of a normal fetal thyroid hormone state to ensure normal brain development is a complex issue. High levels of antibody transmission are associated with the occurrence of fetal thyrotoxicosis. Fetal hyperthyroidism may develop when fetal TSH receptors become physiologically responsive to TSH and TRAbs during the second half of gestation, at around week 20, mostly in women with high levels of TRAbs. It may also occur in the children of mothers treated years before for hyperthyroidism who still have circulating TRAbs. Thus, all pregnant women with GD and euthyroid pregnant women with a history of GD should undergo TRAb determinations at the beginning and throughout pregnancy. If TRAbs are detected, the fetus should be considered at risk of developing thyrotoxicosis and monitored accordingly.[39,41]

Nonautoimmune neonatal hyperthyroidism caused by McCune-Albright syndrome (activating mutation of the *Gsα* gene)[42] or an activating mutation of the TSH receptor gene is a rare disease. Molecular abnormalities of the TSH receptor, leading to its constitutive activation, may be responsible for severe, permanent, congenital fetal and postnatal hyperthyroidism. Germline mutations are found in cases of hereditary autosomal dominant hyperthyroidism, and de novo mutations may cause sporadic congenital hyperthyroidism. The clinical course of these diseases requires careful management. Even with high doses of ATDs to control severe congenital thyrotoxicosis, thyroid nodules and goiter enlargement develop early in life, requiring subtotal thyroidectomy followed by radioiodine therapy.[43-45]

During gestation, transient hyperthyroidism may be observed in pregnant women with a hydatidiform mole. Surgical removal of the mole cures the hyperthyroidism. Familial gestational hyperthyroidism caused by a mutant thyrotropin receptor hypersensitive to human chorionic gonadotropin has also been reported in exceptional cases.[46]

Clinical Manifestations

Fetal hyperthyroidism precedes neonatal hyperthyroidism. Neonatal autoimmune hyperthyroidism is generally transient, occurring in only about 2% of the offspring of mothers with GD. However, it is associated with a mortality rate of up to 25% and immediate and long-term morbidity. Fetal and neonatal thyroid function may be disturbed to a varying degree by the presence of TRAbs, use of ATDs, and maternal thyroid hormone state. In cases in which maternal disease is untreated or poorly controlled, intrauterine growth retardation, oligoamnios, prematurity, and fetal death commonly occur. Tachycardia, hyperexcitability, poor weight gain contrasting with a normal or large appetite, goiter, stare, eyelid retraction and/or exophthalmia, small anterior fontanelle, advanced bone age, and hepatomegaly and/or splenomegaly are the most frequently observed clinical features during the neonatal period. Cardiac insufficiency is one of the major risks in these infants. Biologic abnormalities of the liver may also be observed in the absence of cardiac insufficiency. Craniostenosis, microcephaly, and psychomotor disabilities may occur in severely affected infants.[47]

Diagnosis and Treatment During Pregnancy and the Neonatal Period

The early diagnosis and treatment of fetal hyperthyroidism or hypothyroidism are crucial and highlight the importance of TRAb determination throughout pregnancy in women with Graves' disease. The experience of the ultrasound operator also has an impact on the management of pregnancy in women with GD. Fetal thyroid width and circumference should be defined from 20 weeks of gestation.[48] In fetuses with goiter, the main clinical issue is determining whether the cause is maternal treatment that is appropriate for achieving normal maternal thyroid function but inappropriate and excessive for the fetus, leading to fetal hypothyroidism, or fetal thyroid stimulation by maternal Graves' disease, with the presence of TRAbs causing fetal thyroid stimulation and hyperthyroidism.

Fetal ultrasound scans are a noninvasive tool for detecting fetal thyroid dysfunction. Such scans should be taken monthly after 20 weeks of gestation to screen for goiter and/or evidence of fetal thyroid dysfunction in women with GD testing positive for TRAbs and/or receiving ATDs. Thyroid gland enlargement is the starting point for the diagnosis of thyroid dysfunction and ultrasonography is used to assess the presence and vascularity of the goiter. The determination of fetal bone maturation (delayed bone maturation in cases of fetal hypothyroidism) and fetal heart rate (higher than 160/min in cases of fetal hyperthyroidism) may also facilitate the diagnosis of hypo- or hyperthyroidism, guiding the choice of the most appropriate treatment. Invasive fetal blood collection and amniotic fluid sampling are usually not required and should be reserved for cases in which the diagnosis is dubious or intra-amniotic thyroxine injection is required to treat a secondary fetal hypothyroid state.[41,49-52] A combination of maternal criteria (e.g., TRAbs titer, ATD use and dosage) and fetal criteria (e.g., thyroid Doppler signal, fetal heart rate, and bone maturation) is used to distinguish between fetal hypothyroidism and hyperthyroidism.[52]

The prenatal response to treatment, based on fetal status and the results of thyroid function tests carried out on cord blood at birth, may validate the prenatal treatment strategy, but probably cannot predict subsequent neonatal thyroid dysfunction.[53,54] Remarkably, only a minority of newborns from mothers with gestational autoimmune thyroid disease have a disturbed thyroid hormone state.[52,53] Within 2 to 5 days of birth, hyperthyroidism may develop when TRAbs continue to be present in the neonate after the clearance of transplacentally transmitted ATDs from the mother. Thyroid function tests should therefore be repeated in the first week of life, even when normal (or high TSH levels caused by excessive ATD in late gestation) results have been obtained with cord blood. Strong suspicion of neonatal autoimmune hyperthyroidism, when TRAbs are detectable in cord blood and free thyroid hormone levels are high in the 2 to 4 days following birth (FT_4 levels > 35 pmol/L), should lead to the initiation of ATD treatment in the infant shortly after birth to prevent the development of clinical hyperthyroidism, thereby protecting infants from the serious consequences of this condition.[41]

Treatment

During gestation, fetal hyperthyroidism can be prevented by administering antithyroid drugs to the mother. PTU and MMI both cross the placenta and are equally effective for treating hyperthyroidism in pregnancy.[55] However, PTU is more commonly used because the administration of MMI during organogenesis has been associated with neonatal aplasia cutis (a scalp defect), tracheoesophageal fistula, and embryopathy.[56] The fetus benefits directly from the maternal ingestion of these drugs, which cross the placenta and act on the fetal thyroid gland. These drugs may also expose the fetus to the risk of hypothyroidism, so small doses (usually 100 to 150 mg PTU or less daily, 10 to 15 mg MMI or less daily) are therefore recommended to the mother.

During the neonatal period, MMI is preferred (1 mg/kg/day, in three doses). Propanolol (2 mg/kg/day, in two divided doses) can also be used to control tachycardia during the first 1 to 2 weeks of treatment. It is usually possible to decrease the ATD dosage progressively, according to thyroid hormone levels. The disease is transient and may last 2 to 4 months, until TRAbs are eliminated from the infant's circulation. Mothers can breast-feed while taking ATDs, with no adverse effects on the thyroid status of their infants.[57]

References

1. Lavard L, Perrild H, Ranlov I, et al: Incidence of juvenile thyrotoxicosis in Denmark 1982-88. A nationwide study. Eur J Endocrinol 130:565-568, 1994.
2. Brix TH, Kyvik KO, Hegedus L: What is the evidence of genetic factors in the etiology of Graves'disease? A brief review. Thyroid 8:627-634, 1998.
3. Brix TH, Kyvik KO, Christensen K, Hegedus L: Evidence for a major role of heredity in Graves' disease: A population-based study of two Danish twin cohorts. J Clin Endocrinol Metab 86:930-934, 2001.
4. Saitoh O, Nagayama Y: Regulation of Graves' hyperthyroidism with naturally occurring CD4+ CD25+ regulatory T cells in a mouse model. Endocrinology 147:417-2422, 2006.
5. Weetman AP: Graves' disease. N Engl J Med 343: 1236-1248, 2000.
6. Cooper DS: Hyperthyroidism. Lancet 362:459-68, 2003.
7. Wong GW, Cheng PS: Increasing incidence of childhood Graves' disease in Hong Kong: A follow-up study. Clin Endocrinol 54:547-50, 2001.
8. Yang F, Shan Z, Teng X, Li Y, et al: Chronic iodine excess does not increase the incidence of hyperthyroidism: A prospective community-based epidemiological survey in China. Eur J Endocrinol 156:403-408, 2007.
9. Lucidarme N, Ruiz JC, Czernichow P, Léger J: Reduced bone mineral density at diagnosis and bone mineral recovery during treatment in children with Graves' disease. J Pediatr 137:56-62, 2000.
10. Birrell G, Cheetham T: Juvenile thyrotoxicosis; can we do better? Arch Dis Child 89:745-750, 2004.
11. Glaser NS, Styne DM: Predictors of early remission of hyperthyroidism in children. J Clin Endocrinol Metab 82:1719-1726, 1997.
12. Rivkees SA, Dinauer C: An optimal treatment for pediatric Graves' disease is radioiodine. J Clin Endocrinol Metab 92:797-800, 2007.
13. Lee JA, Grumbach MM, Clark OH: The optimal treatment for pediatric Graves' disease is surgery. J Clin Endocrinol Metab 92:801-803, 2007.
14. Cooper DS: Antithyroid drugs in the management of patients with Graves' disease: An evidence-based approach to therapeutic controversies. J Clin Endocrinol Metab 88:3474-3481, 2003.
15. Cooper DS: Antithyroid drugs. N Engl J Med 352: 905-17, 2005.
16. Nakamura H, Noh JY, Itoh K, et al: Comparison of methimazole and propylthiouracil in patients with hyperthyroidism caused by Graves' disease. J Clin Endocrinol Metab 92:2157-2162, 2007.
17. Laurberg P: Remission of Graves' disease during anti-thyroid drug therapy. Time to reconsider the mechanism? Eur J Endocrinol 155:783-786, 2006.
18. Wang SH, Baker JR: Targeting B cells in Graves' disease. Endocrinology 147:4559-4560, 2006.
19. El Fassi D, Nielsen CH, Hasselbalch HC, Hegedües L: The rationale for B lymphocyte depletion in Graves' disease. Monoclonal anti-CD20 antibody as a novel treatment option. Eur J Endocrinol 154:623-632, 2006.
20. Hamburger JI: Management of hyperthyroidism in children and adolescents. J Clin Endocrinol Metab 60:1019-1024, 1985.
21. Zimmerman D, Gan-Gaisano M: Hyperthyroidism in children and adolescents. Pediatr Clin North Am 37:1273-1295, 1990.
22. Boiko J, Léger J, Raux-Demay MC, et al: Maladie de Basedow chez l'enfant: Aspects Cliniques et évolutifs. [Basedow disease in children: Clinical and evolutive aspects.] Arch Pediatr 5:722-730, 1998.
23. Lazar L, Kalter-Leibovici O, Pertzelan A, et al: Thyrotoxicosis in prepubertal children compared with pubertal and postpubertal patients. J Clin Endocrinol Metab 85:3678-3682, 2000.
24. Erbil Y, Ozluk Y, Giriş, M, et al: Effect of lugol solution on thyroid gland blood flow and microvessel density in the patients with Graves' disease. J Clin Endocrinol Metab 92:2182-2189, 2007.
25. Rivkees SA, Cornelius EA: Influence of iodine-131 dose on the outcome of hyperthyroid children. Pediatrics 111:745-9, 2003.
26. Read CH, Tansey MJ, Menda Y: A 36-year retrospective analysis of the efficacy and safety of radioactive iodine in treating young Graves' patients. J Clin Endocrinol Metab 89:4229-4233, 2004.
27. Metso S, Jaatinen P, Huhtala H, et al: Increased cardiovascular and cancer mortality after radioiodine treatment for hyperthyroidism. J Clin Endocrinol Metab 92:2190-2196, 2007.
28. Weetman AP: Graves' hyperthyroidism: How long should antithyroid drug therapy be continued to achieve remission? Nat Clin Pract Endocrinol Metab 2:2-3, 2006.
29. Collen RJ, Landau E, Kaplan SA, Lippe BM: Remission rates of children and adolescents with thyrotoxicosis treated with antithyroid drugs. Pediatrics 65:550-556, 1980.
30. Lippe BM, Landaw EM, Kaplan SA: Hyperthyroidism in children treated with long term medical therapy: Twenty-five percent remission every two years. J Clin Endocrinol Metab 64:1241-1245, 1987.
31. Shulman DI, Muhar I, Jorgensen EV, et al: Autoimmune hyperthyroidism in prepubertal children and adolescents: Comparison of clinical and biochemical features at diagnosis and response to medical therapy. Thyroid 7:755-760, 1997.
32. Mussa GC, Corrias A, Silvestro L, et al: Factors at onset predictive of lasting remission in pediatric patients with Graves' disease followed for at least three years. J Pediatr Endocrinol Metab 12:537-541, 1999.
33. Glaser NS, Styne DM: for the Organisation of Pediatric Endocrinologists of Northern California Collaborative Graves' Disease Study Group: Predicting the likelihood of remission in children with Graves' disease: A prospective, multicenter study. Pediatrics 121:e481-e488, 2008.
34. Kaguelidou F, Alberti C, Castanet M, et al: Predictors of autoimmune hyperthyroidism relapse in children after discontinuation of antithyroid drug treatment. J Clin Endocrinol Metab 93:3817-3826, 2008.

35. Allahabadia A, Daykin J, Holder RL, et al: Age and gender predict the outcome of treatment for Graves' hyperthyroidism. J Clin Endocrinol Metab 85:1038-1042, 2000.
36. Nedrebo B, Holm PI, Uhlving S, et al: Predictors of outcome and comparison of different drug regimens for the prevention of relapse in patients with Graves'disease. Eur J Endocrinol 147:583-589, 2002.
37. Kim TY, Park YJ, Park DJ, et al: Epitope heterogeneity of thyroid-stimulating antibodies predicts long term outcome in Graves' patients treated with antithyroid drugs. J Clin Endocrinol Metab 88:117-124, 2003.
38. Abraham-Nordling M, Wallin G, Lundell G, Törring O: Thyroid hormone state and quality of life at long term follow-up after randomized treatment of Graves' disease. Eur J Endocrinol 156:173-179, 2007.
39. Glinoer D: The regulation of thyroid function in pregnancy: Pathways of endocrine adaptation from physiology to pathology. Endocrinol Rev 18:404-433, 1997.
40. Amito N, Izumi Y, Hidaka Y, et al: No increase of blocking type anti-thyrotropin receptor antibodies during pregnancy in patients with Graves' disease. J Clin Endocrinol Metab 88:5871-5874, 2003.
41. Polak M, Le Gac I, Vuillard E, et al: Fetal and neonatal thyroid function in relation to maternal Graves' disease. Best Pract Res Clin Endocrinol Metab 18:289-302, 2004.
42. Yoshimoto M, Nakayama M, Baba T, et al: A case of neonatal McCune-Albright syndrome with Cushing syndrome and hyperthyroidism. Acta Paediatr Scand 80:984-987, 1991.
43. Kopp P, Van Sande J, Parma J, et al: Congenital hyperthyroidism caused by a mutation in the thyrotropin-receptor gene. N Engl J Med 332: 150-154, 1995.
44. De Roux N, Polak M, Couet J, et al: A neomutation of the thyroid-stimulating hormone receptor in a severe neonatal hyperthyroidism. J Clin Endocrinol Metab 81:2023-6, 1996.
45. Gelwane G, De Roux N, Van den Abbeele AD, et al: 13 years' follow-up of severe congenital nonautoimmune hyperthyroidism due to an activating neomutation of the TSH receptor gene. Horm Res 68:220, 2007.
46. Rodien P, Bremont C, Sanson ML, et al: Familial gestational hyperthyroidism caused by a mutant thyrotropin receptor hypersensitive to human chorionic gonadotropin. N Engl J Med 339:1823-1826, 1998.
47. Daneman D, Howard NJ: Neonatal thyrotoxicosis: Intellectual impairment and craniosynostosis in later years. J Pediatr 97:257-259, 1980.
48. Ranzini AC, Ananth CV, Smulian JC, et al: Ultrasonography of the fetal thyroid: Normograms based on biparietal diameters and gestational age. J Ultrasound Med 20:613-617, 2001.
49. Polak M, Léger J, Luton D, et al: Fetal cord blood sampling in the diagnosis and the treatment of fetal hyperthyroidism in the offsprings of a euthyroid mother, producing thyroid stimulating immunoglobulins. Ann Endocrinol 58:338-342, 1997.
50. Singh PK, Parvin CA, Gronowski AM: Establishment of reference intervals for markers of fetal thyroid status in amniotic fluid. J Clin Endocrinol Metab 88:4175-4179, 2003.
51. Volumenie JL, Polak M, Guibourdenche J, et al: Management of fetal thyroid goitres: A report of 11 cases in a single perinatal unit. Prenat Diagn 20:799-806, 2000.
52. Luton D, Le Gac I, Vuillard E, et al: Management of Graves' disease during pregnancy: The key role of fetal thyroid gland monitoring. J Clin Endocrinol Metab 90:6093-6098, 2005.
53. Skuza KA, Sills IN, Stene M, Rapaport R: Prediction of neonatal hyperthyroidism in infants born to mothers with Graves' disease. J Pediatr 128:264-267, 1996.
54. Kempers MJE, Van Tijn DA, Van Trotsenburg SP, et al: Central congenital hypothyroidism due to gestational hyperthyroidism: Detection where prevention failed. J Clin Endocrinol Metab 88:5851-5857, 2003.
55. Momotani N, Noh JH, Ishikawa N, Ito K: Effects of propylthiouracil and methimazole on fetal thyroid status in mothers with Graves' hyperthyroidism. J Clin Endocrinol Metab 82:3633-3636, 1997.
56. Foulds N, Walpole I, Elmslie F, Mansour S: Carbimazole embryopathy: An emerging phenotype. Am J Med Genet 132:130-135, 2005.
57. Momotani N, Yamashita R, Makino F, et al: Thyroid function in wholly breast-feeding infants whose mothers take high doses of propylthiouracil. Clin Endocrinol 53:177-181, 2000.

PART

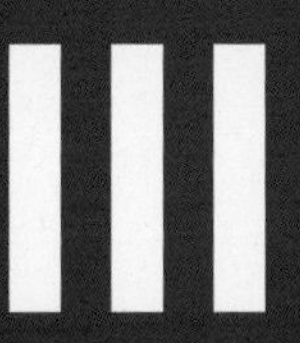

Adult Thyroid Disease

HYPERFUNCTION

Chapter 12

Graves' Disease

Jason M. Hollander and Terry F. Davies

Key Points

- Graves' disease is the commonest cause of hyperthyroidism in young women.
- Treatment can be non-thyroid ablative with antithyroid drugs or ablative with radiodioine or surgery. Most patients are best treated first with antithyroid drugs, and methimazole is the drug of choice.
- TSH receptor antibody measurements may help predict recurrence after antithyroid drugs. When there is a recurrence, patients may opt to continue antithyroid drugs or receive radioiodine ablation therapy.
- Radioiodine is contraindicated in moderate to severe Graves' ophthalmopathy whose primary therapy remains corticosteroids.

HISTORY

Caleb Hillier Parry was the first to describe the features of Graves' disease (GD) in 1825.[1] The disease, however, continues to bear the name of Robert Graves, who in 1835 proposed an association between exophthalmos, goiter, and palpitations. Over a century later, evidence of a thyroid-stimulating factor offered a cause for the disease.[2] In 1964, the stimulator was identified as an IgG antibody.[3] Currently, it is clear that the binding of these antibodies to the thyroid-stimulating hormone (TSH) receptor is the causative factor in GD. These antibodies stimulate thyroid growth and function by mimicking pituitary TSH. The cause of Graves' ophthalmopathy and dermopathy, although less well defined, is also intimately involved with the TSH receptors on orbital and dermal fibroblasts and adipocytes.[4,5]

EPIDEMIOLOGY

The prevalence of GD depends largely on the level of iodine sufficiency in the region in question. In the United States, autoimmune thyroid disease is the most prevalent autoimmune disease, outnumbering other common disorders, such as diabetes mellitus and rheumatoid arthritis.[6] A historical cohort from the United Kingdom has found the incidence of GD in women over a 20-year period to be about 1 in 1000, with a prevalence of approximately 2%.[7] As is true of most autoimmune diseases, men are affected at a much lower rate than women.[8] In patients younger than about 40 years, GD is the most common cause of hyperthyroidism, accounting for 60% to 80% of cases.[9]

CLINICAL PRESENTATION AND DIAGNOSIS

The signs and symptoms of GD can be divided into those that manifest a state of hyperthyroidism (Table 12-1) indistinguishable from other forms of thyrotoxicosis and those that are unique to GD—specifically orbitopathy, ophthalmopathy, and occasionally dermopathy. Ophthalmopathy may rarely occur alone or with Hashimoto's thyroiditis, but most commonly it presents before, at the same time, or after the onset

Table 12–1 Common Manifestations of Thyrotoxicosis

Symptoms	Signs
Palpitations	Tachycardia
Nervousness	Goiter
Easy fatigability	Weight loss
Hyperkinesias	Tremor
Diarrhea	Atrial fibrillation
Excessive sweating	Muscle weakness
Heat intolerance	Stare
Increased appetite	Lid lag

of thyroid hyperfunction. Certainly, when they occur simultaneously, the diagnosis of GD is straightforward.

Laboratory data will invariably reveal a low or suppressed TSH with elevated levels of triiodothyronine (T_3) and thyroxine (T_4), frequently in a ratio higher than 20:1.[10] In areas of relative iodine deficiency, T_3 may be elevated in the face of a normal T_4, a pattern known as T_3 thyrotoxicosis.

On presentation, most patients have diffusely enlarged glands of variable consistency, mostly soft but varying to firm and rubbery. Graves' glands are typically smooth but occasionally may feel nodular. In severe cases, a thrill may be felt over the upper poles, with an associated bruit. Often, the specific diagnosis of GD can be deduced from the clinical picture and family history of autoimmune disease, which is present in 50% of patients. In practice, the measurement of TSH receptor antibodies (TSH-R Abs) is routinely made to document the diagnosis and possibly offer prognostic information. Additionally, in unclear cases, a normal or elevated radioiodine uptake can corroborate the diagnosis by excluding subacute thyroiditis.

This chapter will review the mainstays of GD therapy, including the use of antithyroid drugs (ATDs), radioiodine (RAI), and surgery. Each modality has proven efficacy in the treatment of GD, and the choice of therapy is often dictated by the needs and preference of the individual patient rather than by evidence-based outcome data.[11,12] The goal here is to provide, as much as possible, an evidence-based rationale for the use of each of the three treatment modalities, considering measurable end points such as cure (remission) and weighing them against the real and theoretical risks of each form of treatment. Ultimately, the decision to pursue one form of therapy rather than another represents a complex interplay of facts and factors, including disease severity, age of patient, access to a qualified thyroid surgeon, presence of ophthalmopathy, previous reaction to ATDs, patient compliance, and patient's wishes in regard to childbearing. Fortunately, more than 90% of patients express satisfaction with their chosen therapy.[13]

The second half of the chapter will focus on the therapeutic options for the infiltrative orbitopathy and ophthalmopathy of GD, the management of GD in pregnancy, and an evidence-based approach to treating so-called thyroid crises.

TREATMENT

The main treatment options for GD include ATDs, radioiodine, and surgery.

Antithyroid Drugs

THIONAMIDES

Mechanism of Action

In the United States, thyroidologists have two commonly prescribed ATDs in their armamentarium, propylthiouracil (PTU) and methimazole (MMI). Carbimazole is used widely in England and other countries; once ingested, carbimazole is rapidly converted to MMI.[14] PTU and MMI are known as thionamides, a class of drugs capable of inhibiting thyroid hormone synthesis. The thionamides are actively concentrated by the thyroid gland[15] and subsequently act by interfering with the enzyme thyroid peroxidase (TPO), disrupting the iodination of tyrosine residues on the thyroglobulin molecule. Ultimately, this thionamide-induced inhibition of iodination leads to decreased intrathyroidal stores of T_4 and T_3. The thionamides have proved to possess a number of other salutary effects (see later).

Inhibition of Deiodination. PTU in large doses, but not MMI, decreases peripheral T_4 deiodination, thereby decreasing T_3 levels more rapidly than MMI.[16] This is probably of little clinical importance in most cases of GD; however, when rapid control of thyrotoxicosis is necessary, this property of PTU can be exploited.

Immunosuppression. There has been some controversy over the years surrounding the importance of the immunomodulatory properties of thionamides. It was first argued by some that observed changes in the immune system could be attributed to normalization of thyroid function,[17,18] but convincing data of immunosuppressive effects have been found by many investigators.[19-29] Whether these immunomodulatory effects are caused by the intrathyroidal actions of thionamides or by a direct effect on local immune elements may be a matter for debate, but there is no dispute that a number of immunologically important events accompany thionamide treatment. First, the serum antibodies directed against the TSH receptor, thyroglobulin, and thyroid peroxidase all decrease with thionamide treatment (Fig. 12-1).[19-23] Furthermore, a number of

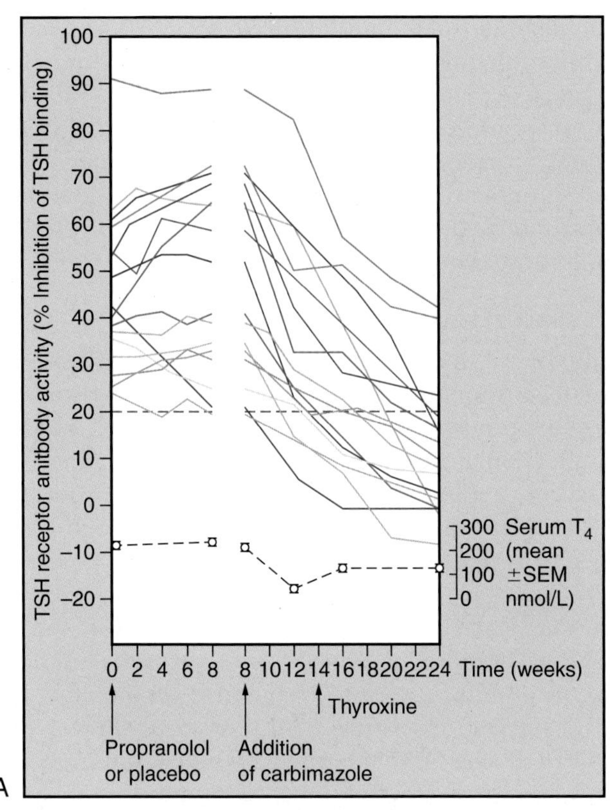

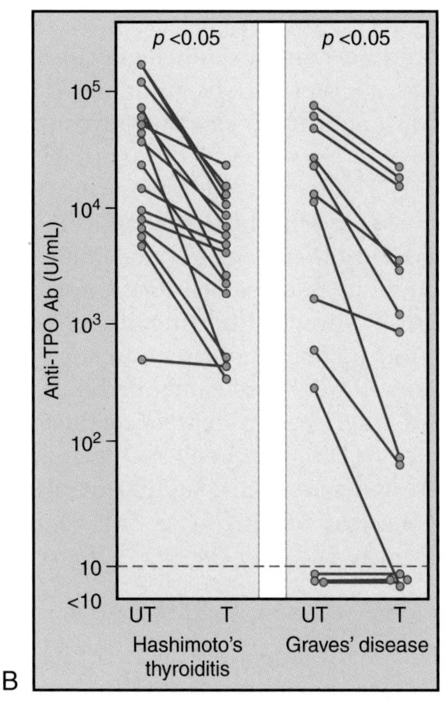

Figure 12–1 Thyroid antibodies after thionamide treatment. **A,** Antibody activity toward the thyroid-stimulating hormone (TSH) receptor during treatment of 16 patients with hyperthyroidism from Graves' disease with propranolol followed by carbimazole and thyroxine (T_4). **B,** Variation in thyroid peroxidase (TPO) antibodies after treatment with methimazole (MMI). Assays were performed after 6 to 8 months of MMI therapy in the Graves' disease patients. *(A adapted from McGregor AM, Petersen MM, McLachlan SM, et al: Carbimazole and the autoimmune response in Graves' disease. N Engl J Med 303:302-307, 1980; B from Mariotti S, Caturegli P, Piccolo P, et al: Antithyroid peroxidase autoantibodies in thyroid diseases. J Clin Endocrinol Metab 71:661-669, 1990.)*

other immune molecules decrease with treatment. Soluble intracellular adhesion molecule-1 (sICAM-1) was found to be elevated in newly diagnosed GD patients and was noted to fall with thionamide therapy.[24] Similarly, soluble interleukin-2 (IL-2) receptor and soluble IL-6 levels were significantly lower in patients treated with MMI than untreated individuals.[25,26] Additionally, thionamides appear to upregulate the expression of Fas ligand (Fas-L) in thyrocytes, inducing Fas-L–mediated apoptosis of infiltrating lymphocytes.[27] Thionamides also inhibit the aberrant follicular cell expression of the major histocompatibility complex, HLA-DR, believed to be a factor in the perpetuation of the autoimmune process.[28] Finally, a number of changes have been observed in immune cell subsets during treatment with ATDs. In particular, suppressor-inducer T-cell subsets are upregulated whereas helper T-cell numbers return to normal during ATD-induced remission.[29] Furthermore, natural killer cells[30] and intrathyroidal lymphocyte numbers decrease during thionamide therapy.[21]

The clinical significance of these immunologic observations remains unclear. Whether immune modulation or simply the restoration of a euthyroid state accounts for the efficacy of thionamide therapy remains unclear. However, the breadth of evidence suggests an effect much greater than the inhibition of iodination and organification discussed earlier.

Pharmacokinetics

Both PTU and MMI are readily absorbed from the gastrointestinal tract and have a bioavailability that exceeds 80%.[31] After a single oral dose, PTU reaches a maximum concentration approximately 1 hour after ingestion and has a half-life of 40 to 120 minutes.[32] Peak plasma concentrations of MMI are achieved between 30 minutes and 3 hours after ingestion,[33] and the half-life is much longer than PTU, from 3 to 6 hours.[31] The plasma half-lives, however, can be deceiving when discussing the activity of these medications. It is clear that both MMI and PTU are concentrated by the thyroid and remain partly unmetabolized for long periods of time. It follows that the drug continues to exert its effect on thyroid hormone metabolism, even after serum concentrations wane.[31] To illustrate this, Jansson and colleagues[34] have demonstrated that intrathyroidal concentrations of MMI are identical in surgically resected thyroids, regardless of whether the last dose of MMI was taken 3 to 6 hours versus 17 to 20 hours prior to surgery. However, the serum concentrations of the drug were significantly higher in the former. Both drugs can therefore be given on a daily basis, although MMI appears to exert better control at this dose frequency.

MMI and PTU are excreted in the urine, but available evidence suggests that no dosage adjustment is required for renal insufficiency[35] or renal failure.[36] Some authors have suggested a sensible empirical dosage adjustment in advanced hepatic dysfunction because elimination half-life increases with degree of liver impairment. Others have contended that no dosage adjustment is necessary.[37] In practice, the lowest dose possible of ATD is used in all such patients. Additionally, there appears to be no significant difference in pharmacokinetics relating to age[38] or degree of thyrotoxicosis.[31]

Differences Between Propylthiouracil and Methimazole

MMI and PTU share many similarities but have important differences. MMI circulates unbound in serum and is highly lipid-soluble, whereas PTU is 80% to 90% bound to albumin, with a very low lipid solubility.[39] These properties suggest that MMI but not PTU would readily cross the placenta as well as enter the lacteals of lactating women. In fact, current evidence debunks this assertion. A recent study has demonstrated equal placental transfer kinetics for PTU and MMI.[40] More importantly, thyroid studies in infants exposed to MMI in utero are indistinguishable from those exposed to PTU.[41] Both medications appear in breast milk at very low concentrations (MMI[42] more than PTU[43]) and are considered safe in lactation.[44,45]

SIDE EFFECTS

Side effects associated with ATDs range from benign nuisance reactions such as rash or gastrointestinal upset to severe, life-threatening reactions such as hepatic failure or agranulocytosis. Although the clinician must be mindful of the toxicities associated with thionamide therapy, the likelihood a patient will experience any side effect is merely 5%,[39] with the most severe reactions occurring less than 0.5% of the time.[46,47] Side effects (Table 12-2) can be categorized in a number of ways, but in practice one must be clear on those toxicities that require cessation of therapy and those that do not.

Cutaneous Effects

In general, most cutaneous reactions do not necessitate termination of ATD therapy. It is reasonable to coadminister an antihistamine provided neither angioedema nor bronchospasm accompanies the rash or pruritus.[37] Alternatively, changing from one ATD to another may provide relief, although cross-reactivity may be as high as 50%.

Hepatotoxicity

This is a more complex topic because elevations in transaminase levels frequently accompany the hyperthyroid state itself.[48] Moreover, subclinical liver injury during PTU therapy may be common, affecting almost 30% of patients by 2 months. In most patients, liver enzyme levels normalize while on continued therapy.[49] We suggest checking liver function at the start of therapy to establish a baseline and on a regular basis thereafter, because serious effects may occur at any time. It is important to note that baseline elevations do not preclude thionamide therapy. To the contrary, PTU has been demonstrated to reduce mortality and improve liver function in patients with alcoholic hepatitis.[50] Marked elevations in aminotransferase levels developing after the start of therapy warrant cessation of the drug. Finally, extant data have suggested little relationship between hepatic necrosis and dose of PTU, indicating the idiosyncratic nature of such reactions.[51] In contrast to PTU, reports of MMI hepatotoxicity are infrequent in the medical literature. When they do manifest, the process is typically cholestatic in nature. Unlike PTU-induced hepatocellular injury, which appears

Table 12–2 Side Effects of Antithyroid Drugs

Hypersensitivity	Hematologic	Liver	Rheumatologic
Rash	Leukopenia	Hepatitis (PTU)	DIL (rare)
Pruritus	Agranulocytosis (<0.5%)	Fulminant	ANCA-positive vasculitis (rare)
Urticaria		Cholestasis (MMI)	Arthralgias

ANCA, antineutrophil cytoplasmic antibody; DIL, drug-induced lupus; MMI, methimazole; PTU, propylthiouracil.

unrelated to dose, the cholestasis associated with MMI occurs more commonly at higher doses and in older individuals.[52] Resolution of MMI-induced cholestasis is the rule once the medication is stopped. Of note, necroinflammatory liver disease has been reported with MMI therapy albeit rarely.

Autoimmune Phenomena

Drug-induced lupus (DIL) associated with PTU has been described, but is exceedingly rare. Of the 12 cases in the literature meeting strict diagnostic criteria, musculoskeletal symptoms predominated and resolution of the illness required nothing more than withdrawal of the ATD in most patients.[53] In contrast, antineutrophil cytoplasmic antibody (ANCA)–positive vasculitis carries a less favorable prognosis. There is considerable overlap in symptomatology between ANCA-positive vasculitis and DIL, including mucocutaneous lesions, fever, and serositis. However, renal dysfunction and serious pulmonary symptoms occur primarily in ANCA-positive vasculitis. At least 50% of patients with PTU-induced vasculitis require immunosuppressive therapy, with the most severe cases requiring plasmapheresis. Although most case reports have implicated PTU, ANCAs have also been identified in GD patients treated with MMI.[54] Prompt recognition of these syndromes is paramount to the safe administration of these medications.

Agranulocytosis

This remains the most feared complication of ATD therapy. A pretreatment white cell count can prevent confusion during therapy because a mild leukopenia can be associated with GD itself.[37] Most cases of agranulocytosis occur within weeks to months of the initiation of ATD therapy but can occur after more than 1 year.[55,56] Fever and sore throat are the most common presenting symptoms. Should these symptoms develop, thionamide therapy should be discontinued immediately and a cell blood count and differential determined. A granulocyte count less than $1000/mm^3$ dictates that thionamide therapy be permanently discontinued. A level between 1000 and $1500/mm^3$ will likely be approached differently by each physician. It is probably safe to continue the ATD provided that the number does not represent a precipitous fall from a previous cell count and that a follow-up test can be done within 1 to 2 days. Perhaps greater caution should be exercised with those older than 40 years; studies have shown a greater frequency of agranulocytosis in this age group (6.4 times higher; $P < .001$).[55] Moreover, one study has found the risk of a fatal reaction to be much higher in those older than 65 years (odds ratio, 12.9; 5% to 95% confidence interval [CI], 1.45 to 114.92).[56] If agranulocytosis does occur, broad-spectrum antibiotics should be initiated. Additionally, granulocyte colony-stimulating factor (G-CSF) may hasten marrow recovery,[57] although definitive evidence is lacking at this time.[58]

MAKING THE CHOICE TO USE ANTITHYROID DRUGS

When surveyed in the early 1990s, most American thyroidologists preferred radioiodine therapy to ATDs and surgery for the treatment of GD.[11,12] Since then, their use has increased but remains in contrast to the practice in Europe, where ATDs tend to be used as first-line therapy.[12] ATDs remain a viable, rationale, and cost-effective[59] first-line therapy for GD. Depending on the study, ATDs effectively induced remission in 30% to 50% of patients, probably reflecting differences in the iodine content of the local diet.[60,61] Moreover, in those who recur, there is no compelling reason that destructive therapy must be used; rather, a recent randomized controlled trial has demonstrated the safety and efficacy of long-term MMI therapy. As would be expected, over 90% of MMI-treated patients remained euthyroid for over 10 years, while just 39% of patients treated with RAI remained euthyroid. Overall, MMI was well tolerated and, in this particular study, surprisingly cheaper than RAI and its consequences.[62]

There are a handful of circumstances that deserve mention when thionamides are clearly preferred, at least as initial therapy. These include the following:

1. ATDs are first-line therapy in pregnancy; this will be reviewed in detail later in this chapter.
2. Current evidence also suggests that moderate to severe active Graves' ophthalmopathy (GO) may worsen, although often transiently, with RAI in about 15% of patients, whereas no progression is observed during ATD therapy.[63]
3. ATDs are encouraged prior to RAI in older patients and in those with suspected or established coronary artery disease to deplete intrathyroidal T_3 and T_4 stores, because the rapid rise in plasma hormone levels that follows thyroid cell breakdown induced by RAI ablation can have serious consequences.[64] Whether pretreatment actually prevents worsening of cardiac status has not been demonstrated in prospective trials. However, there is a clear reduction in posttreatment biochemical parameters of thyroid function in pretreated individuals following RAI compared with those who were not pretreated.[65]

When the decision to use ATDs is finally reached, the clinician is next challenged with other questions in regard to the optimal use of these medications. Which ATD is "best"? At what dose? For how long? The following sections address the clinical controversies surrounding the use of ATDs.

Propylthiouracil or Methimazole

To determine which should be used, the following must be considered:

1. Which drug is more efficacious?
2. Which drug is safer?
3. Which drug is associated with greater compliance?

Unfortunately, there are few head to head trials to answer these questions definitively. A total of four prospective trials and one retrospective trial have compared PTU with MMI. Two of the trials compared 15 mg of MMI daily to 150 mg of PTU daily.[66,67] Both studies strongly favored MMI, likely because of its longer half-life and greater efficacy when dosed once daily. A third trial randomized 22 patients with GD to 30 mg of MMI daily or 100 mg of PTU every 8 hours. There was no difference in thyroid indices or clinical markers detected between these groups.[68] Another study randomized 94 patients to 100 mg PTU every 6, 8, or 12 hours or 10 mg of MMI every 6, 8, or 12 hours.[69] The primary outcome measure was the lowest free T_4 achieved within 3 months of the initiation of the antithyroid treatment. By 3 months, almost every patient achieved a euthyroid state, except those in the every 12-hour dosing arm. It was concluded that PTU and MMI demonstrate similar efficacy. Finally, a retrospective study, including 73 Japanese GD patients, found that by 5 weeks, only 1 of 17 patients receiving PTU, 100 mg every 8 hours, was euthyroid versus 34 of 66 patients on MMI, 10 mg every 8 hours.[70] Although the preponderance of the data available favors the efficacy of MMI, high-quality evidence does not support the routine use of one ATD over the other.

Safety is another important consideration when choosing a treatment. A study by Pearce[56] has found that the per prescription event rate for the following occurred at a significantly higher rate in PTU-treated individuals: (1) agranulocytosis ($P = 0.0016$); (2) neutropenia ($P = 0.0018$); (3) respiratory disorders ($P = 6 \times 10^{-5}$); (4) renal and urinary disorders ($P = 0.0190$); (5) gastrointestinal disorders ($P = 0.0310$); (6) endocrine and reproductive disorders, excluding hypothyroidism ($P = 0.0038$); and (7) psychiatric disorders ($P = 0.0002$). These data, although provocative, must be taken in context. This was a retrospective study using adverse events voluntarily reported to a national registry compared with the number of prescriptions written. Older and perhaps less reliable studies do not support these findings. Werner and coworkers[71] have examined patients on both high (MMI 60 ± 19 mg; PTU 728 ± 216 mg) and low-dose ATDs (MMI 23 ± 10 mg; PTU 255 ± 85 mg). They found no significant difference in adverse events between the medications, although most side effects reported occurred in the high-dose MMI group, suggesting that side effects are dose-related with MMI. This dose-response effect was also noted by Cooper and colleagues.[55] In this study, the records of 50 patients treated with ATDs who developed agranulocytosis were compared with those of 50 patients treated with ATDS with no untoward reactions. There were no cases of agranulocytosis in those taking less than 30 mg of MMI daily; moreover, there was an 8.6-fold increase in agranulocytosis when the dose exceeded 40 mg daily ($P < .01$). In contrast, agranulocytosis occurred at all doses of PTU. Finally, drug-induced hepatitis and some of the rarer rheumatologic manifestations of ATD toxicity occurred almost exclusively in patients treated with PTU.[72] Although the evidence in regard to safety is not definitive, at least two important conclusions can be drawn: (1) serious adverse events are unlikely at low doses of MMI; and (2) rare but serious reactions, including hepatitis and ANCA-positive vasculitis, are more often associated with PTU. Overall, in our opinion, there is a strong suggestion in the literature that MMI is a safer medication.

Compliance has never been a primary outcome measure in studies comparing PTU with MMI. MMI is effective when dosed daily,[68] PTU much less so.[66]For this reason alone, one would infer superior compliance with MMI. Furthermore, one study comparing daily MMI with PTU three times daily found compliance (assessed by pill count) to be 83.3% in the MMI group versus 53.3% in the PTU group.[69]

In conclusion, efficacy, safety, and compliance favor the routine use of MMI in the treatment of GD, particularly if a patient can be maintained on a low dose.

DOSING CONSIDERATIONS

When considering the dose of ATD to be used, the following must also be addressed—whether higher doses of ATDs render patients euthyroid sooner, and whether the dose of ATD influences the remission rate.

When considering an initial dose of medication, the clinical scenario must be carefully evaluated. How symptomatic is the patient? Biochemically, how severe is the disease? What risk does thyrotoxicosis pose to this patient? A euthyroid state can be achieved more rapidly with higher doses of ATDs in exchange for an increased likelihood of adverse events. Reinwein and associates[73] have demonstrated in a randomized controlled trial that at 6 weeks, 68.4% of patients on MMI, 10 mg daily, were euthyroid compared with 83.1% on 40 mg daily. Kallner and coworkers[69] have similarly demonstrated a dose-response effect for PTU and MMI; in their study, almost every patient in the highest dose group (MMI, 10 mg every 6 hours; PTU, 100 mg every 6 hours) achieved a euthyroid state by 6 weeks but only 14% on MMI, 10 mg twice daily, and 29% on PTU, 100 mg twice daily. Finally, Page and colleagues[74] have found that patients randomized to 40 mg of carbimazole daily (about 30 mg MMI) had significantly lower free T_4 values at 4 weeks compared with those randomized to 20 mg of carbimazole (19.4 vs. 35.2 pmol/L; $P < .001$). Despite these biochemical differences, clinical response was not significantly different (weight, pulse, symptom score) between the groups, suggesting that lower doses of ATDs may be preferable in many patients. Additional studies have confirmed the efficacy of initiating ATD therapy at a decidedly low dose (e.g., MMI 15 mg daily) in most patients with mild to moderate GD.[75,76] Conversely, in patients with more severe disease or in those for whom more rapid normalization of thyroid function is required, the evidence supports initiating ATD therapy at a higher dose (e.g., MMI, 20 mg twice daily). Even higher doses are unlikely to be of benefit and carry a much greater risk of side effects.

The second question to be considered is whether ATD dose influences remission. A number of prospective randomized controlled trials have attempted to answer this question. With the exception of one study (by Romaldini and associates), the data have consistently demonstrated no relationship between initial dose and remission rate. Their study[77] randomized patients to either high-dose ATD therapy (693 ± 73 mg PTU; 60 ± 14.5 mg MMI) plus supplemental T_3 or T_4 (so-called block-replace therapy) or standard therapy (PTU, 180 ± 58 mg; MMI, 13.6 ± 5.9 mg). Patients were treated for just over 1 year and followed for almost 2 years after drug discontinuation. Of the patients in the high-dose arm, 75.4% experienced a remission versus 41.6% in the low-dose arm ($P < 0.001$). Based on other studies,[78,79] one would hypothesize that relapse rates in the Romaldini study would converge over time. Jorde and colleagues[78] randomized patients to 60 mg MMI (with levothyroxine [L-T_4] to maintain a euthyroid state) or a titration regimen using methimazole alone. MMI was stopped after 6 months. At 12 months, patients in the high-dose arm were significantly more likely to be in remission (42.1 vs. 77.3%; $P < .02$); however, by 24 months, the remission rate was no longer different, suggesting that higher doses of ATDs delay but do not prevent relapse. Grebe and associates[79] have confirmed this observation, demonstrating a significantly longer median relapse-free interval in patients treated with high-dose carbimazole plus L-T_4 compared with those treated with a traditional dose; 2-year relapse rates were the same. Additional studies, with follow-up ranging from 2 to 4 years, have confirm that high-dose ATD therapy does not influence recurrence rate.[80-82] Furthermore, in most studies, patients randomized to high-dose ATDs experienced a greater number of adverse events.[73,77,79] These data imply that there is no role for prolonged courses of high-dose thionamides.

Block-Replace-Replace

Beginning in 1991, with a study by Hashizume and coworkers[83] demonstrating an astonishingly low 1.7% recurrence rate after ATD treatment, researchers have tested the concept of suppressing TSH with exogenous L-T_4 to prevent the recurrence of GD. The theory was that TSH itself contributed to the perpetuation of TSH-R Ab concentrations by stimulating the release of thyroid antigens. How this could occur in the presence of TSHR-Abs was never explained. Nevertheless, this theory was tested by randomizing patients after 6 months of MMI to placebo plus MMI or L-T4, 100 μg, plus MMI. [83] After an additional year, MMI, but not L-T_4 or placebo, was discontinued. The TSH-R Ab concentrations were significantly lower in the L-T_4 group; moreover, the recurrence rate at 3 years was just 1.7% compared with 34.7% in the placebo group. Unfortunately, these results have not been replicated. No less than seven additional trials have failed to corroborate these results.[84-90] At least one trial has demonstrated an increased rate of recurrence with L-T_4 administration following successful ATD therapy.[91] There is, therefore, currently no role for the use of L-T_4 therapy after discontinuation of ATDs for the GD treatment.

Block-Replace

A rational argument, however, can be made for the addition of a small amount of L-T_4 to an ATD instead of titrating the ATD to bring the patient to euthyroidism, the more traditional approach referred to as block and replace discussed earlier. Although of no advantage in achieving greater remission rates, this approach has been touted as simple and predictable and especially useful in patients difficult to control on ATDs alone.[9] In this scenario, the goal is to normalize the TSH rather than suppress it.

DURATION

The evidence in regard to duration of therapy remains sparse and inconclusive, but most clinicians have supported the concept that the longer the duration of therapy, the lower the relapse rate. Two small uncontrolled studies have concluded that short-term (4 months) ATD therapy is as effective as 12 to 18 months of therapy,[92,93] but a more recent study by Allannic and colleagues[94] has refuted this assertion. The study randomized patients to 6 and 18 months of ATD therapy. Two years after drug withdrawal, significantly more patients in the 18-month arm remained in remission compared with those in the 6-month arm (61.8% vs. 41.7%; $P < 0.05$). Other studies comparing 12- and 24-month,[95] 18- and 42-month,[96] and 6- and 12-month[97] treatment durations have been unable to confirm these data. The evidence, therefore, suggests that ATDs be continued for at least 12 months, with little additional benefit from treatment extending to 18 months or longer unless long-term thionamide therapy is contemplated.

PREDICTORS OF REMISSION

ATDs induce a sustained remission in between 30% and 50% of individuals. However, it is often difficult to predict which patients are likely to benefit from ATDs as primary therapy—that is, if a patient is certain to relapse, destructive therapy would be a more appropriate early intervention. Moreover, once patients have completed a course of ATDs, it remains unclear in many of them who will relapse and when.

A number of retrospective studies have sought to identify laboratory and clinical predictors to stratify patients as being likely to respond to ATDs or unlikely to respond (Table 12-3).[98-102] Age and gender lack sensitivity and specificity but, in general, women are more likely to achieve remission than men and individuals older than 40 years are more likely than those younger than 40 to evidence a lasting response to ATDs. Finally, a smaller goiter and milder hyperthyroidism at baseline increase the likelihood of remission.[103]

Table 12–3 Predictors of Antithyroid Drug–induced Remission

Likely to Remit	Unlikely to Remit
Female	Male
Age > 40 yr	Age < 40 yr
Small goiter	Large goiter
Mild hyperthyroidism	More severe thyrotoxicosis
Low TSH-R Ab titers	High TSH-R Ab titers

TSH-R Ab, thyroid-stimulating hormone receptor antibody.

After 12 to 18 months of ATDs, most thyroidologists will begin withdrawal therapy and observe. Inevitably, more than 50% of patients will relapse. A number of studies have sought to identify predictors of relapse upon cessation of ATD therapy. Since the first study to observe the usefulness of TSH-R Ab levels in the prediction of outcome after ATDs,[104] multiple studies have affirmed the significance of TSH-R Ab levels at the end of ATD therapy, demonstrating that high levels predict failure to achieve remission whereas undetectable levels are generally unhelpful.[102,105,106] The new generation of highly sensitive assays for TSH-R Abs may improve these results. Unfortunately, TSH-R Ab levels normalize in most people during ATD treatment and, therefore, at present offer prognostic information in only a minority of people. Nevertheless, the test is worth performing at the time of ATD withdrawal. The T_3/T_4 ratio has also been suggested as a predictor of relapse. Khanna and colleagues[107] have found that when the T_3/T_4 ratio exceeds 20, there is a more than an 80% chance of relapse. Larger studies are needed to confirm the importance of the T_3/T_4 ratio. When combined with other indices, thyroglobulin may also provide important information and may be the most sensitive index of relapse available, although its specificity is poor.[108,109] TSH itself has been shown to be predictive of relapse. Quadbeck and associates[105] have found that a low TSH level 4 weeks after ATD withdrawal has a positive predictive value of 70% for relapse. More recently, the quantification of thyroidal blood flow with Doppler ultrasound has demonstrated its potential as a tool to predict outcome following ATD treatment.[110] One small prospective trial has found that Doppler sonography could predict recurrence with a sensitivity of 71% and a specificity of 100%.[111] A strong correlation was found between thyroid volume and blood flow ($r = 0.79$ to 0.96), affirming what is already known—larger goiters predict recurrence.

Predicting response to ATDs remains imperfect and often frustrating. Therefore, most patients desiring a therapeutic trial of ATDs should be afforded that chance, even when the clinical predictors are unfavorable. After thionamide withdrawal, all patients must be followed closely for relapse. About 75% of relapses occur in the 3 months following ATD withdrawal. A low TSH level will often be the earliest harbinger of recurrence. Following a relapse, serious consideration should be given to destructive therapy because a second course of ATDs is unlikely to induce a lasting remission. Alternatively, long-term use of ATDs can be discussed with the patient.

Radioiodine

In 1942, Hertz and Roberts published a study evaluating the thyroidal absorption of radiolabeled iodine in 12 GD patients, remarking that 80% to 90% of a small dose of RAI was concentrated in the Graves' thyroid.[112] Within 10 years, experience with RAI grew, offering patients ablative thyroid therapy without the risks of surgery.[113] Today, RAI is one of the preferred treatments for GD because of its safety and efficacy.[11] However, despite the half-century of experience with RAI, a number of clinical conundrums persist. The following sections will review the best evidence in an attempt to resolve outstanding controversies.

EFFICACY

To discuss efficacy, the goal of therapy must be delineated. Traditionally, thyroidologists have aimed to avoid post-therapy hypothyroidism using dosimetry to deliver a set number of millicuries (mCi) to the gland (80 to 160 μCi/gram thyroid tissue). A common method for determining radioiodine dose is as follows:

$$\text{RAI dose} = 80 \text{ to } 160\ \mu\text{Ci} \times \text{thyroid tissue (g)} / \text{uptake (\%)}$$

So, to deliver 160 μCi/g of thyroid tissue to a 30-g thyroid with a 60% uptake:

$$160\,\mu\text{Ci} \times 30\text{ g} \div 0.6 = 8\text{ mCi}$$

Thyroid volume may be estimated or measured using ultrasonography. However, this has proven difficult, probably because of the unpredictable variables in the measurements used to determine dose. Others have long accepted hypothyroidism as inevitable and have strived to ablate the gland, thereby obviating the need for long-term close follow-up. In practice, most patients will end up hypothyroid regardless of the physician's intentions,[114-116] so hypothyroidism must be viewed as a measure of cure rather than as an adverse event. Conversely, the requirement of additional doses of RAI must be viewed as a treatment failure. In one large prospective cohort study of over 2000 patients treated with a fixed 7-mCi dose, the cumulative incidence of hypothyroidism at 1, 10, and 25 years was 24%, 59%, and 82%, respectively. At this dose, 25% of patients required additional doses of RAI (two to six) to achieve control of hyperthyroidism. A retrospective analysis of 186 GD patients treated with between 10.81 and 14.86 mCi found a cumulative incidence of hypothyroidism of 47.1%, 67.1%, 78.3%, 82.3%, and 88.2% at 6 months and 1, 3, 5, and 10 years, respectively.[117] Of these patients, 9.7% remained hyperthyroid following a single treatment of RAI. A recent prospective trial has confirmed these numbers, demonstrating a 2-year incidence of hypothyroidism of 74.2% and a treatment failure rate of 12.9%.[118]

Because hypothyroidism will eventually occur in at least 75% of those treated with RAI, regardless of dosing strategy, a greater focus should be placed on identifying those less likely to respond to a single dose of RAI with the intention of treating them more aggressively at the outset to save the time, discomfort, and expense of additional treatments. A number of studies have identified specific characteristics of nonresponders, including the following: (1) male gender, (2) younger than 40 years, (3) severe hyperthyroidism, (4) medium to large goiter, and (5) concomitant ATD therapy (see later).[114,119] In patients with these characteristics, consideration should be given to delivering larger doses of RAI (approximately 20 mCi) to ensure resolution of hyperthyroidism with a single treatment.

In general, RAI will cure (euthyroid or hypothyroid) 75% to 90% of individuals with GD after a single treatment, a number much greater than the 30% to 50% of remissions induced by ATDs. Finally, at least one large retrospective study with a 24-month follow-up period has found RAI to be the most cost-effective therapy when compared with surgery or thionamides,[120] particularly when higher, ablative doses of RAI were used, maximizing potential for cure.[121]

SIDE EFFECTS

For more than 50 years, RAI has been used to treat hyperthyroid conditions. Despite concern that the radiation exposure might predispose patients to leukemia, chromosomal damage, and thyroid carcinoma, akin to the dramatic rise in childhood thyroid cancer following the Chernobyl disaster,[122] no such adverse events have been observed in adults.[123] This section will review studies on the safety of RAI for the treatment of GD.

Radiation Thyroiditis

After ingestion, ^{131}I is concentrated in thyrocytes, inducing necrosis and ultimately fomenting a potent inflammatory response.[124] As a result, some patients will experience transient anterior neck pain and tenderness (radiation thyroiditis),[125] amenable to nonsteroidal anti-inflammatory drugs. With time, chronic inflammation and fibrosis result in substantial reductions in gland size.[126] Of note, RAI has been shown to distort nuclear architecture and promote cellular atypia leading to erroneous diagnoses of malignancy in fine-needle aspiration (FNA) specimens, suggesting that nodular disease should be adequately addressed prior to ^{131}I therapy.[127]

Perhaps the most immediate concern following administration of RAI is potential worsening of thyroid function as the necrotic cells release preformed thyroid hormone. Transient thyrotoxicosis[128] and, rarely, thyroid storm,[64] have occurred following the administration of ^{131}I. Fortunately, the rise in hormone concentrations is clinically silent in most patients. However, pretreatment with ATDs should be the rule in older patients, those with arrhythmias, and those with coronary disease or at high risk for coronary disease (see later).

Exacerbation of Graves' Ophthalmopathy

In the days to months following RAI, a number of studies have warned that GO may worsen.[63,129] Bartalena and colleagues[63] have demonstrated that in GD patients with slight or no GO randomized to RAI alone, 23 of 150 patients (15%) experienced new-onset or worsening GO compared with 4 of 148 (3%) treated with MMI alone. Similarly, Tallstedt and associates[129] have demonstrated that in individuals between 35 and 55 years old treated with RAI for GD, 13 of 39 patients (33%) experienced exacerbations of existing eye disease or developed eye disease de novo. The incidence of worsening eye disease in the RAI arm was significantly greater ($P = .02$) than in the other arm, a combination of surgically treated and medically treated patients.

A number of other investigators have also reexamined the association between RAI and deterioration of GO.[130,131] Perros and coworkers[130] have evaluated 72 patients with minimally active GO; 12 months following ^{131}I therapy, none of the subjects with minimal disease in this uncontrolled study experienced an exacerbation of GO. In addition, most (60 of 72) patients in their study had been on months of high-dose MMI therapy with replacement L-T_4 (block-replace) prior to RAI, whereas in the original study by Bartalena and associates,[63] therapy consisted of 4 months of MMI, presumably dosed by titration. Furthermore, the subjective ophthalmologic grading systems differed by protocol; in other words, there are significant factors that preclude comparison among studies. Gupta and coworkers[131] eliminated the subjective measurement of eye disease, opting to measure total muscle volume (TMV) in the superior, inferior, and medial rectus muscles of newly diagnosed GD patients with magnetic resonance imaging (MRI). At baseline, 10 patients (50%) showed evidence of mild GO. There was no significant change in TMV following RAI therapy in this small group, although the sensitivity of this technique to change in volume or degree of inflammation is unclear.

In light of the disparity in these data, all patients with GD considering RAI should be counseled that GO may worsen, although the likelihood is small with inactive or mild GO. Prudence dictates that RAI be avoided in patients with moderate to severe GO; if not based on the data presented, then based on the observation that following RAI, TSH-R Ab production rises dramatically.[132,133] Because GO is likely driven by crossover specificity between thyroid and retro-orbital antigens, it follows that sudden increases in TSH-R Abs following ^{131}I could herald exaggeration of the orbital immune response. If RAI is to be administered in more severe cases of GO, most evidence suggests the use of concomitant high-dose glucocorticoids (see later).[63]

Thyroid Cancer

The potential for RAI to induce carcinogenesis continues to trouble some, despite years of experience and mounting evidence attesting to its safety. The Chernobyl experience provided irrefutable evidence that exposure to radioiodine in childhood caused an epidemic of thyroid cancer.[134] However, such exposure was to low doses of radioiodine, already known to be thyrodangerous, in great contrast to the relatively large doses used in GD. Except for a handful of case reports,[135,136] the weight of the evidence refutes an association between therapeutic RAI and cancer-related mortality.[137,138] Similarly, reassuring data refutes an association between ^{131}I and leukemia.[139] In general, the doses of RAI used in the treatment of GD do not appear to be carcinogenic. Interestingly, whereas it likely has little impact on cancer mortality in patients with GD, a population-based cohort study, including over 7000 hyperthyroid individuals treated with RAI, has demonstrated increased all-cause mortality and mortality caused by cardiovascular disease, cerebrovascular disease, and fracture.[140] Whether these findings are attributable to the disease itself or to the RAI is unknown.

Genetic Changes

Finally, reports from the 1960s demonstrating chromosomal abnormalities in leukocytes from patients treated with ^{131}I raised concern that RAI may lead to chromosomal damage and pose a genetic risk to the offspring of treated individuals.[141,142] The literature does not support this assertion. Multiple studies have demonstrated healthy offspring born to individuals previously treated with RAI.[143,144]

Decreased Spermatogenesis

Although changes in spermatogenesis have been reported after large doses of RAI used in the treatment of thyroid cancer,[145] there is no evidence to suggest that this occurs after the relatively small doses used to treat GD. Even with high doses, the effect is transient and of no physiologic significance.[145,146]

In conclusion, more than 50 years of experience with RAI have confirmed its safety and efficacy in the treatment of adult GD when used appropriately for selected patients.

DOSING CONSIDERATIONS

Fixed Dosing

There is still, after 50 years, an ongoing debate as to whether ^{131}I is best delivered in fixed doses or if elaborate calculations based on thyroid size and uptake (dosimetry) improve outcome. Ultimately, the goal of therapy must be to achieve euthyroidism or hypothyroidism in the largest number of GD patients at the lowest possible dose. With spiraling per capita health care costs, a corollary to the goal of therapy could be to provide definitive treatment for GD at the lowest cost. A number of studies have demonstrated impressive efficacy data when ^{131}I is administered in fixed doses ranging from 5 to 15 mCi.[147-150] Doses between 10 and 15 mCi rendered 88.5% to 97.5% of GD patients euthyroid or hypothyroid after a single dose. Lower doses, particularly 5 mCi or less, were associated with a greater number of treatment failures (48.5% euthyroid or hypothyroid).[148,151] Alexander and colleagues[152] have evaluated a unique dosing strategy based on a 24-hour thyroid ^{123}I uptake, with the goal of delivering a fixed 8 mCi to the thyroid gland. The average 24-hour uptake was 58% and the average dose of ^{131}I was 15.6 mCi. At 1 year, 226 patients (86%) were euthyroid or hypothyroid and 36 (14%) remained hyperthyroid; these patients were younger, with a larger thyroid gland, higher serum T_4 concentration at diagnosis, higher 24-hour uptake, and higher prevalence of GO. The dose of ^{131}I per estimated gram of thyroid tissue was significantly lower in the treatment failure patients compared with those who evidenced cure.

Dosimetry

No data exist demonstrating an advantage for dosimetry over fixed dosing in the treatment of GD.[153] Leslie and associates[154] randomized 88 individuals with GD to four dosing strategies: 5 mCi fixed, 10 mCi fixed, low-adjusted (80 µCi/g of thyroid adjusted for 24-hour uptake), and high-adjusted (120 µCi/g of thyroid adjusted for 24-hour uptake). After a mean follow-up of 80 months, 76.1% were euthyroid or hypothyroid; the study could not identify any advantage to using an adjusted-dose method. Jarlov and coworkers[155] have compared an inexpensive practical dosing strategy based on thyroid volume as assessed by palpation to a more traditional approach using an accurate thyroid volume measurement and 24-hour uptake. No significant difference in outcome between groups could be demonstrated, leading the authors to conclude that a semiquantitative approach to ^{131}I dosing is likely to be as effective as more complicated dosing strategies.

Clinical Approach to Dosing

In general, a fixed dose between 15 and 20 mCi will cure (hypothyroid or euthyroid) almost all patients. The literature also supports the cost-effectiveness and simplicity of fixed-dose regimens.[120] Larger doses should be reserved for younger individuals with a larger goiter and more severe disease at diagnosis. Higher doses may also be considered for those who have already failed a dose of RAI and those who may suffer untoward effects from a treatment failure. Patients pretreated with thionamides may also require larger doses because the failure rate has been reported to be higher in these patients unless the ATDs are discontinued for 4 to 7 days prior to RAI therapy (see later).

ADJUNCTIVE TREATMENTS

Thionamides

Thionamides are frequently used to restore a euthyroid state prior to RAI.[11] Moreover, thionamides are frequently restarted after RAI.[11] This practice raises a number of important questions:

1. Should individuals with GD be pretreated with ATDs?
2. If so, who derives the most benefit from pretreatment ATDs?
3. When should ATDs be withdrawn prior to RAI therapy?
4. When can ATDs be resumed following RAI?
5. What is the net effect of ATDs on cure rates following RAI?

Pretreatment with ATDs has not been proven to reduce post-RAI exacerbation of thyrotoxicosis.[156] However, there is an evidence-based rationale to use this strategy in high- risk individuals. Two randomized trials have clearly demonstrated that individuals pretreated with MMI have significantly lower free T_4 and T_3 levels at all time points after RAI administration (Fig. 12-2).[65,157] Although most people in both studies experienced a gradual decline in free T_4 and T_3 following RAI, a small subset in both had progressive increases in thyroid hormone concentrations. Without exception, even in this small subset, pretreated patients had lower hormone levels than non–pretreated individuals. The participants in both studies were not older patients and, despite rises in thyroid hormone, no clinically significant events occurred.

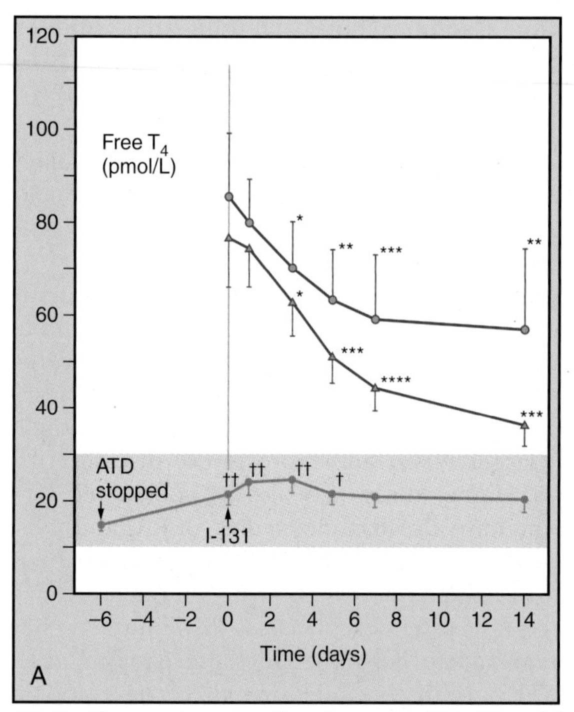

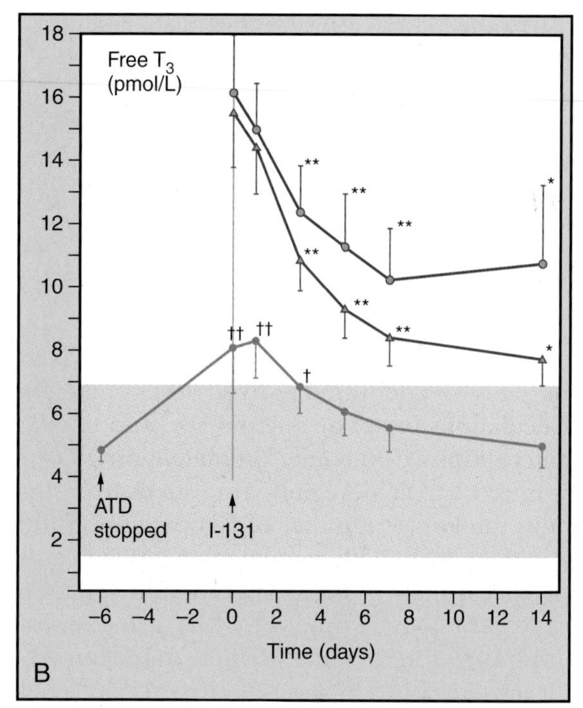

Figure 12–2 Changes in serum free thyroxine (T_4) **(A)** and free triiodothyronine (T_3) **(B)** levels in 21 antithyroid drug–pretreated patients, 21 nonpretreated patients, and a subgroup of 19 nonpretreated patients not experiencing worsening thyrotoxicosis after radioiodine (RAI). Values shown represent the mean and the bars indicate standard error of the mean (SEM). **A,** *, $P < .05$; **, $P < 0$; ***, $P < .005$; ****, $P < .0005$ (compared with T = 0, the day of RAI treatment), †, $P < .005$; ††, $P < .0005$ (compared with day 6, the day of antithyroid drug discontinuation). **B,** *, $P < 0.005$; **, $P < .0005$ (compared with T = 0); †, $P < .01$; ††, $P < .005$ (compared with day 6). ATD, antithyroid drug. *(Adapted from Burch HB, Solomon BL, Cooper DS, et al: The effect of antithyroid drug pretreatment on acute changes in thyroid levels after 131I ablation for Graves' disease. J Clin Endocrinol Metab 86:3016-3021, 2001.)*

Extrapolating these data to older at-risk individuals, pretreatment should be considered to blunt the rise in thyroid hormone post-RAI, thereby preventing post-treatment exacerbations of thyrotoxicosis.

The effect of post-treatment ATDs remains controversial. Three prospective studies have considered the effect of post-RAI ATDs on thyroid function. One study demonstrated no difference in thyroid function 6 weeks after the administration of RAI in a group of patients treated with PTU (beginning 5 days after RAI) versus the control group.[158] Of interest, those randomized to PTU experienced a higher treatment failure rate. The second study randomized 159 patients to RAI alone or RAI followed by MMI and L-T_4 (block-replace).[159] The time to achieve euthyroidism was significantly shorter in the treatment group (2 vs. 8 weeks; $P < .02$). Moreover, treatment with MMI did not affect the one-dose cure rate with RAI. The final study randomized 149 patients to post-therapy MMI beginning 7 days after RAI versus no treatment.[160] There was no significant difference in rate of cure, but MMI slightly but significantly reduced goiter shrinkage. In the MMI group, free T_4 was significantly lower at 3 weeks than in the control arm ($P < .001$). Further studies are needed to clarify the role of ATDs following the administration of RAI, although the clinical situation may drive the decision making in some patients.

It is customary to stop ATDs 4 to 7 days prior to RAI therapy. Is this an evidence-based practice or a theory driven anachronism? The evidence that MMI needs to be withdrawn is relatively weak. One study randomized 30 patients with GD to continue MMI until 4 weeks after RAI or to stop MMI 8 days prior to RAI.[161] Of 19 patients in the MMI-positive arm, 12 recurred and 6 of 11 patients in the MMI arm recurred, a nonsignificant difference ($P = .71$). In contrast, another small but retrospective study found that treatment failures were significantly more likely in individuals taking carbimazole at the time of RAI,[162] and two randomized clinical trials found that this effect disappeared when MMI was discontinued 4 to 6 days prior to RAI therapy.[163,164] The data on pretreatment with PTU are much clearer and support a marked reduction in RAI treatment success, even when discontinued 15 days prior to RAI therapy.[165-167] Santos and coworkers[165] compared 100 GD patients treated with 10 mCi of RAI. Patients were randomized into the groups, MMI, PTU, and no treatment. ATDs were withdrawn 15 days before RAI administration. At 12 months, the no-treatment arm and the MMI arm demonstrated similar rates of cure, 73.3% and 77.8%, respectively (P = NS [not significant]). The PTU group showed a rate of cure of 32%, significantly lower than in the other arms ($P < .05$).

In summary, ATDs are warranted in high-risk individuals prior to RAI. The evidence supports the use of MMI over PTU in this case. MMI should be discontinued at least 4 days prior to therapy but, in very high-risk individuals, it can be resumed 5 to 7 days after RAI.

Beta Blockers

No prospective studies exist evaluating the use of beta blockers with RAI. In younger patients with no cardiac disease, they are probably of little benefit. However, there are no theoretical reasons why beta blockade should interfere with cure and, in high-risk patients undergoing RAI, beta blockers should be added to MMI to ameliorate the potential for post-RAI adrenergic symptoms.

Glucocorticoids

There are two scenarios in which glucocorticoids might be administered concomitantly with RAI: (1) a patient with a concurrent glucocorticoid-dependent illness develops GD; and (2) to prevent the worsening of GO. Glucocorticoids have a number of direct effects on the pituitary-thyroid axis, including suppression of TSH and reduced peripheral monodeiodination of T_4 in addition to their immunosuppressive action. Do these actions affect the outcome of RAI treatment for GD?

Little prospective data exist to answer this question. One study, by Gamstedt and Karlsson,[168] randomized patients to betamethasone 3 weeks before RAI and 4 weeks after RAI or placebo. Interestingly, only 9 of 20 betamethasone-treated patients required thyroid replacement at 1 year compared with 17 of 20 patients in the placebo group ($P < .001$), indicating that glucocorticoids may have a radioprotective effect. Bartalena and colleagues,[169] however, demonstrated that steroids started after RAI have no appreciable impact on the prevalence of hypothyroidism or persistent hyperthyroidism. Finally, a large retrospective study by Jensen and associates[170] reviewed outcome in GD patients treated with prednisolone beginning 2 days prior to RAI compared with patients not receiving steroids. In this study, glucocorticoids had no impact on the final outcome of GD patients treated with RAI. The role of the immunosuppressive effects of corticosteroids has been widely recognized and is the reason for their use with RAI in patients with marked ophthalmopathy.[63,169] Corticosteroids may reduce the levels of TSH-R Abs,[171] thus lowering the RAI uptake in the gland and reducing its effectiveness. However, because the half-life of IgG is prolonged, this effect is not seen in the short term. In contrast, corticosteroids, which are lympholytic, can induce apoptosis in the local immune infiltrate and reduce the effectiveness of RAI-induced immune-mediated thyroid cell destruction.

Therefore, available evidence implies that glucocorticoids started after RAI are not radioprotective and therefore no dosage adjustment is required. Glucocorticoids started prior to RAI may theoretically reduce the cure rate, but there are only limited data to support this.

Lithium

Although the antithyroid effects of lithium are well documented, the exact mechanism of action is not clearly defined. Lithium prevents the release of T_4 and T_3 from the thyroid and may actually inhibit their formation. Additionally, lithium enhances the intrathyroidal retention of iodine, an effect that theoretically could augment the actions of RAI. However, randomized controlled trials have generally been unable to demonstrate that lithium used concomitantly with RAI affects cure.[172,173] This is not to say that lithium is without potential usefulness. When thionamides are held prior to RAI, thyroid hormone levels increase. Following RAI, hormone levels can increase further, exposing frailer patients to risk. High-quality studies have demonstrated the following with respect to lithium and RAI: (1) Lithium prevents the rise in thyroid hormone that follows thionamide withdrawal in preparation for RAI; (2) lithium results in prompter control of post-RAI hyperthyroidism; (3) 2 weeks of lithium therapy significantly reduces post-RAI elevations in thyroid hormone; and (4) lithium may result in more rapid and effective reduction in goiter size.[172,174] Hence, a dose of lithium, 300 mg every 8 hours, can be considered in those individuals whose condition may deteriorate after thionamide withdrawal, although ATDs tend to have a prolonged effect. Lithium can also be continued after ^{131}I to prevent a rise in thyroid hormone level; this may be preferable to restarting a thionamide in high-risk patients because some evidence has suggested that post-RAI ATD therapy may reduce the cure rate. However, the evidence does not support the routine use of lithium to augment the already impressive cure rate of GD with RAI.

Thyroidectomy

For many years, thyroidectomy represented the only treatment available for GD. However, with the discovery of ATDs and RAI, surgery in the United States has been relegated to select situations: (1) patient preference; (2) urgent control of thyrotoxicosis; (3) pregnant patient intolerant of ATDs; (4) child or adolescent intolerant of ATDs (although RAI is used in this age group, many continue to be cautious because of the fear of neoplasia formation[123,174]); (5) large goiter, with or without compressive symptoms; (6) severe Graves' ophthalmopathy[175]; and (7) the presence of suspicious nodules. In general, thyroidologists worldwide concur that there is little role for thyroidectomy in mild GD patients.[12] However, as the surgical community continues to perfect the procedure, making the surgery faster, safer, and less invasive, a salient argument can be made that thyroidectomy is an underused, safe, and extremely effective therapy.[176] Because not all the thyroid tissue is removed, even in the best hands, one could expect the TSH-R Abs in GD to induce thyroid cell growth and disease recurrence. This occurs in up to 15% of patients, but 85% of patients are cured. How such surgery effects cure of an autoimmune disease is unclear. It has been suggested that removal of the gland takes away the vast majority of thyroid-specific T cells and B cells[177] and that thyroid-specific clonal suicide of the remaining thyroid-specific immune cells is induced by the large amount of thyroid antigen released into the circulation at the time of surgery.

TOTAL VERSUS SUBTOTAL THYROIDECTOMY

A subtotal thyroidectomy is typically defined as the removal of most of the gland, sparing about 2 g from the posterior portion bilaterally, because this might minimize the risk of recurrent laryngeal nerve (RLN) damage, hypothyroidism, and hypoparathyroidism. The prevention of hypothyroidism, or more specifically the establishment of a euthyroid state following subtotal thyroidectomy, has proven difficult to predict and is surgeon-dependent; its pursuit explains the unacceptably high recurrence rate following this procedure (Table 12-4). Available evidence suggests that the rate of hypothyroidism ranges from less than 10% to almost 80%, depending on the size of the thyroid remnant left by the surgeon,[178-182] duration of follow-up,[183] and presence or absence of thyroid antibodies.[182] The incidence of recurrence depends on the size of the thyroid remnant as well as the preoperative TSH-R Ab concentration[184] and can be as high as 15%.[185]

RLN injury and hypoparathyroidism are the two major risks of surgery. A meta-analysis including over 7000 surgically treated GD patients has found that the rate of hypoparathyroidism and RLN injury is not significantly different in those patients treated with total thyroidectomy, for whom the surgeon tries to remove all thyroid tissue, versus subtotal thyroidectomy.[186] The rate of permanent RLN injury was 0.7%. The rate of permanent hypoparathyroidism was similarly low, 1%. There were no perioperative mortalities reported. A growing body of evidence supports the assertion that in an experienced endocrine surgeon's hands, the absolute risk of an adverse outcome following a total thyroidectomy is no different than that of a subtotal thyroidectomy.[187-189] Furthermore, the risk of recurrence is zero following a total thyroidectomy. All patients will require L-T_4 replacement indefinitely. Ultimately, the decision to pursue a subtotal versus a total thyroidectomy will involve a number of factors, including the skill and preference of the surgeon. When one considers that as many as 15% of patients recur following a subtotal procedure, we suggest that total thyroidectomy be considered the treatment of choice for GD.

Table 12–4 Cure and Complication Rates of Thyroidectomy (%)

Complicaton/Cure	Subtotal Thyroidectomy	Total Thyroidectomy
Recurrence	7.9	0
Euthyroid	59.7	0
Hypothyroid	25.6	100
RLN injury		
Permanent	0.7	0.9
Temporary	2.8	7.7
Hypoparathyroidism	0.9	1

RLN, recurrent laryngeal nerve.

Data from Palit TK, Miller CC, Miltenburg DM: The efficacy of thyroidectomy for Graves' disease: A meta-analysis. J Surg Res 90:161-165, 2000.

Newer minimally invasive procedures are being developed to improve cosmesis.[190] A recent case series has demonstrated the efficacy and safety of video-assisted subtotal or near-total thyroidectomy for GD using a subclavicular approach.[191] Minimally invasive thyroidectomy via an axillary approach has also been reported.[192] These procedures are not currently performed routinely in the United States.

PREPARING FOR SURGERY

Preoperative therapy is aimed at restoring a euthyroid state prior to surgery. When thyroidectomy is truly elective, this is best accomplished with antithyroid medications titrated as discussed earlier. Inorganic iodide is typically initiated (saturated solution of potassium iodide [SSKI], 1 drop twice daily or Lugol's solution, 3 to 5 drops twice daily) several days prior to the procedure to decrease the vascularity of the gland,[193,194] although the benefit of this maneuver is unproven.[195]

Some small studies have evaluated the use of beta blockers, with or without inorganic iodide, as the sole preoperative treatment modality.[196-200] Naturally, these patients remain hyperthyroid at the time of surgery. Overall, outcome was good, likely because of the younger age and milder disease of most of the GD patients. A small number of patients, however, encountered postoperative problems, including tachycardia and fever, somewhat reminiscent of the profound thyroid crises that followed the introduction of thyroid surgery.[197,198] Restoring a euthyroid state prior to surgery with ATDs forestalls this sort of postoperative complication.

In our practice, we always strive to achieve preoperative euthyroidism with ATDs. Inorganic iodide is then added 1 week prior to the planned procedure. If an urgent or emergent thyroidectomy is warranted, rapid control of thyroid status can be achieved with a combination of thionamides, SSKI, dexamethasone (1 to 2 mg twice daily), and beta blockers.[201,202] The usefulness of this combination was recently demonstrated in an uncontrolled prospective study involving 17 severely hyperthyroid patients. The average T_3 level fell from 500 ± 48 (normal range, 60 to 180) to 143 ± 13 ng/dL in 7 days; all subjects were clinically euthyroid at the time of surgery. A discussion of accelerated hyperthyroidism and thyroid storm, as well as the mechanism of action and clinical application of corticosteroids, iodine, and iodinated radiographic contrast agents, can be found later in this chapter.

OTHER MANIFESTATIONS OF THYROID HYPERFUNCTION

Graves' Ophthalmopathy

EPIDEMIOLOGY

GO represents the most common extrathyroidal manifestation of GD.[203] Approximately 50% of patients will have some degree of clinically evident eye disease, although newer imaging modalities can demonstrate anatomic changes consistent with GO in more than 75% of patients.[204] Severe ophthalmopathy accounts for no more than 3% to 5% of cases.[205] Eye disease is usually bilateral and frequently asymmetrical. The peak incidence of GO demonstrates a bimodal distribution, affecting those in their fifth and seventh decades.[206] The disease tends to be more aggressive in older individuals and in men, with men older than 60 years at the highest risk for developing severe GO.[207] The natural history of the disease is such that watchful waiting and supportive care will be all that most patients will require. Perros and colleagues[208] followed a cohort of 59 patients with GO, who had not received immunosuppressants or surgical treatment, for a median of 12 months; 22% of patients (13) improved substantially, 42.2% of patients (25) showed minor improvement, 22% (13) did not change, and 13.5% of patients (8) deteriorated, ultimately requiring medical intervention. A Swiss study has suggested that the rate of progressive disease may be even lower.[209] Of 196 consecutive patients with newly diagnosed GD, 81 had GO (41%) and 53 patients (65%) received no therapy other than supportive local care. Of these patients, 49% improved substantially, 50% did not change, and 1% worsened. These data support the merits of conservative management in patients with GO.

SMOKING AND GRAVES' OPHTHALMOPATHY

Smoking increases the risk of GD (odds ratio [OR], 3.3; 95% CI, 2.09 to 5.22).[210] Stopping ameliorates this risk.[210] More patients with GO smoke compared with individuals with thyrotoxicosis alone and patients with the worst GO smoke the most.[211] Hence, smoking greatly increases the risk of developing GO (OR, 7.7; 95% CI, 4.3 to 13.7).[212] In contrast, smoking does not appear to be related to other thyroid disorders. Moreover, cigarette smoking increases the risk of progression of GO after RAI and decreases the efficacy of orbital radiation and glucocorticoid therapy.[213] Smoking thus profoundly affects the course of GO and blunts the efficacy of proven therapies. The mechanism whereby smoking exacts this effect has yet to be elucidated, but nicotine is known to influence nitric oxide formation, possibly exacerbating any inflammatory response.[214] Patient education is paramount; unfortunately, education alone is unlikely to deter most smokers.[215] Despite the frustrations of tobacco addiction, smoking cessation must be aggressively addressed in GD patients with eye disease. Pharmacotherapy (e.g., bupropion, varenicline, and nicotine replacement) as well as counseling may be necessary to overcome the inertia of nicotine addiction.

CAUSE

The genetics of Graves' ophthalmopathy appears to be indistinguishable from that of Graves' thyroid disease,[216] despite other statements in the literature.[217] Hence, there is concern about external insults such as smoking, trauma, or pressure buildup in smaller orbits.[203] The result is that autoreactive T lymphocytes infiltrate orbital tissues and the perimysium and endomysium of extraocular muscles, invited by an antigen shared by the thyroid and orbit.[218] The culprit antigen appears to be the TSH receptor, which is overexpressed in retro-orbital fibroblasts and adipocytes.[219] After antigen recognition, the immune system is locally upregulated by the release of a number of inflammatory mediators. Additionally, cytokines, particularly interferon-γ, stimulate fibroblasts to secrete glycosaminoglycans (GAGs), which accumulate in the extracellular matrix.[220] Subsequent fibroblast stimulation results in further accumulation and deposition of GAGs between extraocular muscle fibers, promoting edema and fibril disruption and impairing muscle function (Fig. 12-3). A subset of fibroblasts, preadipocytes, coerced by the inflammatory milieu, matures into adipocytes, increasing the volume of orbital fat and adding to the developing pressure buildup.[221] In more severe cases, as the orbital fat and muscle volumes increase, extraocular muscle impairment and/or proptosis may develop. With time, as inflammation decreases and the disease burns out, the damaged extraocular muscles become fibrosed, causing permanent disability necessitating corrective surgery.

MANAGEMENT OF UNDERLYING HYPERTHYROIDISM AND PROGRESSION OF GRAVES' OPHTHALMOPATHY

Should the presence of GO influence the choice of treatment for Graves' hyperthyroidism? Does removing the thyroid and thus eliminating the source of autoreactive T cells and the bulk of the putative antigen result in regression of GO? A number of studies have evaluated the course of GO following the three treatment modalities for Graves' hyperthyroidism—surgery, thionamides, and RAI. The literature is not definitive. Furthermore, the discussion is complicated by the natural history of untreated GO in that most patients stabilize or improve whereas only a small minority progress. Thus, the effect observed in clinical studies may reflect the natural history of the disease rather than the influence of a particular treatment.

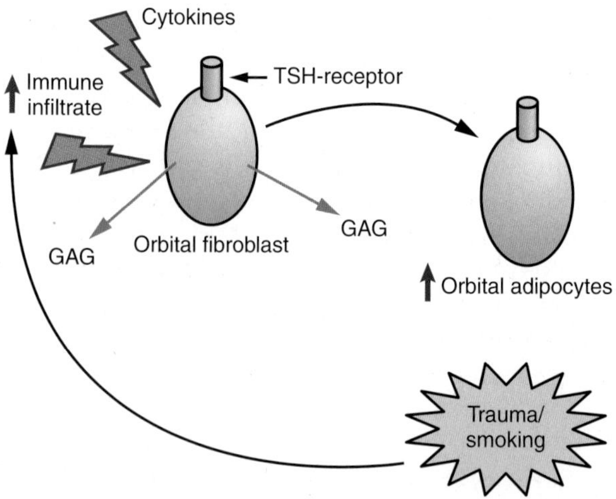

Figure 12–3 Pathophysiology of Graves' ophthalmopathy. In response to the putative antigen, the thyroid-stimulating hormone (TSH) receptor, the immune system is locally upregulated. Cytokines stimulate orbital fibroblasts to secrete glycosaminoglycans (GAGs), promoting edema and fibril disruption. A subset of orbital fibroblasts, preadipocytes, in response to the local immune response, mature into adipocytes, further increasing orbital fat and muscle volumes. Trauma and smoking likely worsen the disease by reducing regulatory T-cell function, further upregulating the aberrant immune response.

Thionamides

There is no evidence that thionamides aggravate or ameliorate GO, although there is a suggestion that the restoration of euthyroidism favorably influences Graves' eye disease.[222] The trouble with ATD therapy remains the high rate of recurrence, with reactivation of thyroid autoimmunity and an elevation of TSH-R Ab levels. There is a well-known relationship between TSH-R Ab and GO, ever since the first description of TSH-R Ab; this was again confirmed in more recent studies.[223] Whether the antibodies are the cause or merely a reflection of ongoing T-cell activity is unclear.

Thyroid Surgery

Similarly, most studies have suggested that surgery has little effect on the course of the disease.[224,225] Moreover, the extent of the thyroid resection (total versus subtotal) appears to have no impact on the progression of GO.[226] Some have contended that a thyroidectomy followed by a remnant ablation, effectively eliminating the culprit antigen along with the source of the culpable T cells, provides patients with the greatest protection against worsening GO.[227,228] There are no prospective data to support or refute this assertion. However, there are abundant data to show the loss of thyroid autoantibodies after thyroid surgery, including the loss of TSH-R Abs.[229] This is reflective of disease dissipation and why many suggest that thyroid surgery is the best way to manage Graves' patients with severe eye disease,[230] a practice we endorse.

Radioiodine Therapy

The association between RAI and the progression of GO remains controversial. The large increase in TSH-R Ab levels after RAI treatment is well documented and thought to be secondary to regulatory T-cell sensitivity to radiation.[231] Hence, the immune response of GD is exacerbated by RAI, which may affect extrathyroidal activity of this immune response in the eyes and skin, and pretibial myxedema has also been shown to exacerbate after RAI.[232] As noted, some prospective randomized trials have demonstrated that GO worsens following RAI.[63,169] Other studies, however, do not support this. Furthermore, the available studies only evaluate individuals with absent to mild eye disease, so the actual impact of RAI on severe GO is less well documented. Some investigators have speculated that untreated post-RAI hypothyroidism may contribute to deterioration in eye symptoms.[129,233] A prospective study by Perros and coworkers[130] and a retrospective study by Tallstedt and colleagues [233] have concluded that prompt treatment of post-RAI hypothyroidism prevents the deterioration of GO observed in other studies.

CLINICAL APPROACH

In general, the presence of mild GO should not influence the choice of treatment for hyperthyroidism. Although destructive therapy with RAI or surgery offers theoretical benefits (e.g., removal of autoreactive T cells), clinical trials have been unable to demonstrate this convincingly. Thionamides are effective at restoring a euthyroid state but probably have little influence on the natural history of GO. Finally, conflicting data exist in regard to the use of RAI in those with more severe GO. Patients with mild to moderate GO can likely be treated with RAI, with little risk of progression. We suggest that patients with GO who opt for RAI be informed that the therapy may exacerbate the disease. We generally will not recommend RAI for patients with severe GO, although this approach is not evidence-based. If RAI is to be used in this setting, prompt treatment of post-RAI hypothyroidism is paramount. Additionally, the evidence strongly supports the use of concomitant glucocorticoids before and after RAI.[63]

ASSESSING DISEASE SEVERITY

The most widely used classification system for GO was the NOSPECS system, introduced in 1969 by the American Thyroid Association.[234] NOSPECS is an acronym (***n**o* signs or symptoms, ***o**nly* symptoms, no signs, **s**oft tissue involvement, ***p**roptosis* of 3 mm or more, **e**xtraocular muscle involvement and restriction, **c**orneal involvement, **s**ight loss). At best, NOSPECS is a helpful guide for physical examination; at worst, it is a cumbersome mnemonic that lacks intraobserver reproducibility.

Defining the severity of disease rather than disease activity can be inherently arbitrary. Certainly, marked proptosis with lagophthalmos and corneal ulceration or sight-threatening optic neuropathy constitutes severe disease. Persistent diplopia caused by extraocular muscle dysfunction does not threaten sight but frequently leads to significant disability and should constitute severe disease as well. On the other hand, periorbital soft tissue edema has an impact on cosmesis but tends to have little impact on binocular vision and acuity. Thus, soft tissue edema should not define disease severity. Finally, the global assessment of ocular involvement may indicate severe disease, although individual parameters may be less marked (Table 12-5).[235]

DISEASE ACTIVITY

The concept of disease activity must be differentiated from that of disease severity. An individual may have severe disease, as defined earlier, but the disease may be inactive, representing burned out GO. This distinction is not semantic; rather, disease activity dictates the therapeutic modality most likely to ameliorate signs and symptoms. A patient with mild GO requires supportive care, whereas severe disease warrants intervention. Active GO responds well to glucocorticoids, orbital radiotherapy, and possibly other immune modulating agents; inactive GO will respond poorly to these therapies. Ultimately, severe inactive disease requires surgery.

To assess activity, various clinical activity scores (CAS) have been introduced (Table 12-6).[236,237] By assigning one point to each of seven items, a CAS is generated. The CAS, although not a perfect indicator of disease activity, can guide therapeutic decision making and often can help predict outcome. Mourits

Table 12–5 Assessment of Severity of Graves' Ophthalmopathy

Degree of Involvement	Proptosis (mm)	Diplopia[a]	Optic Neuropathy[b]
Mild	19-20	Intermittent	Subclinical[c]
Moderate	21-23	Inconstant	Visual acuity 8/10-5/10
Marked	>23	Constant	Visual acuity <5/10

Severe ophthalmopathy: at least one marked or two moderate or one moderate and two mild manifestations.[d]

[a]Normal values show racial variations; accordingly, abnormal values should be considered those 4mm or more above the respective median value.

[b] Diplopia: Intermittent, present only when fatigued; inconstant, present in secondary positions of gaze; constant, present in primary and reading positions.

[c]Abnormal visual evoked potentials or other tests, with normal or slightly reduced (9/10) visual acuity.

[d]Patients with severe GO will need either medical or surgical treatment depending on the activity of eye disease.

Data from Bartalena L, Pinchera A, Marcocci C: Management of Graves' ophthalmopathy: Reality and perspectives. Endocr Rev 21:168-199, 2000.

Table 12–6 Clinical Activity Score (CAS)*

Spontaneous retrobulbar pain
Pain on eye movements
Eyelid erythema
Conjunctival injection
Chemosis
Swelling of the caruncle
Eyelid edema or fullness

*The CAS is calculated by assigning one point to each manifestation and summing the points.
From Pinchera A, Wiersinga W, Glinoer D, et al: Classification of eye changes of Graves' disease. Thyroid 2:235-236, 1996.

and associates[238] have evaluated 43 patients with moderate to severe GO prior to prednisone or orbital irradiation. Those who responded to therapy had significantly higher CAS scores than nonresponders, affirming the assertion that disease activity predicts the outcome of immunosuppressive treatment in GO. Hence, it is important that a patient with severe ocular involvement be assessed for disease activity. Highly active disease is likely to respond to medical treatment, whereas glucocorticoids and/or orbital irradiation are unlikely to benefit those with inactive burned-out disease. These patients will likely require corrective surgery at specialized centers to improve visual and cosmetic deficits.

TREATMENT OPTIONS

Supportive Care

For most patients with mild disease, symptomatic therapy and reassurance that the disease is unlikely to progress should be the foundation of treatment. Patients suffering from photophobia or hyperesthesia to wind or cold air should be instructed to wear dark glasses. Methylcellulose 1% can be instilled in the eyes throughout the day to assuage the foreign body or gritty sensation commonly described by patients with GO and secondary to the stare.

Individuals with lagophthalmos should be instructed to tape their eyes shut in the evenings to prevent xero-ophthalmia and ulceration. Elevating the head of the bed is an additional measure that may reduce swelling and improve eyelid approximation. Even mild diplopia is unpleasant, but may be correctable with prism lenses. Finally, modifiable risk factors, most notably smoking, should be addressed. Smoking cessation should be strongly encouraged.

Corticosteroids

Corticosteroids are the mainstay of therapy for severe active disease. Aside from their immunosuppressive properties, they exert a modulating effect on orbital fibroblasts, reducing the production of GAGs.[239] Moderately high doses are required for several months, and recurrence is not uncommon when the corticosteroids are tapered or withdrawn. The side effects of glucocorticoids are well known and represent a significant drawback to their use. Nonetheless, corticosteroids are efficacious, with optic neuropathy and inflammatory changes responding well, but with exophthalmos and restrictive myopathy demonstrating greater resistance to therapy.

A number of uncontrolled trials have demonstrated the therapeutic merit of oral[240-242] and intravenous[243-246] corticosteroids for the treatment of GO. To date, the work of Bartalena and coworkers[63,169] serves as the best evidence that glucocorticoids alter the course of GO compared with no treatment. Their study in 1989[169] randomized 52 patients with mild or absent GO to RAI or RAI plus prednisone. Of those with mild disease randomized to RAI alone, 56% experienced worsening GO compared with none of those in the prednisone arm. Furthermore, 52% of patients in the treatment arm experienced improvement in their disease. Similarly impressive results were generated by this group in 1998[63]; in this study, 443 patients were randomized to RAI, RAI plus prednisone, or methimazole alone for 18 months. In the RAI arm, 23% of patients experienced new-onset or worsening ophthalmopathy but none displayed regression of disease. This was in marked contrast to the prednisone arm, in which no patients experienced deterioration of eye disease and a remarkable 67% demonstrated clinically significant improvement. These results were also better than those in the MMI arm. Of patients treated with MMI alone, 3% worsened, 2% improved, and eye disease was static in the remaining 95%. These data strongly support the notion that glucocorticoids alter the natural history of GO.

Newer data comparing intravenous with oral therapy suggest that intravenous pulsed steroids offer even superior results, with fewer side effects.[247,248] Marcocci and colleagues[248] randomized 82 patients with moderate to severe GO who were treated with orbital radiotherapy to 22 weeks of an oral steroid taper (beginning at 100 mg; total dose, about 6 g) or pulsed IV steroids for 14 weeks (total dose, from 9 to 12 g; 15 mg/kg × 4 cycles followed by 7.5 mg/kg × 4 cycles). Overall, both treatments produced favorable effects, although the total number of responders was significantly greater in the intravenous group (87.8% vs. 63.4%; $P < .02$). Furthermore, side effects occurred in significantly fewer subjects in the IV arm (56.1% vs. 85.4 %; $P < .01$); in particular, cushingoid features developed in 5 of the subjects in the IV arm compared with 35 of those in the orally treated group. A recent randomized, single-blind trial has confirmed these data.[247] In this study, 70 patients with severe GO were randomized to once-weekly intravenous methylprednisolone (0.5 g, then 0.25 g, 6 weeks each) or to oral prednisolone (100 mg/day, tapering by 10 mg/week). At 3 months, 77% of patients in the intravenous group had a treatment response compared with 51% of patients in the oral group ($P < .01$). Improvements in disease severity compared with baseline, quality of life, and disease activity were also significantly higher in the intravenous group. Additionally, adverse events were significantly less common in the intravenously treated patients ($P < .001$), with marked differences between groups in weight gain and bone loss (by DEXA scan) at the lumbar spine.

Local therapy with periocular glucocorticoid injections could theoretically offer the most favorable risk-to-benefit ratio. A randomized controlled trial has evaluated the efficacy of periocular triamcinolone injections, demonstrating a reduction in diplopia and a significant decrease in extraocular muscle size.[249] Other studies have yielded less promising results.[250] At this time, there is too little experience to recommend local therapy routinely; however, it can be considered in patients with active disease who have strong contraindications to systemic glucocorticoids.

To summarize, glucocorticoids dramatically alter the natural history of GO and should be considered in moderate to severe cases. They exert their greatest effect on inflammatory changes and optic neuropathy. However, extraocular muscle dysfunction may improve, particularly when the disease is very active. A notable response can be expected in two thirds of patients.[251] Steroids are effective, but recurrence is not uncommon after withdrawal, so long tapers (usually 3 to 4 months) are customary. If steroids are selected, a recent study has suggested that IV steroids are superior to oral steroids.[247] Finally, steroids clearly abrogate the progression of GO that may be associated with RAI.[63] Thus, definitive therapy for hyperthyroidism with RAI should be considered on steroid initiation. Although not evidence-based, an ablative dosing strategy (20 mCi) may be beneficial in the long run.[227] In addition, it is good practice to start calcium, cholecalciferol, and a potent bisphosphonate such as alendronate on initiation of prolonged steroid therapy.

Orbital Radiotherapy

Orbital radiotherapy has also been widely used for the treatment of moderate to severe GO. As with glucocorticoids, orbital radiotherapy has no role in the treatment of inactive disease. Most evidence supports the safety of orbital radiotherapy,[252] although there are older reports of vision loss (believed to be caused by dosing errors by inexperienced operators)[253] and more recent observations of retinal vessel proliferation.[254] With the exception of patients with diabetes and/or hypertension, the risk of retinopathy and cataracts has been claimed not to exceed that of the general population. Orbital radiotherapy does not promote tumorigenesis.[252,255]

The efficacy of orbital irradiation has been demonstrated by a number of high-quality randomized trials. Prummel and associates[256] randomized 88 people with mild GO to sham irradiation or orbital irradiation. At 12 months, 52% of irradiated patients evidenced improvement compared with 27% in the sham group (RR [relative risk], 1.9; 95% CI, 1.1 to 3.4; $P = .02$). In the irradiation group, there was significantly less need for additional therapy than in the sham group ($P = 0.049$). The authors found that radiotherapy was particularly effective at improving muscle motility and decreasing the severity of diplopia. A similarly designed study by Mourits and coworkers[257] have confirmed these findings. Kahaly and colleagues[258] have compared different doses of orbital irradiation and demonstrated favorable outcomes in about two thirds of patients. Finally, a randomized double-blind trial comparing orbital irradiation with prednisone demonstrated similar response rates in both groups.[259] In contrast, Gorman and associates[260] irradiated one eye of patients with mild to moderate GO and used the other eye as an internal control. After 6 months, no evidence of clinical benefit could be attributed to orbital radiotherapy in the treated eye versus the untreated eye, leading the authors to conclude that the role of radiotherapy in GO must be reassessed.

In summary, with a few exceptions,[261] extant data support the efficacy and safety of orbital irradiation when performed by adequately trained personnel. As many as two thirds of patients with significant disease will respond to orbital radiotherapy. Extraocular muscle dysfunction, particular of new onset, as well as inflammatory signs, respond well to orbital irradiation. Orbital radiotherapy does not exact an effect for days to weeks, and therefore is an inappropriate choice for optic neuropathy with worsening visual acuity.

Orbital Radiotherapy and Corticosteroids

Is there an advantage to combining these two accepted therapies? Theoretically, the combination might exploit the rapid onset of action of glucocorticoids and the sustained action of irradiation, thereby controlling disease acutely and preventing recurrence upon steroid withdrawal. Marcocci and associates[262] randomized 30 patients with active GO to orbital radiotherapy or orbital radiotherapy plus glucocorticoids. The decrease in a mean ophthalmopathy index was significantly greater in the radiotherapy plus steroid group compared with the radiotherapy-only group. Other studies have been unable to identify a therapeutic benefit from combining these treatment modalities.[263]

The data do not definitively support the routine use of orbital irradiation and glucocorticoids, although a cogent argument could support this combination when presented with severe GO. Combining these agents may exploit the rapid onset of action of corticosteroids as well as the sustained effects of the irradiation, effectively rescuing the patient acutely and preventing relapse on steroid withdrawal.

Orbital Decompression

Unlike glucocorticoids or orbital radiotherapy, orbital decompression is aimed at increasing the orbital space to accommodate increased orbital contents. This is achieved by removing one or more of the orbital walls. Originally a treatment for exposure keratitis, compressive optic neuropathy, and severe orbital inflammation with pain, rehabilitative surgery to correct disfiguring proptosis represents a more recent indication.[264] Common complications of surgery include postoperative muscle imbalance and diplopia. Rarely, blindness, bleeding, periorbital numbness, sinusitis, and lid or globe malposition may occur. Several techniques are currently used,[265] including orbital fat decompression without bony removal.[266] A discussion of the various procedures is beyond our scope here. Suffice it to say, orbital decompression is a safe and effective procedure when performed by an experienced surgeon, preserving or improving vision in over 90% of those with optic neuropathy and reducing proptosis by almost 5 mm.[267] About 30% of patients will develop new or worsening diplopia following the procedure and will require corrective muscle surgery. Finally, surgery on active GO should be avoided, if at all possible, unless the sight is to be saved. The best results are obtained after the disease has run its course and corrective surgery is needed. We suggest that medical management of severe active GO constitute first-line therapy, with surgery reserved for treatment failures leading to progressive disease and later cosmetic correction for marked proptosis.

Rehabilitative Surgery

Diplopia is the debilitating result of extraocular muscle fibrosis. Rehabilitative surgery is aimed at restoring single binocular vision in primary gaze and downward gaze for reading.[264] As many as 20% to 70% of those treated for severe GO will require extraocular muscle surgery to improve diplopia.[205] Generally, surgery is postponed until disease inactivity is certain, although this practice has recently been called into question.[268] Overall, extraocular muscle surgery offers visually debilitated patients a chance at normal binocular vision; in one series, a single surgery yielded acceptable results in 71% of patients, with a second surgery raising the number to 89%.[269]

Finally, botulinum toxin may be of some benefit in patients with small-angle diplopia[270] or upper eyelid retraction.[271] Further evaluation of this noninvasive approach is warranted.

Immunosuppressive Agents

The widespread acceptance of GO as an autoimmune phenomenon has prompted researchers to investigate the usefulness of several immunosuppressive agents, including the calcineurin inhibitor cyclosporine (CSA). There is now little substantive evidence to support the use of CSA as monotherapy for GO.[272] CSA administered concomitantly with glucocorticoids may lead to greater improvement in GO than steroids alone and may result in fewer relapses.[273] Larger studies are needed to confirm these findings. At this time, the use of CSA should be reserved for severe glucocorticoid-resistant disease.

Three inhibitors of tumor necrosis factor α (TNF-α) are commercially available, etanercept, adalimumab, and infliximab. One small uncontrolled study[274] and one case report[275] have suggested that these medications may prove to be effective steroid-sparing therapies in the future.

Rituximab is a monoclonal antibody directed against anti-CD20–positive B cells. Evidence is emerging to suggest that this medication may be particularly effective for GO by depleting the total lymphocyte population in the orbit.[276] Large randomized trials are needed before these medications can be recommended to patients with GO, but preliminary studies have suggested that this antibody can produce results equal to corticosteroids, without the side effects, after one treatment.

Intravenous Immunoglobulin

The experience with IV immunoglobulin (IVIG) for this indication is limited. Two small randomized studies[277,278] and one prospective nonrandomized study[279] have evaluated IVIG in comparison to standard therapy with glucocorticoids. All three studies found IVIG to be at least as effective as steroids in treating moderate to severe GO, with many fewer side effects. These results were not confirmed by a fourth study.[280] However, few patients were included in these studies. Moreover, the risk of disease transmission remains a legitimate concern. There is no role for IVIG therapy in GO at this time.

Plasmapheresis

There are no high-level data to support the use of plasmapheresis for GO. Some studies have reported positive results[281] but other studies were unable to demonstrate any benefit.[282] There is currently no role for plasmapheresis in the routine management of GO.

Somatostatin Analogues

Somatostatin receptors can be visualized on the orbital tissue of patients with GO,[283] offering the possibility that somatostatin analogues might offer disease-modifying potential (Fig. 12-4). A few small uncontrolled studies have yielded conflicting results. More recently, a large prospective, randomized, controlled trial has demonstrated that lanreotide, a slow-release somatostatin analogue, offered no effect on GO beyond that of placebo.[284] Another randomized controlled trial yielded results that were equally as disappointing.[285] In light of these results, somatostatin analogues also have no role in the management of GO, although muscle scanning remains of interest as a marker of disease activity.[286]

Graves' Disease and Pregnancy

Hyperthyroidism complicates about 2 in 1000 pregnancies in the United States.[287] GD is the most common cause of hyperthyroidism in young women and pregnancy is no exception. Hyperemesis gravidarum and gestational trophoblastic disease account for most cases not attributable to GD. Human chorionic gonadotropin (hCG) is a glycoprotein hormone that shares structural similarity to TSH. Several studies have demonstrated a TSH-like effect of hCG at the level of the thyroid, accounting for gestational hyperthyroidism of normal pregnancy, and it is by this mechanism that hyperemesis and trophoblastic disease trigger inappropriate release of thyroid hormone.[288,289] Other causes of hyperthyroidism, such as nodular disease or thyroiditis, are much less common during pregnancy.

Severe thyrotoxicosis is uncommonly encountered during pregnancy, in part because hyperthyroidism is associated with impaired fertility[290] and fetal loss.[291] For patients with milder disease who do conceive, untreated hyperthyroidism poses significant maternal-fetal risk.[292,293] If GD is treated appropriately, however, the risk appears to be no greater than that in the euthyroid population.[292]

Pregnancy dramatically alters the course of many autoimmune diseases as the immune suppression of pregnancy becomes established. Most studies have suggested that thyrotoxicosis wanes or remits entirely during pregnancy, particularly in the latter half of gestation.[294] This is supported by the observation that TSH-R Abs decline throughout pregnancy.[295] Therefore, pregnant women with GD must be followed closely with the expectation that ATDs will be tapered or discontinued in the last trimester of pregnancy.

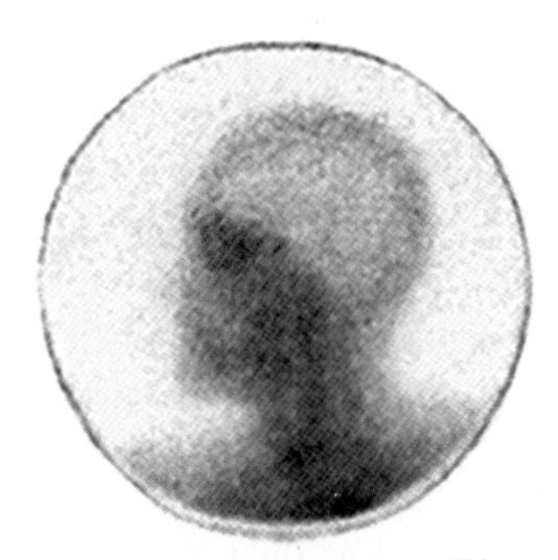

Figure 12–4 Orbital scintigraphy with (^{111}In-DPTA-D-Phe1)-octreotide in a patient with Graves' ophthalmopathy, demonstrating the presence of somatostatin receptors in the orbit. *(From Calao A, Lastoria S, Ferone D, et al: Orbital scintigraphy with [^{111}In-diethylenetriamine pentaacetic acid-D-phe1]-octreotide predicts the clinical response to corticosteroid therapy in patients with Graves' ophthalmopathy. J Clin Endocrinol Metab 83:3790-3794, 1998.)*

Choice of Therapy

With few exceptions, ATDs are considered first-line therapy for pregnant women with GD. Radioiodine readily crosses the placenta and is concentrated in the fetal thyroid, effectively ablating the fetal thyroid tissue.[296] For this reason, RAI is absolutely contraindicated in pregnancy. Surgery should be reserved for the rare cases when ATDs cannot be tolerated, hyperthyroidism cannot be controlled, or ATD requirements are unacceptably high. In the event that surgery is necessary, it is preferable to wait for the second trimester to obviate the risk of early pregnancy loss or later premature labor.

In the United States, PTU has been the drug of choice to manage GD during pregnancy. In the past, it was believed that PTU crossed the placenta to a lesser degree than MMI.[297] However, newer data have questioned this assertion.[40] If PTU crosses the placenta as readily as MMI, what advantage does PTU offer during pregnancy? In fact, MMI is as effective as PTU and is widely used worldwide to treat GD in pregnancy.[298] Of concern, however, has been the growing number of case reports associating the use of MMI during pregnancy with aplasia cutis, a rare scalp defect[299] and a self-proclaimed MMI embryopathy, which includes aplasia cutis, choanal atresia, tracheoesophageal fistula, hypoplastic nipples, psychomotor delay, and characteristic facies.[300] However, larger studies have failed to support this association because such defects also appear in the general population.[292] Consequently, it seems reasonable to use PTU as first-line therapy in pregnancy, considering the rare but possibly real association between MMI and certain congenital anomalies.

Occasionally, ATDs will be contraindicated and/or the thyrotoxicosis too symptomatic to wait for the onset of ATDs, necessitating the use of other agents. Beta blockers are frequently used in nonpregnant patients to quell adrenergic signs and symptoms of thyroid hormone excess until definitive therapy restores a euthyroid state. The safety of beta blockers in pregnancy, however, remains controversial.[301,302] In general, if beta blockade is necessary during pregnancy, we suggest using the lowest dose possible for the shortest duration possible.

Rarely, iodine will be necessary to control hyperthyroidism.[303] Although iodine can rapidly normalize plasma thyroid hormone levels, it should not be relied on for long periods during pregnancy because it may induce obstructive goiter in the neonate.

GOALS OF THERAPY

The goal of GD therapy in pregnancy is to mimic physiologic thyroid hormone levels. As noted, thyrotoxicosis poses a risk to the mother and fetus and therefore must be treated. Conversely, overtreatment, yielding hypothyroidism, can impair the neuropsychological development of the fetus.[304,305] Thus, it is recommended that the free T_4 level be maintained at or just above the upper limit of normal, effectively negating the risk of unintentional fetal hypothyroidism.[306]

In general, PTU, 100 mg three times daily, can be initiated in pregnant women with moderate to severe GD. Lower doses may be appropriate for less severe cases. Free T_4 should be monitored monthly and PTU titrated appropriately. If dosages of 50 to 100 mg daily can maintain euthyroidism, discontinuation may be possible in up to 30% of patients in the third trimester.[307] Occasionally, larger doses will be required to gain control of the disease. If high ATD dosage requirements persist, consideration must be given to a thyroidectomy rather than risk prolonged fetal hypothyroidism and the resultant neuropsychological ramifications.[308]

THYROID-STIMULATING HORMONE RECEPTOR ANTIBODIES AND PREGNANCY

TSH-R Abs pass across the placenta and can influence fetal thyroid function. In fact, high titers of TSH-R Abs remain the best predictor of neonatal hyperthyroidism.[309,310] Furthermore, the specificity of TSH-R Abs can change from stimulatory to blocking,[311] resulting in neonatal *hypo*thyroidism.[312] This conundrum emphasizes the value of laboratory tests that measure the stimulating or inhibitory capacity of TSH-R Abs using bioassays. Hence, the more expensive bioassays offer a clear theoretical advantage under certain circumstances when compared with receptor-based competitive assays.[313]

In practice, three clinical scenarios arise: (1) a euthyroid pregnant woman with GD in remission after a course of ATDs; (2) a euthyroid pregnant woman on L-T_4 after destructive therapy for GD (RAI or surgery); and (3) a pregnant woman currently on PTU for GD (initiated before or during pregnancy).

With this framework in mind, consider the euthyroid pregnant woman with GD who is in remission following a course of ATDs. Her euthyroidism is suggestive that her TSH-R Ab titers are low to absent but the presence of concomitant thyroiditis may actually be restricting the action of stimulating TSH-R Abs. Hence, their measurement is an important part of the evaluation. A receptor assay is the first choice and a bioassay in the last trimester should only be performed if TSH-R Abs are present. Her thyroid function should be followed throughout pregnancy, but as mentioned, she is unlikely to recur during gestation.

A pregnant patient started on PTU prior to or during pregnancy will need her PTU dosed as discussed earlier. The TSH-R Ab level should be measured in the last trimester. A bioassay may not be necessary in this case because the mother is serving as the bioassay. If levels are low or undetectable, the risk of neonatal thyrotoxicosis is negligible. If levels remain elevated, then a bioassay is of interest but not essential; however, the neonate must be evaluated for hyperthyroidism at birth and after 4 to 7 days with a thorough physical examination and laboratory studies.

The pregnant patient on L-T_4 after destructive therapy for GD poses a unique challenge. The TSH-R Ab level should be measured early in pregnancy and, if positive, a formal bioassay should be performed. Inhibitory antibodies should reinforce the importance of maintaining maternal free T_4 in the high-normal range; presumably, this will be adequate therapy to ensure normal growth and development based on the observation that infants with congenital hypothyroidism are born healthy. When high titers of stimulating TSH-R Abs are detected, the fetus must be followed carefully for signs of hyperthyroidism. Fetal heart rate monitoring, assessment of growth and, most recently, ultrasonographic evaluation for fetal goiter are invaluable tools to assess fetal thyroid status.[314,315] The use of ATDs may be considered if signs of fetal thyrotoxicosis are evident. In this situation, ATD therapy cannot be titrated to maternal thyroid status, but must be titrated to certain fetal parameters, such as normalization of tachycardia or reduction in goiter, or to a biochemical measure of fetal thyroid status obtained by cordocentesis.[316]

In general, when GD in pregnancy is managed properly, maternal and neonatal outcome are excellent.

POSTPARTUM GRAVES' DISEASE

The relative immunosuppression of pregnancy rebounds in the postpartum period, often resulting in the reactivation of quiescent autoimmune diseases. A large retrospective study of women ages 18 to 39 years with GD found that 45% were diagnosed in the postpartum period.[317] Moreover, patients in remission during pregnancy frequently relapse in the postpartum period at a rate that has been reported to be as high as 70%.[318] Recurrences occur most commonly within 4 to 6 months after delivery.[318]

To complicate the discussion, silent thyroiditis or Hashitoxicosis occurs commonly in the postpartum period. A retrospective study has examined the course of 96 cases of postpartum hyperthyroidism in women with a history of GD.[319] Radioiodine uptake (RAIU) values fell into three categories: (1) low RAIU, <10%; (2) normal RAIU, 10% to 40%; and (3) elevated RAIU, >40%. Of 96 patients, 26 demonstrated a low RAIU consistent with thyroiditis and 33 demonstrated normal RAIU, suggesting that silent thyroiditis might overlap with the reactivation of GD in some people. Finally, 37 of 96 people demonstrated high RAIU consistent with reactivation of typical GD itself. Most patients in the low and normal group did not require treatment, with 75% experiencing resolution of hyperthyroidism. Several subsequently developed transient hypothyroidism, with 50% ultimately becoming hyperthyroid again by 9 months. These data indicate that autoimmune thyroiditis commonly accompanies the reactivation of GD in the postpartum period, complicating the natural history and interpretation of thyroid function following parturition.

When GD does recur, thionamides are the treatment modality of choice for breast-feeding mothers. ATDs can be taken safely while breast-feeding.[320] Studies have demonstrated that thyroid function in breast-fed infants is not affected by large doses of PTU or MMI.[45,44] Destructive therapy with RAI can be considered after breast-feeding has ceased.

Accelerated Hyperthyroidism (Thyroid Storm)

Accelerated hyperthyroidism, often poorly named thyroid storm, is an uncommon complication of a common disease. Fatality rates have been as high as 20% to 50%, depending on the series.[321] When thyroid surgery was first performed on GD patients, accelerated thyrotoxicosis was common following the release of massive amounts of preformed thyroid hormone into the circulation. Other types of biostress such as infection, trauma, and surgery also may precipitate the crisis in an individual with untreated or incompletely treated hyperthyroidism. It is unclear how these stressors aggravate the thyrotoxic state, because T_3 levels are not appreciably higher than in patients with uncomplicated thyrotoxicosis, and it is likely that cytokine mediation is involved.[322]

There are no formal criteria to diagnose thyroid storm, and often it is only noted by the inexperienced physician rather than the patient. Most would agree that some of the following symptoms in a patient with suspected hyperthyroidism would suggest rapid acceleration: fever, diaphoresis, tachycardia or tachyarrhythmia (perhaps accompanied by pulmonary edema), tremulousness, restlessness, delirium, nausea, vomiting, diarrhea, jaundice, and abdominal pain. If left untreated, coma and circulatory collapse may supervene.

Treatment is aimed at stabilizing and supporting the patient, reducing thyroid hormone levels, and addressing the underlying illness. The following sections will review agents that may be beneficial when rapid control of hyperthyroidism is required. The final section will provide a practical approach to managing the patient presenting with accelerated hyperthyroidism.

BETA BLOCKERS AND CALCIUM CHANNEL BLOCKERS

Beta blockers (BBs) are routinely used in thyrotoxicosis to ameliorate symptoms attributable to enhanced adrenergic sensitivity. Nonselective BBs such as propranolol and cardioselective BBs such as atenolol and metoprolol have long been used to provide symptomatic relief pending primary therapy with RAI, ATDs, or surgery. Tremor, tachycardia, muscle weakness, lid lag, palpitations, anxiety, heat intolerance, and excess sweating generally improve soon after beta blockade is initiated.[323,324,325]

Propranolol is frequently touted as the beta blocker of choice for thyrotoxicosis because of its ability to block peripheral T_4 to T_3 conversion.[326] Moreover, T_3 levels drop significantly faster in patients treated with propranolol compared with those treated with cardioselective beta-blocking agents.[327] The clinical significance of this finding, however, remains uncertain.[328] Additionally, BBs enhance nitrogen retention,[329] reverse thyrotoxic periodic paralysis,[330] and normalize hypercalcemia in the thyrotoxic patient.[331] Propranolol must be dosed every 6 to 8 hours; for this reason, once-daily BBs such as atenolol or metoprolol (Toprol XL) may improve patient compliance.

When BBs are contraindicated, particularly in the setting of obstructive lung disease, two approaches can be considered. An intravenous esmolol infusion can be attempted and rapidly titrated off in the event that the patient develops bronchospasm. Alternatively, a nondihydropyridine calcium channel blocker (e.g., diltiazem or verapamil) may provide symptomatic relief equivalent to propranolol.[332]

Iodides

Iodine produces a rapid reduction in circulating thyroid hormone, primarily by inhibiting hormonal release.[333,334] The T_4 level falls by 50% after 4 days[335] and normalizes in all patients by day 9.[336] A similarly dramatic reduction in T_3 occurs, with normalization in almost all subjects between days 5 and 10. A secondary effect of iodine may be attributable to the inhibition of iodine oxidation and organification (Wolff-Chaikoff effect),[337] although this mechanism cannot explain the rapid onset of action observed with iodine.

Subsequent to the rapid reduction in circulating thyroid hormone, many patients "escape" from the inhibitory effects of iodine. Therefore, iodine is generally not used as monotherapy. In addition, the enrichment of thyroidal iodine stores can blunt the effect of thionamides and, theoretically, under the right circumstances, iodine can inflame an already tenuous hyperthyroid state (Jod-Basedow phenomenon). Finally, the use of iodine precludes definitive therapy with RAI for several weeks.

Nevertheless, iodine is an important tool in patients with actual or impending thyroid crisis. Iodine should be administered with large doses of a thionamide (PTU, 300 to 400 mg every 4 to 6 hours) in the absence of a contraindication. Typical doses are 3 to 5 drops of Lugol's solution twice daily or 1 drop of SSKI twice daily. Doses larger than this increase the likelihood of an adverse reaction. Possible adverse reactions include metallic taste, sialadenitis, rhinitis, conjunctivitis, headache, gastritis, acneiform rash, vasculitis, and leukemoid eosinophilic granulocytosis.[39] Sialadenitis may remit with a dosage reduction; more serious adverse events should prompt discontinuation of the medication.

Corticosteroids

Corticosteroids produce a rapid fall in T_3 and T_4 and a rise in reverse T_3 when administered to hyperthyroid GD patients,[338,339] suggesting a direct inhibition of glandular secretion of thyroid hormone as well as the inhibition of peripheral monodeiodination. Moreover, corticosteroids exert important immunosuppressive (lympholytic) effects, greatly suppressing TSH-R Abs.[171] Finally, steroids may augment the effects of ATDs in reducing goiter size.[340]

Needless to say, corticosteroids have a number of untoward side effects and should be reserved for impending or actual thyroid crisis. In general, steroids are an effective adjunct to thionamides and iodine (or cholecystographic agents) when rapid control of hyperthyroidism is required.[201]

Oral Cholecystographic Agents

Sodium ipodate (Oragrafin) and sodium iopanoate (Telepaque) are iodine-containing cholecystographic agents and, as such, rapidly reduce levels of T_3 and T_4 in part by blocking the release of thyroid hormone. Unlike iodine, ipodate also blocks the peripheral conversion of T_4 to T_3, thereby yielding significantly greater reductions in T_3 levels.[334] After 24 hours, a reduction in T_3 can reach 54% to 62%.[341,342] Furthermore, ipodate combined with MMI may provide more rapid reduction of T_3 as well as more rapid normalization of clinical parameters such as heart rate compared with MMI and SSKI.[343]

Ipodate, 500 to 1000 mg daily, rapidly restores euthyroidism in patients with GD. However prolonged use is associated with an unacceptable recurrence rate.[344] For this reason, ipodate should not be used as monotherapy. In general, ipodate is well tolerated, with few side effects, and should be considered (if available) when rapid control of thyrotoxicosis is required.

Lithium Carbonate

Lithium acts by inhibiting the release of T_3 and T_4, thereby rapidly reducing circulating hormone levels in much the same manner as iodide.[345,346] Unlike iodide, lithium does not interfere with the accumulation of ^{131}I and may even enhance its effect.[172,173] Prolonged use is discouraged because of the relative toxicity of the medication as well as a tendency for the thyroid to escape the inhibitory effects of lithium. Although lithium is rarely used in practice, it may be considered when rapid control of thyrotoxicosis is required and iodide therapy is contraindicated. A reasonable dose is 300 to 450 mg every 8 hours to achieve a serum concentration of 1 mEq/L. A 30% reduction in T_3 and T_4 can be expected by 2 weeks.[347]

Cholestyramine

Thyroxine is conjugated in the liver and excreted in the bile. Free hormone is released and reabsorbed in the gut. Cholestyramine is an anionic exchange resin that binds iodothyronines, preventing their absorption; 4 g, two to four times daily, taken with PTU or MMI, contributed to a more rapid and complete decline in thyroid hormone levels in hyperthyroid GD patients.[348,349] Cholestyramine is an effective adjunct to the treatment of hyperthyroidism. It is safe and well tolerated, although abdominal discomfort, constipation, and flatulence may preclude higher doses. Cholestyramine impairs the absorption of a number of medications; this should be considered prior to initiating treatment.

Perchlorate

Perchlorate prevents thyroidal iodide uptake[350] and may be as effective at normalizing thyroid function as thionamides.[351] Perchlorate is now rarely recommended, with the possible exception of type 1 amiodarone-induced thyrotoxicosis.[352] Initially believed to be safe and inexpensive, a number of reports of fatal aplastic anemia surfaced in the 1960s, and perchlorate fell out of favor.[353-355]

PRACTICAL MANAGEMENT OF ACCELERATED THYROTOXICOSIS

The initial management of thyroid crisis must proceed as follows (in this order): (1) protect airway, obtain vascular access, and stabilize hemodynamics; (2) initiate specific therapy aimed at ameliorating the proximate cause of the crisis (e.g., antibiotics for pneumonia); and (3) reduce thyroid hormone levels and treat the adrenergic signs of thyrotoxicosis.

Once the patient is stabilized and the precipitating illness addressed, large doses of ATDs should be initiated orally, via a nasogastric tube, or rectally if necessary.[356] PTU (300 to 400 mg every 4 to 6 hours) is probably preferable because of its ability to block the peripheral conversion of T_4 to T_3. Although the thionamide will provide little immediate relief, it will prevent the enrichment of thyroid hormone stores following iodide (or ipodate) administration.

Iodine (SSKI, 1 drop twice daily; Lugol's, 3 to 5 drops twice daily) blocks the release of preformed thyroid hormone and should follow the administration of the thionamide. Sodium ipodate is superior to iodine, blocking both the release of preformed thyroid hormone and the peripheral conversion of T_4 to T_3. If available, ipodate, 1 g daily (or 500 mg, twice daily) can be used rather than iodine.

The addition of dexamethasone, 2 mg every 6 hours, will further inhibit the peripheral conversion of T_4 to T_3 and blunt the release of preformed thyroid hormone. The combination of iodine, dexamethasone, and PTU restores T_3 levels to normal in 1 to 2 days.[357]

In the absence of congestive heart failure, BBs can be initiated to blunt the adrenergic symptoms of thyrotoxicosis. Propranolol, 40 to 60 mg every 6 hours, is frequently used because of its effect on peripheral conversion of T_4 to T_3. The clinical implications of this are unknown, however, and cardioselective BBs such as metoprolol, 25 to 50 mg twice daily, may prove as efficacious. When BBs are contraindicated because of obstructive pulmonary disease, a nondihydropyridine calcium channel blocker can be used.

Accelerated thyrotoxicosis is a devastating event. Prompt diagnosis and aggressive treatment are vital to ensure a favorable outcome (Table 12-7).

Table 12–7 Treatment of Accelerated Thyrotoxicosis

Medication	Dosage	Therapeutic Effect	Considerations
Propylthiouracil (PTU)	300-400 mg q4-6h	Inhibits T_3 and T_4 production; decreases peripheral $T_4 \rightarrow T_3$	Contraindicated if previous serious reaction conversion
Iodine		SSKI, 1 drop bid; Lugol's solution, 3-5 drops bid	Blocks the release of preformed thyroid hormone
Ipodate	500 mg bid; 1000 mg qd	Blocks the release of preformed thyroid hormone; decreases peripheral $T_4 \rightarrow T_3$ conversion	Probably more effective than iodine, but unlikely to be available
Dexamethasone	2 mg q6h	Decreases peripheral $T_4 \rightarrow T_3$ conversion; blunts the release of preformed thyroid hormone	
Propranolol	40-60 mg q6h	Blunts adrenergic signs; decreases peripheral conversion of $T_4 \rightarrow T_3$	Caution in obstructive lung disease, heart failure
Diltiazem	30-60 mg q6h	Reduces heart rate	Used as an alternative to beta blockers, caution in heart failure

SSKI, saturated solution of potassium iodide.

References

1. Parry CH: Disease of the Heart. Collections from the Unpublished Writings, vol 2. London, Underwoods, 1825, pp 111–125.
2. Adams DD, Purves HD: Abnormal responses in the assay of thyrotrophin. Proc Univ Otago Med Sch 34:11-12, 1956.
3. Kriss JP, Pleshakov V, Chien JR: Isolation and identification of the long-acting thyroid stimulator and its relation to hyperthyroidism and circumscribed pretibial myxedema. J Clin Endocrinol 24:1005-1028, 1964.
4. Bahn RS: TSH receptor expression in orbital adipose/connective tissues from patients with thyroid-associated ophthalmopathy. Thyroid 12: 193-195, 2002.
5. Wiersinga WM, Prummel MF: Pathogenesis of Graves' ophthalmopathy: Current understanding. J Clin Endocrinol Metab 86:501-503, 2001.
6. Jacobson DL, Gange SJ, Rose NR, Graham NM: Epidemiology and estimated population burden of selected autoimmune diseases in the United States. Immunol Immunopathol 84:223-243, 1997.
7. Vanderpump MPJ, Tunbridge WMG, French JM, et al: The incidence of thyroid disorders in the community: A twenty-year follow-up of the Whickham survey. Clin Endocrinol 43:55-68, 1995.
8. Hollowell JG, Staehling NW, Flanders WD, et al: Serum TSH, T-4, and thyroid antibodies in the United States population (1988 to 1994): National Health and Nutrition Examination Survey (NHANES III). J Clin Endocrinol Metab 87:489-499, 2002.
9. Weetman AP: Graves' disease. N Engl J Med 343:1236-4128, 2000.
10. Yanagisawa T, Sato K, Kato Y, et al: Rapid differential diagnosis of Graves' disease and painless thyroiditis using total T3/T4 ration, TSH, and total alkaline phosphatase activity. Endocr J 52:29-36, 2005.
11. Solomon B, Glinoer D, Lagrasses R, Wartofsky L: Current trends in the management of Graves' disease. J Clin Endocrinol Metab 80:1518-1524, 1990.
12. Wartofsky L, Glinoer D, Solomon B, et al: Differences and similarities in the diagnosis and treatment of Graves' disease in Europe, Japan, and the United States. Thyroid 1:129-135, 1991.
13. Torring O, Tallstedt L, Wallin G, et al: Graves' hyperthyroidism: Treatment with antithyroid drugs, surgery, or radioiodine—a prospective, randomized study. Thyroid Study Group. J Clin Endocrinol Metab 81:2986-2993, 1996.
14. Jansson R, Dahlberg PA, Lindstom B: Comparative bioavailability of carbimazole and methimazole. Int J Clin Pharmacol Ther Toxicol 21:505-510, 1983.
15. Marchant B, Alexander WD, Robertson JWK, Lazarus JH: Concentration of ^{35}S-propylthiouracil by the thyroid gland and its relationship to anion trapping mechanism. Metabolism 20:989-999, 1971.
16. Abuid J, Larsen PR: Comparison of the acute changes during therapy with antithyroid agents. J Clin Invest 54:201-208, 1974.
17. Wenzel KW, Lente JR: Similar effects of thionamide drugs and perchlorate on thyroid-stimulating immunoglobulins in Graves' disease: Evidence against an immunosuppressive action of thionamide drugs. J Clin Endocrinol Metab 58:62-69, 1984.
18. Volpe R: The immunomodulatory effects of antithyroid drugs are mediated via actions on thyroid cells, affecting thyrocyte-immunocyte signaling: A review. Curr Pharm Des 7:451-460, 2001.
19. McGregor AM, Petersen MM, McLachlan SM, et al: Carbimazole and the autoimmune response in Graves' disease. N Engl J Med 303:302-307, 1980.
20. Weetman AP, McGregor AM, Hall R: Evidence for an effect of antithyroid drugs on the natural history of Graves' disease. Clin Endocrinol (Oxf) 21:163-172, 1984.
21. Totterman TH, Karlsson FA, Bengtsson M, Mendel-Hartvig I: Induction of circulating activated suppressor-like T cells by methimazole therapy for Graves' disease. N Engl J Med 16:15-22, 1987.
22. Marcocci C, Chiovato L, Mariotti S, Pinchera A: Changes of circulating thyroid autoantibody levels during and after the therapy with methimazole in patients with Graves' disease. J Endocrinol Invest 5:13-19, 1982.
23. Davies TF, Weiss I, Gerber MA: Influence of methimazole on murine thyroiditis. J Clin Invest 73:397-404, 1984.
24. Sonnet E, Massart C, Gibassier J, et al: Longitudinal study of soluble intercellular adhesion molecure-1 (ICAM-1) in sera of patients with Graves' disease. J Endocrinol Invest 22:430-435, 2000.
25. Tsatsoulis A, Vlachoyiannopoulos PG, Dalekos GN, et al: Increased serum interleukin 1 beta during treatment of hyperthyroidism with antithyroid drugs. Eur J Clin Invest 25:654-658, 1996.
26. Salvi M, Girasole G, Pedrazzoni M, et al: Increased serum concentrations of interleukin-6 and soluble IL-6 receptor in patients with Graves' disease. J Clin Endocrinol Metab 81:2976-2979, 1996.
27. Mitsiades N, Poulaki V, Tseleni-Balafouta S, et al: Fas ligand expression in thyroid follicular cells from patients with thionamide-treated Graves' disease. Thyroid 10:527-532, 2000.
28. Zantut-Wittmann DE, Tambascia MA, da Silva Trevisan MA, et al: Antithyroid drugs inhibit in vivo HLA-DR expression in thyroid follicular cells in Graves's disease. Thyroid 11:575-580, 2001.
29. Ohashi H, Okugawa T, Itoh M: Circulating activated T cell subsets in autoimmune thyroid diseases: Differences between untreated and treated patients. Acta Endocrinol (Copenh) 125:502-509, 1991.
30. Wang PW, Luo SF, Huang BY, et al: Depressed natural killer activity in Graves' disease and during antithyroid medication. Clin Endocrinol (Oxf) 28:205-214, 1988.

31. Kampmann JP, Hansen JM: Clinical pharmacokinetics of antithyroid drugs. Clin Pharmacokinet 6:401-428, 1981.
32. Cooper DS, Saxe VC, Maloof F, Ridgeway EC: Studies of propylthiouracil using a newly developed radioimmunoassay. J Clin Endocrinol Metab 52:204-213, 1981.
33. Melander A, Hallengren B, Rosendal-Helgesen S, et al: Comparative in vitro effects and in vivo kinetics of antithyroid drugs. Eur J Clin Pharmacol 17:295-299, 1980.
34. Jansson R, Dahlberg PA, Johansson H, Lindstrom B: Intrathyroidal concentrations of methimazole in patients with Graves' disease. J Clin Endocrinol Metab 57:129-132, 1983.
35. Jansson R, Lindstom B, Dahlberg PA: Pharmacokinetic properties and bioavailability of methimazole. Clin Pharmacokinet 10:443-450, 1985.
36. Cooper DS, Steigerwalt S, Migdal S: Pharmacology of propylthiouracil in thyrotoxicosis and chronic renal railure. Arch Intern Med 62:217-220, 1987.
37. Cooper DS: Antithyroid drugs. N Engl J Med 352:905-917, 2005.
38. Kampmann JP, Mortensen HB, Bach B, et al: Kinetics of propylthiouracil in the elderly. Acta Med Scand Suppl 624:93-98, 1979.
39. Mechanick JI, Davies TF: Medical management of hyperthyroidism: Theoretical and practical aspects. In Falk SA (ed): Thyroid Disease: Endocrinology, Surgery, Nuclear Medicine, and Radiotherapy, 2d ed. Philadelphia, Lippincott, Williams & Wilkins, 1997, pp 257-258.
40. Mortimer RH, Cannell GR, Addison RS, et al: Methimazole and propylthiouracil equally cross the perfused human term placental lobule. J Clin Endocrinol Metab 82:3099-3102, 1997.
41. Momotani N, Noh JY, Ishikawa N, Ito K: Effects of propylthiouracil and methimazole on fetal thyroid status in mothers with Graves' hyperthyroidism. J Clin Endocrinol Metab 82:3633-3636, 1997.
42. Johansen K, Andersen AN, Kampmann JP, et al: Excretion of methimazole in human milk. Eur J Clin Pharmacol 23:339-341, 1982.
43. Kampmann JP, Johansen K, Hansen JM, Helweg J: Propylthiouracil in human milk. Revision of a dogma. Lancet 1:736-737, 1980.
44. Azizi F, Hedayati M: Thyroid function in breast-fed infants whose mothers take high dose methimazole. J Endocrinol Invest 25:493-496, 2002.
45. Momotani N, Yamashita R, Makino F, et al: Thyroid function in wholly breast-feeding babies whose mothers take high doses of propythiouracil. Clin Endocrinol (Oxf) 53:177-181, 2000.
46. Tajiri J, Noguchi S: Antithyroid drug-induced agranulocytosis: Special reference to normal white blood cell count agranulocytosis. Thyroid 27:227-229, 2004.
47. Ichiki Y, Akahoshi M, Yamashita N, et al: Propylthiouracil-induced severe hepatitis: A case report and review or the literature. J Gastroenterol 33:747-750, 1998.
48. Huang MJ, Li KL, Wei JS, et al: Sequential liver and bone biochemical changes in hyperthyroidism: Prospective controlled follow-up study. Am J Gastroenterol 89:1071-1076, 1994.
49. Liaw YF, Huang MJ, Fan KD, et al: Hepatic injury during propylthiouracil therapy in patients with hyperthyroidism. Ann Intern Med 118:424-428, 1993.
50. Orrego H, Blake JE, Blendis LM, et al: Long-term treatment of alcoholic liver disease with propylthiouracil. N Engl J Med 17:1421-1427, 1987.
51. Williams KV, Nayak S, Becker D, et al: Fifty years of experience with propylthiouracil-associated hepatoxicity: What have we learned?. J Clin Endocrinol Metab 82:1727-1733, 1997.
52. Woeber KA: Methimazole-induced hepatotoxicity. Endocr Pract 8:222-224, 2002.
53. Aloush V, Litinsky I, Caspi D, Elkayam O: Propylthiouracil-induced autoimmune syndromes: Two distict clinical presentations with different course and management. Semin Arthritis Rheum 36:4-9, 2006.
54. Harper L, Chin L, Daykin J, et al: Propythiouracil and carbimazole associated-antineutrophil cytoplasmic antibodies (ANCA) in patients with Graves' disease. Clin Endocrinol 60:671-675, 2004.
55. Cooper DS, Goldminz D, Levin AA, et al: Agranulocytosis associated with antithyroid drugs: Effects of patient age and drug dose. Ann Intern Med 98:26-29, 1983.
56. Pearce SHS: Spontaneous reporting of adverse reactions to carbimazole and propylthiouracil in the UK. Clin Endocrinol 61:589-594, 2004.
57. Balkin MS, Buchholtz M, Ortiz J, Green AJ: Propythiouracil-induced agranulocytosis treated with recombinant human granulocyte colony-stimulating factor. Thyroid 3:305-309, 1993.
58. Fukata S, Kuma K, Sugawara M: Granulocyte colony-stimulating factor (G-CSF) does not improve recovery from antithyroid drug-induced agranulocytosis: A prospective study. Thyroid 9:29-31, 1999.
59. Ljunggren JG, Torringo O, Wallin G, et al: Quality of life aspects and costs in treatment of Graves' hyperthyroidism with antithyroid drugs, surgery, or radioiodine: Results from a prospective, randomized study. Thyroid 8:653-659, 1998.
60. Carella C, Mazziotti G, Sorvillo F, et al: Serum TSH receptor antibodies concentrations in patients with Graves' disease before, at the end of methimazole treatment, and after drug withdrawal: Evidence that the activity of TSH receptor antibody and/or thyroid response modify during the observation period. Thyroid 16:295-302, 2006.
61. Nedrebo BG, Holm PI, Uhlving S, et al: Predictors of outcome and comparison of different drug regimens for the prevention of relapse in patients with Graves' disease. Eur J Endocrinol 147:583-589, 2002.
62. Azizi F, Ataie L, Hedayati M, et al: Effect of long-term continuous methimazole treatment of hyperthyroidism: Comparison with radioiodine. Eur J Endocrinol 152:695-701, 2005.

63. Bartalena L, Macocci C, Bogazzi F, et al: Relation between therapy for hyperthyroid and the course of Graves' ophthalmopathy. N Engl J Med 338:73-78, 1998.
64. McDermott MT, Kidd GS, Dodson LE, Hofeldt FD: Radioiodine-induced thyroid storm. Case report and literature review. Am J Med 75:353-359, 1983.
65. Andrade VA, Gross JL, Maia AL: Effect of methimazole pretreatment on serum thyroid hormone levels after radioiodine treatment in Graves' hyperthyroidism. J Clin Endocrinol Metab 84:4012-4016, 1999.
66. He CT, Hsieh AT, Hung YJ, et al: Comparison of single daily dose of methimazole and propylthiouracil in the treatment of Graves' hyperthyroidism. Clin Endocrinol (Oxf) 60:676-681, 2004.
67. Homsanit M, Sriussadaporn S, Vannasaeng S, et al: Efficacy of single daily dosage of methimazole vs. propylthiouracil in the induction of euthryoidism. Clin Endocrinol (Oxf) 54:385-390, 2001.
68. Nicholas WC, Fischer RG, Stevenson RA, Bass JD: Single daily dose of methimazole compared with every 8 hours propylthiouracil in the treatment of hyperthyroidism. South Med J 88:973-976, 1995.
69. Kallner G, Vitols S, Ljunggren JG: Comparison of standardized initial doses of two antithyroid drugs in the treatment of Graves' disease. J Intern Med 239:525-529, 1996.
70. Okamura K, Ikenoue H, Shiroozu A, et al: Reevaluation of the effects of methylmercaptoimidazole and propylthiouracil in patients with Graves' hyperthyroidism. J Clin Endocrinol Metab 65:719-723, 1987.
71. Werner MC, Romaldini JH, Bromber N, et al: Adverse effects related to thionamide drugs and their dose regimen. Am J Med Sci 297:216-219, 1989.
72. Cooper DS: Antithyroid drugs in the management of patients with Graves' disease: An evidence-based approach to therapeutic controversies. J Clin Endocrinol Metab 88:3474-3781, 2003.
73. Reinwein D, Benker G, Lazarus JH, Alexander WD: A prospective randomized trial of antithyroid drug dose in Graves' disease therapy. European multicenter study group on antithyroid drug treatement. J Clin Endocrinol Metab 76:1516-1521, 1993.
74. Page SR, Sheard CE, Herbert M, et al: A comparison of 20 or 40 mg per day of carbimazole in the initial treatment of hyperthyroidism. Clin Endocrinol (Oxf) 45:511-516, 1996.
75. Shiroozu A, Okamura K, Ikenoue H, et al: Treatment of hyperthyroidism with a small single daily dose of methimazole. J Clin Endocrinol Metab 63:125-128, 1986.
76. Mashio Y, Beniko M, Matsuda A, et al: Treatment of hyperthyroidism with a small single daily dose of methimazole: A prospective long-term follow-up study. Endocr J 44:553-558, 1997.
77. Romaldini JH, Bromberg N, Werner RS, et al: Comparison of effects of high and low dosage regimens of antithyroid drugs in the management of Graves' hyperthyroidism. J Clin Endocrinol Metab 57:563-570, 1983.
78. Jorde R, Ytre-Anre K, Stormer J, Sundsfjord J: Short-term treatment of Graves' disease with methimazole in high versus low doses. J Intern Med 238:161-165, 1995.
79. Grebe Sk, Feek CM, Ford HC, et al: A randomized trial of short-term treatment of Graves' disease with high-dose carbimazole plus thyroxine versus low-dose carbimzale. Clin Endocrinol (Oxf) 48:585-592, 1998.
80. Benker G, Reinwein D, Kahaly G, et al: Is there a methimazole dose effect on remission rate in Graves' disease? Results from a long-term prospective study. The European multicentre trial group of the treatment of hyperthyroidism with antithyroid drugs. Clin Endocrinol (Oxf) 49:451-457, 1998.
81. Edmonds CJ, Tellez M: Treatment of Graves' disease by carbimazole: High dose with thyroxine compared with titration dosing. Eur J Endocrinol 131:120-124, 1994.
82. Lucas A, Salinas J, Rius F, et al: Medical therapy of Graves' disease: Does thyroxine prevent recurrence of hyperthyroidism. J Clin Endocrinol Metab 82:2410-2413, 1997.
83. Hashizume K, Ichikawa K, Sakurai A, et al: Administration of thyroxine in treated Graves' disease. Effects on the level of antibodies to thyroid-stimulating hormone receptor and on the risk of recurrence of hyperthyroidism. N Engl J Med 324:947-953, 1991.
84. Nedrebo BG, Holm PI, Uhlving S, et al: Predictors of outcome and comparison of different drug regimens for the prevention of relapse in patients with Graves' disease. Eur J Endocrinol 147:583-589, 2002.
85. Hoermann R, Quadbeck B, Roggenbuck U, et al: Relapse of Graves' disease after successful outcome of antithyroid drug therapy: Results of a prospective randomized study on the use of levothyroxine. Thyroid 12:1119-1128, 2002.
86. Raber W, Kmen E, Waldhausl W, Vierhapper H: Medical therapy of Graves' disease: Effect on remission rates of methimazole alone and in combination with triiodothyronine. Eur J Endocrinol 142:117-124, 2000.
87. Rittmaster RS, Abbott EC, Douglas R, et al: Effect of methimazole, with or without L-thyroxine, on remission rates in Graves' disease. J Clin Endocrinol Metab 83:814-818, 1998.
88. McIver B, Rae P, Beckett G, et al: Lack of effect of thyroxine in patients with Graves' hyperthyroidism who are treated with an antithyroid drug. N Engl J Med 25:220-224, 1996.
89. Rittmaster RS, Zwicker H, Abbott EC, et al: Effect of methimazole with or without exogenous L-thyroxine on serum concentrations of TSH receptor antibodies in patients with Graves' disease. J Clin Endocrinol Metab 81:3283-3288, 1996.
90. Tamai H, Hayaki I, Kawai K, et al: Lack of effect of thyroxine administration on elevated thyroid-stimulating hormone receptor antibody levels in treated Graves' disease patients. J Clin Endocrinol Metab 80:1481-1484, 1995.

91. Mastorakos G, Doufas AG, Mantzos E, et al: T4 but not T3 administration is associated with increased recurrence of Graves' disease after successful medical therapy. J Endocrinol Invest 26:979-984, 2003.
92. Greer MA, Kammer H, Bouma DJ: Short-term antithyroid drug therapy for the thyrotoxicosis of Graves' disease. N Engl J Med 297:173-176, 1977.
93. Bing, RF, Rosenthal FD. Early remission in thyrotoxicosis produced by short courses of treatment. Acta Endocrinol (Copenh) 100:221-223, 1982.
94. Allannic H, Fauchet R, Orgaiazzi J, et al: Antithyroid drugs and Graves' disease: A prospective randomized evaluation of the efficacy of treatment duration. J Clin Endocrinol Metab 70:675-679, 1990.
95. Garcia-Mayor RV, Paramo C, Luna CR, et al: Antithyroid drug and Graves' hyperthyroidism. Significance of treatment duration and TRAb determination on lasting remission. J Endocrinol Invest 15:815-820, 1992.
96. Maugendre D, Gatel A, Campion L, et al: Antithyroid drugs and Graves' disease—prospective randomized assessment of long-term treatment. Clin Endocrinol 50:127-132, 1999.
97. Weetman AP, Pickerill AP, Watson P, et al: Treatment of Graves' disease with block-replace regimen of antithyroid drugs: The effect of treatment duration and immunogenetic susceptibility on relapse. QJ Med 87:337-341, 1994.
98. Chowdhury TA, Dyer PH: Clinical, biochemical and immunological characteristics of relapsers and non-relapsers of thyrotoxicosis treated with antithyroid drugs. J Intern Med 244:293-297, 1998.
99. Vitti P, Rago T, Chiovato L, et al: Clinical features of patients with Graves' disease undergoing remission after antithyroid drug treatment. Thyroid 7:369-375, 1997.
100. Allahabadia A, Daykin J, Holder RL, et al: Age and gender predict the outcome of treatment for Graves' hyperthyroidism. J Clin Endocrinol Metab 85:1038-1042, 2000.
101. Kawai K, Tamai H, Matsubavashi S, et al: A study of untreated Graves' patients with undetectable TSH binding inhibitor immunoglobulins and the effect of anti-thyroid drugs. Clin Endocrinol (Oxf) 43:551-556, 1995.
102. Michelangeli V, Poon C, Taft J, et al: The prognostic value of TSH receptor antibody measurement in early stages of treatment of Graves' disease with antithyroid drugs. Thyroid 8:119-124, 1998.
103. Benker G, Vitti P, Kahaly G, et al: Response to methimazole in Graves' disease. The European Multicenter Study Group. Clin Endocrinol (Oxf) 43:257-263, 1995.
104. Davies TF, Yeo PP, Evered DC, et al: Value of thyroid-stimulating-antibody determinations in predicting short-term thyrotoxic relapse in Graves' disease. Lancet 1:1181-1182, 1977.
105. Quadbeck B, Hoermann R, Roggenbuck U, et al: Sensitive thyrotropin and thyrotropin-receptor antibody determination one month after discontinuation of antithyroid drug treatment as predictors of relapse in Graves' disease. Thyroid 15: 1047-1054, 2005.
106. Schleusener H, Schwander J, Fischer C, et al: Prospective multicentre study on the prediction of relapse after antithryoid drug treatment in patients with Graves' disease. Acta Endocrinol (Copenh) 121:689-701, 1989.
107. Khanna CM, Shankar LR, Jaffi CB, et al: Predictor of outcome of hyperthyroidism due to Graves' disease: Serum trioodothyronine/thyroxine ratio. J Assoc Physicians India 44:98-101, 1996.
108. Ikenoue H, Okamura K, Sato K, et al: Prediction of relapse in drug-treated Graves' disease using thyroid stimulation indices. Acta Endocrinol (Copenh) 125:643-650, 1991.
109. Talbot JN, Duron F, Feron R, et al: Thyroglobulin, TSH and TSH binding inhibiting immunoglobulins assayed at the withdrawal of antithyroid drug therapy as predictors of relapse of Graves' disease within one year. J Endocrinol Invest 12:589-595, 1989.
110. Varsamidis K, Varsamidou E, Mavopoulos G: Doppler ultrasound in predicting relapse of hyperthyroidism in Graves' disease. Acta Radiol 41:54-58, 2000.
111. Saleh A, Cohnen M, Furst G, et al: Prediction of relapse after antithyroid drug therapy of Graves' disease: Value of color Doppler sonogrophy. Exp Clin Endocrinol Diabetes 112:510-513, 2004.
112. Hertz S, Roberts A, Salter WT: Radioactive iodine as an indicator in thyroid physiology. IV. The metabolism of iodine in Graves' disease. J Clin Invest 21:25-29, 1942.
113. Werner SC, Coelho B, Quimby EH: Ten-year results of I-131 therapy of hyperthyroidism. Bull NY Acad Med 33:783-806, 1957.
114. Metso S, Jaatinen P, Huhtala H, et al: Long-term follow-up study of radioiodine treatment of hyperthyroidism. Clin Endocrinol (Oxf) 61:641-648, 2004.
115. Cunnien AJ, Hay ID, Gorman CA, et al: Radioiodine-induced hypothyroidism in Graves' disease: Factors associated. J Nucl Med 23:978-983, 1982.
116. Holm LE, Lundell G, Israelsson A, Dahlqvist I: Incidence of hypothyroidism occurring long after iodine-131 therapy for hyperthyroidism. J Nucl Med 23:103-107, 1982.
117. Ahmad AM, Ahmad M, Young ET: Objective estimates of the probability of developing hypothyroidism following radioactive iodine treatment of thyrotoxicosis. Eur J Endocrinol 146:767-775, 2002.
118. Tarantini B, Ciuoli C, Di Cairano G, et al: Effectiveness of radioiodine (131-I) as definitive therapy in patients with autoimmune and non-autoimmune hyperthyroidism. J Endocrinol Invest 29:594-598, 2006.

119. Allahabadia A, Daykin J, Sheppard MC, et al: Radioiodine treatment of hyperthyroidism—prognostic factors for outcome. J Clin Endocrinol Metab 86:3611-3617, 2001.
120. Patel NN, Abraham P, Buscombe J, Vanderpump MPJ: The cost effectiveness of treatment modalities for thyrotoxicosis in a UK center. Thyroid 16:593-598, 2006.
121. Hardisty CA, Jones SJ, Hedley AJ, et al: Clinical outcomes and costs of care in radioiodine treatment of hyperthyroidism. J R Coll Physician Lond 24:36-42, 1990.
122. Likhtarov I, Kovgan L, Vavilov S, et al: Post-chernobyl thyroid cancers in Ukraine. Report 2: Risk analysis. Radiat Res 166:375-386, 2006.
123. Read CH Jr, Tansey MJ, Menda Y: A 36-year retrospective analysis of the efficacy and safety of radioactive iodine in treating young Graves' patients. J Clin Endocrinol Metab 89:4229-4233, 2004.
124. Jones BM, Kwok CC, Kung AW: Effect of radioactive iodine therapy on cytokine production in Graves' disease: Transient increases in interleukin-4, IL-6, IL-10, and tumor necrosis factor-alpha, with longer term increases in interferon gamma production. J Clin Endocrinol Metab 84:4106-4110, 1999.
125. Burmeister LA, du Cret RP, Mariash CN: Local reactions to radioiodine in treatment of thyroid cancer. Am J Med 90:217-222, 1991.
126. Gomez-Arnaiz N, Andia E, Guma A, Abos R, et al: Ultrasonographic thyroid volume as a reliable prognostic index of radioiodine-131 treatment outcome in Graves' disease hyperthyroidism. Horm Metab Res 35:492-497, 2003.
127. Centeno BA, Szyfelbein WM, Daniels GH, et al: Fine-needle aspiration biopsy of the thyroid gland in patients with prior Grave' disease treated with radioactive iodine. Morphologic findings and practical pitfalls. Acta Cytol 40:1189-1197, 1996.
128. Nakajo M, Tsuchimochi S, Tanabe H, et al: Three basic patterns of changes in thyroid hormone levels in Graves' disease during the one-year period after radioiodine therapy. Ann Nucl Med 19:297-308, 2005.
129. Tallstedt L, Lundell G, Torring O, et al: Occurrence of ophthalmopathy after treatment for Graves' hyperthyroidism. The thyroid study group. N Engl J Med 25:1733-1738, 1992.
130. Perros P, Kendall-Taylor P, Neoh C, et al: A prospective study of the effects of radioiodine therapy for hyperthyroidism in patients with minimally active Graves' ophthalmopathy. J Clin Endocrinol Metab 90:5321-5323, 2005.
131. Gupta MK, Perl J, Beham R, et al: Effect of 131 iodine therapy on the course of Graves' ophthalmopathy: A quantitative analysis of extraocular muscle volumes using orbital magnetic resonance imaging. Thyroid 11:959-965, 2001.
132. McGregor AM, Petersen MM, Capiferri R, et al: Effects of radioiodine on thyrotrophin binding inhibiting immunoglobulins in Graves' disease. Clin Endocrinol (Oxf) 11:437-444, 1979.
133. Fenzi F, Hashizume K, Roudebush CP, DeGroot LJ: Changes in thyroid-stimulating immunoglobulins during antithyroid therapy. J Clin Endocrinol Metab 48:572-576, 1979.
134. Ito M, Yamashita S, Ashizawa K, et al: Childhood thyroid diseases around Chernobyl evaluated by ultrasound examination and fine-needle aspiration cytology. Thyroid 5:365-368, 1995.
135. Kolade VO, Bosinski TJ, Ruffy EL: Acute promyelocytic leukemia after iodine-131 therapy for Graves' disease. Pharmacotherapy 25:1017-1020, 2005.
136. Shimon I, Kneller A, Olchovsky D: Chronic myeloid leukemia following ^{131}I treatment for thyroid carcinoma: A report of two cases and review of the literature. Clin Endocrinol (Oxf) 43:651-654, 1995.
137. Dickman PW, Holm LE, Lundell G, et al: Thyroid cancer risk after thyroid examination with ^{131}I: A population-based cohort study in Sweden. Int J Cancer 106:580-587, 2003.
138. Ron E, Doody MM, Becker DV, et al: Cancer mortality following treatment for adult hyperthyroidism. Cooperative thyrotoxicosis therapy follow-up study group. JAMA 280:347-355, 1998.
139. Hall P, Boice JD Jr., Berg G, et al: Leukaemia incidence after iodine-131 exposure. Lancet 340:1-4, 1992.
140. Franklyn JA, Maisonneuve P, Sheppard MC, et al: Mortality after the treatment of hyperthyroidism with radioactive iodine. N Engl J Med 338:712-718, 1998.
141. Cantolino SJ, Schmickel RD, Ball M, Cisar CF: Persistent chromosomal aberrations following radioiodine therapy for thyrotoxicosis. N Engl J Med 275:739-745, 1966.
142. Nofal MM, Beierwaltes WH: Persistent chromosomal aberrations following radioiodine therapy. J Nucl Med 5:840-850, 1964.
143. Safa AM, Schumacher OP, Rodriguez-Antunez A: Long-term follow-up results in children and adolescents treated with radioactive iodine(^{131}I) for hyperthyroidism. N Engl J Med 292:167-171, 1975.
144. Einhorn J, Hulten M, Lindsten J, et al: Clinical and cytogenetic investigation in children of parents treated with radioiodine. Acta Radiol Ther Phys Biol 11:193-208, 1972.
145. Esfahani AF, Eftekhari M, Zenooz N, Saghari M: Gonadal function in patients with differentiated thyroid cancer treated with (^{131})I. Hell J Nucl Med 7:52-55, 2004.
146. Wichers M, Benz E, Palmedo H, et al: Testicular function after radioiodine therapy for thyroid cancer. Eur J Nucl Med 27:503-507, 2000.
147. Nebesio TD, Siddiqui AR, Pescovitz OH, Eugster EA: Time course to hypothyroidism after fixed-dose radioablation therapy of Graves' disease in childen. J Pediatr 141:99-103, 2002.

148. Esfahani AF, Kakhki CR, Fallahi B, et al: Comparative evaluation of two fixed doses of 185 and 370 MBq ^{131}I, for the treatment of Graves' disease resistant to antithyroid drugs. Hell J Nucl Med 8: 158-161, 2005.
149. Erem C, Kandemir N, Hacihasanoglu A, et al: Radioiodine treatment of hyperthyroidism: Prognostic factors affecting outcome. Endocrine 25:55-60, 2004.
150. Razvi S, Basu A, McIntyre EA, et al: Low failure rate of fixed administered activity of 400 MBq ^{131}I with pre-treatment with carbimazole for thyrotoxicosis: The Gateshead Protocol. Nucl Med Commun 25:675-682, 2004.
151. Sankar R, Sekhri T, Sripathy G, et al: Radioactive iodine therapy in Graves' hyperthyroidism: A prospective study from a tertiary referral centre in north India. J Assoc Physicians India 53:603-606, 2005.
152. Alexander EK, Larsen PR: High-dose ^{131}I therapy for the treatment of hyperthyroidism caused by Graves' disease. J Clin Endocrinol Metab 87:1073-1077, 2002.
153. Peters H, Fischer C, Bogner U, et al: Radioiodine therapy of Graves' hyperthyroidism: Standard vs. calculated 131 iodine activity. Results from a prospective, randomized, multicentre study. Eur J Clin Invest 25:883-884, 1995.
154. Leslie WD, Ward L, Salamon EA, et al: A randomized comparison of radioiodine doses in Graves' hyperthyroidism. J Clin Endocrinol Metab 88:978-983, 2003.
155. Jarlov AE, Heqedus L, Kristensen LO, et al: Is calculation of the dose in radioiodine therapy of hyperthyroidism worthwhile? Clin Endocrinol (Oxf) 43:325-329, 1995.
156. Aro A, Huttunen JK, Lamberg BA, et al: Comparison of propranolol and carbimazole as adjuncts to iodine-131 therapy of hyperthyroidism. Acta Endocrinol (Copenh) 96:321-327, 1981.
157. Burch HB, Solomon BL, Cooper DS, et al: The effect of antithyroid drug pretreatment on acute changes in thyroid levels after ^{131}I ablation for Graves' disease. J Clin Endocrinol Metab 86:3016-3021, 2001.
158. Bazzi MN, Bagchi N: Adjunctive treatment with propylthiouracil or iodine following radioiodine therapy for Graves' disease. Thyroid 3:269-272, 1993.
159. Kung AW, Yau CC, Cheng AC: The action of methimazole and L-thyroxine in radioiodine therapy: A prospective study on the incidence of hypothyroidism. Thyroid 5:7-12, 1995.
160. Bonnema SJ, Bennedbaek FN, Gram J, et al: Resumption of methimazole after 131I therapy of hyperthyroid disease. Effect on thyroid function and volume evaluated by a randomized clinical trial. Euro J of Endocrinol 149:485-492, 2003.
161. Bonnema SJ, Bennedbaek FN, Veje A, et al: Continuous methimazole therapy and its effect on the cure rate of hyperthyroidism using radioactive iodine: An evaluation by a randomized trial. J Clin Endocrinol Metab 91:2946-2951, 2006.
162. Sabri O, Zimny M, Schrechenberger M, et al: Radioiodine therapy in Graves' disease patients with or without carbimazole at the time of radioiodine therapy. Thyroid 9:1181-1188, 1999.
163. Braga M, Walpert N, Burch HB, et al: The effect of methimazole on cure rates after radioiodine treatment for Graves' hyperthyroidism: A randomized clinical trial. Thyroid 12:135-139, 2002.
164. Andrade VA, Gross JL, Maia AL: The effect of methimazole pretreatment on the efficacy of radioactive iodine therapy in Graves' hyperthyroidism: One-year follow-up of a prospective, randomized study. J Clin Endocrinol Metab 86:3488-3493, 2001.
165. Santos RB, Romaldini JH, Ward LS: Propylthiouracil reduces the effectiveness of radioiodine treatment in hyperthyroid patients with Graves' disease. Thyroid 14:525-530, 2004.
166. Tuttle RM, Patience T, Budd S: Treatment with propylthiouracil before radioactive iodine therapy is associated with a higher treatment failure rate than therapy with radioactive iodine alone in Graves' disease. Thyroid 5:243-247, 1995.
167. Bonnema SJ, Bennedbaek FN, Veje A, et al: Propythiouracil before ^{131}I therapy of hyperthyroid disease: Effect on cure rate evaluated by a randomized clinical trial. J Clin Endocrinol Metab 89:4439-4444, 2004.
168. Gamstedt A, Karlsson A: Pretreatment with betamethasone of patients with Graves' disease given radioiodine therapy: Thyroid autoantibody responses and outcome of therapy. J Clin Endocrinol Metab 73:125-131, 1991.
169. Bartalena L, Marcocci C, Bogazzi F, et al: Use of corticosteroids to prevent progression of Graves' ophthalmopathy after radioiodine therapy for hyperthyroidism. N Engl J Med 321:1349-1352, 1989.
170. Jensen BE, Bonnema SJ, Heqedus L: Glucocorticoids do not influence the effect of radioiodine therapy in Graves' disease. Eur J Endocrinol 153:13-14, 2005.
171. Kubota S, Ohye H, Nichihara E, et al: Effect of high-dose methylprednisolone pulse therapy followed by oral prednisolone administration of the production of anti-TSH receptor antibodies and clinical outcome in Graves' disease. Endocr J 52:735-741, 2005.
172. Bogazzi F, Bartalena L, Brogioni S, et al: Comparison of radioiodine with radioiodine plus lithium in the treatment of Graves' hyperthyroidism. J Clin Endocrinol Metab 84:499-503, 1999.
173. Bal CS, Kumar A, Pandey RM: A randomized controlled trial to evaluate the adjuvant effect of lithium on radioiodine treatment of hyperthyroidism. Thyroid 12:399-405, 2002.
174. Barrio R, Lopez-Capape M, Martinez-Badas I, et al: Graves' disease in children and adolescents: Response to long-term treatment. Acta Paediatr 94:1583-1589, 2005.

175. Winsa B, Rastad J, Larsson E, et al: Total thryoidectomy in therapy-resistant Graves' disease. Surgery 116:1068-1074, 1994.
176. Weber KJ, Solorzano CC, Lee JK, et al: Thyroidectomy remains an effective treatment option for Graves' disease. Am J Surg 191:400-405, 2006.
177. Martin A, Goldsmith NK, Friedman EW, et al: Intrathyroidal accumulation of T cell phenotypes in autoimmune thyroid disease. Autoimmunity 6:269-281, 1990.
178. Patwardhan NA, Monont M, Rao S, et al: Surgery still has a role in Graves' hyperthyroidism. Surgery 114:1108-1112, 1993.
179. Ozoux JP, de Calan L, Portier G, et al: Surgical treatment of Graves' disease. Am J Surg 156:177-181, 1988.
180. Sugino K, Mimura T, Toshima K, et al: Follow-up evaluation of patients with Graves' disease treated by subtotal thyroidectomy and risk factor analysis for post-operative thyroid dysfunction. J Endocrinol Invest 16:195-199, 1993.
181. Cusick EL, Krukowski ZH, Matheson NA: Outcome of surgery for Graves' disease re-examined. Br J Surg 74:780-783, 1987.
182. Reid DJ: Hyperthyroidism and hypothyroidism complicating the treatment of thyrotoxicosis. Br J Surg 74:1060-1062, 1987.
183. Hedley AJ, Bewsher PD, Jones SJ, et al: Late onset hypothyroidism after subtotal thyroidectomy for hyperthyroidism: Implications for long term follow-up. Br J Surg 70:740-743, 1983.
184. Sugino K, Mimura T, Ozaki O, et al: Early recurrence of hyperthyroidism in patients with Graves' disease treated by subtotal thyroidectomy. World J Surg 19:648-652, 1995.
185. Sugrue DD, Drury MI, McEvoy M, et al: Long term follow-up of hyperthyroid patients treated with subtotal thyroidectomy. Br J Surg 70:408-411, 1983.
186. Palit TK, Miller CC, Miltenburg DM: The efficacy of thyroidectomy for Graves' disease: A meta-analysis. J Surg Res 90:161-165, 2000.
187. Gaujoux S, Leenhardt L, Tresallet C, et al: Extensive thyroidectomy in Graves' disease. J Am Coll Surg 202:868-873, 2006.
188. Lal G, Ituarte P, Kebebew E, et al: Should total thyroidectomy become the preferred procedure for surgical management of Graves' disease? Thyroid 15:569-574, 2005.
189. Ku CE, Lo CY, Chan WF, et al: Total thryoidectomy replaces subtotal thyroidectomy as the preferred surgical treatment for Graves' disease. ANZ J Surg 75:528-531, 2005.
190. Inabnet WB 3rd, Jacob BP, Gagner M: Minimally invasive endoscopic thyroidectomy by cervical approach. Surg Endosc 17:1808-1811, 2003.
191. Maeda S, Uga T, Hayashida N, et al: Video-assisted subtotal or near-total thyroidectomy for Graves' disease. Br J Surg 93:61-66, 2006.
192. Takami HE, Ikeda Y: Minimally invasive thyroidectomy. Curr Opin Oncol 18:43-47, 2006.
193. Change DC, Wheeler MH, Woodcock JP, et al: The effect of preoperative Lugol's iodine on thyroid blood flow in patients with Graves' hyperthyroidism. Surgery 102:1055-1061, 1987.
194. Rangaswamy M, Padhy AK, Gopinath PG, et al: Effect of Lugol's iodine on vascularity of thyroid gland in hyperthyroidism. Nucl Med Commun 10:679-684, 1989.
195. Coyle PJ, Mitchell JE: Thyroidectomy: Is Lugol's iodine necessary? Ann R Coll Surg Engl 64:334-335, 1982.
196. Gerst PH, Fildes J, Baylor P, Zonszein J: Long-acting beta-adrenergic antagonists as preparation for surgery in thyrotoxicosis. Arch Surg 121:838-840, 1986.
197. Lee KS, Kim K, Hur KB, Kim CK: The role of propranolol in the preoperative preparation of patients with Graves' disease. Surg Gynecol Obstet 162:365-369, 1986.
198. Peden NR, Browning MC, Feely J, et al: The clinical and metabolic responses to early surgical treatment for hyperthyroid Graves' disease: A comparison of three pre-operative treatment regimens. QJ Med 56:579-591, 1985.
199. Feek CM, Sawers JS, Irvine WJ, et al: Combination of potassium iodide and propranolol in preparation of patients with Graves' disease for thyroid surgery. N Engl J Med 302:883-885, 1980.
200. Tevaarwerk GJ, Boyd D: Propranolol in thyrotoxicosis: II. Serum thyroid hormone concentrations during subtotal thyroidectomy. Can J Surg 22:264-266, 1979.
201. Panzer C, Beazley R, Braverman L: Rapid preoperative preparation for severe hyperthyroid Graves' disease. J Clin Endocrinol Metab 89:2142-2144, 2004.
202. Baeza A, Aquavo J, Barria M, Pineda G: Rapid preoperative preparation in hyperthyroidism. Clin Endocrinol (Oxf) 35:439-442, 1991.
203. Wiersinga WM, Bartalena L: Epidemiology and prevention of Graves' ophthalmopathy. Thyroid 12:855-860, 2002.
204. Ozgen A, Alp MN, Ariyurek M, et al: Quantitative CT of the orbit in Graves' disease. Br J Radiol 72:757-762, 1999.
205. Burch HB, Wartofsky L: Graves' ophthalmopathy: Current concepts regarding pathogenesis and management. Endocrin Rev 14:747-793, 1993.
206. Bartley GB: The epidemiologic characteristics and clinical course of ophthalmopathy associated with autoimmune thyroid disease in Olmsted County, Minnesota. Trans Am Ophthalmol Soc 92:477-588, 1994.
207. Perros P, Crombie AL, Matthews JN, et al: Age and gender influence the severity of thyroid-associated ophthalmopathy: A study of 101 patients attending a combined thyroid-eye clinic. Clin Endocrinol (Oxf) 38:367-372, 1993.

208. Perros P, Crombie AL, Kendall-Taylor P: Natural history of thyroid associated ophthalmopathy. Clin Endocrinol (Oxf) 42:45-50, 1995.
209. Noth D, Gebauer M, Muller B, et al: Graves' ophthalmopathy: Natural history and treatment outcomes. Swiss Med Wkly 131:603-609, 2001.
210. Vestergaard P: Smoking and thyroid disorders—a meta-analysis. Eur J Endocrinol 146:153-161, 2002.
211. Shine B, Fells P, Edwards OM, Weetman AP: Association between Graves' ophthalmopathy and smoking. Lancet 335:1251-1253, 1990.
212. Pummel MF, Wiersinga WM: Smoking and risk of Graves' disease. JAMA 269:479-482, 1993.
213. Bartalena L, Marcocci C, Tanda ML, et al: Cigarette smoking and treatment outcomes in Graves' ophthalmopathy. Ann Intern Med 129:632-635, 1998.
214. Argentin G, Cicchetti R: Evidence for the role of nitric oxide in antiapoptotic and genotoxic effect of nicotine on human gingival fibroblasts. Apoptosis 11:1887-1897, 2006.
215. Karadimas P, Bouzas EA, Mastorakos G: Advice against smoking is not effective in patients with Graves' ophthalmopathy. Acta Med Austriaca 30:59-60, 2003.
216. Villanueva R, Inzerillo AM, Tomer Y, et al: Limited genetic susceptibility to severe Graves' ophthalmopathy: No role for CTLA-4 but evidence for an environmental cause. Thyroid 10:791-798, 2000.
217. Bartalena L, Marcocci C, Pinchera A: Graves' ophthalmopathy: A preventable disease? Eur J Endocrinol 146:457-461, 2002.
218. Garrity JA, Bahn RS: Pathogenesis of Graves' ophthalmopathy: Implications for prediction, prevention, and treatment. Am J Ophthalmol 142:147-153, 2006.
219. McGregor AM: Has the autoantigen for Graves' ophthalmopathy been found? Lancet 352:595-596, 1998.
220. Smith TJ, Bahn RS, Gorman CA, Cheavens M: Stimulation of glycosaminoglycan accumulation by interferon-gamma in cultured human retroocular fibroblasts. J Clin Endocrinol Metab 72: 1169-1171, 1991.
221. Sorisky A, Pardasani D, Gagnon A, Smith TJ: Evidence of adipocyte differentiation in human orbital fibroblasts in primary culture. J Clin Endocrinol Metab 81:3428-3431, 1996.
222. Prummel MF, Wiersinga WM, Mourits MP, et al: Effect of abnormal thyroid function on the severity of Graves' ophthalmopathy. Arch Intern Med 150:1098-1101, 1990.
223. Eckstein AK, Plicht M, Lax H, et al: TSH receptor autoantibodies are independent risk factors for Graves' ophthalmopathy and help to predict severity and outcome of the disease. J Clin Endocrinol Metab 91:3464-3470, 2006.
224. Marcocci C, Bartalena L, Bogazzi F, et al: Relationship between Graves' ophthalmopathy and type of treatment of Graves' hyperthyroidism. Thyroid 2:171-178, 1992.
225. Marcocci C, Bruno-Bossio G, Manetti L, et al: The course of Graves' ophthalmopathy is not influenced by near total thyroidectomy: A case-control study. Clin Endocrinol 51:503-506, 1999.
226. Jarhult J, Rudberg C, Larsson E, et al: Graves' disease with moderate-severe endocrine ophthalmopathy—long-term results of a prospective, randomized, study of total or subtotal thyroid resection. Thyroid 15:1157-1164, 2005.
227. DeGroot L: Radioiodine and the immune system. Thyroid 7:259-264, 1997.
228. Moleti M, Mattina F, Salamone I, et al: Effects of thyroidectomy alone or followed by radioiodine ablation of thyroid remnants on the outcome of Graves' ophthalmopathy. Thyroid 13:653-658, 2003.
229. Chiovato L, Latrofa F, Braverman LE, et al: Disappearance of humoral thyroid autoimmunity after complete removal of thyoid antigens. Ann Intern Med 139:346-351, 2003.
230. Oertli D: Graves' ophthalmopathy. Swiss Med Wkly 132:48, 2002.
231. McGregor AM, McLachlan SM, Smith BR, Hall R: Effect of irradiation on thyroid-autoantibody production. Lancet 2:442-444, 1979.
232. Harvey RD, Metcalfe RA, Morteo C, et al: Acute pretibial myxoedema following radioiodine therapy for thyrotoxic Graves' disease. Clin Endocrinol 42:657-660, 1995.
233. Tallstedt L, Lundell G, Blomgren H, Bring J: Does early administration of thyroxine reduce the development of Graves' ophthalmopathy after radioiodine treatment? Eur J Endocrinol 130:494-7, 1994.
234. Werner S: Classification of the eye changes of Graves' disease. J Clin Endocrinol Metab 29:982-984, 1969.
235. Bartalena L, Pinchera A, Marcocci C: Management of Graves' ophthalmopathy: Reality and perspectives. Endocr Rev 21:168-199, 2000.
236. Mourits MP, Koornneef L, Wiersinga WM, et al: Clinical criteria for the assessment of disease activity in Graves' ophthalmopathy: A novel approach. Br J Ophthalmol 73:639-644, 1989.
237. Pinchera A, Wiersinga W, Glinoer D, et al: Classification of eye changes of Graves' disease. Thyroid 2:235-236, 1992.
238. Mourits MP, Prummel MF, Wiersinga WM, Koornneef L: Clinical activity score as a guide in the management of patients with Graves' ophthalmopathy. Clin Endocrinol (Oxf) 47:9-14, 1997.
239. Smith TJ: Dexamethasone regulation of glycosaminoglycan synthesis in cultured human skin fibroblasts. J Clin Invest 74:2157-2164, 1984.
240. Kinsell LW, Partridge JW, Foreman N: The use of ACTH and cortisone in the treatment and the differential diagnosis of malignant exophthalmos: A preliminary report. Ann Intern Med 38:913-917, 1953.

241. Werner SC: Prednisone in emergency treatment of malignant exophthalmos. Lancet 1:10004-10007, 1966.
242. Day RM, Carroll FD: Corticosteroids in the treatment of optic nerve involvement associated with thyroid dysfunction. Arch Ophthalmol 79:279-282, 1968.
243. Nagayama Y, Izumi M, Kiriyama T, et al: Treatment of Graves' ophthalmopathy with high-dose intravenous prednisolone pulse therapy. Acta Endocrinol 116:513-518, 1987.
244. Kendall-Taylor P, Crombie AL, Stephenson AM, et al: Intravenous methylprednisolone in the treatment of Graves' ophthalmopathy. BMJ 297:1574-1578, 1988.
245. Hiromatsu Y, Tanaka K, Sato M, et al: Intravenous methylprednisolone pulse therapy for Graves' ophthalmopathy. Endocr J 40:63-72, 1993.
246. Matejka G, Verges B, Vaillant G, et al: Intravenous methylprednisolone pulse therapy in the treatment of Graves' ophthalmopathy. Horm Metab Res 30:93-98, 1998.
247. Kahaly GJ, Pitz S, Hommel G, Dittmar M: Randomized, single blind trial of intravenous versus oral steroid monotherapy in Graves' orbitopathy. J Clin Endocrinol Metab 90:5234-5240, 2005.
248. Marcocci C, Bartalena L, Tanda ML: Comparison of the effectiveness and tolerability of intravenous or oral glucocorticoids associated with orbital radiotherapy in the management of severe Graves' ophthalmopathy: Results of a prospective, single-blind, randomized study. J Clin Endocrinol Metab 86:3562-3567, 2001.
249. Ebner R, Devoto MH, Bordaberry M, et al: Treatment of thyroid-associated ophthalmopathy with periocular injections of triamcinolone. Br J Ophthalmol 88:1380-1386, 2004.
250. Marcocci C, Bartalena L, Panicucci M, et al: Orbital cobalt irradiation combined with retrobulbar or systemic corticosteroids for Graves' ophthalmopathy: A comparative study. Clin Endocrinol (Oxf) 27:33-42, 1987.
251. Perros P, Kendall-Taylor P: Medical treatment for thyroid-associated ophthalmopathy. Thyroid 12:241-244, 2002.
252. Marcocci C, Bartalena L, Rocchi R, et al: Long-term safety of orbital radiotherapy for Graves' ophthalmopathy. J Clin Endocrinol Metab 88:3561-3566, 2003.
253. Kinyoun JL, Kalina RE, Brower SA, et al: Radiation retinopathy after orbital irradiation for Graves' ophthalmopathy. Arch Ophthalmol 102:1473-1476, 1984.
254. Wakelkamp IM, Tan H, Saeed P, et al: Orbital irradiation for Graves' ophthalmopathy: Is it safe? A long-term follow-up study. Ophthalmology 111:1557-1562, 2004.
255. Schaefer U, Hesselmann S, Micke O, et al: A long-term follow-up study after retro-orbital irradiation for Graves' ophthalmopathy. Int J Radiat Oncol Biol Phys 52:192-197, 2002.
256. Prummel MF, Terwee CB, Gerding MN, et al: A randomized controlled trial of orbital radiotherapy versus sham irradiation in patients with mild Graves' ophthalmopathy. J Clin Endocrinol Metab 89:15-20, 2004.
257. Mourits MP, van Kempen-Harteveld ML, Garcia MB, et al: Radiotherapy for Graves' orbitopathy: Randomized placebo-controlled study. Lancet 355:1505-1509, 2000.
258. Kahaly GJ, Rosler HP, Pitz S, Hommel G: Low-versus high-dose radiotherapy for Graves' ophthalmopathy: A randomized, single blind trial. J Clin Endocrinol Metab 85:102-108, 2000.
259. Prummel MF, Mourits MP, Blank L, et al: Randomized double-blind trial of prednisone versus radiotherapy in Graves' ophthalmopathy. Lancet 342:949-954, 1993.
260. Gorman CA: Radiotherapy for Graves' ophthalmopathy: Results at one year. Thyroid 12:251-255, 2002.
261. Gorman CA, Garrity JA, Fatourechi V, et al: A prospective, randomized, double-blind, placebo-controlled study of orbital radiotherapy for Graves' ophthalmopathy. Ophthalmology 108:1523-1534, 2001.
262. Marcocci C, Bartalena L, Bogazzi F, et al: Orbit radiotherapy combined with high-dose systemic glucocorticoids for Graves' ophthalmopathy is more effective than radiotherapy alone: Results of a prospective randomized study. J Endocrinol Invest 14:853-860, 1991.
263. Ohtsuka K, Sato A, Kawaguchi S, et al: Effect of steroid pulse therapy with and without orbital radiotherapy on Graves' ophthalmopathy. Am J Ophthalmol 135:285-290, 2003.
264. Rose JG, Burkat CN, Boxrud CA: Diagnosis and management of thyroid orbitopathy. Otolaryngol Clin North Am 38:1043-1074, 2005.
265. Boulos PR, Hardi I: Thyroid-associated orbitopathy: A clinicopathologic and therapeutic review. Curr Opin Ophthalmol 15:389-400, 2004.
266. Adenis JP, Robert PY, Lasundry JG, Dolloul Z: Treatment of proptosis with fat removal orbital decompression in Graves' ophthalmopathy. Eur J Ophthalmol 8:246-252, 1998.
267. Goh MS, McNab AA: Orbital decompression in Graves' orbitopathy: Efficacy and safety. Intern Med J 35:586-591, 2005.
268. Coats DK, Paysse EA, Plager DA, Wallace DK: Early strabismus surgery for thyroid ophthalmopathy. Ophthalmology 106:324-329, 1999.
269. Mourits MP, Koorneef L, van Mourik-Noordenbos AM, et al: Extraocular muscle surgery for Graves' ophthalmopathy: Does prior treatment influence surgical outcome? Br J Ophthalmol 74:481-483, 1990.
270. Gair EJ, Lee JP, Khoo BK, Maurino V: What is the role of botulinum toxin in the treatment of dysthyroid strabismus? J AAPOS 3:272-274, 1999.

271. Shih MJ, Liao SL, Lu HY: A single transcutaneous injection with Botox for dysthyroid lid retraction. Eye 18:466-469, 2004.
272. Prummel MF, Mourits MP, Berghout A, et al: Prednisone and cyclosporine in the treatment of severe Graves' ophthalmopathy. N Engl J Med 321:1353-1359, 1989.
273. Kahaly G, Schrezenmeir J, Krause U, et al: Ciclosporin and prednisone v. prednisone in treatment of Graves' ophthalmopathy: A controlled, randomized and prospective study. Eur J Clin Invest 16:415-422, 1986.
274. Paridaens D, van den Bosch WA, van der Loos TL, et al: The effect of etanercept on Graves' ophthalmopathy: A pilot study. Eye 19:1286-1289, 2005.
275. Durrani OM, Reuser TO, Murray PI: Infliximab: A novel treatment for sight-threatening thyroid associated ophthalmopathy. Orbit 24:117-119, 2005.
276. Salvi M, Vannucchi G, Campi I, et al: Efficacy of rituximab treatment for thyroid-associated ophthalmopathy as a result of intraorbital B-cell depletion in one patient unresponsive to steroid immunosuppression. Eur J Endocrinol 154:511-517, 2006.
277. Kahaly G, Pitz S, Muller-Forell W, Hommel G: Randomized trial of intravenous immunoglobulins versus prednisolone in Graves' ophthalmopathy. Clin Exp Immunol 106:197-202, 1996.
278. Antonelli A, Saracino A, Alberti B, et al: High-dose intravenous immunoglobulin treatment in Graves' ophthalmopathy. Acta Endocrinol (Copenh) 126:13-23, 1992.
279. Baschieri L, Antonelli A, Nardi S, et al: Intravenous immunoglobulin versus corticosteroid in treatment of Graves' ophthalmopathy. Thryoid 7:579-585, 1997.
280. Seppel T, Schlagheche R, Becker A, et al: High-dose intravenous therapy with 7S immunoglobulins in autoimmune endocrine ophthalmopathy. Clin Exp Rheumatol 14(Suppl 15):S109-S114, 1996.
281. Glinoer D, Schrooyen M: Plasma exchange therapy for severe Graves' ophthalmopathy. Horm Res 26:184-189, 1987.
282. Kelly W, Longson D, Smithard D, et al: An evaluation of plasma exchange for Graves' ophthalmopathy. Clin Endocrinol (Oxf) 18:485-493, 1983.
283. Calao A, Lastoria S, Ferone D, et al: Orbital scintigraphy with [^{111}In-diethylenetriamine pentaacetic acid-D-phe1]-octreotide predicts the clinical response to corticosteroid therapy in patients with Graves' ophthalmopathy. J Clin Endocrinol Metab 83:3790-3794, 1998.
284. Chang TC, Liao SL: Slow-release lanreotide in Graves' ophthalmopathy: A double-blind randomized, placebo-controlled clinical trial. J Endocrinol Invest 29:413-422, 2006.
285. Wemeau JL, Caron P, Bechers A, et al: Octreotide (long-acting release formulation) treatment in patients with Graves' orbitopathy: Clinical results of a four-month, randomized, placebo-controlled, double-blind study. J Clin Endocrinol Metab 90:841-848, 2005.
286. Kahaly GJ: Recent developments in Graves' ophthalmopathy. J Endocrinol Invest 27:254-258, 2004.
287. Inzucchi S, Comite F, Burrow G: Graves' disease and pregnancy. Endocr Pract 1:186-192, 1995.
288. Linoer D, de Nayer P, Bourdoux P, et al: Regulation of maternal thyroid during pregnancy. J Clin Endocrinol Metab 71:276-287, 1990.
289. Tomer Y, Huber GK, Davies TF: Human chorionic gonadotropin (hCG) interacts directly with recombinant human TSH receptor. J Clin Endocrinol Metab 74:1477-1479, 1992.
290. Poppe K, Velkeniers B: Female infertility and the thyroid. Best Pract Res Clin Endocrinol Metab 18:153-165, 2004.
291. Anselmo J, Cao D, Karrison T, et al: Fetal loss associated with excess thyroid hormone exposure. JAMA 292:691-695, 2004.
292. Momotani N, Ito K, Hamada N, et al: Maternal hyperthyroidism and congenital malformations in the offspring. Clin Endocrinol 20:695-700, 1984.
293. Davis LE, Lucas MJ, Hankins GDV, et al: Thyrotoxicosis complicating pregnancy. Am J Obster Gynecol 160:63-70, 1989.
294. Shah MS, Davies TF, Stagnaro-Green A: The thyroid during pregnancy: A physiological and pathological stress test. Minerv Endocrinol 28:233-245, 2003.
295. González-Jiménez A, Fernández-Soto ML, Escobar-Jiménez F, et al: Thyroid function parameters and TSH-receptor antibodies in healthy subjects and Graves' disease patients: A sequential study before, during and after pregnancy. Thyroidology 5:13-20, 1993.
296. Gorman CA: Radioiodine and pregnancy. Thyroid 9:721-726, 1999.
297. Marchant B, Brownlie BE, Hart DM, et al: The placental transfer of propylthiouracil, methimazole and carbimazole. J Clin Endocrinol Metab 45:1187-1193, 1977.
298. Wing DA, Millar LK, Koonings PP, et al: A comparison of propylthiouracil versus methimazole in the treatment of hyperthyroidism in pregnancy. Am J Obstet Gynecol 170:90-95, 1994.
299. Milham S: Scalp defects in infants of mothers treated for hyperthyroidism with methimazole or cabimazole during pregnancy. Teratology 32:321, 1985.
300. Foulds N, Walpole I, Elmslie F, Mansour S: Carbimazole embryopathy: An emerging phenotype. Am J Med Genet A 132:130-135, 2005.
301. Petit KP, Nielsen HC: Chronic in utero beta-blockade alters fetal lung development. Dev Pharmacol Ther 19:131-140, 1992.
302. Ray JG, Vermeulen MJ, Burrows EA, Burrows RF: Use of antihypertensive medications in pregnancy and the risk of adverse perinatal outcomes: McMaster Outcome Study of Hypertension in Pregnancy 2 (MOS HIP 2). BMC Pregnancy Childbirth 1:6, 2001.
303. Jamieson A, Semple CG: Successful treatment of Graves' disease in pregnancy with Lugol's iodine. Scot Med J 85:536-539, 2000.

304. Klein RZ, Sargent JD, Larsen PR, et al: Relation of severity of maternal hypothyroidism to cognitive development of offspring. J Med Screen 7:127-130, 2000.
305. Haddow ME, Palomaki GE, Allan WC, et al: Maternal thyroid deficiency during pregnancy and subsequent neuropsychological development of the child. N Engl J Med 341:549-555, 1999.
306. Momotani N, Noh J, Oyanagi H, et al: Antithyroid drug therapy for Graves' disease during pregnancy. Optimal regimen for fetal thyroid status. N Engl J Med 315:24-28, 1986.
307. Hamburger JI: Diagnosis and management of Graves' disease in pregnancy. Thyroid 2:219-224, 1992.
308. Mandel SJ, Cooper DS: The use of antithyroid drugs in pregnancy and lactation. J Clin Endocrinol Metab 86:1853-1860, 2001.
309. Clavel S, Madec AM, Bornet H, et al: Anti TSH-receptor antibodies in pregnant patients with autoimmune thyroid disorder. Br J Obstet Gynaecol 11:1003-1008, 1990.
310. Tamaki H, Amino N, Aozasa M, et al: Universal predictive criteria for neonatal over thyrotoxicosis requiring treatment. Am J Perinatol 5:152-158, 1988.
311. Kung AW, Jones BM: A change from stimulatory to blocking antibody activity in Graves' disease during pregnancy. J Clin Endocrinol Metab 83:514-518, 1998.
312. Connors MH, Styne DM: Transient neonatal 'athyreosis' resulting from TSH-binding inhibitory immunoglobulins. Pediatrics 78:287-290, 1986.
313. Brown RS, Bellisario RL, Botero D, et al: Incidence of transient congenital hypothyroidism due to maternal TSH receptor-blocking antibodies in over one million babies. J Clin Endocrinol Metab 81:1147-1151, 1996.
314. Luton D, Le Gac I, Vuillard E, et al: Management of Graves' disease during pregnancy: The key role of fetal thyroid gland monitoring. J Clin Endocrinol Metab 90:6093-6098, 2005.
315. Cohen O, Pinhas-Hamiel O, Sivan E, et al: Serial in utero ultrasonographic measurements of the fetal thyroid: A new complementary tool in the management of maternal hyperthyroidism during pregnancy. Pregnat Diagn 23:740-742, 2003.
316. McNab T, Ginsberg J: Use of anti-thyroid drugs in euthyroid pregnant women with previous Graves' disease. Clin Invest Med 28:127-131, 2005.
317. Benhaim Rochester D, Davies TF: Increased risk of Graves' disease after pregnancy. Thyroid 15:1287-1290, 2005.
318. Nakagawa Y, Mori K, Hoshikawa S, et al: Postpartum recurrence of Graves' hyperthyroidism can be prevented by the continuation of antithyroid drugs during pregnancy. Clin Endocrinol (Oxf) 57:467-471, 2002.
319. Momotani N, Noh J, Ishikawa N, Ito K: Relationship between silent thyroiditis and recurrent Graves' disease in the postpartum period. J Clin Endocrinol Metab 79:285-289, 1994.
320. American Academy of Pediatrics Committee on Drugs: Transfer of drugs and other chemical into human milk. Pediatrics 108:776-789, 2001.
321. Burch HB, Wartofsky L: Life-threatening thyrotoxicosis. Thyroid storm. Endocrinol Metab Clin North Am 22:263-277, 1993.
322. Brooks MH, Waldstein SS, Bronsky D, Sterling K: Serum triiodothyronine concentration in thyroid storm. J Clin Endocrinol Metab 40:339-341, 1975.
323. Henderson JM, Portmann L, Van Melle G, et al: Propranolol as an adjunct therapy for hyperthyroid tremor. Eur Neurol 37:182-185, 1997.
324. Olson BR, Klein I, Benner R, et al: Hyperthyroid myopathy and the response to treatment. Thyroid 1:137-141, 1991.
325. Grossman W, Robin NI, Johnson LW, et al: Effects of beta blockade on the peripheral manifestations of thyrotoxicosis. Ann Intern Med 74:875-879, 1971.
326. Harrower AD, Fyffe JA, Horn DB, Strong JA: Thyroxine and triiodothyronine levels in hyperthyroid patients during treatment with propranolol. Clin Endocrinol (Oxf) 7:41-44, 1977.
327. Jones MK, Birtwell J, Owens DR, et al: Beta-adrenoreceptor blocking drugs and thyroid hormones in hyperthyroid subjects. Postgrad Med J 57:207-209, 1981.
328. McDevitt DG, Nelson JK: Comparative trial of atenolol and propranolol in hyperthyroidism. Br J Clin Pharmacol 6:233-237, 1978.
329. Georges LP, Santangelo RP, Mackin JF, Canary JJ: Metabolic effects of propranolol in thryotoxicosis. I. Nitrogen, calcium, and hydroxyproline. Metabolism 1:11-21, 1975.
330. Lin SH, Lin YF: Propranolol rapidly reverses paralysis, hypokalemia, and hypophosphatemia in thyrotoxic periodic paralysis. Am J Kidney Dis 37:620-623, 2001.
331. Feely J: Propranolol and the hypercalcaemia of thyrotoxicosis. Acta Endocrinol (Copenh) 98:528-532, 1981.
332. Milner MR, Gelman KM, Phillips RA, et al: Double-blind crossover trial of diltiazem versus propranolol in the management of thyrotoxic symptoms. Pharmacotherapy 12:100-106, 1990.
333. Emerson CH, Anderson AJ, Howard WJ, et al: Serum thyroxine and triidothyronine concentrations during iodide treatment of hyperthyroidism. J Clin Endocrinol Metab 40:33-36, 1975.
334. Robuschi G, Manfredi A, Salvi M, et al: Effect of sodium ipodate and iodide on free T4 and free T3 concentrations in patients with Graves' disease. J Endocrinol Invest 9:287-291, 1986.
335. Wartofsky L, Ransil BJ, Ingbar SH: Inhibition by iodine of the release of thyroxine from the thyroid glands of patients with thyrotoxicosis. J Clin Invest 49:78-86, 1970.
336. Roti E, Robuschi G, Manfredi A, et al: Comparative effects of sodium ipodate and iodide on serum thyroid hormone concentrations in patients with Graves' disease. Clin Endocrinol (Oxf) 22:489-496, 1985.

337. Wolff J, Chaikoff IL: The inhibitory action of excess iodide upon the synthesis of diiodotyrosine and of thyroxine in the normal rat. Endocrinology 43:174-179, 1948.
338. Bános C, Takó J, Salamon F, et al: Effect of ACTH-stimulated glucocorticoid hypersecretion on the serum concentrations of thyroxine-binding globulin, thyroxine, triiodothyronine, reverse triiodothyronine and on the TSH-response to TRH. Acta Med Acad Sci Hung 36:381-394, 1979.
339. Williams DE, Chopra IJ, Orgiazzi J, Solomon DH: Acute effects of corticosteroids on thyroid activity in Graves' disease. J Clin Endocrinol Metab 41:354-361, 1975.
340. Mori T, Sugawa H, Kosugi S, et al: Effectiveness of short-term steroid treatment on the reduction in goiter size in antithyroid drug-treated patients with Graves' disease. Endocr J 44:575-580, 1997.
341. Shen DC, Wu SY, Chopra IJ, et al: Long-term treatment of Graves' hyperthyroidism with sodium ipodate. J Clin Endocrinol Metab 61:723-727, 1985.
342. Wu SY, Chopra IJ, Solomon DH, Johnson DE: The effect of repeated administration of ipodate in hyperthyroidism. J Clin Endocrinol Metab 47:1358-1362, 1978.
343. Roti E, Robuschi G, Gardini E, et al: Comparison of methimazole, methimazole and sodium ipodate, and methimazole and saturated solution of potassium iodide in the early treatment of hyperthyroid Graves' disease. Clin Endocrinol (Oxf) 28:305-314, 1988.
344. Martino E, Balzano S, Bartalena L, et al: Therapy of Graves' disease with sodium ipodate is associated with high recurrence rate of hyperthyroidism. J Endocrinol 14:847-851, 1991.
345. Berens SC, Bernstein RS, Robbins J, Wolff J: Antithyroid effects of lithium. J Clin Invest 49:1357-1367, 1970.
346. Temple R, Berman M, Robbins J, Wolff J: The use of lithium in the treatment of thyrotoxicosis. J Clin Invest 51:2746-2756, 1972.
347. Kristensen O, Andersen HH, Pallisgaard G: Lithium carbonate in the treatment of thyrotoxicosis. A controlled trial. Lancet 1:603-605, 1976.
348. Solomon BL, Wartofsky L, Burman KD: Adjunctive cholestyramine therapy for thyrotoxicosis. Clin Endocrinol (Oxf) 38:39-43, 1993.
349. Tsai WC, Pei D, Wang TF, et al: The effect of combination therapy with propylthiouracil and cholestyramine in the treatment of Graves' hyperthyroidism. Clin Endocrinol (Oxf) 62:521-524, 2005.
350. Stanbury JB, Wyngaarden JB: Effect of perchlorate on the human thyroid gland. Metabolism 1:533-539, 1952.
351. Wenzel KW, Lente JR: Similar effects of thionamide drugs and perchlorate on thyroid-stimulating immunoglobulins in Graves' disease: Evidence against an immunosuppressive action of thionamide drugs. J Clin Endocrinol Metab 58:62-69, 1984.
352. Bartalena L, Wiersinga WM, Tanda ML, et al: Diagnosis and management of amiodarone-induced thyrotoxicosis in Europe: Results of an international survey among members of the European thyroid association. Clin Endocrinol (Oxf) 61:494-502, 2004.
353. Johnson RS, Moore WG: Fatal aplastic anaemia after treatment of thyrotoxicosis with potassium perchlorate. Br Med J 1:1369-1371, 1961.
354. Krevans JR: Asper SP Jr, Rienhoff WF JF: Fatal aplastic anemia following use of potassium perchlorate in thyrotoxicosis. JAMA 181:162-164, 1962.
355. Gjemdal N: Fatal aplastic anemia following use of potassium perchlorate in thyrotoxicosis. Acta Med Scand 174:129-131, 1963.
356. Jongiaroenprasert W, Akarawut W, Chantasart D, et al: Rectal administration of propylthiouracil in hyperthyroid patients: Comparison of suspension enema and suppository form. Thyroid 12:627-631, 2002.
357. Croxson MS, Hall TD, Nicoloff JT: Combination drug therapy for treatment of hyperthyroid Graves' disease. J Clin Endocrinol Metab 45:623-630, 1977.

Chapter 13

Thyroiditis

Masanobu Yamada, Tetsuro Satoh, and Koshi Hashimoto

Key Points

- Silent thyroiditis occurs during Hashimoto's thyroiditis or Graves' disease in remission; often occurs in postpartum women several months after delivery; thyrotoxicosis is usually mild; transient hypothyroidism may occur after thyrotoxicosis phase; rare patients have positive anti–thyroid-stimulating hormone receptor antibody.
- Subacute thyroiditis represents destructive thyroiditis; despite presence of thyrotoxicosis, radioactive iodine uptake suppressed in acute phase; following initial thyrotoxic phase, thyroid status generally falls into mild hypothyroidism, finally recovers to euthyroid; corticosteroids empirically effective for rapid relief of severe neck pain, should be gradually tapered to avoid early relapse.
- Acute supportive thyroiditis should be suspected in any febrile patient with acute, painful, anterior neck swelling; *Staphylococcus* and *Streptococcus* most often isolated; pyriform sinus fistula (PSF) difficult to detect, can lead to recurrent episodes; antimicrobial therapy can lead to complete cure but in presence of PSF, surgical excision required; immunocompromised hosts at high risk.

Thyrotoxicosis (hyperfunction) can be seen in some of the types of thyroiditis listed in Table 13-1. Thyroid pain and tenderness are characteristic features of subacute thyroiditis, but are rare in sporadic silent thyroiditis or postpartum thyroiditis. Thyrotoxicosis results from excessive release of thyroid hormone from the thyroid grand caused by the destructive changes of various types of thyroiditis. These disorders are therefore referred to as destruction-induced thyrotoxicosis. Radioactive iodine uptake (RAIU) is depressed in the hyperthyroid phase of the disease. This situation contrasts markedly with the elevated RAIU in patients with Graves' disease. In the typical case, differential diagnosis can be performed (Fig. 13-1). However, these types of thyroiditis mimic other diseases as well as each other. Differentiation of the types of thyroiditis requires an understanding of their unique clinical presentations, radiologic studies, laboratory data, and indications for pharmacotherapy.

Acute exacerbation of Hashimoto's thyroiditis or painful chronic thyroiditis has also been reported to be associated with thyroid pain and fever, but only in rare cases. The three common thyroiditides with hyperfunction of the thyroid gland will be described in this chapter.

SILENT THYROIDITIS (SPORADIC AND POSTPARTUM THYROIDITIS)

Sporadic silent thyroiditis, also called painless thyroiditis or sporadic thyroiditis, and postpartum thyroiditis are frequent causes of transient thyrotoxicosis. Both are probably variants of the same disorder, and postpartum thyroiditis is essentially silent thyroiditis in the postpartum period.[1-4] Postpartum thyroiditis develops during the first 12 months postpartum in 5% to 9% of all women who have given birth.[5-8]

Thyrotoxicosis without pain of the thyroid gland and spontaneous improvement of thyrotoxicosis usually occur within 3 months. Differential diagnosis from other disorders showing thyroid dysfunction and appropriate treatment should be performed. Although silent thyroiditis is a temporary and benign disorder, it may easily be misdiagnosed, and some cases may evolve into permanent hypothyroidism.

Epidemiology, Risk Factors, and Pathogenesis

Silent thyroiditis occurs in women with an approximately a sevenfold higher rate than in men.[4,7] Two peaks of age are found, 20 to 30 and 40 to 50 years old. The former period coincides with the major period for pregnancy and delivery, and thus corresponds to postpartum thyroiditis; it comprises approximately

Table 13–1 Classification of Thyroiditis

Type	Also Known As
Hashimoto's thyroiditis	Chronic lymphocytic thyroiditis
Postpartum thyroiditis	Painless postpartum thyroiditis
Silent thyroiditis	Sporadic thyroiditis Painless thyroiditis
Subacute thyroiditis	Painful subcute thyroiditis, de Quervain's thyroiditis, giant cell thyroiditis
Acute suppurative thyroiditis	Infectious thyroiditis, pyogenic thyroiditis, bacterial thyroiditis
Drug-induced thyroiditis (amiodarone, lithium, interferon alfa, interleukin-2)	
Riedel's thyroiditis	Fibrous thyroiditis

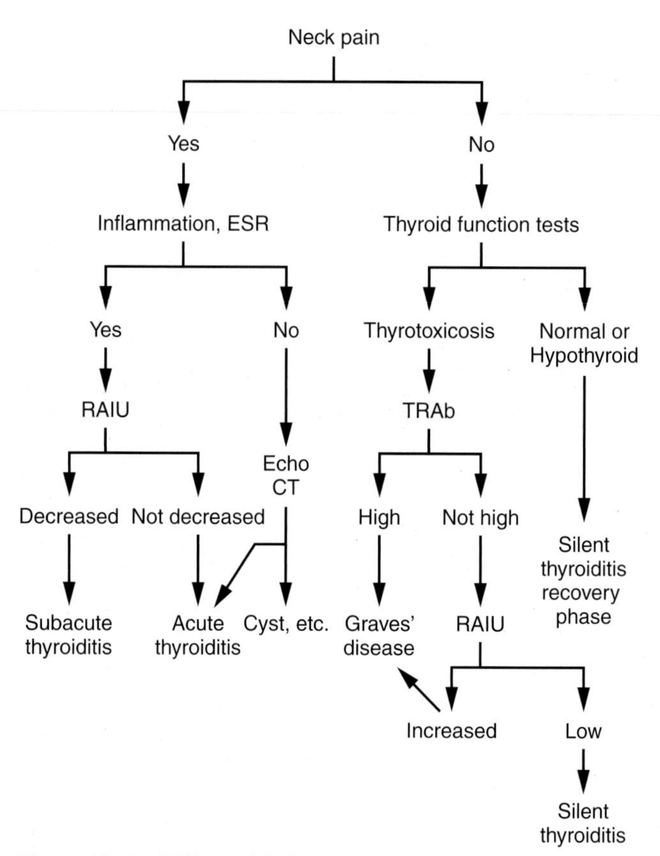

Figure 13–1 Differential diagnosis of thyroiditis. ESR, erythrocyte sedimentation rate; RAIU, radioactive iodine uptake; TRAb, thyroid-stimulating hormone (TSH) receptor antibody.

20% of all cases of silent thyroiditis. The latter is compatible with the peak of chronic thyroiditis. However, patients as young as 5 and as old as 93 years old have been reported. Some patients have been identified following an operation for Cushing's syndrome, after changing the dose or termination of glucocorticoid therapy, or after receiving interferon therapy for other disorders.[2,9,10]

There is abundant evidence that sporadic and postpartum thyroiditis are immunologically related diseases. Biopsy of the thyroid gland shows focal or diffuse extensive lymphocytic infiltration and collapsed follicles, degeneration of follicular cells, and multinucleated giant cells (Fig. 13-2A to E). About half of silent thyroiditis patients show lymphoid follicles. Unlike Hashimoto's thyroiditis, oxyphilic changes and severe fibrotic changes are absent. During the recovery phase, there are still lymphoid follicles and lymphocytic infiltration; however, no collapsed follicles or degeneration of follicular cells is observed (see Fig 13-2F). The histologic changes of postpartum thyroiditis are comparable to those of silent thyroiditis.

The mechanisms involved in the disruption of the thyroid gland and subsequent improvements remain unclear. However, many patients are positive for antithyroid antibody, and antithyroid peroxidase antibodies are present in almost all patients. Therefore, silent thyroiditis has been considered to develop from chronic thyroiditis (Hashimoto's disease) and is also found in patients with a history of Graves' disease.

During pregnancy, the maternal immune reaction is regulated to prevent rejection of the fetal allograft, and it returns to the normal immune state in the postpartum period. Therefore, gestation and the postpartum period are characterized by fluctuations in the immune response. Reflecting this situation, postpartum thyroiditis is accompanied by a significant elevation of circulating thyroid antibodies. It has recently been reported that fetal microchimerism may be a factor in developing postpartum thyroiditis.

Genes that confer a high degree of susceptibility to the development of sporadic or postpartum thyroiditis have not been identified. Several studies have demonstrated that human leukocyte antigen (HLA) haplotypes associated with autoimmune thyroid disease has also been found to be associated with silent thyroiditis and postpartum thyroiditis. For example, HLA-DR4, -DR5, and -DR3, in combination with HLA-A1 and -B8, have been reported to have a weak association with postpartum thyroiditis in certain populations.[11-14] The CTLA-4 gene polymorphism that is reported to be associated with Graves' disease and autoimmune hypothyroidism is negative in postpartum thyroiditis.[15]

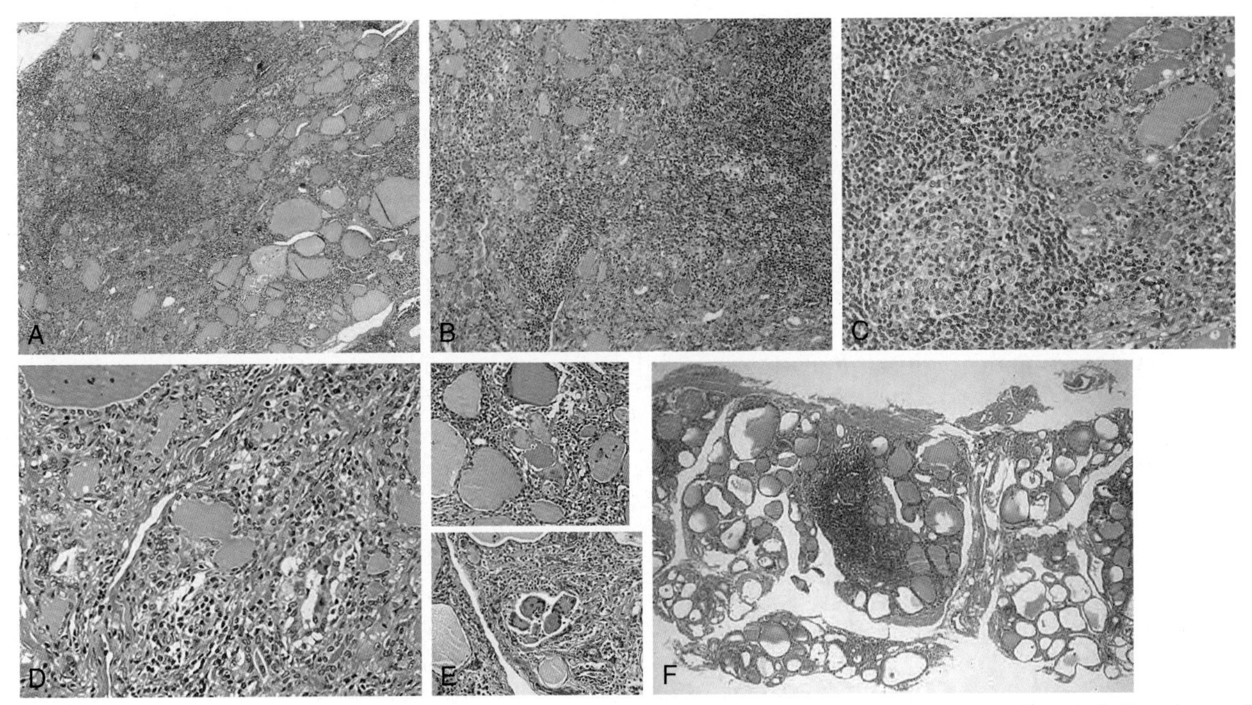

Figure 13–2 Histologic views of silent thyroiditis. **A-E,** Late thyrotoxic phase. **F,** Recovery phase. Lymphocytic infiltration and collapsed follicles are seen **(A-D),** as are giant cells **(E).** *(Courtesy Dr. Keiichi Kamijo, Thyroid Research Institution, Japan.)*

Clinical Features

The onset and severity of silent thyroiditis are variable. In one series, about 8% of patients were asymptomatic and were found by routine thyroid testing. In the acute phase, the thyroid follicles are collapsed, and thyroid hormones leak into the blood and cause thyrotoxicosis. Therefore, frequent symptoms are palpitations, shortness of breath, tachycardia, weight loss, fatigability, diarrhea, and sweating. In Asians, paresis is rarely observed. Because thyrotoxicosis occurs suddenly, some patients show anxiety and nervousness. Compared with Graves' disease, most of these symptoms of silent thyroiditis generally are mild and short term, but a small number of patients show severe thyrotoxicosis similar to that seen in Graves' disease.

Many patients go to the hospital after symptoms start to improve in the euthyroid or hypothyroid phase, so sometimes they have experienced a previous period with severe symptoms. This self-improvement and the short duration of the symptoms suggest silent thyroiditis. In the recovery phase, the patient may show symptoms of severe hypothyroidism, including fatigue, coldness, edema, and sometimes goiter.

The physical signs of silent thyroiditis are similar to those in thyrotoxicosis. However, unlike in Graves' disease, exophthalmos, localized myxedema, and thyroid acropathy do not occur. The goiter is generally palpable, with slight to mild swelling in about half of patients.

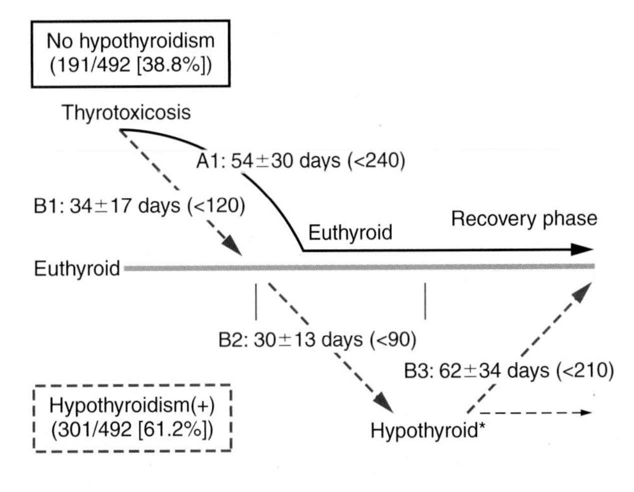

Figure 13–3 Clinical course of silent thyroiditis.

A schematic representation of the clinical course of silent thyroiditis is shown in Figure 13-3 (Dr. Keiichi Kamijo, personal communication, 2007).[16] Of 492 patients, 191 patients (38.8%) returned to the euthyroid phase without hypothyroidism, whereas 301 patients (61.2%) developed hypothyroidism following the thyrotoxicosis and euthyroid phases. The duration of the thyrotoxicosis phase was variable, but was usually 54 ± 30 days (240 days maximum) in the patients who did not develop a hypothyroid phase and 34 ± 17 days (120 days maximum) in patients who developed hypothyroidism. Intriguingly, this difference of duration was significant. The euthyroid period lasted 30 ± 13 days (90 days maximum). The hypothyroid interval lasted 62 ± 34 days (210 days maximum). However, 42 of the 301 patients developed permanent hypothyroidism (14.0%). In another study, 30% of patients with silent thyroiditis and subacute thyroiditis developed a hypothyroid phase.[7,12,17] It has also been reported that half of patients who have an episode of silent thyroiditis eventually develop permanent thyroid disease.

In postpartum thyroiditis, transient thyrotoxicosis presents at about postpartum week 14, followed by transient hypothyroidism at a median of 19 weeks.[4] Postpartum thyroiditis is almost always associated with the presence of antithyroid antibodies, usually anti–thyroid peroxidase (TPO) antibodies that rise in titer after postpartum week 6. Conversely, thyroid dysfunction occurs in up to 50% of the antibody-positive women. Of patients with thyroid dysfunction, 19% showed thyrotoxicosis alone, 49% hypothyroidism alone, and the remaining 32% were biphasic.

Diagnosis

Diagnosis is based on history, physical examination, and thyroid function tests. If a patient has Hashimoto's thyroiditis, physical examination generally reveals a firm, irregular, and nontender goiter.

In the thyrotoxic phase, serum thyroid hormone levels, including free thyroxine (T_4) and free triiodothyronine (T_3) are elevated, and the serum thyroid-stimulating hormone (TSH) level is decreased. Compared to that in Graves' disease, the elevation of serum thyroid hormones is generally mild. In typical cases, the serum T_4 level increases disproportionately relative to the serum T_3 level, and the T_3/T_4 ratio is lower than that in Graves' disease. However, it is difficult to distinguish silent thyroiditis from Graves' disease based only on the T_3/T_4 ratio.[18]

The serum thyroglobulin (TG) concentration may be high, reflecting destruction of thyroid follicules. Anti-TPO antibodies are high in about 60% and anti-TG antibodies in 25% of patients.[19] Although the anti-TSH receptor antibody is generally specific for Graves' disease, it is slightly elevated in approximately 5% to 10% of patients with sporadic thyroiditis. Conversely, negativity for this antibody, particularly when tested using a recently developed assay system, strongly suggests some disease other than Graves' disease.

Ultrasonography of the thyroid gland shows low blood flow, whereas in Graves' disease is very high. A bruit sound on the thyroid gland, eye symptoms, and other symptoms, including localized myxedema or acropachy, may be helpful for the differential diagnosis from Graves' disease. However, patients who have a history of Graves' disease sometimes have sporadic thyroiditis.

The most critical examination is ^{131}I or ^{99m}-Tc pertechnetate uptake (RAIU) in the thyroid grand. Whereas high and diffuse uptake in the thyroid grand is observed in Graves's disease, an extremely low uptake (generally less than 3%) is observed in silent thyroiditis. This examination should be done in the period with high serum thyroid hormone levels (thyrotoxic phase) and after stopping breast-feeding in postpartum thyroiditis.

There is no specific blood marker indicating sporadic thyroiditis. The erythrocyte sedimentation rate (ESR) and white blood cell count are generally normal. It has been reported that the zinc ion concentration in red blood cells and urine deoxypyridinoline and the ratio of eosinophils and monocytes may be useful for the diagnosis, but further studies are necessary to confirm this.[20]

Treatment

Treatment of many patients with silent thyroiditis may not be required. However, when the patient shows symptoms caused by severe thyrotoxicosis, acute symptoms can be managed with β-adrenergic blockers or sedatives.

It has also been reported that prednisone, 30 to 50 mg/day, decreases the size of the thyroid gland and the duration of the thyrotoxic phase to 7 to 10 days.[7,21] Although subtotal thyroidectomy or ^{131}I therapy for silent thyroiditis has also been reported, these modalities are not generally required.[22]

In severe thyrotoxicosis, sodium ipodate therapy, 500 mg/day, is effective for rapid control of the thyrotoxicosis by inhibiting peripheral deiodination of thyroxine and reducing the serum T_3 concentration.[23]

In the hypothyroidism phase, if the patient's symptoms are severe or of long duration, replacement of thyroid hormones such as levothyroxine may be indicated. However, as noted, most cases of hypothyroidism improve within 6 months, and it is therefore necessary to appropriately decrease dose and withdraw the drugs. When levothyroxine therapy is withdrawn, if the serum T_4 concentration falls and the serum TSH concentration rises, and hypothyroidism lasts for longer than 6 months, it is probably permanent. In such cases, thyroid hormone replacement therapy should be continued.

Clinical Course and Prevention

Sporadic thyroiditis sometimes relapses several months or years later.[24] Detailed analysis of patients has revealed that two thirds of the patients experienced relapse.[25] All patients should be followed at 1- to 2-year intervals for evidence of goiter or hypothyroidism. Women with postpartum thyroiditis have a 70% risk of developing the syndrome after a subsequent pregnancy. When a patient has repeated thyrotoxicosis, differential diagnosis with Graves' disease should be done each time. Conversely, when a patient with Graves' disease has repeated thyrotoxicosis, the possibility of sporadic thyroiditis should be considered.

Pitfalls, Complications, and Controversies

Patients with silent thyroiditis may receive inappropriate treatment such as an antithyroid drugs because of failure to recognize the disorder. Antithyroid drugs are not indicated for the management of patients with thyrotoxicosis, because the symptoms are caused by the release of thyroid hormone from the damaged thyroid grand.

SUBACUTE THYROIDITIS

Subacute thyroiditis (SAT) also referred to de Quervain's thyroiditis, giant cell thyroiditis, and subacute granulomatous thyroiditis, is a self-limited inflammatory thyroid disease usually lasting for weeks to several months.[26] SAT is the most common cause of painful thyroid in adults and may account for up to 5% of clinical thyroid abnormalities.[26] Common viral infection is highly suspected to be related to the pathogenesis of SAT. The clinical course of SAT is typically composed of three phases: (1) an initial thyrotoxic phase caused by the leakage of reserve thyroid hormone as a result of destruction of thyroid follicles; (2) a subsequent transient hypothyroid phase; and (3) the final recovery phase to euthyroid.

Epidemiology, Risk Factors, and Pathogenesis

SAT most often occurs between the second and fifth decades of life and appears to be rare in children and older adults.[26] As in autoimmune thyroid diseases, women are preferentially affected by SAT compared with men (female-to-male ratio, 5:1). SAT is the most common cause of tender thyroid glands in adults and may account for up to 5% of clinical thyroid abnormalities.[26] In all ethnic groups studied, there is obvious genetic susceptibility to SAT in patients who carry the histocompatibility antigen HLA Bw35.[26]

SAT is known to occur following infection of the upper respiratory tract and sometimes begins with a prodrome of viral infection. SAT has been reported to be associated with infection with several viruses, including mumps, measles, adenovirus, coxsackie, Epstein-Barr, parvovirus B19, and influenza viruses.[27] SAT has also been observed during interferon therapy of hepatitis B and C.[28,29] Although these clinical findings strongly suggest that SAT is caused by viral infection, conclusive evidence—for example, that specific viral pathogens have been directly isolated from the thyroid of SAT patients—is limited.[26] Familial and regional incidence of SAT appear to be rare, and there seem to be seasonal outbreaks in summer and autumn.[30]

Histopathologic findings of SAT are primarily destruction of the follicular epithelium and loss of follicular integrity.[26] The affected lesions show a patchy distribution, with noncaseous granulomas comprised of colloid, small lymphocytes, neutrophils, macrophages with or without epithelial features, and multinucleated giant cells of the foreign body type. Immunohistochemical studies of biopsy specimens have been reported.[31] These pathohistologic changes revert to normal, with minimal residual fibrosis, once the disease subsides.[26]

Clinical Features

SAT may be preceded by an upper respiratory tract infection and begins with a general prodrome of viral infection such as fatigue, malaise, low-grade fever, pharyngitis, myalgia, and arthralgia.[26] Fever occasionally reaches as high as 40° C. The severity of the anterior neck pain, as well as tenderness and enlargement of the thyroid gland, vary widely, depending on the case. In a few cases, neck pain is entirely absent.[26] The neck pain may initially occur in one lobe and later move to the opposite lobe (creeping thyroiditis). The pain may be exacerbated by turning the head, swallowing, or coughing, and may radiate to the jaw, ear, or occiput on the ipsilateral side. The affected thyroid gland can be palpated as a tender and firm nodular goiter or as a diffuse goiter when both glands are involved. Physical findings of thyrotoxicosis such as palpitation, finger tremor, and sweating may be present during the acute phase. The clinical features of SAT in children appear to be similar to those in adults.[32]

Diagnosis

Clinical diagnosis of SAT can be made by the presence of the following: (1) painful thyroid; (2) elevation of inflammatory parameters such as ESR and C-reactive protein (CRP); (3) thyrotoxicosis (elevated free T_4, with undetectable TSH) with suppressed RAIU by scintigraphy; and/or (4) maplike hypoechoic regions in affected thyroid glands by neck ultrasonography (US).[26] The ESR may be extremely accelerated and sometimes exceed 100 mm/hr, and CRP values may also be highly elevated in the acute phase.[26] The serum TG level may increase as a reflection of follicular destruction. The white blood cell count (WBC) may be normal or slightly elevated with no left shift in neutrophils.[26] The peripheral eosinophil-to-monocyte ratio is reported to be significantly lower in SAT patients compared with patients with Graves' disease.[33] Biochemical thyrotoxicosis is present in the acute phase in approximately 50% of SAT patients.[26] In contrast to Graves' disease, with a marked elevation of serum free T_3 compared with free T_4, the free T_3/T_4 ratio is reported to be significantly lower in SAT patients.[33] As a rule, antithyroid antibodies may be undetectable in SAT but, in some cases, weak elevation of anti-TG, anti-TPO, or anti-TSH receptor antibodies may be observed.[26] These autoantibodies may be generated in response to leakage of substantial thyroid antigens as a result of follicular destruction.[26] Typical findings in neck US may reveal varying degrees of irregular hypoechoic areas in the affected thyroid regions (Fig. 13-4).

These hypoechoic regions appear as low to normal vascularity by color flow Doppler US.[34] The diagnosis of SAT is confirmed by specific cytologic findings of biopsy specimens showing granuloma containing multinucleated giant cells, as noted.

Differential diagnosis should rule out other disorders involving anterior neck pain, including the following:

1. Acute suppurative thyroiditis
2. Hemorrhage into preexisting thyroid cyst or nodule
3. Acute exacerbation of (painful) Hashimoto's thyroiditis or
4. Thyroid malignancies such as anaplastic cancer and malignant lymphoma

Radiation- and drug (amiodarone)-induced thyroiditis and globus hystericus should also be excluded.[26] Computed tomography (CT) and magnetic resonance imaging (MRI) of the neck may be useful to rule out other thyroid disorders or conditions causing anterior neck pain.[35]

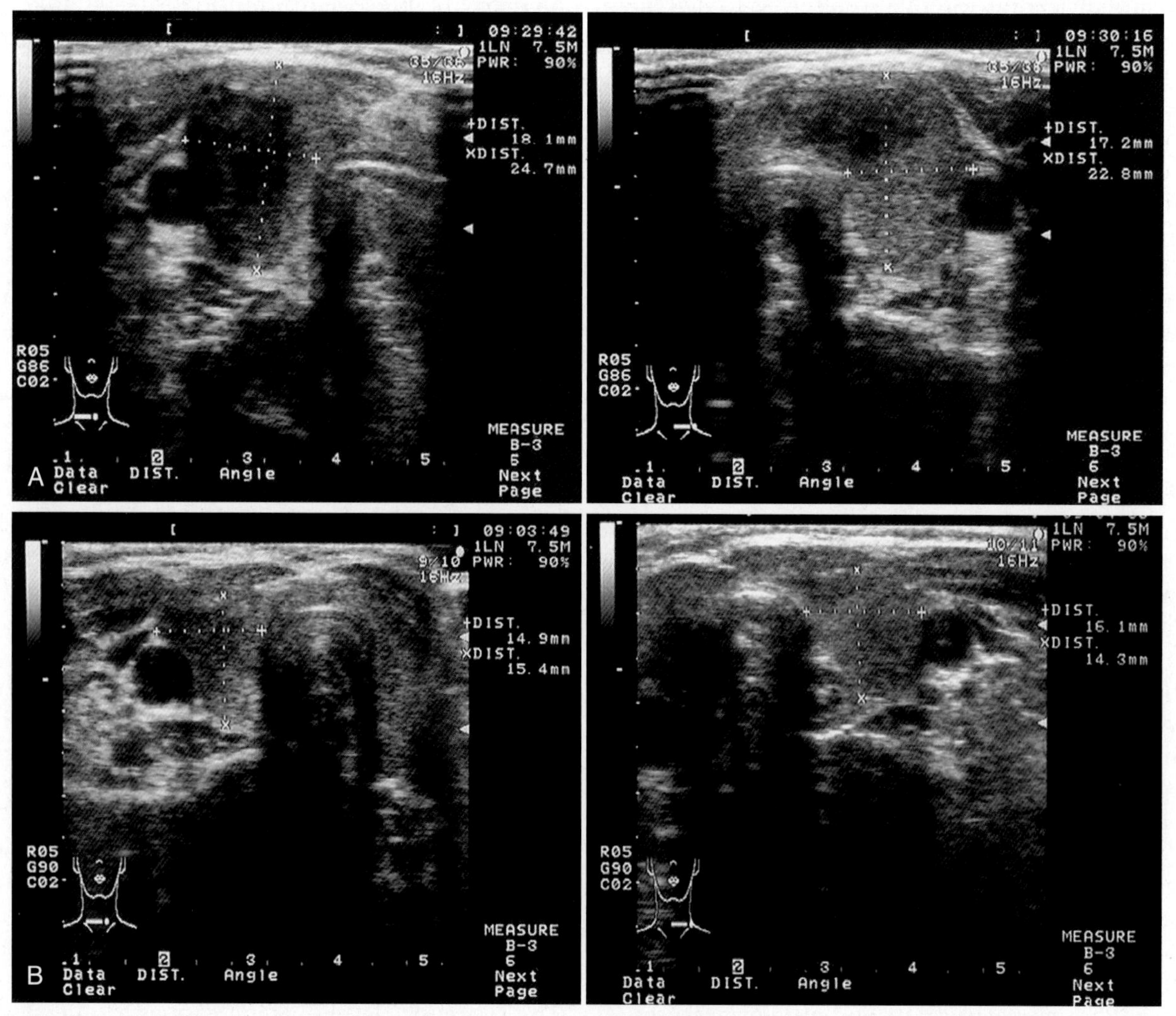

Figure 13–4 Neck findings in subacute thyroiditis (SAT) shown by ultrasonography (US). **A,** Initial US revealed swelling of both lobes and the presence of irregular hypoechoic regions. **B,** Same patient after a 2-week administration of prednisolone showed marked improvement of thyroid swelling and reduction of hypoechoic areas.

Treatment

It appears reasonable that treatment for SAT should aim for quick relief of thyroid inflammation and prevention of permanent hypothyroidism caused by massive destruction of the thyroid gland. However, because the pathogenesis of SAT has not yet been established, options of treatment for SAT are empirical. Neither antibiotics nor antithyroid drugs are useful for the treatment of SAT. To reduce mild to moderate anterior neck pain, salicylates and other nonsteroidal anti-inflammatory drugs (NSAIDs) may be adequate. For more severe neck pain associated with high fever, corticosteroid (prednisolone, 20 to 40 mg/day) may be administered. Corticosteroids may dramatically improve neck pain and general symptoms within 24 to 48 hours in most SAT cases. Because the initial levels of serum sialic acid, ESR, CRP, thyroglobulin, free T_3, and free T_4 in SAT patients appear not to be useful for predicting early relapse during corticosteroid therapy,[36] it is recommended that corticosteroids be gradually tapered, with cautious evaluation of physical symptoms, inflammatory markers, and US findings. Too rapid discontinuation of corticosteroids may result in early exacerbation of SAT and require repetitive administration of large doses of steroids.[26] Overall, corticosteroids may be effective for dramatic relief of symptoms, but may not prevent the development of transient hypothyroidism.[26]

Clinical Course and Prevention

The clinical courses of SAT is typically composed of three phases with respect to thyroid dysfunction—a first acute thyrotoxic phase caused by leakage of thyroid hormone from the destruction of thyroid follicles, a subsequent transient hypothyroid phase, and a final recovery phase to euthyroid. Thyrotoxic symptoms in the early phase may generally be milder than those in Graves' disease.[26] Transient hypothyroidism in the second phase lasting for several weeks to months may be mild and rarely requires replacement therapy with T_4.[26] Treatment with T_4 appears to be helpful for preventing early exacerbation of SAT.[27]

Pitfalls, Complications, and Controversies

Permanent hypothyroidism in SAT is relatively rare, but is reported to occur in up to 5% to 31% of cases.[37] Recurrence of SAT after long-term latency is also rare (4%). In addition, there have been rare case reports of Graves' disease occurring after SAT[38] and of thyroid storm caused by SAT.[39]

ACUTE SUPPURATIVE THYROIDITIS

Acute suppurative thyroiditis (AST), also known as acute infectious, bacterial, or pyogenic thyroiditis, is a rare disease. In most cases, it occurs in children or young people, in which the pyriform sinus fistula (PSF) is the most common route of infection.[40] The PSF is a congenital, third pharyngeal pouch remnant, which is hard to detect. Unless it is detected, it can cause recurrent AST.

Epidemiology, Risk Factors, and Pathogenesis

AST is a rare disorder; only about 300 and 100 cases have been reported in adults and children, respectively.[41-46] In most cases, AST occurs in adolescents or in those between 20 and 40 years of age.[47,48] There are no gender differences in AST. The thyroid gland is rarely infected because of its complete fibrous encapsulation, ample vascular and lymphatic supply, and high concentration of iodine and peroxidase in the gland.[44] Several potential routes of origin of thyroid infection have been suggested. The presence of previous thyroid disease, such as nodular goiter, adenoma, or carcinoma, is a predisposing factor for infection.[41] It has been reported that patients who have had previously diseased areas of the thyroid gland could be compromised hosts who are vulnerable to *Aspergillus* and *Pneumocystis jiroveci* (formerly called *P. carinii*) infection.[49,50] Other routes of infection are hematogenous or by direct spread from an adjacent site or thyroglossal cyst or fistula, including congenital anomalies.[51,52] The most common source is a regional infection, including group A beta-hemolytic streptococcal pharyngitis.[41] Other preceding infections, such as tonsillitis, parotitis, otitis, and mastoiditis, can cause AST via direct inoculation. Interestingly, only one case of AST has been reported as a complication of thyroid surgery.[53]

It is of note that AST caused by *Streptococcus aureus* in a patient with atopic dermatitis after fine-needle aspiration, suggesting that special care is required in patients with atopic dermatitis to avoid bacterial infection.[54] Infective organisms may reach the thyroid via the bloodstream or lymphatics from other sites of infection in the body, such as the respiratory tract, urinary tract, and gastrointestinal tract.[42]

It has been reported that a pyriform sinus fistula (PSF) (Fig. 13-5) is the most common route of infection in AST, especially in children. The fistula is located on the left side in up to 90% of patients.[55,56] AST caused by fistula infection is often preceded by an upper respiratory infection, which may lead to inflammation of the fistula and transmit the causative organisms to the thyroid.[57] PSF is considered an embryonic remnant related to the migration of the C cells from their anlage, the ultimobranchial body, located caudal to the fourth pharyngeal pouch to the developing thyroid lobe.[58,59] The fistula is lined by squamous, columnar, or ciliated epithelium and sometimes forms branches in the thyroid lobe (Fig. 13-6A, B). Immunostaining for calcitonin reveals aggregates of many C cells in the thyroid near the fistula (see Fig. 13-6C). Therefore, it is considered that the PSF is a remnant related to the ultimobranchial body, and that the fistulae trace the migration route of the ultimobranchial body to the thyroid gland.[58]

Clinical Features

Most patients with AST present with a sudden onset of thyroidal (neck) pain; fever; firm tenderness, redness, and warm swelling in the anterior neck, especially on the left side; pharyngeal pain; and difficulty in swallowing. The location of the pain does not become relocated during the clinical course, which is a key point to differentiate subacute thyroiditis from AST. Unilateral or bilateral lobar enlargement can be present. Subsequent changes, including a firm nodule, which indicates abscess formation, may develop in the course of 1 to 3 days.

It is known that AST caused by PSF has some variable clinical features (Table 13-2). One is what is termed *pseudothyroid malignant tumor type*, in which local inflammation is mild. It manifests by swelling of the anterior neck, resembling thyroid malignancy. This type is often seen in adults and older children and the diameter of the fistula is usually extremely narrow.[60] The other one is termed *cystic enlargement type*, in which patients often show dyspnea. It is seen in infants and newborns. Cystic enlargement of the fistula causes pressure on the trachea and dyspnea.[45,61]

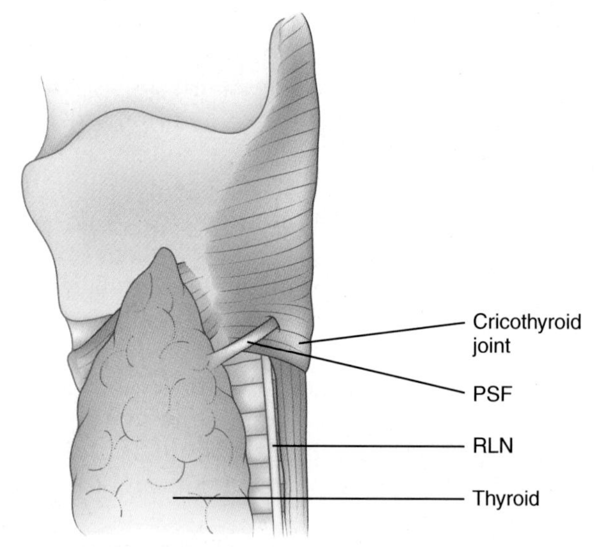

Figure 13–5 Lateral view of the left pyriform sinus fistula (PSF). RLN, recurrent laryngeal nerve.

Diagnosis

For patients who complain of erythema, warmth, swelling, and pain in the anterior neck region and demonstrate pharyngeal pain, difficulty in swallowing, and severe inflammation, AST should be a differential diagnosis. In most cases in which the symptoms are prominent in the left side of the neck and there are recurrent episodes of similar inflammation, especially in children and young people, AST via inferior PSF should be considered first in the differential diagnosis. US study shows an uneven mass of unclear margin, with heterogeneous echogenicity in the thyroid or adjacent tissues (Fig. 13-7A). The abscess lesion is seen as an image of low accumulation in the thyroid scintigram and low intensity in the CT scan (see Fig. 13-7B). Aspiration of the mass followed by bacterial culture and Gram staining should be performed. It is important to determine the location of the inferior PSF to achieve a complete cure.

After local inflammation is cured by appropriate antibiotic therapy, a barium swallow should be performed to examine the inferior pharynges and esophagus (Fig. 13-8). The sensitivity of the barium swallow for detecting a fistula is about 80%.[56] A pharyngeal scope can help detect the fistula. A new

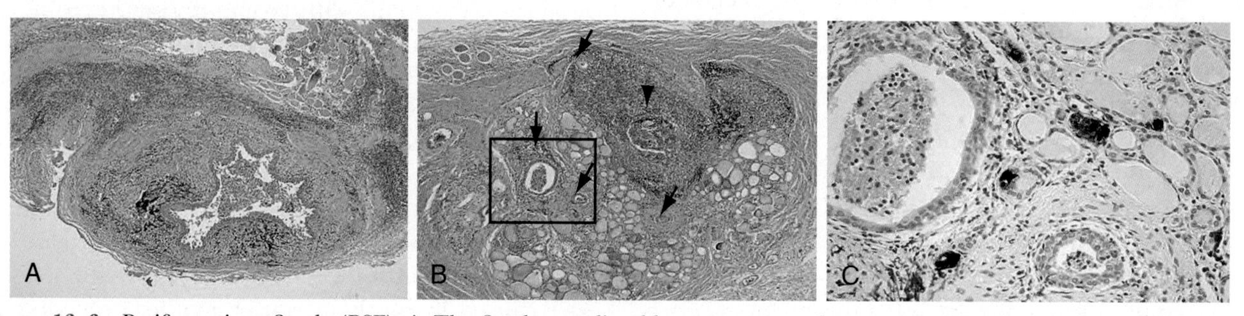

Figure 13–6 Pyriform sinus fistula (PSF). **A,** The fistulae are lined by squamous, columnar, or ciliated epithelium. **B,** PSF forms branches in the thyroid. Arrows indicate branches of the PSF. The arrowhead indicates the main duct of the fistula. The boxed region is shown at higher power. **C,** Anticalcitonin immunostaining shows many C cells surrounding the branches. *(Courtesy A. Miyauchi, Kuma Hospital, Kobe, Japan, 2007.)*

Table 13–2 Clinical Subtypes of Acute Suppurative Thyroiditis (AST) Caused by Pyriform Sinus Fistula

Parameter	Typical AST	Clinical Subtype Pseudothyroid Malignant Tumor Type	Cystic Enlargement Type
Symptom	Acute inflammation in thyroid lesion	Swelling in thyroid lesion, mimics thyroid malignancy; mild inflammation and/or mild neck pain	Cystic swelling in neck; dyspnea
Age	Mainly children, some adults	Adults or older children	Infants or newborns
Diameter of fistula	Narrow, usually 0.5-3 mm	Extremely narrow, less than 1 mm	Bold and cystic
Recurrence	Repeatable	Rare	

From A. Miyauchi, Kuma Hospital, Kobe, Japan, personal communication, 2007.

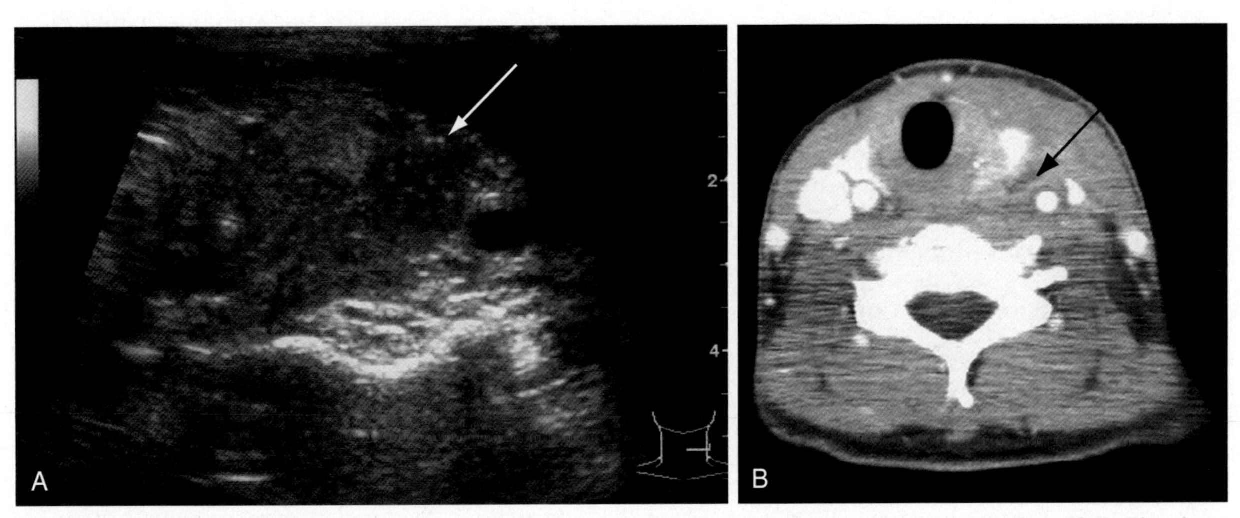

Figure 13–7 **A,** Ultrasonography demonstrates a low-echoic area (arrow) indicating an abscess in the thyroid. **B,** The abscess is shown as a nonenhanced low-intensity area (arrow) in a computed tomography (CT) scan.

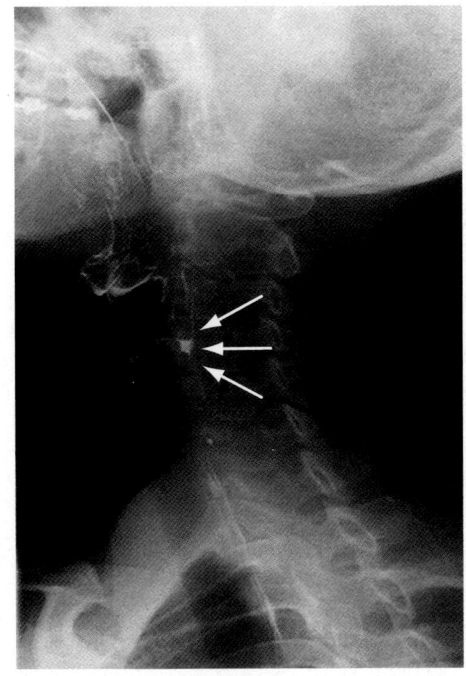

Figure 13–8 A barium swallow (lateral view) demonstrates a pyriform sinus fistula (arrows).

method has been introduced involving CT scanning, MRI, and an ultrasound examination done using a trumpet maneuver with the aim of using air as a contrast agent.[62,63] Subacute thyroiditis should be considered a differential diagnosis. Pain in the thyroid lesion is observed in both AST and subacute thyroiditis; however, systemic inflammation is more severe in AST. Pharyngeal pain is observed in most AST patients. Inflammation in subacute thyroiditis often relocates from one side to another, called creeping thyroiditis. In the early stage of subacute thyroiditis, patients show thyrotoxicosis, with suppressed serum TSH levels and increased free T_3 and free T_4 levels, whereas this is rarely found in AST patients. Steroid administration is effective for subacute thyroiditis but harmful for AST, so an accurate diagnosis is required.

Infection of intrinsic cysts, including thyroglossal duct cyst, cystic hygroma, and branchial cleft cyst, is another differential diagnosis of AST. Internal hemorrhage in the thyroid nodules and painful Hashimoto's disease could also be on the list of differential diagnosis of AST.

Treatment

Empirical antibiotic therapy usually leads to a complete cure of AST. It should eliminate *S. aureus* and *S. pyogenes,* which are the most common pathogens in more than 80% of child and more than 70% of adult patients, respectively.[42] In children, AST is attributed to hemolytic streptococcal infection or a variety of anaerobes in most cases (about 70%), whereas mixed pathogens are identified in over 50% of cases.[41,45,46] On determination of the pathogens, appropriate parenteral antibiotics should be prescribed. Patients with abscesses require surgical drainage. In the case of PSF infection, total excision with closure of the sinus should be performed. Thyroid lobectomy is done if the tract passes through the thyroid lobe.[56,57]

Clinical Course and Prevention

When appropriate antibacterial therapy is administered, AST is usually a self-limited disease, lasting weeks to months.[64] Patients with recurrent episodes of AST require intensive examination to detect the PSF for prevention of further episodes.

Pitfalls, Complications, and Controversies

Complications are rare and, if they occur, the prognosis is excellent in most cases if patients receive appropriate medical and surgical treatment. Local complications include paralysis of the vocal cords, disruption of regional sympathetic nerves, abscess rupture and/or extension into adjacent tissues, internal jugular vein thrombosis (Lemierre's syndrome), and compression of the trachea by the abscess.[65]

Transient or prolonged hypothyroidism can occur in the case of severe and diffuse inflammation and/or necrosis in the thyroid gland. Infection can become systemic and death may occur if the diagnosis or therapy is delayed or is inappropriate. Moreover, rupture of a thyroid abscess may cause mediastinitis, pericarditis, or pneumonia, which can be life-threatening.[41] Rheumatic fever has been reported to be caused by group A beta-hemolytic streptococcal thyroiditis. Without a complete cure by appropriate antibiotics, the pyriform sinus fistula could be missed, because local inflammation induces edema and closure of the entrance of the fistula.

References

1. Muller AF, Drexhage HA, Berghout A: Postpartum thyroiditis and autoimmune thyroiditis in women of childbearing age: Recent insights and consequences for antenatal and postnatal care. Endocr Rev 22:605-630, 2001.
2. Roti E, Minelli R, Giuberti T, et al: Multiple changes in thyroid function in patients with chronic active HCV hepatitis treated with recombinant interferon-alpha. Am J Med 101:482-487, 1996.
3. Stagnaro-Green A: Clinical review 152: Postpartum thyroiditis. J Clin Endocrinol Metab 87:4042-4047, 2002.
4. Lazarus JH, Parkes AB, Premawardhana LD: Postpartum thyroiditis. Autoimmunity 35:169-173, 2002.
5. Amino N, Mori H, Iwatani Y, et al: High prevalence of transient post-partum thyrotoxicosis and hypothyroidism. N Engl J Med 306:849-852, 1982.
6. Amino N, Tada H, Hidaka Y, et al: Postpartum autoimmune thyroid syndrome. Endocr J 47:645-655, 2000.
7. Nikolai TF, Turney SL, Roberts RC: Postpartum lymphocytic thyroiditis. Prevalence, clinical course, and long-term follow-up. Arch Intern Med 147:221-224, 1987.
8. Gerstein HC: How common is postpartum thyroiditis? A methodologic overview of the literature. Arch Intern Med 150:1397-1400, 1990.
9. Takasu N, Komiya I, Nagasawa Y, et al: Exacerbation of autoimmune thyroid dysfunction after unilateral adrenalectomy in patients with Cushing's syndrome due to an adrenocortical adenoma. N Engl J Med 322:1708-1712, 1990.
10. Nikolai TF, Brosseau J, Kettrick MA, et al: Lymphocytic thyroiditis with spontaneously resolving hyperthyroidism (silent thyroiditis). Arch Intern Med 140:478-482, 1980.
11. Vargas MT, Briones-Urbina R, Gladman D, et al: Antithyroid microsomal autoantibodies and HLA-DR5 are associated with postpartum thyroid dysfunction: Evidence supporting an autoimmune pathogenesis. J Clin Endocrinol Metab 67:327-333, 1988.
12. Tachi J, Amino N, Tamaki H, et al: Long term follow-up and HLA association in patients with postpartum hypothyroidism. J Clin Endocrinol Metab 66:480-484, 1988.
13. Kologlu M, Fung H, Darke C, et al: Postpartum thyroid dysfunction and HLA status. Eur J Clin Invest 20:56-60, 1990.
14. Weetman AP, McGregor AM: Autoimmune thyroid disease: Further developments in our understanding. Endocr Rev 15:788-830, 1994.
15. Waterman EA, Watson PF, Lazarus JH, et al: A study of the association between a polymorphism in the CTLA-4 gene and postpartum thyroiditis. Clin Endocrinol (Oxf) 49:251-255, 1998.
16. Kamijo K: Painless thyroiditis. Nippon Rinsho Suppl 1:430-433, 2006.
17. Othman S, Phillips DI, Parkes AB, et al: A long-term follow-up of postpartum thyroiditis. Clin Endocrinol (Oxf) 32:559-564, 1990.
18. Yoshimura Noh J, Momotani N, Fukada S, et al: Ratio of serum free triiodothyronine to free thyroxine in Graves' hyperthyroidism and thyrotoxicosis caused by painless thyroiditis. Endocr J 52:342-537, 2005.

19. Woolf PD: Transient painless thyroiditis with hyperthyroidism: A variant of lymphocytic thyroiditis? Endocr Rev 1:411-420, 1980.
20. Izumi Y, Hidaka Y, Tada H, et al: Simple and practical parameters for differentiation between destruction-induced thyrotoxicosis and Graves' thyrotoxicosis. Clin Endocrinol (Oxf) 57:51-58, 2002.
21. Nikolai TF, Coombs GJ, McKenzie AK, et al: Treatment of lymphocytic thyroiditis with spontaneously resolving hyperthyroidism (silent thyroiditis). Arch Intern Med 142:2281-2283, 1982.
22. Gorman CA, Duick DS, Woolner LB, et al: Transient hyperthyroidism in patients with lymphocytic thyroiditis. Mayo Clin Proc 53:359-365, 1978.
23. Arem R, Munipalli B: Ipodate therapy in patients with severe destruction-induced thyrotoxicosis. Arch Intern Med 156:1752-1757, 1996.
24. Lazarus JH, Ammari F, Oretti R, et al: Clinical aspects of recurrent postpartum thyroiditis. Br J Gen Pract 47:305-308, 1997.
25. Dahlberg PA, Jansson R: Different aetiologies in post-partum thyroiditis? Acta Endocrinol (Copenh) 104:195-200, 1983.
26. Farwell AP: Subacute thyroiditis and acute infectious thyroiditis. In Braverman LE, Utiger RD (eds): The Thyroid. Philadelphia, Lippincott-Raven, 2006, pp 536-547.
27. Volpe R: Subacute thyroiditis and sclerosing thyroiditis. In DeGroot LG (ed): Endocrinology, 3rd ed. Philadelphia, WB Saunders, 1995, pp 742-751.
28. Osmur O, Daglyoz G, Akarca U, et al: Subacute thyroiditis during interferon therapy for chronic hepatitis B infection. Clin Nucl Med 13:643-648, 2003.
29. Parana R, Cruz M, Lyra L, et al: Subacute thyroiditis during treatment with combination therapy (interferon plus ribavirin) for hepatitis C virus. J Viral Hepat 7:393-395, 2000.
30. Fatourechi V, Aniszewski JP, Eghbali Fatourechi GZ, et al: Clinical features and outcome of subacute thyroiditis is an incidence cohort: Olmsted County, Minnesota, study. J Clin Endocrinol Metab 88:2100-2105, 2003.
31. Kojima M, Nakamura S, Oyama T, et al: Cellular composition of subacute thyroiditis. An immunohistochemical study of six cases. Pathol Res Pract 198:833-837, 2002.
32. Ogawa E, Katsushima Y, Fujiwara I, et al: Subacute thyroiditis in children: Patient report and review of the literature. J Ped Endcrinol Metab 16:897-900, 2003.
33. Izumi Y, Hidaka Y, Tada H, et al: Simple and practical parameters for differentiation between destruction-induced thyrotoxicosis and Graves' disease. Clin Endocrinol 57:51-58, 2002.
34. Hiromatsu Y, Ishibashi M, Miyake I, et al: Color Doppler urtrasonography in patients with subacute thyroiditis. Thyroid 9:1189-1193, 1999.
35. Jhaveri K, Shroff MM, Fatterpekar GM, et al: CT and MR imaging findings associated with subacute thyroiditis. Am J Neuroradiol 24:143-146, 2003.
36. Mizukoshi T, Noguchi S, Murakami T, et al: Evaluation of recurrence in 36 subacute thyroiditis patients managed with predonisolone. Int Med 40:292-295, 2001.
37. Iitaka M, Momotani N, Ishii J, et al: Incidence of subacute thyroiditis recurrences after a prolonged latency: 24-year survey. J Clin Endocrinol Metab 81:466-469, 1996.
38. Bartalena L, Bogazzi F, Pecori F, et al: Graves' disease occurring after subacute thyroiditis: Report of a case and review of the literature. Thyroid 6:345-348, 1996.
39. Swinburne JL, Kreisman SH: A rare case of subacute thyroiditis causing thyroid storm. Thyroid 17:73-76, 2007.
40. Takai S, Miyauchi A, Matsuzaka F, et al: Internal fistula as a route of infection in acute suppurative thyroiditis. Lancet 1:751-752, 1979.
41. Brook I: Microbiology and management of acute suppurative thyroiditis in children. Int J Pediatr Otorhinolaryngol 67:447-451, 2003.
42. Berger SA, Zonszein J, Villamena P, et al: Infectious diseases of the thyroid gland. Rev Infect Dis 5:108-122, 1983.
43. Shah SS, Baum SG: Diagnosis and management of infectious thyroiditis. Curr Infect Dis Rep 2:147-153, 2000.
44. Farwell AP: Infectious thyroiditis. In Braverman LE, Utiger RD (eds): The Thyroid. Philadelphia, Lippincott, Williams & Wilkins, 2000, pp 1044-1050.
45. Rich EJ, Mendelman PM: Acute suppurative thyroiditis in pediatric patients. Pediatr Infect Dis J 6:936-940, 1987.
46. Chi H, Lee YJ, Chiu NC, et al: Acute suppurative thyroiditis in children. Pediatr Infect Dis J 21:384-387, 2002.
47. Sekiyama R: Thyroiditis: A clinical review. Am Fam Physician 48:615-621, 1993.
48. Singer PA: Thyroiditis: Acute, subacute, and chronic. Med Clin North Am 75:61-77, 1991.
49. Young RC, Bennett JE, Vogel CL, et al: Aspergillosis. The spectrum of the disease in 98 patients. Medicine 49:147-173, 1970.
50. Gallant JE, Enriquez RE, Cohen KL, et al: Pneumocystis carinii thyroiditis. Am J Med 84:303-306, 1988.
51. Higbee D: Acute thyroiditis in relation to deep infectious of the neck. Ann Otol Rhinol Laryngol 52:620-626, 1943.
52. Bussman YC, Wong ML, Bell MJ, et al: Suppurative thyroiditis with gas formation due to mixed anaerobic infection. J Pediatr 90:321-322, 1977.
53. Miyauchi A, Matsuzaka F, Kuma K, et al: Piriform sinus fistula: An underlying abnormality common in patients with acute suppurative thyroiditis. World J Surg 14:400-405, 1990.
54. Nishihara E, Miyauchi A, Matsuzuka F, et al: Acute suppurative thyroiditis after fine-needle aspiration causing thyrotoxicosis. Thyroid 15:1183-1187, 2005.

55. Miyauchi A, Matsuzuka F, Takai S, et al: Piriform sinus fistula. Arch Surg 116:66-69, 1981.
56. Cases JA, Wenig BM, Silver CE, et al: Recurrent acute suppurative thyroiditis in an adult due to a fourth branchial pouch fistula. J Clin Endocrinol Metab 85:953-956, 2000.
57. Chaudhary N, Gupta A, Motwani G, et al: Fistula of the fourth branchial pouch. Am J Otolaryngol 24:250-252, 2003.
58. Miyauchi A, Matsuzuka F, Kuma K, et al: Piriform sinus fistula and the ultimobranchial body. Histopathology 20:221-227, 1992.
59. Miyauchi A, Yokozawa T, Matsuzuka F, et al: Acute suppurative thyroiditis: Infection in thyroid nodules or infection through apiriform sinus fistula. Thyroidol Clin Exp 10:75-79, 1998.
60. Kodama T, Ito Y, Obara T, et al: Acute suppurative thyroiditis in appearance of unusual neck mass. Endocrinol J 34:427-430, 1987.
61. Miller D, Hill JL, Sun CC, et al: The diagnosis and management of pyriform sinus fistulae in infants and young children. J Pediatr Surg 18:377-381, 1983.
62. Miyauchi A, Tomoda C, Uruno T, et al: Computed tomography scan under a trumpet maneuver to demonstrate piriform sinus fistulae in patients with acute suppurative thyroiditis. Thyroid 15:1409-1413, 2005.
63. Wang HK, Tiu CM, Chou YH, et al: Imaging studies of pyriform sinus fistula. Pediatr Radiol 33:328-333, 2003.
64. Szabo SM, Allen DB: Thyroiditis: Differentiation of acute suppurative and subacute. Clin Pediatr (Phila) 28:171-173, 1989.
65. Lough DR, Ramadan HH, Aronoff SC: Acute suppurative thyroiditis in chidren. Otolaryngol Head Neck Surg 114:462-465, 1996.
66. Sultany GL, Kahalah MB: Acute rheumatic fever after thyroid abscess in an adult. South Med J 76:810-812, 1983.

Chapter 14

Toxic Nodular Goiter: Toxic Adenoma and Toxic Multinodular Goiter

Pamela R. Schroeder and Paul W. Ladenson

Key Points

- Toxic adenoma and toxic multinodular goiter are common causes of hyperthyroidism, especially in women and older adults.
- Diagnosis is made by symptoms, signs, and laboratory data consistent with hyperthyroidism; confirmed by radionuclide imaging.
- Known pathogenetic mechanisms are somatic activating mutations of thyroid-stimulating hormone receptor and guanine nucleotide stimulatory alpha subunit.
- Recommended treatment is usually with iodine-131.
- Risks of not treating even mild associated hyperthyroidism include atrial fibrillation and bone loss.

Thyrotoxicosis refers to the constellation of symptoms and signs caused by excess circulating and tissue free triiodothyronine (T_3), free thyroxine (T_4), or both. These result in hypermetabolism and other excessive tissue-specific thyroid hormone effects, as well as their secondary complications. The term *hyperthyroidism*, when used most properly, refers to an increase in endogenous thyroid hormone synthesis, and represents one set of conditions causing thyrotoxicosis. This chapter will focus on two related causes of hyperthyroidism, toxic adenoma and toxic multinodular goiter, both of which are also known as Plummer's disease.[1]

TOXIC ADENOMA, TOXIC MULTINODULAR GOITER, AND AUTONOMOUS THYROID FUNCTION

A toxic adenoma is a benign monoclonal tumor consisting of thyroid follicular cells, which produce excessive amounts of T_3 and/or T_4. Similarly, a toxic multinodular goiter is comprised of more than one functioning thyroid nodule or glandular region without full consolidation into a nodule. In toxic adenomas, the excessive thyroid hormone autonomously produced can suppress the function of remaining thyroid tissue. Thus, in toxic adenoma and toxic multinodular goiter, thyroid hormone production is no longer controlled by the hypothalamic-hypophyseal-thyroid axis, leading to thyroid hormone excess and the resulting clinical symptoms, signs, and potential complications.

OVERVIEW OF MOLECULAR PATHOGENESIS

Thyroid-stimulating hormone (TSH) binds to its receptor on the basolateral surface of thyroid follicular cells. The TSH receptor is a member of the seven-transmembrane–spanning, G protein–coupled receptor family. When TSH binds to the extracellular amino terminus of the TSH receptor, the intracellular carboxyl terminal domain interacts with the guanine nucleotide stimulatory alpha subunit (Gs), which stimulates adenylyl cyclase conversion of adenosine triphosphate (ATP) to cyclic adenosine monophosphate (cAMP). Activation of this pathway leads to cell growth and thyroid hormone secretion. When TSH concentrations are five- to tenfold higher, TSH binding to its receptor leads to its interaction with Gq, activating phospholipase C, which in turn leads to increased intracellular calcium, diacylglycerol, and inositol phosphate. Activation of this pathway regulates iodination and thyroid hormone production (Fig. 14-1).[2,3]

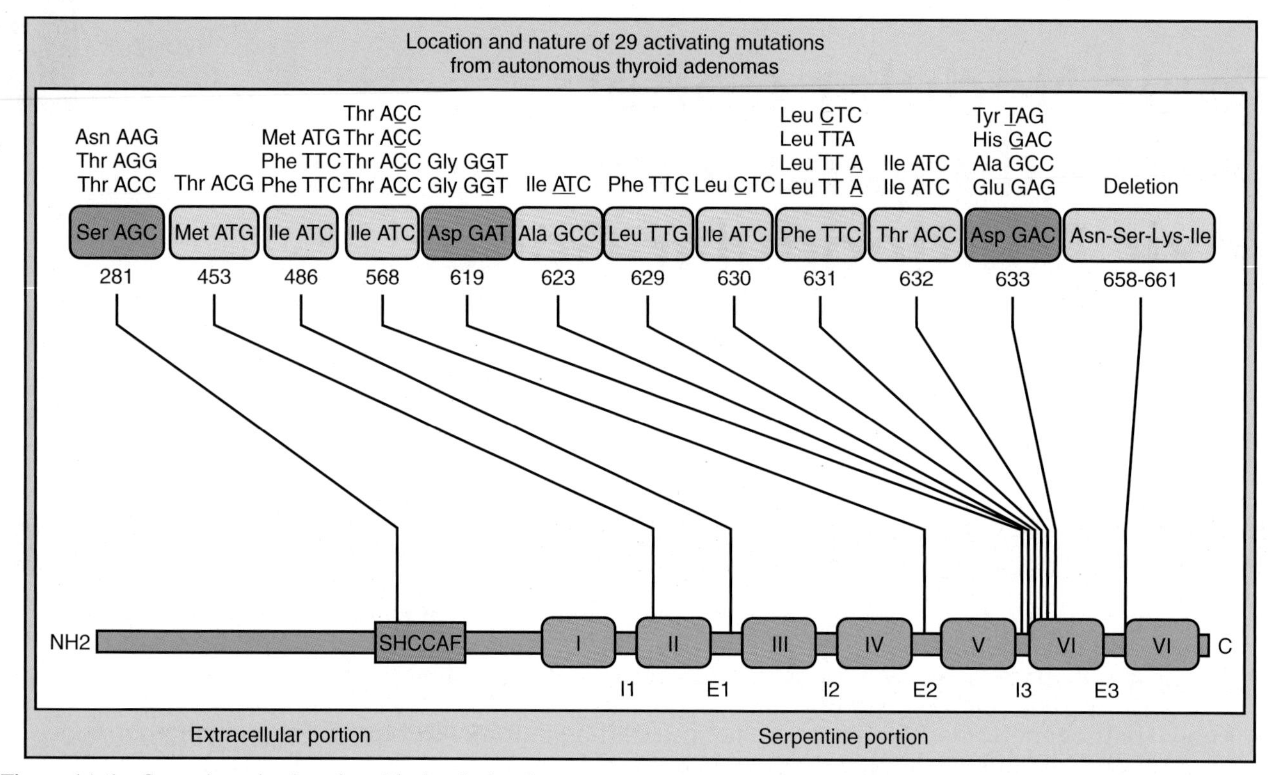

Figure 14–1 Somatic activating thyroid-stimulating hormone receptor mutations. Shown are the locations of 29 activation mutations found in toxic adenomas. Most of the mutated residues are found in the third cytoplasmic loop or sixth transmembrane portion of the receptor. *(Courtesy of Dr. Leslie J. DeGroot, Brown University, Providence, RI.)*

EPIDEMIOLOGY

Incidence and Prevalence

Toxic adenomas are fivefold more common in women than men and their incidence increases with advancing age. In one study, autonomously functioning thyroid nodules were seen in 57% of patients older than 60 years, whereas they were present in only 13% of younger patients.[4] An epidemiologic study in New Zealand has confirmed an increasing incidence of toxic adenoma and toxic multinodular goiter with age.[5]

Reported frequencies of toxic adenoma and toxic multinodular goiter vary widely, from 2% to 45% in various populations. Their prevalence is inversely related to a population's dietary iodine sufficiency—higher in iodine-deficient areas, such as some parts of Europe, than in regions with an iodine-replete diet. The incidence of toxic multinodular goiter has also been reported to increase with sudden dietary iodine supplementation.[6] This phenomenon was first described when the incidence of hyperthyroidism rose sharply following the rapid introduction of supplemental iodine into the Tasmanian diet in the 1960s.[7] Similarly, in Spain, Switzerland, Zimbabwe, and Congo, after abrupt increases in dietary iodine,[8,9] the incidence of hyperthyroidism, including toxic multinodular goiter, initially increased with supplementation and then subsequently declined.[10,11] This form of hyperthyroidism can be severe, even fatal, as the result of cardiovascular complications. This occurs most commonly in those older than 40 years with preexisting multinodular goiters and intrinsic heart disease. Such iodine-induced hyperthyroidism can be largely avoided by the careful introduction and vigilant monitoring of an appropriate increase in the dietary iodine for deficient populations, as has been demonstrated by programs in Iran, Switzerland, and Romania.[11-13]

Natural History

In the United States, among 349 patients with autonomously functioning thyroid nodules seen over an 18-year period, 62 (18%) became thyrotoxic.[4] Similarly, a study from Germany examining the natural history of toxic adenomas found that 67 of 375 patients (18%) with euthyroid solitary autonomous nodules developed hyperthyroidism over a mean of 53 months, for an incidence of 4%/year. In this German study, the incidence of new thyrotoxic cases accelerated with time, with a 3% annual incidence over the first 7 years, increasing to 10% in subsequent years.[14]

Nodule size is a strong predictor of whether thyrotoxicosis will develop in solitary adenomas. Most autonomously functioning thyroid nodules that become thyrotoxic are larger than 2.5 to 3 cm in diameter.[4,15,16] In Hamburger's study,[4] 20% of patients with a nontoxic autonomously functioning thyroid nodules 3 cm or larger developed thyrotoxicosis, even though nodule size did not change in most of these patients during 1 to 15 years of follow-up. Conversely, the spontaneous resolution of autonomously functioning thyroid nodules can occur uncommonly because of hemorrhage, cystic degeneration, and loss of autonomous function. For example, Hamburger saw spontaneous degeneration in 6 of 159 patients (4%) with autonomously functioning thyroid nodules during follow-up.

Toxic multinodular goiters develop gradually over time from nontoxic multinodular goiters. Factors that have an impact on this progression include genetic changes in the nodule, degree of dietary iodine sufficiency, and exposure to certain other environmental factors. Smoking, which generates thiocyanate, could adversely affect the thyroid gland's ability to use iodine, which could particularly contribute to the evolution of toxic multinodular goiter in region of iodine deficiency. However, evidence from epidemiologic studies of whether smoking is a risk factor for toxic multinodular goiter has been controversial. Smoking was associated with an increased prevalence of toxic multinodular goiter in Danish women from an iodine deficient area (odds ratio [OR], 1.7; 95% confidence interval [CI], 1.1 to 2.5), but no higher prevalence was seen in men who smoked.[17] In contrast, two studies, one of which was from an iodine-replete area, failed to find an association between smoking and toxic multinodular goiter, even in women.[18,19]

Consequences of not treating a toxic multinodular goiter include clinical hyperthyroidism, including increased risks of atrial fibrillation, heart failure, and decreased bone mineral density in postmenopausal women. In individuals with subclinical hyperthyroidism studied in Great Britain, 10-year all-cause and cardiovascular mortalities were increased.[20] Similarly, the Leiden 85-plus study found higher all-cause and cardiovascular mortalities over 5 years in those 85-year-olds with low TSH levels.[21]

Incidence of Thyroid Cancer in Toxic Adenomas and Toxic Multinodular Goiters

Autonomously functioning thyroid tissues rarely harbor malignancy, but cancers may coexist in the thyroid gland and rare exceptions of malignancies in autonomously functioning nodules have been reported. Surgical series of patients treated for thyrotoxicosis have revealed an overall prevalence of thyroid cancer, ranging from 5.5% to 7.5%.[22-24] In one Italian study, in which 179 of 1832 patients with thyrotoxicosis were treated surgically, the overall prevalence of thyroid cancer was 6.1%, with incidences of 7.5% and 2.5% in those with toxic multinodular goiter and toxic adenoma, respectively. However, a retrospective study of 333 patients with hyperthyroidism has revealed that only 2 of 77 (2.6%) functioning nodules in the toxic adenoma group were themselves malignant and none of the 402 functioning nodules in the toxic multinodular group were malignant.[24]

Similar genetic mutations, such as Ras mutations and rearrangements in PPAR gamma, have been found in benign follicular neoplasms and thyroid cancers, leading to the hypothesis that autonomously functioning nodules can be a precursor to thyroid cancer. However, clinical follow-up studies have not revealed an increased incidence of thyroid cancer in patients with autonomously functioning nodules. In fact, the rates of thyroid cancer in patients with autonomously functioning nodules are similar to those found in autopsy studies, most of which demonstrate a prevalence of 5% to 10% for occult thyroid cancer.[25-32] This coexisting cancer prevalence has been reported to vary from 2% to 35%, depending on factors such as geographic location, age of the patient, thoroughness of the sectioning of the thyroid gland, and histologic criteria for the diagnosis of thyroid cancer.[33-41]

CAUSE AND PATHOGENESIS

Genetic Pathogenesis

Theoretically, activating germline or somatic mutations in any of the critical elements of the TSH receptor–cAMP signal transduction system could lead to the development of autonomous thyroid gland growth and hormonogenesis. These could include the TSH receptor, guanine nucleotide regulatory subunits, adenylyl cyclase, and protein kinase A. Conversely, an inactivating mutation in a protein that negatively regulates the cascade—for example, cAMP phosphodiesterases—could also activate the primary pathway regulating thyrocyte growth and function.

SOMATIC ACTIVATING GS ALPHA MUTATIONS

Toxic adenomas represent a clone of proliferating follicular epithelial cells that grow and produce thyroid hormone autonomously. Toxic multinodular goiter can be the result of one or more benign nodules becoming autonomous in a gland with many of these benign neoplasms. At the same time, multinodular goiters can contain monoclonal and polyclonal nodules within the same gland. A study of 25 nodules from 9 multinodular goiters has revealed that 9 were polyclonal and 16 were monoclonal; polyclonal and monoclonal nodules were seen in 3 goiters, with 3 goiters containing only polyclonal nodules and 3 goiters containing only monoclonal nodules.[42] Human multinodular goiters have been shown to be heterogeneous in both morphology and function. In another study, 300 samples from cold and hot regions of 20 human multinodular goiters were transplanted onto nude mice and radiolabeled with ^{3}H-thymidine to assess proliferation and with radioactive iodine to assess function. There was no correlation between iodine uptake and size or other morphologic features of these tissues, demonstrating that autonomous growth and autonomous function can be independent.[43]

The first mutations identified in toxic adenomas were somatic activating point mutations in Gs alpha, which were identified after similar mutations were found in pituitary somatotroph adenomas.[44,45] Mutations located at arginine 201 and glutamine 227 lead to constitutive activation of the G protein, with consequent stimulation of the cAMP signaling cascade. The reported prevalences of such Gs alpha gain-of-function mutations has varied widely in various series, ranging from 0% to 75% of autonomously functioning thyroid nodules; however, they are probably responsible for less than 10% of all toxic adenomas.[3,46] Another special example of Gs alpha mutation causing hyperthyroidism is the McCune-Albright syndrome, in which there is a sporadic activating mutation in arginine 201 in a mosaic distribution.[47] In addition to thyrotoxicosis, which occurs in 33% of these patients, constitutive activation of the cAMP cascade in other tissues can cause polyostotic fibrous dysplasia (98%), café-au-lait skin hyperpigmentation (85%), and other endocrine gland hyperfunction, including gonadotropin-independent precocious puberty (62%), acromegaly (27%), and adrenocortical hyperfunction (6%).[48,49]

SOMATIC ACTIVATING THYROID-STIMULATING HORMONE RECEPTOR MUTATIONS

The only other mutations found to date in toxic adenomas have been in the TSH receptor. Most of the mutated residues are located in the third cytoplasmic loop or the sixth transmembrane portion of the receptor. Distinct TSH receptor mutations have also been found in different nodules in the same multinodular goiter.[3,46] These are the most frequent mutations identified in toxic adenomas, with reported prevalences varying from 8% to 82%. This broad range of reported prevalences may be due to the result of a number of factors. First, the various experimental methods used to detect TSH receptor mutations—direct sequencing, single-strand conformation polymorphism, and denaturing gradient gel electrophoresis—differ in their ability to detect point mutations.[46,50-56] For example, one group using the more sensitive denaturing gradient gel electrophoresis to identify TSH receptor mutations in 75 toxic nodules found 6 cases of TSH receptor mutations that had been missed by direct sequencing.[54-56] The quality of the DNA sample also contributes to this variability, because degradation of the DNA is more likely to occur with tissue embedded in paraffin[57,58] than with tissue that has been frozen.[50-55] Other factors that contribute to this broad range of reported TSH receptor mutation prevalences are distinct populations[58,59] and their dietary iodine content.[53,54,60,61] In countries with a moderate iodine deficiency, TSH receptor mutations are found in up to 80% of toxic adenomas.

GERMLINE ACTIVATING THYROID-STIMULATING HORMONE RECEPTOR MUTATIONS

Germline mutations that activate the TSH receptor are rare. Such generalized defects would not be expected to cause solitary toxic adenoma, but rather diffuse gland involvement. Examples of this disorder have been described as hereditary toxic thyroid hyperplasia or familial nonautoimmune hyperthyroidism. Affected individuals develop a toxic multinodular goiter that can have its onset from infancy to adult; transmission of the disorder is autosomal dominant. Among the multiple families that have been investigated, each has had a different mutation in the TSH receptor.[62-64] Mutations in the TSH receptor have also been described in children with congenital hyperthyroidism and unaffected parents, indicating a new germline mutation.[65-69] These patients typically have a diffuse goiter and more severe thyrotoxicosis than those with hereditary nonautoimmune hyperthyroidism. Interestingly, the mutations seen in the congenital nonautoimmune thyrotoxicosis are similar to those found in toxic adenomas, whereas the mutations seen in hereditary nonautoimmune hyperthyroidism are different.

Role of Growth Factors

TRANSFORMING GROWTH FACTOR $\beta 1$

Transforming growth factor β1 (TGF-β1) is thought to counteract the stimulatory roles of TSH and other growth factors, blocking uptake and organification of iodine, thyroglobulin expression, and thyroid follicular cell proliferation in vitro.[70-72] TSH actually stimulates thyrocyte TGF-β1 expression in vitro, representing a potential mechanism for modulating its own effects. TGF-β1 alters expression of insulin-like growth factor 1 (IGF-1) and IGF-binding proteins in a manner that would diminish thyrocyte proliferation (see later). Consequently, TGF-β1 appears to inhibit goitrogenesis. Microarray assessments of gene expression in autonomously functioning thyroid nodules, with or without TSH receptor mutations, compared with adjacent normal thyroid tissue, have shown patterns of expression of TGF-β1 signaling pathway elements consistent with inactivation of this physiologic inhibitory pathway. These observations have included decreased expression of TGF-β receptor type III (betaglycan), Smad 1, 3, and 4, ERK 1, and P300, as well as increased expression of inhibin, endoglin, Smad 6 and 7, and PAI-1 in autonomously functioning thyroid nodules.[73] TGF-β1 also decreases production and release of IGF-1, which itself stimulates thyroid cell growth in vitro.[74] In human thyrocyte primary cultures, TGF-β1 also increases IGF binding protein BP-3 and BP-5 production, higher levels of which have been correlated with decreased thyroid function.[75] Finally, plasmin treatment of cultured follicular cells leads to increased TGF-β1 activity in the media, implicating the plasminogen or plasminogen activator system in the activation of TGF-β1.[76] However, derangements of this system have not been associated with the development of toxic nodular goiter to date.

INSULIN-LIKE GROWTH FACTOR 1

Several studies have supported a synergistic role for IGF-1 with TSH in thyroid growth. First, goiter is seen in more than 70% of patients with acromegaly, who have high IGF-1 levels.[77-79] Insulin-like growth factors enhance TSH action and are required for full TSH stimulation of thyroid cell growth and function in vitro.[80] However, the need for both TSH and IGF-1 for normal follicular cell growth is supported by the observation that when hypopituitary patients lacking TSH are treated with growth hormone, there is no increase in thyroid size despite increased IGF-1.[81] IGF-1 appears to act at least partially in an autocrine fashion, as illustrated by a primary culture of follicular cells from a thyroid adenoma that did not require exogenous IGF-1 to grow.[82] Iodide also appears to modulate IGF-1. In cultured thyroid cells, an increased intracellular organified iodide concentration decreased IGF-1 mRNA transcription, protein production, and cell growth.[74,84]

INSULIN-LIKE GROWTH FACTOR–BINDING PROTEINS

IGF BPs bind IGF-1 and control its availability, with some stimulating IGF-I action and others inhibiting it. Mechanisms of their stimulatory effects include enhancing IGF-1 binding to its receptor and prolonging its intracellular half-life. TSH, via the cAMP signaling cascade, decreases IGF BP production, whereas insulin and epidermal growth factor (EGF) increase it.[85] TSH inhibition of IGF BP synthesis leads to a higher level of unbound IGF-1, increasing its availability to stimulate thyroid tissue. It has also been shown that autonomously functioning thyroid nodules express less IGF BP-5 and IGF BP-6 compared with normal thyroid tissue,[73,86] consistent with their constitutively activated cAMP signaling.

FIBROBLAST GROWTH FACTORS AND THEIR RECEPTORS

Cells from multinodular goiters have increased expression of fibroblast growth factors 1 and 2 (FGF-1 and FGF-2), as well as the FGF receptor 1 (FGFR-1). FGF-1–treated rats exhibit an increase in thyroid weight by more than one third within 1 week; however, this effect does not occur in hypophysectomized rats,[87,88] who also have no increase in FGF-2, FGFR-1, IGF-1, IGF BP-2, or IGF BP-3. These responses are restored when hypophysectomized rats are treated with TSH.

FGFs are usually bound to an extracellular matrix and, to be active mitogens, they must be released from the extracellular matrix. Thus, processing of FGFs by proteases represents a mechanism of control similar to that of some IGF BPs and IGF-1. Another mechanism of control is that truncated forms of the FGF receptor bind to FGF and influence its availability. It is likely that TSH is needed in combination with growth factors, such as IGF and FGF, to stimulate growth of the thyroid gland and goitrogenesis.

ANGIOGENIC FACTORS

Vascular endothelial growth factor (VEGF) stimulates growth of blood vessels supplying thyroid follicular cells. Human thyroid follicular cells in vitro produce VEGF in response to TSH. Production of VEGF receptors on endothelial cells, but not follicular cells, is stimulated by TSH in rats in vivo. VEGF then activates the VEGF receptors on endothelial cells in a paracrine fashion, which causes cell proliferation and hypervascularity. These findings are consistent with the hypervascularity seen in the thyroid of patients with Graves' disease.[89,90]

Recently, iodide has been shown to inhibit TSH-induced expression of the angiogenic factors VEGF-A, VEGF-B, and placenta-derived growth factor (PlGF) in cultured human thyroid follicles.[91] Rat thyroid follicular cells produce PlGF. In goitrogen-treated rats, TSH stimulates the binding of PlGF to the vascular endothelial growth factor receptor (VEGFR).[90] Thus, PlGF may have effects similar to those of VEGF.

Furthermore, in rat models of goitrogenesis, which was induced by iodine deficiency, methimazole, and sodium perchlorate, goiter formation was inhibited by the expression of recombinant adenovirus vectors expressing truncated and inhibitory forms of VEGF receptor 1 (VEGFR-1), FGFR-1, and the receptor for angiopoietin 2, Tie2.[92] Thus, multiple growth factor axes are implicated in the formation of goiter.

Thrombospondin has an inhibitory effect on angiogenesis. In vitro, human and porcine thyrocytes secrete thrombospondin, a growth inhibitor.[93-95] TSH decreases the production of thrombospondin.[94] Findings in the in vivo rat goiter model are consistent with this; thrombospondin levels in endothelial cells disappear within 2 weeks after treatment with methimazole and iodine depravation.[96]

ENDOTHELIN-1 AND ATRIAL NATRIURETIC PEPTIDE

Human thyroid follicular cells make endothelin-1 (ET-1), which is a potent vasoconstrictor. ET-1 is mainly produced by the endothelial cells of the vasculature. Endothelins bind to their receptors, ETA and ETB. ETA is located on smooth muscle cells, where activation of this receptor causes vasoconstriction. ETB is located on endothelial cells, where its activation causes the release of nitric oxide, prostacyclin, and atrial natriuretic peptide (ANP). ET-1 has been shown to bind to its high-affinity receptor in cultured human thyrocytes.[97] Homozygous knockout mice lacking ET-1 are smaller than their littermates, have small thyroid glands without midline fusion, and have small thymus glands that are not descended.[98] ET-1 stimulates the proliferation of cultured human thyroid epithelial cells. This effect of ET-1 is inhibited by the calcium channel blocker verapamil.[99] In the rat goiter model, ET-1 mRNA and protein levels increased 3.5- and 5-fold, respectively, during hyperplasia.[100] In human vascular smooth muscle cells in vitro, ET-1 increases the synthesis of VEGF, the angiogenic factor that leads to hypervascularity and proliferation.[101] These results, taken together, suggest that ET-1 functions as a growth-promoting factor for human thyroid cells.

ANP is also produced by thyroid follicular cells. ANP decreases the production of VEGF in cultured endothelial cells in vitro and is thought to act as an antiangiogenic factor.[101,102] Human thyroid cells express ANP receptors, which are thought to signal via a cyclic guanosine monophosphate (cGMP) pathway.[103] TSH has been shown to decrease the number of ANP receptors in thyroid cells.[104] In cultured bovine thyroid follicles, ANP prevents TSH from stimulating iodide uptake and decreases thyroglobulin mRNA.[105] ANP also causes a retracted cell phenotype in cultured human thyrocytes via guanylyl cyclase receptors.[106] Taken together, these data suggest that ANP has an inhibitory action on thyroid hormone synthesis.

CLINICAL FEATURES

The symptoms and signs of toxic adenoma or toxic multinodular goiter may include those classically associated with the hypermetabolic state of thyrotoxicosis. Specifically, patients may complain of fatigue, unintentional weight loss, heat intolerance, diaphoresis, tremor, palpitations, hyperdefecation, anxiety, nervousness, irritability, difficulty with mental concentration, and hair loss. Women may experience oligomenorrhea, and amenorrhea is rarely seen.[107] Men may complain of decrease in libido, erectile dysfunction, and gynecomastia.[15] Signs of thyrotoxicosis can include tachycardia, systolic hypertension, hyperactive or fatigued demeanor, staring gaze and lag, brisk carotid upstrokes, hyperdynamic point of maximal impulse (PMI), systolic flow murmur, proximal muscle weakness, fine hand tremor, velvety or oily skin, and hair thinning. In taking the history of a patient with suspected or known toxic nodular goiter, the possibility of recent iodide exposure—in the form of medication (e.g., amiodarone), radiocontrast dye, or dietary supplements—should be sought because this can provoke transient thyrotoxicosis in a preexisting thyroid nodule or multinodular goiter.

In patients with mild or subclinical hyperthyroidism, which is common with toxic adenoma and toxic multinodular goiter, symptoms and signs of thyrotoxicosis may be absent altogether. In older patients most often afflicted by toxic multinodular goiter, typical symptoms and signs of even severe hyperthyroidism may be absent. Their presentations may be dominated by nonspecific apathy and weight loss, sometimes accompanied by atrial fibrillation and heart failure.

A second set of clinical manifestations arise from the thyroid nodule or goiter itself. Patients with a toxic adenoma may experience related neck discomfort and mild dysphagia, especially when there has been spontaneous hemorrhage into an adenoma. Those with a multinodular goiter may have local cervical compressive symptoms, including dysphagia, odynophagia, neck pressure, and dyspnea, especially when lying down and raising the arms above the head. Hoarseness caused by recurrent laryngeal nerve palsy is a rare manifestation of benign nodular goiter and should raise concern about possible malignancy. On physical examination, thyroid enlargement may be appreciable as a nodule or goiter, which can seem either multinodular or diffuse on palpation. The nodule or nodules are typically rubbery, smooth, mobile, and nontender, unless there has been recent hemorrhage. Compression of local structures may be evidenced by tracheal deviation and external jugular vein engorgement; rarely, a large substernal goiter may compress the superior vena cava, causing facial and cervical plethora and edema. In patients with a goiter on the verge of thoracic outlet obstruction, raising both arms over the head may provoke cervical vein engorgement and facial plethora (Pemberton's sign). Fixation of the gland, regional adenopathy, or vocal cord paresis are not typical findings in benign nodular goiter and should prompt further consideration of malignancy. Signs specifically associated with Graves' disease, such as exophthalmos and pretibial myxedema, are absent.

DIAGNOSIS

Laboratory Findings

Serum TSH measurement is the pivotal initial test that can exclude or lead to further consideration of hyperthyroidism caused by toxic adenoma or multinodular goiter; it should be measured in all patients with a thyroid nodule or goiter. The serum free T_4 and free or total T_3 levels may be elevated or in the upper part of the normal range. Isolated T_3 toxicosis, in which the serum T_3 concentration is elevated but free T_4 is normal, occurs in approximately 1% of patients with hyperthyroidism.[15] When the TSH is low, but both free T_4 and T_3 levels are normal, the patient has subclinical or mild hyperthyroidism, which is common in toxic multinodular goiter, especially in older patients. It is important to remember, however, that a similar constellation of thyroid function test findings—that is, low TSH with serum T_4 and T_3 levels in the lower half of the normal range—can be caused by central hypothyroidism.

Abnormalities in routine laboratory test analytes are infrequently seen in toxic nodular goiter patients compared with those with Graves' disease. However, these can include elevated serum calcium, alkaline phosphatase, and ferritin concentrations and either low or lower than previous total and low-density lipoprotein (LDL) cholesterol levels. Although thyroid function test results can confirm the presence of thyrotoxicosis and the cause suspected based on the presence of a thyroid nodule or goiter, the cause must almost always be confirmed and malignancy excluded with additional testing, as described later.

Radiologic, Ultrasound, and Nuclear Medicine Findings

The presence of a thyroid nodule or nodular goiter may be evident on chest x-ray or tomographic imaging of the neck or chest. It is not uncommon for toxic nodular goiter to be incidentally detected on imaging studies, such as these or carotid ultrasound.

Thyroid sonography can be helpful in the assessment of potential toxic nodular goiter patients in several ways: (1) confirming that a palpable cervical mass is within the thyroid; (2) quantifying the nodule's dimensions to assist with subsequent radioiodine dosimetry and/or follow-up; (3) defining the anatomic relationships of the thyroid nodule(s) to adjacent structures; and (4) demonstrating that a solitary palpable nodule is only the most prominent of more numerous nodules within the gland.

Radionuclide imaging and quantitative radioisotopic uptake studies are almost always required to establish that toxic adenoma or toxic nodular goiter are the specific cause of thyrotoxicosis, exclude the possibility of coexisting malignancy in a nodular thyroid gland, and to acquire functional data that can assist with subsequent ^{131}I dosimetry. Radionuclide imaging may be performed with ^{123}I or ^{99m}Tc-technetium pertechnetate, both of which are trapped by the sodium-iodide symporter in functioning thyroid tissue, although only radioiodine is subsequently organified. In patients with hyperthyroidism caused by a toxic adenoma, there is characteristic restriction of radionuclide uptake to the responsible hyperfunctioning nodule(s), with suppression of radionuclide uptake in the remainder of the gland (Fig. 14-2). In a patient with a low serum TSH concentration, not only does the scan appearance support the diagnosis of toxic adenoma, but in almost all cases it also excludes malignancy in the nodule. It is important to remember that there is a differential diagnosis for this scan appearance, including congenital hemiagenesis of the thyroid with compensatory hypertrophy of the sole lobe, previous hemithyroidectomy, asymmetrical subacute or autoimmune thyroiditis, or a large hypofunctioning nodule in the contralateral lobe. However, in none of these conditions would a low serum TSH concentration and elevated thyroid hormone levels be expected unless the patient coincidentally had another condition causing thyrotoxicosis. In patients with toxic multinodular goiter, the radionuclide scan shows more than one focal area of increased tracer concentration with suppression of extranodular thyroid tissue (see Fig. 14-2). If some thyroid nodules are hypofunctioning (cold), it may be necessary to rule out cancer in them by fine-needle aspiration cytology before defining the optimal plan for treatment of the patient's hyperthyroidism (see later).

The fractional radionuclide uptake by the thyroid gland is determined with a probe to quantify the tracer taken up by the thyroid gland, typically at 24 hours for ^{123}I and 20 minutes for ^{99m}Tc-technetium pertechnetate. In toxic nodular goiter, the fractional

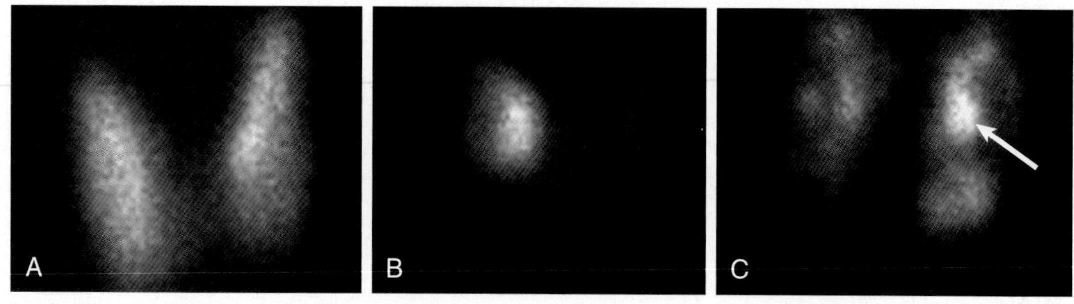

Figure 14–2 Radioactive ^{123}I scans in patients with Graves' disease **(A)**, a toxic adenoma **(B)**, and a toxic multinodular goiter **(C)**. **A,** Graves' disease. A 59-year-old woman presented with a suppressed thyroid-stimulating hormone (TSH) level and elevated free thyroxine (T_4) and triiodothyronine (T_3) levels. ^{123}I images demonstrate diffusely increased accumulation of iodine throughout both lobes of the thyroid gland. ^{123}I uptake at 24 hours was elevated at 54%. These findings are most consistent with Graves' disease. **B,** Toxic adenoma. A 33-year-old woman presented with hyperthyroidism, suppressed TSH, and elevated free T_4. The ^{123}I images demonstrate a focus of intense ^{123}I accumulation in the right lobe of the thyroid gland in the location of a nodule. ^{123}I uptake in the rest of the normal gland is suppressed, which is consistent with toxic adenoma. **C,** Toxic multinodular goiter. A 41-year-old woman presented with hyperthyroidism. The ^{123}I images demonstrate a focus of intense radiotracer accumulation in the left midthyroid lobe (arrow), suggestive of a functioning thyroid nodule. The rest of the gland has a lower level of ^{123}I accumulation, suggesting suppression of normal background thyroid tissue by the functioning nodule. The overall heterogeneity of the ^{123}I uptake throughout the gland suggests an underlying multinodular gland. ^{123}I uptake at 24 hours was 16.1%, which is within the normal range. *(Courtesy of Dr. Heather Jacene.)*

thyroid uptake of radioiodine can be elevated, high-normal or, most infrequently, low-normal, typically ranging from 12% to 60%. In toxic nodular goiter patients who have recently been exposed to a large iodine load, the radioiodine uptake can be low. Thyroid uptake values for ^{99m}Tc-technetium pertechnetate are normally much lower, 0.2% to 3.5% of the dose, but comparable relative thyroid uptake levels can be expected.[108-110] These imaging and quantitative uptake characteristics of toxic nodules and multinodular goiters are distinguished from those seen in other causes of thyrotoxicosis (Table 14-1).

TREATMENT

Hyperthyroidism caused by toxic adenoma or toxic nodular goiter rarely remits spontaneously unless the patient has recently been exposed to a provocative iodine load or a solitary hyperfunctioning nodule undergoes hemorrhagic degeneration. Consequently, optimal treatment for most patients entails a permanent therapy, radioiodine or surgery.

Radioactive Iodine and Antithyroid Drugs

RADIOACTIVE IODINE

For most U.S. patients, where even moderately large does of ^{131}I can be administered on an ambulatory basis, radioiodine represents the most attractive treatment for most patients with toxic adenoma or toxic multinodular goiter. It is generally preferable to surgery when there is no suspicion of coexisting thyroid malignancy, no large goiter threatening local compressive symptoms, no other reason for neck surgery (e.g., primary hyperparathyroidism), no imperative for immediate cure, and whenever the patient's general health makes him or her a poor candidate for surgery.[111] Radioactive iodine treatment is less attractive in children and adolescents, in whom the radiation dose administered to extranodular tissue approximates that known to be associated with subsequent thyroid cancer.[112] ^{131}I therapy is contraindicated in pregnant women.

It is controversial whether the administered ^{131}I dose should be determined by some form of simplified dosimetry or an arbitrary dosage used in all patients. Typical dosimetric schemes consider gland size, its fractional uptake of a preceding tracer dose, and a standard administered dose constant (e.g., 0.16 mCi/g of estimated hyperfunctioning tissue). However, controlled studies have failed to show that calculated administered doses of radioiodine are superior to an empirically chosen constant dose for all patients (e.g., 15 mCi).[113-115] This is probably due to the result of imprecision in the estimated mass and heterogeneous radioisotope distribution within and lack of data about ^{131}I retention time in the functioning thyroid tissue. Although radioiodine is largely cleared from the patient within 14 days, resolution of hyperthyroidism typically requires 4 to 8 weeks. Consequently, it may be prudent to use temporary antithyroid drug treatment to achieve euthyroidism, discontinue it for several days before and after ^{131}I administration, and then resume therapy to maintain normal thyroid function while waiting for the effect of the radioiodine, particularly in older patients and those with cardiac disease. Because propylthiouracil (PTU) has been shown to induce relative resistance to radioiodine in those with Graves' disease and methimazole has not, the latter

Table 14–1 Radionuclide Uptake and Imaging in the Differential Diagnosis of Thyrotoxicosis

Cause of Thyrotoxicosis	Fractional Uptake in 24 hr (%)	Radionuclide Distribution
Graves' disease	35-95	Homogeneous within thyroid
Toxic uni- or multinodular goiter	20-60	Restricted to autonomous regions in thyroid
Subacute thyroiditis	0-2	No or minimal uptake
Silent thyroiditis	0-2	No or minimal uptake
Iodine-induced thyrotoxicosis	0-2	No or minimal uptake
Factitious or iatrogenic thyrotoxicosis	0-2	No or minimal uptake
Struma ovarii	0-2	Uptake in ovary
Follicular carcinoma	0-5	Uptake in cancer metastases
Thyroid-stimulating hormone–induced thyrotoxicosis	30-80	Homogeneous within thyroid

is the antithyroid drug of choice for such adjunctive therapy.[116-123] One randomized controlled trial has also confirmed this effect of PTU in toxic multinodular goiter.[124] With typical administered radioiodine doses, such as 10 to 30 mCi of ^{131}I, hyperthyroidism is cured in 62% to 98% of patients with toxic adenoma or toxic nodular goiter.[125-130] The remainder almost invariably respond to a second radioiodine dose, which is typically given no sooner than 4 to 6 months later. Predictors of relative resistance to radioiodine therapy include large goiters and those with a higher fractional thyroid uptake of radioiodine.[131]

Potential adverse effects of ^{131}I therapy for toxic nodular goiter are essentially limited to radiation thyroiditis and postablative hypothyroidism. Radiation thyroiditis can cause anterior neck pain in the week after therapy and exacerbation of thyrotoxicosis because of the release of preformed thyroid hormone from the gland, which typically occurs 2 to 8 weeks after treatment. Pretreatment with an antithyroid drug has been shown to decrease the severity of thyrotoxicosis caused by radiation thyroiditis in Graves' disease,[132-135] but this has not been established for toxic nodular goiter. Thyroiditis-related gland swelling with potential worsening of compressive symptoms is a concern that has not actually been realized in studies of radioiodine therapy for nodular goiter.[136,137] Long term, thyroid volume typically decreases by about 40% after ^{131}I treatment.[138,139]

The incidence of postablative hypothyroidism after radioiodine therapy has been reported to be 25% to 50%, which is lower than that encountered after treatment of patients with Graves' disease. This is presumably because suppressed extranodular thyroid tissue does not take up radioiodine. Radioisotopic distribution within functioning tissue can also be heterogeneous. Postablative hypothyroidism is more common when higher doses of radioactive iodine are administered.

Other sides effects occur rarely. Symptoms related to sialadenitis (e.g., salivary gland swelling and pain) or gastritis (e.g., nausea or vomiting) are uncommon with the usual administered ^{131}I doses for toxic nodular goiter. Excess risk for other future cancers after radioactive iodine treatment for toxic nodular goiter appears to be absent or extremely low. A Swedish study of 10,552 patients treated for hyperthyroidism (mean dose, 506 MBq), with an average 15-year follow-up, found a standardized incidence ratio of 1.06 (95% CI, 1.01 to 1.11) for any type of cancer occurring 1 year or more after ^{131}I treatment. Among the 10-year survivors, increased risk of stomach, kidney, and brain cancers was seen, but only the risk for stomach cancer increased over time and with increasing radioactive iodine dose. Thus, these investigators concluded that the overall cancer risk does not increase with increasing ^{131}I dose or with time since exposure.[140]

In another retrospective report by the Cooperative Thyrotoxicosis Therapy Follow-up Study of 35,593 patients with hyperthyroidism treated with ^{131}I, there was a standardized cancer mortality ratio of 1.16 (95% CI, 1.03 to 1.30) in those with a toxic multinodular goiter. The number of cancer deaths seen in the study was close to the predicted mortality rates in the general population, but there was a small excess mortality caused by breast, lung, kidney, and thyroid malignancies. Radioactive iodine administration was not linked to total cancer deaths (standard mortality ratio [SMR], 1.02; 95% CI, 0.98 to 1.07) or any specific cancer except for thyroid cancer (SMR, 3.94; 95% CI, 2.52 to 5.86). In this study, however, the authors concluded that "in absolute terms the excess number of deaths was small and the underlying thyroid disease appeared to play a role."[141] Although there are limited data concerning the incidence of infertility, spontaneous abortion, and infants with birth defects in mothers previously treated with radioiodine, there has been no evidence of these deleterious consequences.[142]

RECOMBINANT THYROID-STIMULATING HORMONE–STIMULATED ^{131}I THERAPY

The relatively low fractional uptake of radioiodine by nodular goiters can limit the effectiveness of ^{131}I therapy and increase the administered dose requirement. Consequently, in recent years, recombinant TSH (thyrotropin alfa, rTSH, Thyrogen) has been investigated as an off-label approach to increasing thyroidal radioiodine uptake for the treatment of hyperthyroidism and goiter size in patients with toxic nodular goiter. rTSH has also been used to facilitate goiter shrinkage with ^{131}I in patients with nontoxic nodular goiter, in whom rTSH permits a 50% to 60% reduction in the administered ^{131}I dose[143,144] while producing a more substantial decrease in goiter volume. Studies in nontoxic nodular goiter patients have demonstrated the importance of using a rTSH dose less than that used for thyroid cancer testing (e.g., a single 0.01- to 0.45-mg rTSH dose).[144-146] Larger rTSH doses have been reported to induce severe thyrotoxicosis or gland swelling with increased obstructive symptoms. rTSH-stimulated ^{131}I therapy has also been used for older patients with clinical or subclinical hyperthyroidism caused by large multinodular goiters. In such patients, the relatively low fractional uptake of radioiodine by the thyroid reduces the cure rate after ^{131}I. In one study of 41 patients with clinical or subclinical hyperthyroidism caused by large multinodular goiter, patients who were randomly assigned to receive 0.45 mg rTSH before ^{131}I had a greater reduction in goiter volume at 1 year, 58% versus 40%. However, rTSH pre-treated patients also had a higher rate of postradioiodine hypothyroidism, 65% versus 21%,[147] probably because rTSH enhanced uptake in previously suppressed regions of the gland. Because of its risk of exacerbating hyperthyroidism, rTSH is generally inadvisable when administering a larger ^{131}I dose is an option, especially in older patients and those with underlying heart disease.

ANTITHYROID DRUGS

The thionamide antithyroid drugs—methimazole and propylthiouracil in the United States and carbimazole in Europe and Asia—have limited roles in the management of patients with nontoxic nodular goiter. Unlike hyperthyroid Graves' disease, thyroid autonomy in toxic nodular goiter rarely remits unless it has been provoked by an iodine load. Furthermore, because of the substantial store of previously synthesized thyroid hormone that can be present in the large gland of a patient with toxic nodular goiter, thionamide therapy alone may not control hyperthyroidism completely for weeks or months.

Nonetheless, there remain certain indications for short-term antithyroid drug therapy. First, thionamides can be useful for the initial control of hyperthyroidism that is severe or complicates cardiac or other conditions in a fragile patient. By restoring euthyroidism, such thionamide pretreatment can then make subsequent surgery or radioiodine therapy safer. Second, PTU is the immediate treatment of choice for pregnant patients with hyperthyroidism, although toxic nodular goiter is rare in this population. Third, a time-limited course of antithyroid drugs can sometimes be useful to evaluate the clinical status of patients with subclinical hyperthyroidism who have nonspecific symptoms, such as nervousness or insomnia, that may or may not improve with definitive treatment of mild hyperthyroidism. If a patient experiences an improvement in symptoms or sense of well-being when thyroid function has been restored to normal on thionamide therapy, then the case for radioiodine therapy or surgery is stronger.

The specific mechanisms of action, doses, and side effects of the thionamide antithyroid drugs have been extensively reviewed.[148]

Surgery

Surgery is an effective and prompt treatment for patients with toxic nodular goiter. It has the added advantage of reliably curing both hyperthyroidism and obstructive or cosmetic problems related to goiter size. However, thyroidectomy also has predictable disadvantages for all patients and risks of certain serious injuries in a minority. Surgery requires hospitalization and general anesthesia with its attendant risks, particularly for older patients in whom toxic nodular goiter is more common. Surgery causes temporary pain and leaves a scar, which should usually be modest. Hypothyroidism is almost a certainty after total or near-total thyroidectomy. The proximity of the recurrent laryngeal nerves and parathyroid glands to the thyroid makes them vulnerable to injury, with resulting voice change and airway obstruction, and hypocalcemia, respectively. These complications of thyroid surgery have been described in detail elsewhere.[149]

NOVEL MINIMALLY INVASIVE THERAPIES

Several novel minimally invasive therapies for thyroid nodules have been assessed in recent years, including percutaneous ethanol injection, interstitial laser photocoagulation, radiofrequency ablation, and high-power ultrasound. These techniques are typically used under ultrasound guidance in awake patients.

Percutaneous ethanol injection (PEI) for autonomously functioning thyroid nodules has been performed and reported over the last decade and can be used for both cystic and solid nodules.[150-156] The volume of injected ethanol varies with the nodule's size and, in the case of complex cysts, with the volume of fluid aspirated. Multiple procedures are usually performed over the course of days to weeks. Several studies have shown that PEI can produce complete or partial cure of hyperthyroidism and decrease nodule volume.[151-154,156-158] In one study of PEI therapy for autonomously functioning thyroid nodules followed for 3 years, there was normalization of serum TSH, recovery of extranodular radioiodine uptake in 88% of patients, and a 63% reduction in nodule volume. Most nonresponders had thyroid nodule volumes larger than 60 mL. Complications of PEI include local pain, which is very common, transient dysphonia, exacerbation of thyrotoxicosis, and/or fever (rare), and subcutaneous hematoma.[154-156,158-160]

Successful treatment of autonomously functioning thyroid nodules with ultrasound-guided interstitial laser photocoagulation (ILP) has also been reported in a few patients. In a 17-year-old young woman with subclinical hyperthyroidism, ILP treatment with 3 W for 650 seconds at 1950 J resulted in a normal serum TSH concentration by 2 months and a decrease in nodule volume of 40% at 9 months.[161-164] In another study of thyroidectomy in two ILP-treated patients with large autonomously functioning nodules, surgical histopathology confirmed well-defined tissue ablation.[165] Side effects of ILP included transient thyrotoxicosis and local neck pain.

Percutaneous radiofrequency ablation (RFA) has been used in two preliminary studies, one in cats and the other in humans, for the treatment of hyperthyroidism and benign cold nodules, respectively. RFA treatment of hyperthyroid cats led to a transient decrease of serum total T_4 and free T_4 with subsequent euthyroidism for a mean of 4 months, but hyperthyroidism recurred in all the cats, and adverse effects included Horner's syndrome in two cats and laryngeal paralysis in one cat.[166] The RFA treatment of 35 benign cold thyroid nodules in 30 euthyroid patients required conscious sedation in 77% and led to a reduction in the mean volume of the nodules over 9 months; thyroid function remained normal. Cystic nodules had a significantly better response than solid nodules ($P < .05$), 88% of patients' symptoms improved, and only one patient developed vocal cord palsy.[167] Further studies are needed to evaluate the efficacy and safety of this procedure. One preliminary study has used high-intensity focused ultrasound for localized ablation of thyroid in eight ewes. Although the procedure was successful, with the thyroid histology revealing central coagulative necrosis, one animal died 3 days after the procedure of inhalation pneumonia and three animals died because the ultrasound beam injured adjacent organs.[168] Thus, the safety of the method remains to be defined.

CLINICAL COURSE AND PREVENTION

Typical clinical responses to treatment of toxic adenomas and toxic multinodular goiters have been described for each of the therapies used. Surgery is the quickest approach to cure, but preoperative preparation with antithyroid medication and postoperative recovery prolong the overall time frame of surgical management. Treatment with radioiodine typically requires 1 to 3 months for resolution of hyperthyroidism and as long as 2 years for it maximal effect on goiter size. When antithyroid drugs are used as an interim measure, glandular stores of thyroid preformed thyroid hormone may delay recovery for 4 to 12 weeks.

Hypothyroidism is almost universal after bilateral thyroidectomy and occurs in approximately one third of hemithyroidectomy patients. Although postablative hypothyroidism is less common after radioiodine treatment of toxic nodular goiter than Graves' disease, it still occurs in 25% to 50% of patients. Furthermore, radioiodine-treated patients who remain euthyroid in the months after treatment require lifelong monitoring, because late hypothyroidism can occur.

Prevention of toxic nodular goiter is only effective in regions of the world in which endemic iodine deficiency predisposes the population to nodular goiters that can later become autonomous. In iodine-sufficient regions, there are no known dietary or lifestyle measures that have been shown to prevent toxic nodular goiter.

References

1. Plummer HC, Boothby WM: The value of iodine in exophthalmic goiter. J Iowa State Med Soc 14:66-73, 1924.
2. Van Sande J, Parma J, Tonacchera M, et al: Somatic and germline mutations of the TSH receptor gene in thyroid diseases. J Clin Endocrinol Metab 80:2577-2585, 1995.
3. Corvilain B, Van Sande J, Dumont JE, Vassart G: Somatic and germline mutations of the TSH receptor and thyroid diseases. Clin Endocrinol 55:143-158, 2001.

4. Hamburger JI: Evolution of toxicity in solitary nontoxic autonomously functioning thyroid nodules. J Clin Endocrinol Metab 50:1089-1093, 1980.
5. Brownlie BE, Wells JE: The epidemiology of thyrotoxicosis in New Zealand: Incidence and geographical distribution in north Canterbury, 1983-1985. Clin Endocrinol 33:249-259, 1990.
6. Stanbury JB, Ermans AE, Bourdoux P, et al: Iodine-induced hyperthyroidism: Occurrence and epidemiology. Thyroid 8:83-100, 1998.
7. Connolly RJ, Vidor GI, Stewart JC: Increase in thyrotoxicosis in endemic goiter area after iodation of bread. Lancet I:500-502, 1970.
8. Todd CH, Allain T, Gomo ZAR, et al: Increase in thyrotoxicosis associated with iodine supplements in Zimbabwe. Lancet 346:1563-1564, 1995.
9. Bourdoux P, Ermans AM, Mukalay AMW, et al: Iodine-induced thyrotoxicosis in Kivu, Zaire. Lancet 347:552-553, 1996.
10. Galofre JC, Fernandez-Calvet L, Rios M, Garcia-Mayor RV: Increased incidence of thyrotoxicosis after iodine supplementation in an iodine sufficient area. J Endocrinol Invest 17:23-27, 1994.
11. Baltisberger BL, Minder CE, Burgi H: Decrease of incidence of toxic nodular goitre in a region of Switzerland after full correction of mild iodine deficiency. Eur J Endocrinol 132:546-549, 1995.
12. Azizi F, Daftarian N: Side effects of iodized oil administration in patients with simple goiter. J Endocrinol Invest 24:72-77, 2001.
13. Simescu M, Varciu M, Nicolaescu E, et al: Iodized oil as a complement to iodized salt in schoolchildren in endemic goiter in Romania. Horm Res 58:78-82, 2002.
14. Sandrock D, Olbricht T, Emrich D, et al: Long-term follow-up in patients with autonomous thyroid adenoma. Acta Endocrinol 128:51-55, 1993.
15. Cooper DS: Hyperthyroidism. Lancet 362:459-468, 2003.
16. Pearce EN: LE Braverman LE: Hyperthyroidism: Advantages and disadvantages of medical therapy. Surg Clin N Am 84:833-847, 2004.
17. Vestergaard P, Rejnmark L, Weeke J, et al: Smoking as a risk factor for Graves' disease, toxic nodular goiter, and autoimmune hypothyroidism. Thyroid 12:69-75, 2002.
18. Bartalena L, Martino E, Marcocci C, et al: More on smoking habits and Graves' ophthalmopathy. J Endocrinol Invest 12:733-737, 1989.
19. Prummel MF, Wiersinga WM: Smoking and risk of Graves' disease. JAMA 269:479-482, 1993.
20. Parle JV, Maisonneuve P, Sheppard MC, et al: Prediction of all-cause and cardiovascular mortality in elderly people from one low serum thyrotropin result: A 10-year cohort study. Lancet 358:861-865, 2001.
21. Gussekloo J, Van Exel E, de Craen AJM, et al: Thyroid status, disability and cognitive function, and survival in old age. JAMA 292:2591-2599, 2004.
22. Pacini F, Elisei R, Di Coscio GC, et al: Thyroid carcinoma in thyrotoxic patients treated by surgery. J Endocrinol Invest 11:107-112, 1988.
23. Smith M, McHenry C, Jarosz H, et al: Carcinoma of the thyroid in patients with autonomous nodules. Am Surg 54:448-449, 1988.
24. Sahin M, Guvener ND, Ozer F, et al: Thyroid cancer in hyperthyroidism: Incidence rates and value of ultrasound-guided fine-needle aspiration biopsy in this patient group. J Endocrinol Invest 28:815-818, 2005.
25. Sobrinho-Simoes MA, Sambade MC, Goncalves V: Latent thyroid carcinoma at autopsy: A study from Oporto, Portugal. Cancer 43:1702-1706, 1979.
26. Bondeson L, Ljungberg O: Occult thyroid carcinoma at autopsy in Malmo, Sweden. Cancer 47:319-323, 1981.
27. Siegal A, Modan M: Latent carcinoma of thyroid in Israel: A study of 260 autopsies. Isr J Med Sci 17:249-253, 1981.
28. Lang W, Borrusch H, Bauer L: Occult carcinomas of the thyroid. Evaluation of 1,020 sequential autopsies. Am J Clin Pathol 90:72-76, 1988.
29. Bisi H, Fernandes VS, de Camargo RY, et al: The prevalence of unsuspected thyroid pathology in 300 sequential autopsies, with special reference to the incidental carcinoma. Cancer 64:1888-1893, 1989.
30. Furmanchuk AW, Roussak N, Ruchti C: Occult thyroid carcinomas in the region of Minsk, Belarus. An autopsy study of 215 patients. Histopathology 23:319-325, 1993.
31. Arem R, Padayatty SJ, Saliby AH, Sherman SI: Thyroid microcarcinoma: Prevalence, prognosis, and management. Endocr Pract 5:148-156, 1999.
32. Kovacs GL, Gonda G, Vadasz G, et al: Epidemiology of thyroid microcarcinoma found in autopsy series conducted in areas of different iodine intake. Thyroid 15:152-157, 2005.
33. Bondeson L, Ljungberg O: Occult papillary thyroid carcinoma in the young and the aged. Cancer 53:1790-1792, 1984.
34. Harach HR, Franssila KO, Wasenius VM: Occult papillary carcinoma of the thyroid. A "normal" finding in Finland. A systematic autopsy study. Cancer 56:531-538, 1985.
35. Franssila KO, Harach HR: Occult papillary carcinoma of the thyroid in children and young adults. A systemic autopsy study in Finland. Cancer 58:715-719, 1986.
36. Komorowski RA, Hanson GA: Occult thyroid pathology in the young adult: An autopsy study of 138 patients without clinical thyroid disease. Hum Pathol 19:689-696, 1988.
37. Ottino A, Pianzola HM, Castelletto RH: Occult papillary thyroid carcinoma at autopsy in La Plata, Argentina. Cancer 64:547-551, 1989.
38. Yamamoto Y, Maeda T, Izumi K, Otsuka H: Occult papillary thyroid carcinoma of the thyroid. A study of 408 autopsy cases. Cancer 65:1173-1179, 1990.

39. Martinez-Tello FJ, Martinez-Cabruja R, Fernandez-Martin J, et al: Occult carcinoma of the thyroid. A systematic autopsy study from Spain of two series performed with two different methods. Cancer 71:4022-4029, 1993.
40. Sakorafas GH, Giotakis J, Stafylia V: Papillary thyroid microcarcinoma: A surgical perspective. Cancer Treat Rev 31:423-438, 2005.
41. Solares CA, Penalonzo MA, Xu M, Orellana E: Occult papillary thyroid carcinoma in postmortem species: Prevalence at autopsy. Am J Otolaryngol 26:87-90, 2005.
42. Kopp P, Kimura ET, Aeschimann S, et al: Polyclonal and monoclonal thyroid nodules coexist within human multinodular goiters. J Clin Endocrinol Metab 79:134-139, 1994.
43. Peter HJ, Gerber H, Studer H, Smeds S: Pathogenesis of heterogeneity in human multinodular goiter. A study on growth and function of thyroid tissue transplanted onto nude mice. J Clin Invest 76:1992-2002, 1985.
44. Lyons J, Landis CA, Harsh G, et al: Two G protein oncogenes in human endocrine tumors. Science 249:655-659, 1990.
45. O'Sullivan C, Barton CM, Staddon SL, et al: Activating point mutations of the gsp oncogene in human thyroid adenomas. Mol Carcinog 4:345-349, 1991.
46. Krohn K, Paschke R: Progress in understanding the etiology of thyroid autoimmunity. J Clin Endocrinol Metab 86:3336-3345, 2001.
47. Weinstein LS, Shenker A, Gejman P, et al: Activating mutations of the stimulatory G protein in the McCune-Albright syndrome. N Engl J Med 325:1688-1695, 1991.
48. Ringel MD, Schwindinger WF, Levine MA: Clinical implications of genetic defects in G proteins: The molecular basis of McCune-Albright syndrome and Albright hereditary osteodystrophy. Rev Molec Med 75:171-184, 1996.
49. Spiegel AM: Mutations in G proteins and G protein-coupled receptors in endocrine disease. J Clin Endocrinol Metab 81:2434-2442, 1996.
50. Porcellini A, Ciullo I, Laviola L, et al: Novel mutations of thyrotropin receptor gene in thyroid hyperfunctioning adenomas. Rapid identification by fine needle aspiration biopsy. J Clin Endocrinol Metab 79:657-661, 1994.
51. Paschke R, Tonacchera M, Van Sande J, et al: Identification and functional characterization of two new somatic mutations causing constitutive activation of the thyrotropin receptor in hyperfunctioning autonomous adenomas of the thyroid. J Clin Endocrinol Metab 79:1785-1789, 1994.
52. Russo D, Arturi F, Suarez HG, et al: Thyrotropin receptor gene alterations in thyroid hyperfunctioning adenomas. J Clin Endocrinol Metab 81:1548-1551, 1996.
53. Parma J, Duprez L, Van Sande J, et al: Diversity and prevalence of somatic mutations in the thyrotropin receptor and Gs alpha genes as a cause of toxic thyroid adenomas. J Clin Endocrinol Metab 82:2695-2701, 1997.
54. Fuhrer D, Holzapfel HP, Wonerow P, et al: Somatic mutations in the thyrotropin receptor gene and not in the Gs alpha protein gene in 31 toxic thyroid nodules. J Clin Endocrinol Metab 82:3885-3891, 1997.
55. Fuhrer D, Kubisch C, Scheibler U, et al: The extracellular thyrotropin receptor domain is not a major candidate for mutations in toxic thyroid nodules. Thyroid 8:997-1001, 1998.
56. Trulzsch B, Krohn K, Wonerow P, et al: Detection of thyroid-stimulating hormone receptor and Gs alpha mutations in 75 toxic thyroid nodules by denaturing gradient gel electrophoresis. J Mol Med 78:684-691, 2001.
57. O'Sullivan C, Barton CM, Staddon SL, et al: Activating point mutations of the gsp oncogene in human thyroid adenomas. Mol Carcinog 4:345-349, 1991.
58. Takeshita A, Nagayama Y, Yokoyama N, et al: Rarity of oncogenic mutations in the thyrotropin receptor of autonomously functioning thyroid nodules in Japan. J Clin Endocrinol Metab 80:2607-2611, 1995.
59. Russo D, Arturi F, Wicker R, et al: Genetic alterations in thyroid hyperfunctioning adenomas. J Clin Endocrinol Metab 80:1347-1351, 1995.
60. Tonacchera M, Chiovato L, Pinchera A, et al: Hyperfunctioning thyroid nodules in toxic multinodular goiter share activating thyrotropin receptor mutations with solitary toxic adenoma. J Clin Endocrinol Metab 83:492-498, 1998.
61. Tonacchera M, Vitti P, Agretti P, et al: Functioning and nonfunctioning thyroid adenomas involve different molecular pathogenic mechanisms. J Clin Endocrinol Metab 84:4155-4158, 1999.
62. Duprez L, Parma J, Van Sande J, et al: Germline mutations in the thyrotropin receptor gene cause non-autoimmune autosomal dominant hyperthyroidism. Nat Genet 7:396-401, 1994.
63. Tonacchera M, Van Sande J, Cetani F, et al: Functional characteristics of three new germline mutations of the thyrotropin receptor gene causing autosomal dominant toxic thyroid hyperplasia. J Clin Endocrinol Metab 81:547-554, 1996.
64. Fuhrer D, Wonerow P, Willgerodt H, Paschke R: Identification of a new thyrotropin receptor germline mutation (leu629phe) in a family with neonatal onset of autosomal dominant nonautoimmune hyperthryoidism. J Clin Endocrinol Metab 82:4234-4238, 1997.
65. Kopp P, Van Sande J, Parma J, et al: Congenital hyperthyroidism caused by a mutation in the thyrotropin-receptor gene. N Engl J Med 332:150-154, 1995.

66. De Roux N, Polak M, Coue J, et al: A neomutation of the thyroid-stimulating hormone receptor in a severe neonatal hyperthyroidism. J Clin Endocrinol Metab 81:2023-2026, 1996.
67. Holzapfel HP, Wonerow P, Von Petrykowski W, et al: Sporadic congenital hyperthyroidism due to a spontaneous germline mutation in the thyrotropin receptor gene. J Clin Endocrinol Metab 82:3879-3884, 1997.
68. Kopp P, Muirhead S, Jourdain N, et al: Congenital hyperthyroidism caused by a solitary toxic adenoma harboring a novel somatic mutation (serine281-isoleucine) in the extracellular domain of the thyrotropin receptor. J Clin Invest 100:1634-1639, 1997.
69. Gruters A, Schonenberg T, Biebermann H, et al: Severe congenital hyperthyroidism caused by a germ-line neo mutation in the extracellular portion of the thyrotropin receptor. J Clin Endocrinol Metab 83:1431-1436, 1998.
70. Pang XP, Park M, Hershman JM: Transforming growth factor beta blocks protein kinase-A–mediated iodide transport and protein kinase-C–mediated DNA synthesis in FRTL-5 rat thyroid cells 131:45-50, 1992.
71. Taton M, Lamy F, Roger PP, Dumont JE: General inhibition by transforming growth factor beta 1 of thyrotropin and cAMP responses in human thyroid cells in primary culture. Mol Cell Endocrinol 95:13-21, 1993.
72. Krohn K, Fuhrer D, Bayer Y, et al: Molecular pathogenesis of euthryoid and toxic multinodular goiter. Endocrine Reviews 26:504-524, 2005.
73. Eszlinger M, Krohn K, Frenzel R, et al: Gene expression analysis reveals evidence for inactivation of the TGF- 1 signaling cascade in autonomously functioning thyroid nodules. Oncogene 23:795-804, 2004.
74. Beere HM, Soden J, Tomlinson S, Bidey SP: Insulin-like growth factor-I production and action in porcine thyroid follicular cells in monolayer: Regulation by transforming growth factor-beta. J Endocrinol 130:3-9, 1991.
75. Eggo MC, King WJ, Black EG, Sheppard MC: Functional human thyroid cells and their insulin-like growth factor-binding proteins: Regulation by thyrotropin, cyclic 3′,5′-adenosine monophosphate, and growth factors. J Clin Endocrinol Metab 81:3056-3062, 1996.
76. Cowin AJ, Bidey SP: Transforming growth factor-beta 1 synthesis in human thyroid follicular cells: Differential effects of iodide and plasminogen on the production of latent and active peptide forms. J Endocrinol 141:183-190, 1994.
77. Gasperi M, Martino E, Manetti L, et al: Acromegaly Study Group of the Italian Society of Endocrinology: Prevalence of thyroid diseases in patients with acromegaly: Results of an Italian multi-center study. J Endocrinol Invest 25:240-245, 2002.
78. Wuster C, Steger G, Schmelzle A, et al: Increased incidence of euthyroid and hyperthyroid goiters independently of thyrotropin in patients with acrogmegaly. Horm Metab Res 23:131-134, 1991.
79. Miyakawa M, Saji M, Tsushima T, et al: Thyroid volume and serum thyroglobulin levels in patients with acromegaly: Correlation with plasma insulin-like growth factor I levels. J Clin Endocrinol Metab 67:973-978, 1988.
80. Eggo MC, Bachrach LK, Burrow GN: Interaction of TSH, insulin and insulin-like growth factors in regulating thyroid growth and function. Growth Factors 2:99-109, 1990.
81. Cheung NW, Lou JC, Boyages SC: Growth hormone does not increase thyroid size in the absence of thyrotropin: A study in adults with hypopituitarism. J Clin Endocrinol Metab 81:1179-1183, 1996.
82. Williams DW, Williams ED, Wynford-Thomas D: Loss of dependence on IGF-1 for proliferation of human thyroid adenoma cells. Br J Cancer 57:535-539, 1988.
83. Beere HM, Soden J, Tomlinson S, Bidey SP: Insulin-like growth factor-I production and action in porcine thyroid follicular cells in monolayer: Regulation by transforming growth factor-beta. J Endocrinol 130:3-9, 1991.
84. Hofbauer LC, Rafferzeder M, Janssen OE, Gartner R: Insulin-like growth factor I messenger ribonucleic acid expression in porcine thyroid follicles is regulated by thyrotropin and iodine. Eur J Endocrinol 132:605-610, 1995.
85. Eggo MC, Bachrach LK, Brown AL, Burrow GN: Thyrotropin inhibits, while insulin, epidermal growth factor and tetradecanoyl phorbol acetate stimulate insulin-like growth factor binding protein secretion from sheep thyroid cells. Growth Factors 4:221-230, 1991.
86. Eszlinger M, Krohn K, Paschke R: Complementary DNA expression array analysis suggests a lower expression of signal transduction proteins and receptors in cold and hot thyroid nodules. J Clin Endocrinol Metab 86:4834-4842, 2001.
87. Chanoine JP, Stein GS, Braverman LE, et al: Acidic fibroblast growth factor–modulated gene expression in the rat thyroid in vivo. J Cell Biochem 50:392-399, 1992.
88. DeVito WJ, Chanoine JP, Alex S, et al: Effect of in vivo administration of recombinant acidic fibroblast growth factor on thyroid function in the rat: Induction of colloid goiter. Endocrinology 131:729-735, 1992.
89. Sato K, Yamazaki K, Shizume K, et al: Stimulation by thyroid-stimulating hormone and Graves' immunoglobulin G of vascular endothelial growth factor mRNA expression in human thyroid follicles in vitro and flt mRNA expression in the rat thyroid in vivo. J Clin Invest 96:1295-1302, 1995.
90. Viglietto G, Romano A, Manzo G, et al: Upregulation of the angiogenic factors PlGF, VEGF and their receptors (flt-1, flk-1/KDR) by TSH in cultured thyrocytes and in the thyroid gland of thiouracil-fed rats suggest a TSH-dependent paracrine mechanism for goiter hypervascularization. Oncogene 15:2687-2698, 1997.

91. Yamada E, Yamazaki K, Takano K, et al: Iodide inhibits vascular endothelial growth factor-A expression in cultured human thyroid follicles: A microarray search for effects of thyrotropin and iodide on angiogenesis factors. Thyroid 16:545-554, 2006.
92. Ramsden JD, Buchanan MA, Egginton S, et al: Complete inhibition of goiter in mice requires combined gene therapy modification of angiopoietin, vascular endothelial growth factor, and fibroblast growth factor signaling. Endocrinology 146:2895-2902, 1995.
93. Prabakaran D, Kim P, Kim KR, Arvan P: Polarized secretion of thrombospondin is opposite to thyroglobulin in thyroid epithelial cells. J Biol Chem 268:9041-9048, 1993.
94. Bellon G, Chaquor B, Antonicelli F, et al: Differential expression of thrombospondin, collagen and thyroglobulin by thyroid-stimulating hormone and tumor-promoting phorbol ester in cultured porcine thyroid cells. J Cell Physiol 160:75-88, 1994.
95. Patel VA, Logan A, Watkinson JC, et al: Isolation and characterization of human thyroid endothelial cells. Am J Physiol Endocrinol Metab 284:E168-E176, 2003.
96. Patel VA, Hill DJ, Eggo MC, et al: Changes in the immunohistochemical localization of fibroblast growth factor-2, transforming growth factor-beta 1 and thrombospondin-1 are associated with early angiogenic events in the hyperplastic rat thyroid. J Endocrinol 149:485-499, 1996.
97. Jackson S, Tseng YC, Lahiri S, et al: Receptors for endothelin in cultured human thyroid cells and inhibition by endothelin of thyroglobulin secretion. J Clin Endocrinol Metab 75:388-392, 1992.
98. Kurihara Y, Kurihara H, Maemura K, et al: Impaired development of the thyroid and thymus in endothelin-1 knockout mice. J Cardiovasc Pharmacol 26(Suppl 3):S13-S16, 1995.
99. Eguchi K, Kawakami A, Nakashima M, et al: Stimulation of mitogenesis in human thyroid epithelial cells by endothelin. Acta Endocrinol 128:215-220, 1993.
100. Colin IM, Selvais PL, Rebai T, et al: Expression of the endothelin-1 gene in the rat thyroid gland and changes in its peptid and mRNA levels in goiter formation and iodide-induced involution. J Endocrinol 143:65-74, 1994.
101. Pedram A, Razandi M, Hu RM, Levin ER: Vasoactive peptides modulate vascular endothelial cell growth factor production and endothelial cell proliferation and invasion. J Biol Chem 272:17097-17103, 1997.
102. Pedram A, Razandi M, Levin ER: Natriuretic peptides suppress vascular endothelial cell growth factor signaling to angiogenesis. Endocrinology 142:1578-1586, 2001.
103. Tseng YC, Lahiri S, Sellitti DF, et al: Characterization by affinity cross-linking of a receptor for atrial natriuretic peptide in cultured human thyroid cells associated with reductions in both adenosine 3′,5′-monophosphate production and thyroglobulin secretion. J Clin Endocrinol Metab 70:528-533, 1990.
104. Tseng YL, Burman KD, Lahiri S, et al: Thyrotropin modulated receptor-mediated processing of the atrial natriuretic peptide receptor in cultured thyroid cells. J Clin Endocrinol Metab 72:669-674, 1991.
105. Costamagna ME, Coleoni AH, Pellizas CG, et al: Atrial natriuretic peptide inhibits iodide uptake and thyroglobulin messenger ribonucleic acid expression in cultured bovine thyroid follicles. Regul Pept 106:19-26, 2002.
106. Sellitti DF, Lagranha C, Perrella G, et al: Atrial natriuretic factor and C-type natriuretic peptide induce retraction of human thyrocytes in monolayer culture via guanylyl cyclase receptors. J Endocrinol 173:169-176, 2002.
107. Krassas GE: Thyroid disease and female reproduction. Fertil Steril 74:1063-1070, 2000.
108. Atkins HL, Klopper JF: Measurement of thyroidal technetium uptake with the gamma camera and computer system. Am J Roentgenol 118:831-835, 1973.
109. Hays M, Wesselossky B: Simultaneous measurement of thyroid trapping $(^{99m}TcO4-)$ and binding (^{131}I)clinical and experimental studies in man. J Nuc Med 14:785-792, 1973.
110. Hurley P, Maisey M, Natarajan T, Wagner HJ: A computerized system for rapid evaluation of thyroid function. J Clin Endocrinol Metab 34:354-360, 1972.
111. Reiners C, Schneider P: Radioiodine therapy of thyroid autonomy. Eur J Nuc Med 29(Suppl 2): S471-S478, 2002.
112. Gorman CA, Robertson JS: Radiation dose in the selection of ^{131}I or surgical treatment for toxic thyroid adenoma. Ann Intern Med 89:85-90, 1978.
113. Jarlov AE, Hegedus L, Kristensen LO, et al: Is calculation of the dose in radioiodine therapy of hyperthyroidism worthwhile? Clin Endocrinol 43:325-329, 1995.
114. Peters H, Fischer C, Bogner U, et al: Radioiodine therapy of Graves' hyperthyroidism: Standard vs. calculated 131iodine activity. Results from a prospective, randomized, multicentre study. Eur J Clin Invest 25:186-193, 1995.
115. Catargi B, Leprat F, Guyot M, et al: Optimized radioiodine therapy of Graves' disease: Analysis of the delivered dose and of other possible factors affecting outcome. Eur J Endocrinol 141:117-121, 1999.
116. Koroscil TM: Thionamides alter the efficacy of radioiodine treatment in patients with Graves' disease. South Med J 88:831-836, 1995.
117. Tuttle RM, Patience T, Budd S: Treatment with propylthiouracil before radioactive iodine therapy is associated with a higher treatment failure rate than therapy with radioactive iodine alone in Graves' disease. Thyroid 5:243-247, 1995.
118. Hancock LD, Tuttle RM, LeMar H, et al: The effect of propylthiouracil on subsequent radioactive iodine therapy in Graves' disease. Clin Endocrinol 47:425-430, 1997.

119. Imseis RE, Vanmiddlesworth L, Massie JD, et al: Pretreatment with propylthiouracil but not methimazole reduces the therapeutic efficacy of iodine-131 in hyperthyroidism. J Clin Endocrinol Metab 83:685-687, 1998.
120. Turton DB, Silverman ED, Shakir KM: Time interval between the last dose of propylthiouracil and I-131 therapy influences cure rates in hyperthyroidism caused by Graves' disease. Clin Nucl Med 23:810-814, 1998.
121. Sabri O, Zimny M, Schulz G, et al: Success rate of radioiodine therapy in Graves' disease: The influence of thyrostatic medication. J Clin Endocrinol Metab 84:1229-1233, 1999.
122. Andrade VA, Gross JL, Maia AL: The effect of methimazole pretreatment on the efficacy of radioactive iodine therapy in Graves' hyperthyroidism: One-year follow-up of a prospective, randomized study. J Clin Endocrinol Metab 86:3488-3493, 2001.
123. Braga M, Walpert N, Burch HB, et al: The effect of methimazole on cure rates after radioiodine treatment for Graves' hyperthyroidism: A randomized clinical trial. Thyroid 12:135-139, 2002.
124. Bonnema SJ, Bennedbaek FN, Veje A, et al: Propylthiouracil before 131-I therapy of hyperthyroid diseases: Effect on cure rate evaluated by a randomized clinical trial. J Clin Endocrinol Metab 89:4439-4444, 2004.
125. Huysmans DA, Corstens FH, Kloppenborg PW: Long-term follow-up in toxic solitary autonomous thyroid nodules treated with radioactive iodine. J Nucl Med 32:27-30, 1991.
126. Nygaard B, Hegedus L, Gervil M, et al: Radioiodine treatment of multinodular non-toxic goiter. BMJ 307:828-832, 1993.
127. Huysmans DA, Hermus AR, Corstens FH, Kloppenborg PW: Long-term results of two schedules of radioiodine treatment for toxic multinodular goiter. Eur J Nucl Med 20:1056-1062, 1993.
128. Nygaard B, Hegedus L, Nielsen KG, et al: Long-term effect of radioactive iodine on thyroid function and size in patients with solitary autonomously functioning toxic thyroid nodules. Clin Endocrinol 50:197-202, 1999.
129. Allahabadia A, Daykin J, Sheppard MC, et al: Radioiodine treatment of hyperthyroidism—prognostic factors for outcome. J Clin Endocrinol Metab 86:3611-3617, 2001.
130. Korber C, Schneider P, Korber-Hafner N, et al: Antithyroid drugs as a factor influencing the outcome of radioiodine therapy in Graves' disease and toxic nodular goiter? Eur J Nucl Med 28:1360-1364, 2001.
131. Kristoffersen US, Hesse B, Rasmussen AK, Kjaer A: Radioiodine therapy in hyperthyroid disease: Poorer outcome in patients with high 24 hours radioiodine uptake. Clin Physiol Funct Imaging 26:167-170, 2006.
132. Stensvold AD, Jorde R, Sundsfjord J: Late and transient increases in free T_4 after radioiodine treatment for Graves' disease. J Endocrinol Invest 20:580-584, 1997.
133. Andrade VA, Gross JL, Maia AL: Effect of methimazole pretreatment on serum thyroid hormone levels after radioactive treatment of Graves' hyperthyroidism. J Clin Endocrinol Metab 84:4012-4016, 1999.
134. Burch HB, Solomon BL, Cooper DS, et al: The effect of antithyroid drug pretreatment on acute changes in thyroid hormone levels after (131)I ablation for Graves' disease. J Clin Endocrinol Metab 86:3016-3021, 2001.
135. Cooper DS: Antithyroid drugs in the management of patients with Graves' disease: An evidence-based approach to therapeutic controversies. J Clin Endocrinol Metab 88:3474-3481, 2003.
136. Huysmans DA, Hermus AR, Corstens FH, et al: Large, compressive goiters treated with radioiodine. Ann Intern Med 121:757-762, 1994.
137. Nygaard B, Faber J, Hegedus L: Acute changes in thyroid volume and function following ^{131}I therapy of multinodular goiter. Clin Endocrinol 41:715-718, 1994.
138. Le Moli R, Wesche MF, Tiel-Van Buul MM, Wiersinga WM: Determinants of long-term outcome of radioiodine therapy of sporadic non-toxic goiter. Clin Endocrinol 50:783-789, 1999.
139. Reinhardt MJ, Joe A, von Mallek D, et al: Dose selection for radioiodine therapy of borderline hyperthyroid patients with multifocal and disseminated autonomy on the basis of ^{99m}Tc-pertechnetate thyroid uptake. Eur J Nucl Med Mol Imaging 29:480-485, 2002.
140. Holm LE, Hall P, Wiklund K, et al: Cancer risk after iodine-131 therapy for hyperthryoidism. J Natl Cancer Inst 83:1072-1077, 1991.
141. Ron E, Doody MM, Becker DV, et al: Cancer mortality following treatment for adult hyperthyroidism. Cooperative thyrotoxicosis therapy follow-up study group. JAMA 280:347-355, 1998.
142. Safa AM, Schumacher OP, Rodriquez-Antunez A: Long-term follow-up results in children and adolescents treated with radioactive iodine (^{131}I) for hyperthyroidism. N Engl J Med 292:167-171, 1975.
143. Nieuwlaat WA, Hermus AR, Sivro-Prndelj F, et al: Pretreatment with recombinant human TSH changes the regional distribution of radioiodine on thyroid scintigrams of nodular goiters. J Clin Endocrinol Metab 86:5330-5336, 2001.
144. Nieuwlaat WA, Huysmans DA, van den Bosch HC, et al: Pretreatment with a single, low dose of recombinant human thyrotropin allows dose reduction of radioiodine therapy in patients with nodular goiter. J Clin Endocrinol Metab 88:3121-3129, 2003.
145. Nielsen VE, Bonnema SJ, Hegedus L: Transient goiter enlargement after administration of 0.3 mg of recombinant human thyrotropin in patients with benign nontoxic nodular goiter: A randomized, double-blind, cross-over trial. J Clin Endocrinol Metab 91:1317-1322, 2006.

146. Nielsen VE, Bonnema SJ, Boel-Jorgensen H, et al: Stimulation with 0.3-mg recombinant human thyrotropin prior to iodine 131 therapy to improve the size reduction of benign nontoxic nodular goiter. Arch Intern Med 166:1476-1482, 2006.
147. Silva MN, Rubio IG, Romao R, et al: Administration of a single dose of recombinant human thyrotropin enhances the efficacy of radioiodine treatment of large compressive multinodular goiters. Clin Endocrinol 60:300-308, 2004.
148. Cooper DS: Antithyroid drugs. N Engl J Med 352:905-917, 2005.
149. Sherman SI, Ladenson PW: Endocrine complications of head and neck surgery. In Eisele DW (ed): Complications in Head and Neck Surgery. St. Louis, Mosby, 1993, pp 83-89.
150. Livraghi T, Paracchi A, Ferrari C, et al: Treatment of autonomous thyroid nodules with percutaneous ethanol injection: Preliminary results. Work in progress. Radiology 175:827-829, 1990.
151. Goletti O, Monzani R, Caraccio N, et al: Percutaneous ethanol injection treatment of autonomously functioning single thyroid nodules: Optimization of treatment and short-term outcome. World J Surg 16:784-789, 1992.
152. Paracchi A, Ferrari C, Livraghi T, et al: Percutaneous intranodular ethanol injection: A new treatment for autonomous thyroid adenoma. J Endocrinol Invest 15:353-362, 1992.
153. Martino E, Murtas ML, Loviselli A, et al: Percutaneous intranodular ethanol injection for treatment of autonomously functioning thyroid nodules. Surgery 112:1161-1164, 1992.
154. Monzani F, Goletti O, Caraccio N, et al: Percutaneous ethanol injection treatment of autonomous thyroid adenoma: Hormonal and clinical evaluation. Clin Endocrinol 36:491-497, 1992.
155. Monzani F, Lippi F, Goletti O, et al: Percutaneous aspiration and ethanol sclerotherapy for thyroid cysts. J Clin Endocrinol Metab 78:800-802, 1994.
156. Papini E, Panunzi C, Pacella CM, et al: Percutaneous ultrasound-guided ethanol injection: A new treatment of toxic autonomously functioning thyroid nodules? J Clin Endocrinol Metab 76:411-416, 1993.
157. Mazzeo S, Toni MG, De Gaudio C, et al: Percutaneous injection of ethanol to treat autonomous thyroid nodules. AJR Am J Roentgenol 161:871-876, 1993.
158. Livraghi T, Paracchi A, Ferrari C, et al: Treatment of autonomous thyroid nodules with percutaneous ethanol injection: 4-year experience. Radiology 190:529-533, 1994.
159. Del Prete S, Russo D, Caraglia M, et al: Percutaneous ethanol injection of autonomous thyroid nodules with a volume larger than 40 ml: Three years of follow-up. Clin Radiol 56:895-901, 2001.
160. Brkljacic B, Sucic M, Bozikov V, et al: Treatment of autonomous and toxic thyroid adenomas by percutaneous ultrasound-guided ethanol injection. Acta Radiol 42:477-481, 2001.
161. Dossing H, Bennedbaek FN, Karstrup S, Hegedus L: Benign solitary solid cold thyroid nodules: US-guided interstitial laser photocoagulation—initial experience. Radiology 225:53-57, 2002.
162. Dossing H, Bennedbaek FN, Hegedus L: Ultrasound-guided interstitial laser photocoagulation of an autonomous thyroid nodule: The introduction of a novel alternative. Thyroid 13:885-888, 2003.
163. Dossing H, Bennedbaek FN, Hegedus L: Effect of ultrasound-guided interstitial laser photocoagulation on benign solitary solid cold thyroid nodules—a randomized study. Eur J Endocrinol 152:341-345, 2005.
164. Dossing H, Bennedbaek FN, Hegedus L: Effect of ultrasound-guided interstitial laser photocoagulation on benign solitary solid cold thyroid nodules: One versus three treatments. Thyroid 16:763-768, 2006.
165. Pacella CM, Bizzarri G, Guglielmi R, et al: Thyroid tissue: US-guided percutaneous interstitial laser ablation—a feasibility study. Radiology 217:673-677, 2000.
166. Mallery KF, Pollard RE, Nelson RW, et al: Percutaneous ultrasound-guided radiofrequency heat ablation for treatment of hyperthyroidism in cats. J Am Vet Med Assoc 223:1602-1607, 2003.
167. Kim YS, Rhim H, Tae K, et al: Radiofrequency ablation of benign cold thyroid nodules: Initial clinical experience. Thyroid 16:361-367, 2006.
168. Esnault O, Franc B, Monteil JP, Chapelon JY: High-intensity focused ultrasound for localized thyroid-tissue ablation: Preliminary experimental animal study. Thyroid 14:1072-1076, 2004.

Chapter 15

Thyroid-Stimulating Hormone–Induced Hyperfunction

Paolo Beck-Peccoz and Luca Persani

Key Points

- Hyperthyroidism due to TSH-oma is biochemically characterized by high levels of circulating free thyroid hormones in the presence of normal/high levels of TSH.
- The clinical appearance of hyperthyroidism may be mild, sometimes overshadowed by signs and symptoms of concomitant acromegaly, or by neurologic symptoms (headache, visual field defect) due to compression on the surrounding anatomic structures by the tumor mass.
- T_3 suppression test and TRH test are useful in the differential diagnosis between TSH-omas and syndromes of thyroid hormone resistance.
- The first therapeutic approach to TSH-omas is the surgical removal of the adenoma.
- The medical treatment is based on the administration of long-acting somatostatin analogs, such as octreotide or lanreotide, which are successful in about 95% of patients.

Thyroid hyperfunction induced by endogenous thyroid-stimulating hormone (TSH) hypersecretion is a very rare clinical condition that is secondary to two different disorders, TSH-secreting pituitary adenoma (TSH-oma) and resistance to thyroid hormone action (RTH). The main difference between these two syndromes consists of the presence of signs and symptoms of hyperthyroidism in patients with TSH-oma, whereas RTH patients are in general euthyroid (so-called generalized RTH, GRTH). However, in a minority of RTH patients, features of hyperthyroidism may be present involving some organs and not others, such as heart (tachycardia) and brain (nervousness, insomnia, attention deficit, hyperactivity). This particular form of RTH is known as pituitary RTH (PRTH). Both TSH-omas and RTH are characterized by elevated serum thyroid hormone levels in the presence of normal or high TSH concentrations. TSH secretion from the tumor is autonomous, whereas thyrotropes of patients with RTH are refractory to the action of high levels of circulating thyroid hormones; thus, in both situations, negative feedback mechanism is not operating.[1-4] In keeping with this, Gershengorn and Weintraub[5] have suggested referring to them as inappropriate TSH secretion, in which "inappropriate" refers to the fact that contrary to what happens in the classic hyperthyroidism, TSH is not inhibited in these particular forms of thyroid hyperfunction. Currently, we propose to classify these entities as central hyperthyroidism.

The routine use of ultrasensitive immunometric assays for TSH measurement has greatly improved the diagnostic workup of hyperthyroid patients, allowing the recognition of cases with unsuppressed TSH secretion. As a consequence, central hyperthyroidism is now more often diagnosed earlier and an increased number of patients with normal or elevated TSH levels in the presence of high free thyroid hormone concentrations have been recognized.[2,3] When the diagnosis of central hyperthyrodism has been made, the differential diagnosis between TSH-oma and RTH, particularly PRTH, is mandatory.[1,4] Failure to recognize these different disorders may result in dramatic consequences, such as improper thyroid ablation or unnecessary pituitary surgery in patients with RTH. Conversely, early diagnosis and correct treatment of TSH-omas may prevent the occurrence of neurologic and endocrine complications, such as headache, visual field defects, and hypopituitarism, and should improve the rate of cure.

In this chapter, we will focuse on the pathophysiology, clinical features, diagnostic procedures, differential diagnosis, and treatment of thyroid hyperfunction caused by the presence of TSH-secreting pituitary adenomas.

PATHOPHYSIOLOGY

TSH-omas are almost always benign tumors and up to date transformation of a TSH-oma into a carcinoma with multiple metastases has been reported in only one patient.[6] Most of them (72%) secrete only TSH, although this is often accompanied by the unbalanced hypersecretion of an alpha subunit (pituitary glycoprotein hormone alpha subunit, α-GSU). About one fourth of TSH-omas are mixed adenomas, characterized by concomitant hypersecretion of other anterior pituitary hormones, mainly growth hormone (GH) or prolactin (PRL), which are known to share the common transcription factor Pit-1 with TSH.[7] Hypersecretion of TSH and GH is the most frequent association (16%), followed by hypersecretion of TSH and PRL (10.4%) and occasionally TSH and gonadotropins.

As for the other types of pituitary adenomas, the molecular mechanisms leading to the formation of TSH-omas are presently unknown. Inactivation analysis of X chromosomes has demonstrated that most pituitary adenomas, including the small number of TSH-omas investigated, derive from the clonal expansion of a single, initially transformed cell.[8] Therefore, the presence of a transforming event providing gain of proliferative function, followed by secondary mutations or alterations favoring tumor progression, presumably also apply to TSH-omas. Several proto-oncogenes and tumor suppressor genes, as well as pituitary-specific genes, have been screened for mutations able to confer growth advantage to pituitary cells. As for other pituitary adenomas, no mutations in oncogenes commonly activated in human cancer, particularly *Ras*, have been reported in TSH-omas. In contrast with GH-secreting adenomas in which the oncogene *gsp* in frequently present, none of the screened TSH-omas has been shown to express activating mutations of genes encoding for G protein subunits, such as αs, αq, α11, or αi2, or for TRH receptor.[9] Moreover, the transcription factor Pit-1 exerts a crucial role on cell differentiation and expression of PRL, GH, and TSH genes. Thus, Pit-1 gene has been studied and shown to be overexpressed, but not mutated, in 14 TSH-omas.[2]

As far as the possible loss of antioncogenes is concerned, no loss of p53 was found in one TSH-oma studied, wherease loss of retinoblastoma gene (Rb) was not investigated in TSH-omas. Another candidate gene is menin, the gene responsible for the multiple endocrine neoplasia type 1 (MEN 1). In fact, 3% to 30% of sporadic pituitary adenomas show loss of heterozygosity (LOH) on 11q13, where menin is located; LOH on this chromosome seems to be associated with the transition from the noninvasive to the invasive phenotype. A recent screening study carried out on 13 TSH-omas using polymorphic markers on 11q13 has shown LOH in 3, but none of them showed a menin mutation at sequence analysis.[2] Interestingly, hyperthyroidism caused by TSH-omas has been reported in five cases in a familial setting of MEN 1.

The extreme refractoriness of tumoral thyrotrophs to the inhibitory action of thyroid hormones has led to a search for alterations in thyroid hormone receptor (TR) function. Absence of TRα1, TRα2, and TRβ1 expression was reported in one TSH-oma, but aberrant alternative splicing of TRβ2 mRNA encoding TRβ variant lacking triiodothyronine (T_3) binding activity has been shown as a mechanism for impaired T_3-dependent negative regulation of both TSHβ and α-GSU in tumoral tissue.[10] Moreover, it has been suggested that somatic mutations of TRβ may be responsible for the defect in negative regulation of TSH secretion in some TSH-omas.[11]

Finally, LOH and particular polymorphisms at the somatostatin receptor type 5 gene locus seems to be associated with an aggressive phenotype and resistance to somatostatin analogue treatment, possibly because of lack of somatostatin-induced inhibition of TSH secretion.[12] Moreover, overexpression of basic fibroblast growth factor by some TSH-omas has suggested the possibility that it may play a role in the development of fibrosis and tumor cell proliferation in this unusual type of pituitary neoplasm.[13]

CLINICAL FEATURES

In patients with TSH-oma, signs and symptoms of hyperthyroidism are frequently associated with those related to the compression of the surrounding anatomic structures by expanding tumor, thus causing visual field defects, loss of vision, headhache, and partial or complete hypopituitarism (Table 15-1). Most patients have a long history of thyroid dysfunction, frequently misdiagnosed as Graves' disease, and about 30% of them have had inappropriate thyroidectomy or radioiodine thyroid ablation.[1,2,14] Clinical features of hyperthyroidism are sometimes milder than expected on the basis of circulating thyroid hormone levels. In some acromegalic patients, signs and symptoms of hyperthyroidism may be clinically missed, because they are overshadowed by those of acromegaly. Contrary to what is observed in patients with primary thyroid disorders, cardiotoxicosis with atrial fibrillation and/or cardiac failure and episodes of periodic paralysis are rare events.

The presence of a goiter is the rule, even in previously thyroidectomized patients, because thyroid residue may regrow as a consequence of TSH hyperstimulation. Occurrence of uni- or multinodular goiter is frequent (about 72% of reported cases), whereas differentiated thyroid carcinomas have been documented in only a few cases.[15,16] Progression towards toxic goiter is infrequent.[17] In contrast to Graves' disease, the occurrence of circulating antithyroid autoantibodies is similar to that found in the general population, about 8%. Bilateral exophthalmos has occurred in a few patients who subsequently developed autoimmune thyroiditis; unilateral exophthalmos caused by orbital invasion by pituitary tumor was reported in three patients with TSH-omas.[2,18]

Disorders of the gonadal axis are frequent. Menstrual disorders occur in all females with mixed TSH-PRL tumors and in one third of those with pure TSH-oma. Central hypogonadism, delayed puberty, and decreased libido have also been found in a number of males with TSH-omas and/or mixed TSH-FSH adenomas.

DIAGNOSTIC PROCEDURES

The finding of elevated levels of circulating thyroid hormones in the presence of measurable TSH concentrations is the biochemical feature characteristic of central hyperthyroidism. No difference in basal values of TSH and free thyroid hormone levels was seen between patients with TSH-oma and those with RTH. However, a unbalanced hypersecretion of circulating free α-GSU levels and an elevated α-GSU/TSH molar ratio have been detected in more than 80% of patients with documented TSH-oma.[1,14,19,20] In addition, measurements of several parameters of peripheral thyroid hormone action have been proposed to quantify the degree of tissue hyperthyroidism.[2] In particular, bone (carboxy terminal cross-linked telopeptide of type I collagen, ICTP) and liver (sex hormone–binding globulin, SHBG) parameters may help in differentiating hyperthyroid patients with TSH-oma from those with PRTH.[1,21] Because it occurs in the common forms of hyperthyroidism, patients with TSH-oma have high ICTP and SHBG levels, but these are in the normal range in patients with hyperthyroidism caused by PRTH (Table 15-2).

Stimulatory and inhibitory tests are helpful in the diagnosis of TSH-oma. The T_3 suppression test appear to be important to assess the presence of a TSH-oma. A complete inhibition of TSH secretion after the T_3 suppression test (80 to 100 μg/day for 8 to 10 days) has never been recorded in patients with TSH-oma (see Table 15-2), particularly in those previously thyrodectomized.[1,14,19] In this latter condition, T_3 suppression seems to be the most sensitive and specific test in assessing the presence of a TSH-oma. However, this test is contraindicated in older patients or in those with coronary heart disease. Therefore, TRH test has been widely used in the workup of these adenomas. In the vast majority of patients, TSH and α-GSU levels do not increase after TRH injection (see Table 15-2). In patients with hyperthyroidism, discrepancies between TSH and α-GSU responses to TRH are pathognomonic of TSH-omas cosecreting other pituitary hormones.[20]

Because most TSH-omas maintain the sensitivity to native somatostatin and its analogues (octreotide and lanreotide),[22-25] we have treated a series of patients with TSH-omas or PRTH with these compounds. We documented a marked decrease of free T_3 and T_4 levels in all patients, except one with pituitary adenoma, whereas all patients with PRTH did not respond (Fig. 15-1). Thus, administration of long-acting somatostatin analogues for at least 2 months can be useful in the differential diagnosis of problematic cases of central hyperthyroidism.[26] Nevertheless, because none of these tests is of clear-cut diagnostic value, it is recommend to carry out both T_3 suppression and TRH tests whenever possible, because the combination of their results increases the specificity and sensitivity of the diagnostic workup.[1,14,19]

Finally, high-resolution computed tomography (CT) and nuclear magnetic resonance imaging

Table 15–1 Clinical Manifestations in Patients with Thyroid-Stimulating Hormone (TSH)-oma

Parameter	Patients with TSH-oma
Age range (yr)	8-84
Female-to-male ratio	1.31
Previous thyroidectomy	30%
Severe thyrotoxicosis	22%
Goiter	92%
Thyroid nodule(s)	73%
Macroadenomas	79%
Visual field defects	36%
Headache	20%
Menstrual disorders*	32%
Galactorrhea*	29%
Acromegaly	15%

*Only female patients were considered.

Table 15–2 Differential Diagnosis Between Thyroid-Stimulating Hormone (TSH)–Secreting Pituitary Adenomas (TSH-omas) and Resistance to Thyroid Hormone (RTH)*

Parameter	TSH-omas (*N* = 20)	RTH (*N* = 32)	*P*
Serum TSH mU/L	2.8 ± 0.5	2.7 ± 0.3	NS
High α-GSU levels	70%	3%	<.0001
High α-GSU/TSH m.r.	83%	2%	<.0001
Serum FT_4 (pmol/L)	35.4 ± 4.0	31.2 ± 2.4	NS
Serum FT_3 (pmol/L)	14.0 ± 1.2	12.1 ± 0.9	NS
Serum SHBG (nmol/L)	117 ± 18	61 ± 4	<.0001
Blunted TSH response to TRH test	94%	2%	<.0001
Abnormal TSH response to T_3 suppression†	100%	100%‡	NS

FT_3, free triiodothyronine; FT_4, free thyroxine; α-GSU, glycoprotein hormone alpha subunit; m.r., molar ratio; NS, not significant; SHBG, sex hormone–binding globulin; TRH, thyrotropin-releasing hormone.

*Only patients with an intact thyroid were taken into account. Data were obtained from patients followed at our institute and are expressed as mean ± standard error or as a percentage.

†T_3 suppression test (Werner's test: 80-100 μg T_3 for 8-10 days). Quantitatively normal responses to T_3—that is, complete inhibition of basal and TRH-stimulated TSH levels—have never been recorded in either group of patients.

‡Although abnormal in quantitative terms, the TSH response to the T_3 suppression test was qualitatively normal in most RTH patients.

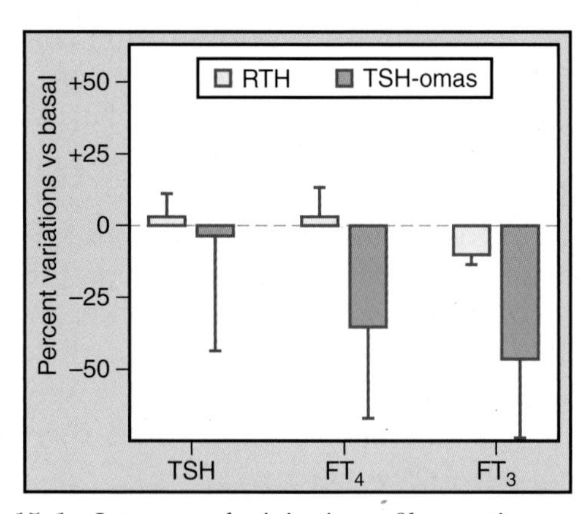

Figure 15–1 Intramuscular injections of long-acting somatostatin analogues (SMS) can be useful in the differential diagnosis between resistance to thyroid hormone (RTH) and thyroid-stimulating hormone (TSH)–secreting pituitary adenomas (TSH-omas). RTH patients are not responsive to chronic (2 to 3 months) SMS administration, whereas this treatment causes normalization or more than a 50% decrease in free thyroxine (FT_4) or free triiodothyronine (FT_3) circulating levels in the large majority of patients with TSH-omas.

(MRI) are currently preferred for the visualization of a TSH-oma. Most TSH-omas were diagnosed at the stage of macroadenomas with frequent suprasellar extension or sphenoidal sinus invasion. Microadenomas are now reported with increasing frequency, accounting for about 15% of all recorded cases in clinical and surgical series. Pituitary scintigraphy with radiolabeled octreotide (OctreoScan) has been shown to localize TSH-omas expressing somatostatin receptors.[27] However, the specificity of octreoscan is low, because positive scans can be seen in the case of a pituitary mass of different types, either secreting or nonsecreting. Such a procedure may be useful in the recognition of the possible ectopic localization of a TSH-oma; two cases of TSH-omas have been found in the nasopharyngeal region.[28,29]

DIFFERENTIAL DIAGNOSIS

The diagnosis of primary hyperthyroidism (i.e., Graves' disease, uni- or multinodular toxic goiter, or activating mutations of TSH receptor), is ruled out by the finding of measurable levels of circulating TSH (Fig. 15-2). However, circulating factors, such as antibodies against TSH or thyroid hormones, as well as abnormal forms of albumin or transthyretin, may interfere in the determination of TSH and thyroid hormone levels, yielding spuriously high hormone levels and possibly simulating the biochemical characteristics of central hyperthyroidism.[4]

Once the existence of central hyperthyroidism is confirmed and the presence of methodologic interferences excluded,[1,4] several diagnostic steps have to be carried out to differentiate a TSH-oma from RTH, particularly PRTH. The possible presence of neurologic signs and symptoms (e.g., visual defects and headache) or clinical features of concomitant hypersecretion of other pituitary hormones (e.g., acromegaly, amenorrhea, galactorrhea) points to the presence of a TSH-oma. Furthermore, the presence of alterations of the

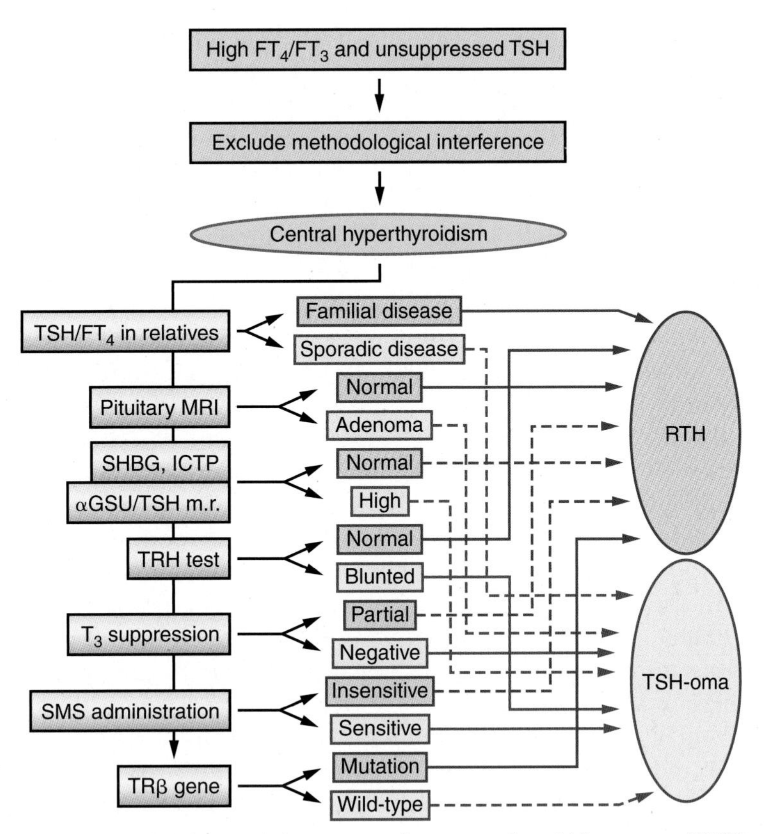

Figure 15–2 Flowchart for the differential diagnosis between resistance to thyroid hormone (RTH) and thyroid-stimulating hormone (TSH)–secreting pituitary adenoma (TSH-oma). After exclusion of methodologic interference, central hyperthyroidism is confirmed. A panel of clinical, biochemical, and genetic tests may be necessary to reach a differential diagnosis. Red findings are more consistent with RTH and blue findings with TSH-oma. Solid lines indicate findings that provide a stronger diagnostic indication. m.r., molar ratio. See text for details.

pituitary gland by MRI or CT scanning strongly supports the diagnosis of a TSH-oma. Nevertheless, the differential diagnosis with PRTH may be difficult when the pituitary adenoma is very small or in the case of confusing lesions, such as ectopic tumors, empty sella, or pituitary incidentalomas, with the latter lesion often found in the general population.[26] In these cases, elevated α-GSU concentrations or a high α-GSU/TSH molar ratio and TSH unresponsiveness to TRH stimulation or T_3 suppression tests, or both, favor the presence of a TSH-oma (see Fig. 15-2). Moreover, the finding of similar biochemical data in relatives definitely indicates the presence of RTH, because familial cases of TSH-omas have not been documented. Finally, an apparent association between TSH-oma and RTH has been reported and somatic mutations in the thyroid-hormone receptor have been found in some tumors.[10,11] Thus, the occurrence of TSH-oma in patients with RTH should be carefully considered.

TREATMENT

The first therapeutic approach to TSH-omas is the trans-sphenoidal or subfrontal adenomectomy, with the choice of route depending on the tumor volume and its suprasellar extension. The primary objectives of the treatment are twofold—that is, the removal of the pituitary tumor and the restoration of euthyroidism. The operation is sometimes difficult because of the marked fibrosis of these tumors, possibly related to high expression of basic fibroblast growth factor,[13] which may lead to adenomas called pituitary stones because of their hardness.[30] In addition, these tumors may be locally invasive, involving the cavernous sinus, internal carotid artery, or other structures, therefore rendering complete resection of the tumor impractical or dangerous. Antithyroid drugs (methimazole or propylthiouracil, 20 to 30 and 200 to 300 mg/day, respectively) or somatostatin analogues, such as octreotide (100 μg subcutaneously, two or three times daily), along with propranolol (80 to 120 mg/day PO) can be administered to restore euthyroidism before surgery. However, this approach may cause TSH secretion from normal nonadenomatous thyrotropes to be reactivated, so that a useful parameter for determining the complete removal of the adenoma—the unmeasurable levels of circulating TSH a few days after surgery—may be lost.[31] If surgery is contraindicated or declined, pituitary radiotherapy (no less than 45 Gy fractionated at 2 Gy/day or 10 to 25 Gy in a single dose if a stereotactic gamma knife is available) should be considered. A successful experience of an invasive TSH-oma associated with an unruptured aneurysm treated by two-stage operation and gamma knife has been reported.[32]

With these therapeutic approaches, normalization of thyroid hormone circulating levels and apparent complete removal of tumor mass was observed in one third of patients, who could therefore be considered apparently cured (follow-up ranged from 2 to 121 months). An additional one third of patients were judged improved; normalization of thyroid hormone circulating levels was achieved in all, although there was no complete removal of the adenoma. Together, these findings indicate that about two thirds of TSH-omas are under control with surgery and/or irradiation. In the remaining patients, TSH hypersecretion was unchanged after treatment, which undoubtedly reflects tumor large mass and invasiveness. Previous thyroid ablation or antithyroid drug treatments did not significantly affect the results of surgery and/or radiotherapy. Postsurgical deaths were reported in few cases. Evaluation of pituitary function, particularly ACTH secretion, should be carefully undertaken soon after surgery and checked again every year, especially in patients treated with radiotherapy. In addition, in the case of surgical cure, postoperative TSH is undetectable and may remain low for many weeks or months, causing central hypothyroidism. A permanent central hypothyroidism may occur because of compression by the tumor or surgical damage of the normal thyrotrophs. Thus, transient or permanent L-T_4 replacement therapy may be necessary. Finally, in a few patients total thyroidectomy was performed after pituitary surgery failure, because the patients were at risk of thyroid storm.

Although the surgical cure rate of TSH-omas is now improved because of early diagnosis, some patients require medical therapy to control the hyperthyroidism. The rationale for medical treatment is based on in vitro studies. Somatostatin (SRIH) binding experiments have indicated that almost all TSH-omas express a variable number of SRIH receptors; the highest SRIH-binding site densities are found in mixed GH/TSH adenomas.[22] Because somatostatin analogues are highly effective in reducing TSH secretion by neoplastic thyrotrophs,[1,14,19,23-26] the inhibitory pathway mediated by somatostatin receptors appears to be intact in these adenomas. There is a consistently good correlation between SRIH-binding capacity and maximal biologic response, as quantified by inhibition of TSH secretion and in vivo restoration of a euthyroid state.[22] The presence of dopamine receptors in TSH-omas was the rationale for therapeutic trials with dopaminergic agonists, such as bromocriptine and cabergoline. Several studies have shown a large heterogeneity of TSH responses to dopaminergic agents in primary cultures or in vivo, with the best results achieved in mixed TSH-PRL adenomas.[2] Effects of these two inhibitory agents should be reevaluated in light of the demonstration of possible heterodimerization of somatostatin receptor type 5 and dopamine D2 receptor.[33] Nonetheless, the medical treatment of TSH-omas is now based on long-acting somatostatin analogues, such as long-acting octreotide (Sandostatin), sustained-release lanreotide, or Lanreotide Autogel.[1,14,19,23-26] Treatment with these analogues leads to a reduction of TSH and α-GSU secretion in almost all cases, with restoration of the euthyroid state in most of them. Circulating thyroid hormone levels normalized in 96% of patients not previously thyroidectomized. Goiter size was significantly reduced by somatostatin analogue therapy in 20% of cases. Vision improvement was documented in 68% of patients and pituitary tumor mass shrinkage occurred in about 40%. Resistance to somatostatin analogue treatment, escape of TSH secretion from the inhibitory effects of the drugs, or discontinuation of treatment because of side effects was documented in a minority of cases. Of interest are the findings of octreotide treatment in pregnant women that was effective in restoring euthyroidism in the mother and had no side effects on development and thyroid function of the fetus.[34,35] Moreover, in almost all patients with mixed TSH-GH hypersecretion, signs and symptoms of acromegaly concomitantly disappeared.

Patients on somatostatin analogues have to be carefully monitored, because untoward side effects, such as cholelithiasis and carbohydrate intolerance, may become manifest. The administered dose should be tailored for each patient, depending on therapeutic response and tolerance, including gastrointestinal side effects. The tolerance is usually good, because gastrointestinal side effects are transient with long-acting analogues. The marked somatostatin-induced suppression of TSH secretion and consequent biochemical hypothyroidism seen in some patients may require L-T_4 substitution. Finally, no studies have reported of somatostatin analogue treatment of TSH-omas in patients who underwent thyroid ablation by thyroidectomy or radioiodine. Because aggressive and invasive macroadenomas are more frequently found in these patients,[1] it is mandatory to treat them to block further growth of a pituitary tumor mass.

In conclusion, whether somatostatin analogue treatment may be an alternative to surgery and/or irradiation in patients with TSH-oma still remains to be established. However, the therapeutic success of both octreotide and lanreotide administration is high, approaching 95% of treated patients. Somatostatin analogues may therefore represent a useful tool for long-term treatment of such rare pituitary tumors.

References

1. Beck-Peccoz P, Brucker-Davis F, Persani L, et al: Thyrotropin-secreting pituitary tumors. Endocr Rev 17:610-638, 1996.
2. Beck-Peccoz P, Persani L: Thyrotropin-secreting pituitary adenomas, 2007. Available at http://www.thyroidmanager.org/Chapter13/chapter13a.html.
3. Refetoff S, Weiss RE, Usala SJ: The syndromes of resistance to thyroid hormone. Endocr Rev 14:348-399, 1993.
4. Gurnell M, Beck-Peccoz P, Chatterjee VK: Resistance to thyroid hormone. In DeGroot LJ, Jameson JL (eds): Endocrinology, 5th ed. Philadelphia, Elsevier Saunders, 2005, pp 2227-2237.
5. Gershengorn MC, Weintraub BD: Thyrotropin-induced hyperthyroidism caused by selective pituitary resistance to thyroid hormone. A new syndrome of "inappropriate secretion of TSH." J Clin Invest 56:633-642, 1975.
6. Mixson AJ, Friedman TC, David AK, et al: Thyrotropin-secreting pituitary carcinoma. J Clin Endocrinol Metab 76:529-533, 1993.
7. Cohen LE, Radovick S: Molecular bases of pituitary hormone deficiencies. Endocr Rev 23:431-442, 2002.
8. Ma W, Ikeda H, Watabe N, et al: A plurihormonal TSH-producing pituitary tumor of monoclonal origin in a patient with hypothyroidism. Horm Res 59:257-261, 2003.
9. Dong Q, Brucker-Davis F, Weintraub BD, et al: Screening of candidate oncogenes in human thyrotroph tumors: Absence of activating mutations of the Gαq, Gα11, Gαs, or thyrotropin-releasing hormone receptor genes. J Clin Endocrinol Metab 81:1134-1140, 1996.
10. Ando S, Sarlis NJ, Krishnan J, et al: Aberrant alternative splicing of thyroid hormone receptor in a TSH-secreting pituitary tumor is a mechanism for hormone resistance. Mol Endocrinol 15:1529-1538, 2001.
11. Ando S, Sarlis NJ, Oldfield EH, Yen PM: Somatic mutation of TRbeta can cause a defect in negative regulation of TSH in a TSH-secreting pituitary tumor. J Clin Endocrinol Metab 86:5572-5576, 2001.
12. Filopanti M, Ballare E, Lania AG, et al: Loss of heterozygosity at the SS receptor type 5 locus in human GH- and TSH-secreting pituitary adenomas. J Endocrinol Invest 27:937-942, 2004.
13. Ezzat S, Horvath E, Kovacs K, et al: Basic fibroblast growth factor expression by two prolactin and thyrotropin-producing pituitary adenomas. Endocr Pathol 6:125-134, 1993.
14. Brucker-Davis F, Oldfield EH, Skarulis MC, et al: Thyrotropin-secreting pituitary tumors: Diagnostic criteria, thyroid hormone sensitivity, and treatment outcome in 25 patients followed at the National Institutes of Health. J Clin Endocrinol Metab 84:476-486, 1999.
15. Gasparoni P, Rubello D, Persani L, Beck-Peccoz P: Unusual association between a thyrotropin-secreting pituitary adenoma and a papillary thyroid carcinoma. Thyroid 8:181-183, 1998.
16. Ohta S, Nishizawa S, Oki Y, Namba H: Coexistence of thyrotropin-producing pituitary adenoma with papillary adenocarcinoma of the thyroid—a case report and surgical strategy. Pituitary 4:271-274, 2001.
17. Abs R, Stevenaert A, Beckers A: Autonomously functioning thyroid nodules in a patient with a thyrotropin-secreting pituitary adenoma: Possible cause-effect relationship. Eur J Endocrinol 131:355-358, 1994.
18. Kourides IA, Pekonem F, Weintraub BD: Absence of thyroid-binding immunoglobulins in patients with thyrotropin-mediated hyperthyroidism. J Clin Endocrinol Metab 51:272-274, 1980.
19. Socin HV, Chanson P, Delemer B, et al: The changing spectrum of TSH-secreting pituitary adenomas: Diagnosis and management in 43 patients. Eur J Endocrinol 148:433-442, 2003.
20. Terzolo M, Orlandi F, Bassetti M, et al: Hyperthyroidism due to a pituitary adenoma composed of two different cell types, one secreting alpha-subunit alone and another cosecreting alpha-subunit and thyrotropin. J Clin Endocrinol Metab 72:415-421, 1991.
21. Persani L, Preziati D, Matthews CH, et al: Serum levels of carboxyterminal cross-linked telopeptide of type I collagen (ICTP) in the differential diagnosis of the syndromes of inappropriate secretion of TSH. Clin Endocrinol (Oxf) 47:207-214, 1997.
22. Bertherat J, Brue T, Enjalbert A, et al: Somatostatin receptors on thyrotropin-secreting pituitary adenomas: Comparison with the inhibitory effects of octreotide upon in vivo and in vitro hormonal secretions. J Clin Endocrinol Metab 75:540-546, 1992.
23. Gancel A, Vuillermet P, Legrand A, et al: Effets of a slow-release formulation of the new somatostatin analogue lanreotide in TSH-secreting pituitary adenomas. Clin Endocrinol 40:421-428, 1994.
24. Chanson P, Weintraub BD, Harris AG: Octreotide therapy for thyroid stimulating-secreting pituitary adenomas. A follow-up of 52 patients. Ann Intern Med 119:236-240, 1993.
25. Kuhn JM, Arlot S, Lefebvre H, et al: Evaluation of the treatment of thyrotropin-secreting pituitary adenomas with a slow-release formulation of the somatostatin analog lanreotide. J Clin Endocrinol Metab 85:1487-1491, 2000.

26. Mannavola D, Persani L, Vannucchi G, et al: Different response to chronic somatostatin analogues in patients with central hyperthyroidism. Clin Endocrinol (Oxf) 62:176-181, 2005.
27. Losa M, Magnani P, Mortini P, et al: Indium-111 pentetreotide single-photon emission tomography in patients with TSH-secreting pituitary adenomas: Correlation with the effect of a single administration of octreotide on serum TSH levels. Eur J Nucl Med 24:728-731, 1997.
28. Cooper DS, Wenig BM: Hyperthyroidism caused by an ectopic TSH-secreting pituitary tumor. Thyroid 6:337-343, 1996.
29. Pasquini E, Faustini-Fustini M, Sciarretta V, et al: Ectopic TSH-secreting pituitary adenoma of the vomerosphenoidal junction. Eur J Endocrinol 148: 253-257, 2003.
30. Webster J, Peters JR, John R, et al: Pituitary stone: Two cases of densely calcified thyrotropin-secreting pituitary adenomas. Clin Endocrinol (Oxf) 40:137-143, 1994.
31. Losa M, Giovanelli M, Persani L, et al: Criteria of cure and follow-up of central hyperthyroidism due to thyrotropin-secreting pituitary adenomas. J Clin Endocrinol Metab 81:3086-3090, 1996.
32. Ohki M, Sato K, Tuchiya D, et al: A case of TSH-secreting pituitary adenoma associated with an unruptured aneurysm: Successful treatment by two-stage operation and gamma knife. No To Shinkei 895-899, 1999.
33. Rocheville M, Lange DC, Kumar U, et al: Receptors for dopamine and somatostatin: Formation of hetero-oligomers with enhanced functional activity. Science 288:154-157, 2000.
34. Blackhurst G, Strachan MW, Collie D, et al: The treatment of a thyrotropin-secreting pituitary macroadenoma with octreotide in twin pregnancy. Clin Endocrinol (Oxf) 57:401-404, 2002.
35. Chaiamnuay S, Moster M, Katz MR, Kim YN: Successful management of a pregnant woman with a TSH-secreting pituitary adenoma with surgical and medical therapy. Pituitary 6:109-113, 2003.

Chapter 16

Hyperthyroidism and Trophoblastic Disease

Emily J. Tan and Jerome M. Hershman

Key Points

- Human chorionic gonadotropin (hCG) has weak thyroid-stimulating hormone (TSH)-like activity and can directly stimulate the thyroid gland in normal pregnancy.
- hCG in serum exists as a mixture of heterologous isoforms.
- Biochemical and clinical hyperthyroidism of varying degrees is associated with conditions of excessive hCG concentration (e.g., gestational transient thyrotoxicosis, multiple-gestation pregnancy, hyperemesis gravidarum, trophoblastic tumors, other hCG-secreting tumors, and hyperplacentosis).
- Hyperthyroidism from excess hCG generally requires symptomatic treatment of thyrotoxicosis and resolves completely with treatment of the underlying disorder as hCG secretion declines.
- A unique familial mutation of the TSH receptor has been identified.

The first case of hyperthyroidism occurring in a woman with hydatidiform mole was described in 1955.[1] Since that time, the role of human chorionic gonadotropin (hCG) as a thyroid stimulator has been an area of great interest. hCG is a glycoprotein hormone that shares structural similarity with pituitary thyroid stimulating hormone (TSH). Studies have shown that hCG acts as a weak thyroid stimulator, with 1/10,000 the potency of human TSH.[2] Physiologically, at this potency, hCG concentrations in the usual normal pregnancy are not sufficient to cause clinically apparent hyperthyroidism. However, in the setting of increased hCG concentration, such as gestational transient thyrotoxicosis, multiple-gestation pregnancy, hyperemesis gravidarum, trophoblastic tumors (hydatidiform mole and choriocarcinoma), other hCG-secreting tumors, or hyperplacentosis, clinically apparent hyperthyroidism may occur. It is important to recognize the possible association of hyperthyroidism induced by hCG stimulation of the TSH receptor, because there are important implications for the practice of clinical medicine.

HUMAN CHORIONIC GONADOTROPIN

hCG belongs to the glycoprotein hormone family, which includes TSH, luteinizing hormone (LH), and follicle-stimulating hormone (FSH). They share a common alpha subunit, coded on chromosome 6,[3] which consists of a polypeptide chain of 92 amino acid residues with two N-linked oligosaccharide side chains. The beta subunit is hormone-specific, coded on chromosome 19 and noncovalently bound to the alpha subunit.

The beta subunit of hCG is comprised of 145 residues, with two N-linked and four O-linked oligosaccharide side chains (Fig. 16-1).[4,5] The beta subunit of TSH is composed of 112 residues, with one N-linked oligosaccharide side chain. Both hCG and TSH share a 12-cysteine residue at highly conserved positions, thus contributing to the similarity in the overall three-dimensional structure of the two molecules and providing a basis for the stimulation of the TSH receptor by hCG.

hCG and LH also have a high degree of structural similarity in the beta subunit, with 85% sequence identity in 114 amino acids.[4,5] They differ, however, in the carboxy terminal sequence (β-CTP), with hCG having an additional 31–amino acid extension.

The glycoprotein hormone receptors are all G protein–coupled receptors that signal through the cyclic adenomonophosphate (cAMP) and inositol phosphate pathways. They share homology of about 70% in their transmembrane domain, which is comprised of a single polypeptide chain with seven

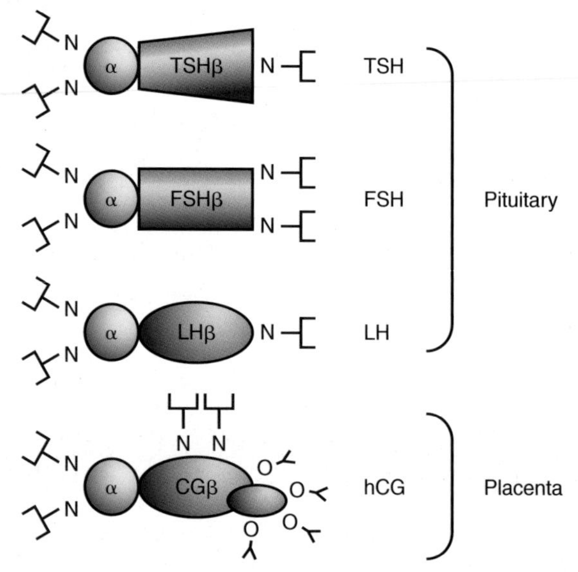

Figure 16–1 Human chorionic gonadotropin (hCG) belongs to the glycoprotein hormone family, which includes thyroid-stimulating hormone (TSH), luteinizing hormone (LH), and follicle-stimulating hormone (FSH). They share a common alpha subunit and a hormone-specific beta subunit. The schematic shows N-linked and O-linked oligosaccharide side chains. *(Adapted from Goodwin T, Hershman JM: Hyperthyroidism due to inappropriate production of human chorionic gonadotropin. Clin Obstet Gynecol 40:32-44, 1997.)*

hydrophilic alpha helices. The specific hormone receptors differ in the large amino terminal extracellular domain that makes up the hormone binding site.[6] However, there is about 45% homology in this extracellular domain between the LH, hCG, and TSH receptors.[5]

Human Chorionic Gonadotropin: Human Thyrotropin

Many patients with hydatidiform mole or choriocarcinoma were found to be hyperthyroid.[7-9] A search for the thyroid stimulator ultimately resulted in the isolation of hCG in 1975.[10] It is believed that the structural similarity between hCG and TSH, as well as the homology in their receptors, is the basis for stimulation of the TSH receptor by hCG. hCG has thyroid-stimulating activity in the McKenzie mouse bioassay and has been shown to increase iodide uptake and cAMP production[11-13] in FRTL-5 rat thyroid cells. Thymidine incorporation and c-myc expression, indicating stimulation of thyroid cell growth, were also induced by hCG in FRTL-5 cells.[14,15] Studies using human thyroid follicles have shown that hCG stimulates adenylate cyclase,[16] iodide uptake, organification, and triiodothyronine (T_3) secretion,[17] supporting the role of hCG as a human thyrotropin. When studied in Chinese hamster ovary (CHO) cells expressing recombinant TSH receptor, hCG increased cAMP production in a dose-dependent manner[18,19] and displaced binding of radiolabeled TSH from its receptor.[20] Other studies have demonstrated that a monoclonal antibody to hCG reduces the thyroid-stimulating activity in serum of pregnant women,[13,21] suggesting that hCG itself is the thyroid stimulator. Supporting this hypothesis is the demonstration that adding anti-TSH receptor antibody results in the inhibition of hCG-mediated thyrotropic stimulation in human thyroid follicles.[22]

Isoforms of Human Chorionic Gonadotropin: Varying Thyrotropic Potential

hCG in serum exists as a mixture of heterologous isoforms containing varying amounts of oligosaccharide side chains. Purified hCG has a molecular weight of 36,700, with 30% carbohydrate and a high content of sialic acid.[9] The half-life of this native hCG is 24 hours and it has an acidic isoelectric point at pH 3.8. Studies with human thyroid follicles have shown that pure hCG has weak thyroid-stimulating activity, with hCG being $1/10{,}000$ as potent as human TSH.[2]

The bioactivity and half-life of hCG are highly influenced by the number and structure of the oligosaccharide side chains, and extensive structural variations in hCG exist. It has been suggested that the carbohydrate side chains interfere with the binding of native hCG to the TSH receptor and that deglycosylation or desialylation enhances the affinity of hCG to the TSH receptor. Deglycosylation or desialylation results in hCG isoforms with more potent thyrotropic activity in vitro.[22-24] Removal of oligosaccharide side chains results in hCG isoforms that become more basic, and basic isoforms have been demonstrated to have a higher thyroid-stimulating activity compared with acidic isoforms (Fig. 16-2).[25] Basic isoforms have increased potency in activating cAMP and a higher bioactivity-to-immunoactivity ratio in CHO cells transfected with the human TSH receptor.[19,25] Asialo-hCG, in which all the carbohydrate side chains have been removed, has been demonstrated to have the highest potency of the hCG isoforms[22,25]; however, in another study, asialo-hCG demonstrated an antagonistic effect on binding of TSH to its receptor.[26]

Deletion of the β-CTP extension from native hCG results in a mutant hCG, with similarity in structure and thyroid-stimulating potency to LH. LH has been shown in in vitro studies to be 10 times more potent than hCG in cAMP stimulation at the TSH receptor.[19] It is believed that the large carboxy terminal extension of the native hCG molecule interferes with binding of the hCG to the TSH receptor and prevents overt hyperthyroidism in normal pregnancy.[27]

Nicked hCG, resulting from enzymatic deactivation and degradation,[28] has missing peptide links at β44-45 or at β47-48 and has been shown to have 1.5 to 2 times the thyrotropic potency of native hCG.[20]

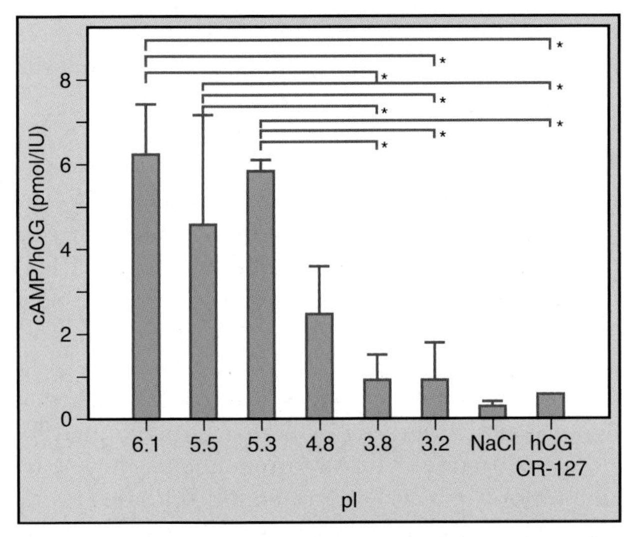

Figure 16–2 Thyrotropic potency of molar human chorionic gonadotropin (hCG) isoforms with different isoelectric points. Basic isoforms (pI, 6.1-5.3) show significantly higher potency than acidic isoforms (pI, 3.8-3.2). *(Adapted from Yoshimura M, Pekary AE, Pang XP, et al: Thyrotropic activity of basic isoelectric forms of human chorionic gonadotropin extracted from hydatidiform mole tissues. J Clin Endocrinol Metab 78:862-864, 1994.)*

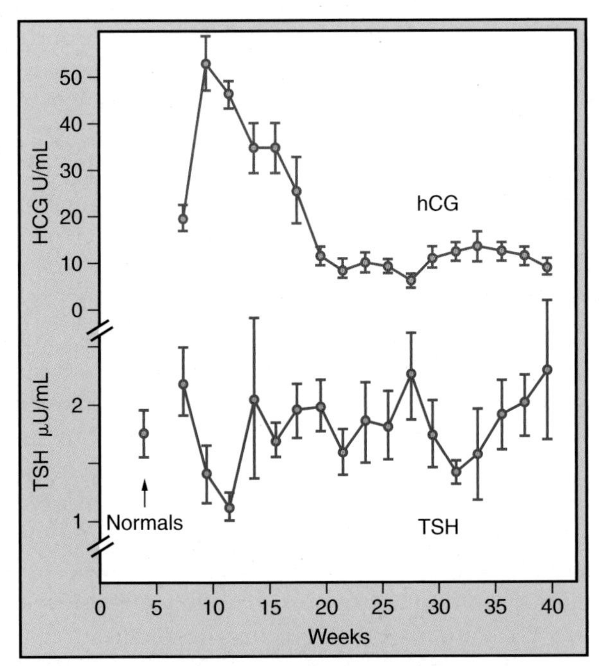

Figure 16–3 Serum human chorionic gonadotropin (hCG) and thyroid-stimulating hormone (TSH) as a function of gestational age. Peak hCG corresponds to a nadir TSH at weeks 8 to 12. TSH returns to baseline with declining hCG levels in the second trimester. *(Adapted from Harada A, Hershman JM, Reed AW, et al: Comparison of thyroid stimulators and thyroid hormone concentrations in the sera of pregnant women. J Clin Endocrinol Metab 48:793-797, 1979.)*

Although hCG isoforms with lower carbohydrate and lower sialic acid content have more potent thyroid stimulating activity in vitro, they have a shorter half-life in vivo. The sialic acid inhibits uptake by hepatic cells,[29] and thus asialo-hCG and desialylated isoforms are more rapidly cleared by hepatic cells in the pathway for degradation. Nicked hCG has also been demonstrated to have a shorter half-life compared with native hCG.[28] In contrast, acidic hCG isoforms that are highly sialated and less potent in vitro have been demonstrated to have delayed clearance in vivo.[30] Therefore, the activity of hCG in vivo is caused by the thyrotropic activity of the isoform and its half-life.

Thyroid Function and Human Chorionic Gonadotropin in Normal Pregnancy

In normal pregnancy, hCG concentration peaks at weeks 8 to 12, with maximum levels of 30 to 100 U/mL. This peak has been shown to correspond with a nadir of TSH concentration (Fig. 16-3).[31] A direct relationship between hCG concentration and free thyroxine (T_4) concentration has been shown, although the free T_4 level generally remains within the normal range.[32] Thyroid-stimulating activity has also been noted to correlate directly with the serum hCG level. It has thus been suggested that hCG secreted from the placenta directly increases secretion of thyroid hormones from the thyroid gland. However, this has been difficult to demonstrate convincingly because of the other effects on thyroid hormone economy during pregnancy—namely, increase in thyroxine-binding globulin (TBG), increased iodide clearance, possibly increased degradation of thyroxine by the placenta, and variations in albumin concentration. Nevertheless, given that hCG has weak thyrotropic activity, it is believed that the higher hCG concentration during the first trimester of gestation is sufficient to induce a mild elevation of thyroid hormone level that blunts secretion of TSH, resulting in a decreased serum TSH level. As the hCG level declines during the second and third trimesters, there is a concurrent rise in the TSH concentration back to baseline (see Fig. 16-3).

The prevalence of subnormal TSH (subclinical hyperthyroidism) associated with first-trimester pregnancy is not known exactly, but has been reported in 18% to 21% of normal pregnancies.[33,34] Most women are asymptomatic, and the subtle thyroid abnormalities usually resolve spontaneously with the declining hCG concentration even before they are recognized. When TSH levels were followed in the second and third trimesters of normal pregnancies, suppression was noted in only 5% and 2%, respectively.

DISORDERS RESULTING FROM INCREASED HUMAN CHORIONIC GONADOTROPIN CONCENTRATION

Gestational Transient Thyrotoxicosis

In a subset of pregnancies, TSH suppression is associated with elevation in free T_4 and T_3 levels, with or without associated clinical features of hyperthyroidism. Often also associated with vomiting, this entity is known as gestational transient thyrotoxicosis (GTT) or nonautoimmune hyperthyroidism. It has been reported to occur in 1% to 3% of pregnancies[33,35] but it is suspected that the prevalence of GTT is higher. Because of the transient nature of this condition and the variable clinical manifestations of hyperthyroidism, the diagnosis of GTT is frequently missed in pregnancy. It has been reported that only 50% of patients with GTT have symptoms consistent with hyperthyroidism, such as tachycardia, fatigue, weight loss, or absence of weight gain. GTT is also found more frequently in women who have some underlying thyroid condition, such as autoimmune thyroiditis or Graves' disease, glandular autonomy, or genetic resistance to thyroid hormone, and these patients generally present with more severe thyrotoxicosis.[36] The cause of GTT is believed to be related to a higher concentration of hCG, generally higher than 75 U/mL, as well as a prolonged duration of hCG elevation (Fig. 16-4). Other causative factors that have been proposed are the presence of hCG variants with a prolonged half-life, dysregulation of beta-hCG production, and hCG isoforms with increased thyrotropic activity.[21,33,37,38] GTT is usually transient, often resolving as hCG levels decline by week 20. Because it is self-limited, GTT rarely requires treatment. Hyperthyroid symptoms may be treated with β-adrenergic blocking drugs for a short time until the thyroid function normalizes. Most severe cases of GTT are associated with hyperemesis gravidarum (see later), and some of these may require antithyroid medications. GTT tends to recur in subsequent pregnancies and is not associated with a less favorable outcome of pregnancy.

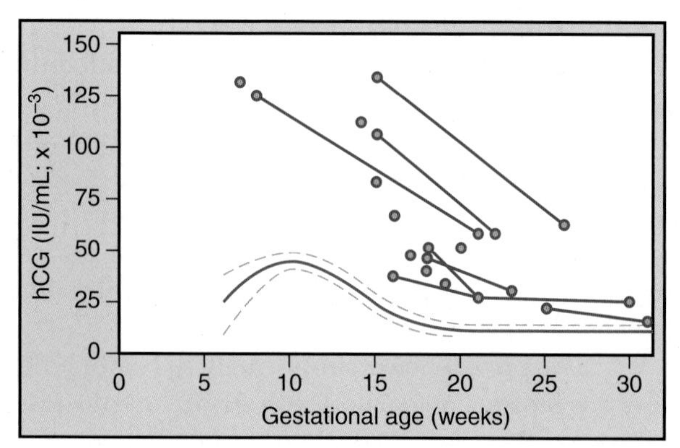

Figure 16–4 Human chorionic gonadotropin (hCG) levels in women with gestational transient thyrotoxicosis (GTT). The curve flanked by the dashed lines represents the mean hCG concentration in normal pregnancy. Individual points represent data from pregnancies complicated by GTT, which is demonstrated to be associated with higher hCG concentration and prolonged duration of hCG elevation. *(Adapted from Glinoer D: The thyroid in pregnancy: A European perspective. Thyroid Today 18:1-11,1995.)*

Multiple-Gestation Pregnancy

In normal pregnancies, the peak concentration of hCG and the duration of the hCG peak both contribute to the degree of thyroid stimulation and TSH suppression. In a normal singleton pregnancy, peak hCG levels higher than 75 U/mL generally persist for no longer than 1 week. Multiple-gestation pregnancies, on the other hand, are associated with a higher concentration of hCG that is maintained for a longer duration.[34] In twin pregnancies, there have been reports of hCG levels remaining elevated for up to 6 weeks, presumably because of the larger placental volume in multiple-gestation pregnancies. Along with this higher hCG concentration and persistence of elevated hCG level, there is a more profound suppression of the TSH level in a higher percentage of these pregnancies. In twin gestation, it was noted that 60% of pregnant women have suppressed TSH in the first trimester compared with 21% of single-gestation pregnancies, and TSH was suppressed to a greater degree in these twin gestations compared with the singletons. Free T_4 was elevated in 30% of twin pregnancies compared with the 1% to 3% of singleton pregnancies. In triplet gestation, the TSH may remain suppressed throughout pregnancy and occasionally even postpartum.[39]

Hyperemesis Gravidarum

Hyperemesis gravidarum is an uncommon condition associated with pregnancy. It is defined as severe nausea and vomiting in women at less than 16 weeks' gestation, resulting in more than 5% weight loss, dehydration, and large ketonuria. Patients may present with hyponatremia, hypokalemia, hypochloremic acidosis, and abnormal liver function. This condition generally begins early in pregnancy (6 to 9 weeks of gestation) and full resolution is usually seen by weeks 18 to 20. Patients often require hospitalization for intravenous fluid hydration, electrolyte repletion, treatment with sedatives, antiemetics, and, depending on severity, corticosteroids.

The prevalence of hyperemesis gravidarum is not known exactly, with reports varying from 0.5% to 1.5% of pregnancies.[40-45] The variations in prevalence are partly caused by the different definitions of hyperemesis gravidarum. The severity of the nausea and vomiting may also be overlooked and considered normal morning sickness. There is a higher prevalence among Asians than whites, and one study has reported that 4.5% of pregnancies in Kuwait were complicated by hyperemesis gravidarum.[46]

The cause of hyperemesis gravidarum is unknown. Excess hCG has been a proposed mechanism, and serum hCG has been found in higher concentrations in patients with increasing severity of vomiting (Fig. 16-5).[47] However, in some reports, hCG concentrations have also been found to be no different in patients with hyperemesis gravidarum when compared with nonhyperemetic patients.[21,48] In patients with hyperemesis gravidarum, hCG isoforms with higher thyrotropic activity have been isolated.[37] Whether there may be some other associated action of hCG in hyperemetic patients is unknown. Some patients with very high concentrations of hCG do not have hyperemesis. A higher estrogen concentration has been suggested as the cause of the vomiting, because there was a direct relationship between the degree of vomiting and estrogen concentration,[47,49] and high levels of estrogen have been known to induce nausea and vomiting. However, the exact cause of hyperemesis gravidarum has yet to be established.

Syndrome of Transient Hyperthyroidism of Hyperemesis Gravidarum

Hyperthyroidism with hyperemesis gravidarum has been well described. Of patients with hyperemesis gravidarum, 30% to 60% have been reported to show some degree of hyperthyroidism.[42-45,47] Hyperthyroidism is usually transient, with spontaneous resolution once the vomiting ceases. The exact frequency of transient hyperthyroidism of hyperemesis gravidarum (THHG) is unclear. The reported frequency may be lower than the actual number; some cases may be missed because the symptoms of hyperthyroidism may be attributed to the hyperemetic state. If thyroid function is not assessed, the hyperthyroidism will not be detected. In addition, the thyroid hyperactivity is often transient, so that thyroid test results and hCG levels may have already normalized by the time they are evaluated.

The degree of hyperthyroidism associated with hyperemesis gravidarum is variable, representing a spectrum of clinical manifestations. Some patients present with isolated biochemical evidence of suppressed TSH and mild elevation of serum T_4 concentration without any thyrotoxic symptoms (subclinical hyperthyroidism). Others may show signs of clinical hyperthyroidism with tachycardia, tremor,

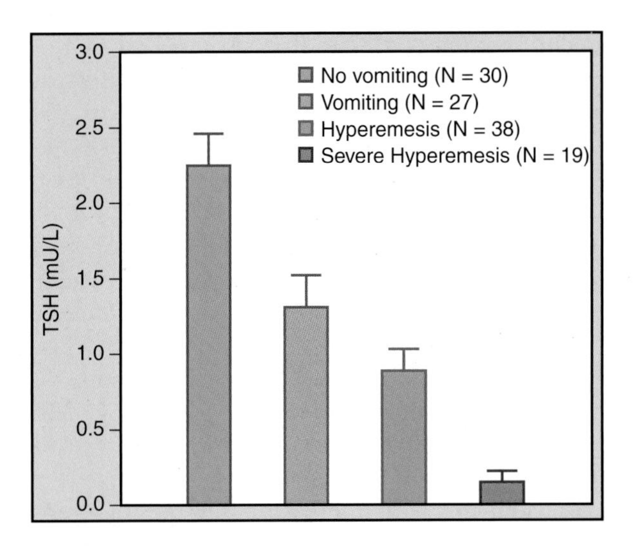

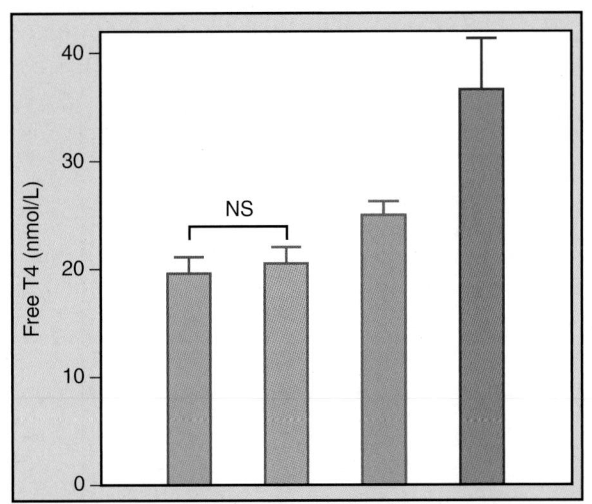

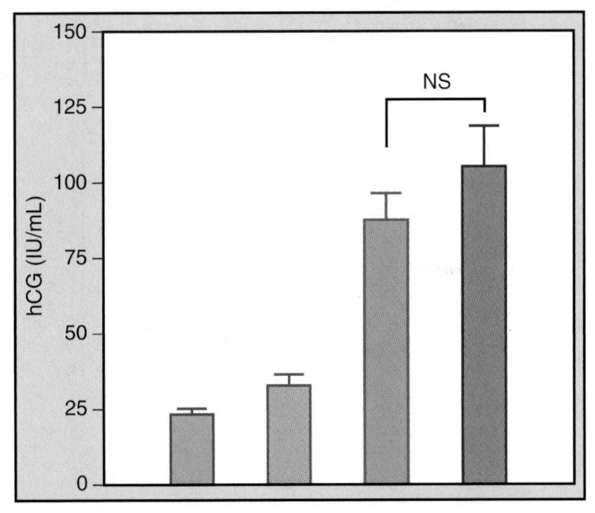

Figure 16–5 Relationship between severity of vomiting and serum levels of thyroid-stimulating hormone (TSH), free thyroxine (T_4), and human chorionic gonadotropin (hCG). With increasing severity of vomiting, there is greater suppression of TSH, more pronounced increase in free T_4, and a higher concentration of hCG. *(Adapted from Goodwin T, Montoro M, Mestman J, et al: The role of chorionic gonadotropin in transient hyperthyroidism of hyperemesis gravidarum. J Clin Endocrinol Metab 75:1333-1337, 1992.)*

heat intolerance, palpitations, anxiety, and nervousness (gestational thyrotoxicosis). Rarely, others may have severe manifestations, with thyroid storm.

The association of hyperthyroidism and hyperemesis gravidarum has been attributed to the stimulatory effect of hCG on the TSH receptor. The underlying cause of both hyperemesis and hyperthyroidism is believed by some to be hCG itself, as thyrotoxicosis of Graves' disease during pregnancy is generally not associated with hyperemesis. hCG concentration was noted to be highest in patients with the most severe degree of vomiting (see Fig. 16-5). The degree of thyroid stimulation correlates with the degree of vomiting in patients with hyperemesis gravidarum; with increasing severity of emesis, there are higher concentrations of free T_4 and free T_3, lower TSH levels, and higher thyroid-stimulating activity (Fig. 16-6; see Fig. 16-5). Excess hCG has been suggested to mediate hyperthyroidism and hyperemesis gravidarum through different mechanisms (Fig. 16-7).[47] It is believed to act at the level of the TSH receptor to stimulate thyroid hormone secretion directly, with resultant hyperthyroidism. At the same time, hCG acts at the hCG receptor on the corpus luteum to stimulate increased production of estrogen and progesterone, with resultant hyperemesis. Elevated estrogen concentrations have been reported in patients with hyperemesis gravidarum.[49] An hCG isoform with high biologic and immunologic activity has been isolated from patients with hyperemesis gravidarum.[37] Patients presenting with gestational thyrotoxicosis were found to have higher amounts of asialo-hCG, which is known to have higher thyrotropic activity.[37] However, other groups have found higher acidic hCG isoforms in patients with hyperemesis gravidarum.[38,50]

In some patients, treatment of the hyperthyroidism cures the hyperemesis. However, in other reports, vomiting continues despite normalization of the hyperthyroid state. In addition, not all hyperthyroid patients are hyperemetic and some hypothyroid patients have also been reported to have severe vomiting. Furthermore, patients with gestational thyrotoxicosis or Graves' disease do not all have associated hyperemesis. One study has shown that patients with hyperemesis gravidarum have a decreased basal metabolic rate[51] which is contrary to the usual finding in hyperthyroidism.

Thyrotoxicosis associated with hyperemesis gravidarum must be clearly distinguished from Graves' hyperthyroidism. The outcomes of pregnancies complicated by hyperemesis gravidarum are generally favorable for a full-term uncomplicated delivery, without an associated increase in preterm labor or increase in malformation, although some reports have described low birth weight.[41,52] In contrast, pregnancies associated with Graves' hyperthyroidism are usually associated with other complications, including spontaneous abortion, premature labor, stillbirth, low birth weight, preeclampsia, maternal heart failure, neonatal hyperthyroidism, and hypothyroidism. Because the thyrotoxicosis resulting from hyperemesis gravidarum is usually transient, there is not sufficient time to induce the

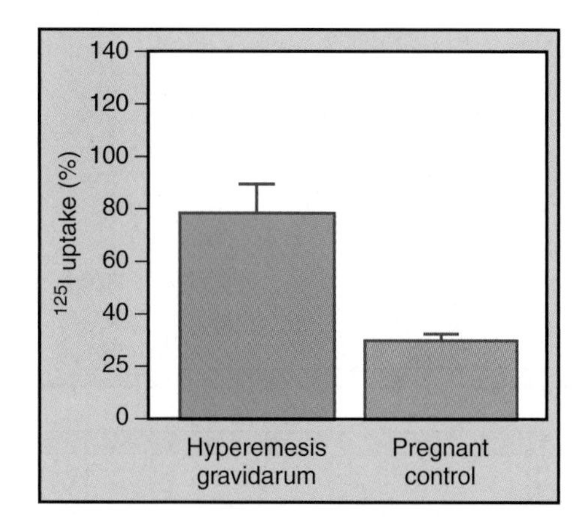

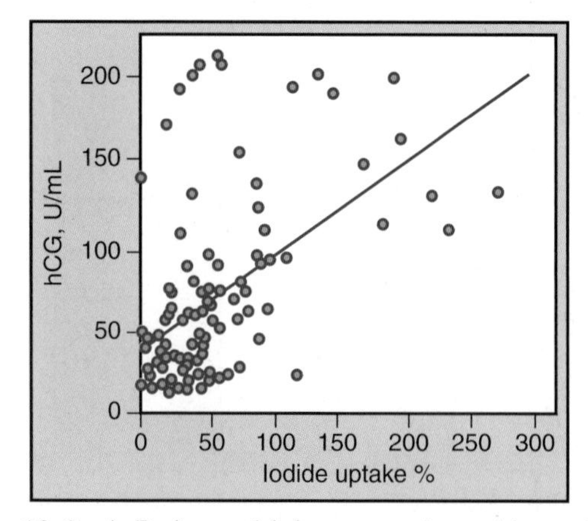

Figure 16–6 **A,** Patients with hyperemesis gravidarum had higher serum thyrotropic activity compared with pregnant controls. **B,** Higher human chorionic gonadotropin (hCG) concentration was associated with increased serum thyrotropic activity. *(Adapted from Goodwin T, Montoro M, Mestman J, et al: The role of chorionic gonadotropin in transient hyperthyroidism of hyperemesis gravidarum. J Clin Endocrinol Metab 75:1333-1337, 1992.)*

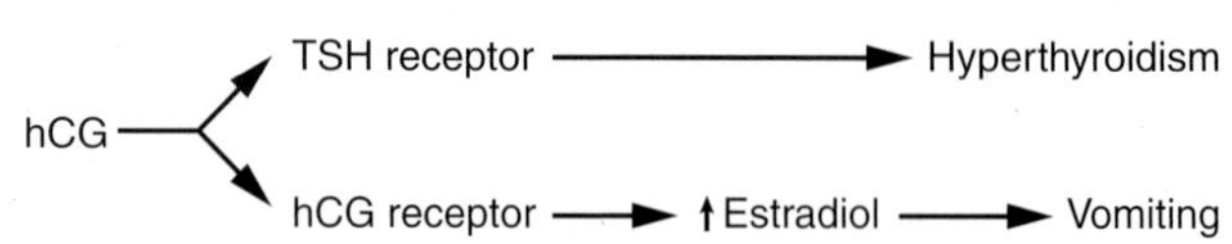

Figure 16–7 Proposed mechanism of the role of human chorionic gonadotropin (hCG) in hyperthyroidism and hyperemesis. TSH, thyroid-stimulating hormone. *(Adapted from Goodwin T, Montoro M, Mestman J, et al: The role of chorionic gonadotropin in transient hyperthyroidism of hyperemesis gravidarum. J Clin Endocrinol Metab 75:1333-1337, 1992.)*

complications generally seen with a more prolonged thyrotoxic state.

Patients with transient hyperthyroidism of hyperemesis gravidarum have no prior history of thyroid disease or symptoms of hyperthyroidism before conception although, rarely, the diagnosis of Graves' disease is first made in pregnancy. The thyroid gland in patients with THHG is generally not enlarged or only mildly enlarged and less than twice the normal size. There are no eye findings of Graves' disease and no muscle wasting. Tachycardia and mild tremor may be present, but the skin is generally not warm or moist. Thyroid antibodies are negative. The free T_4 concentration is elevated to a greater degree compared with the free T_3 concentration, resulting in a higher free T_4/T_3 ratio than that associated with Graves' disease. This may be attributable to the impairment of conversion of T_4 to T_3 because of poor nutrition from the vomiting.

Management of THHG is generally supportive, because this condition is often self-limited and resolves by weeks 18 to 22 of gestation when hCG levels decline. Patients are often hospitalized for hyperemesis gravidarum. Treatment of hyperthyroidism is generally limited to alleviating thyrotoxic symptoms with β-adrenergic blocking drugs. Sedative drugs may be used for symptomatic relief. Antithyroid medication is not usually required; however, for frank thyrotoxicosis or persistent or more severe hyperthyroidism, antithyroid therapy may be necessary. Patients started on an antithyroid drug need to be monitored closely to reduce the dose as the hyperthyroidism resolves with decreasing hCG level. Surgical thyroidectomy is never indicated.

Hydatidiform Mole

Hydatidiform moles have been reported to occur in 0.5 to 2.5/1000 pregnancies,[53] with an increase in prevalence in Asian and Latin American countries. The risk of molar pregnancy is greatest in pregnancies at the extremes of maternal age (younger than 15 years and older than 50 years) and in those with a history of previous molar pregnancy. Hydatidiform moles are characterized as complete or partial. Complete moles are female, consist of 45 paternally derived chromosomes, and are composed of vesicles of swollen hydropic villi without evidence of fetal tissue. Partial moles have some embryonic and fetal tissues and are chromosomally triploid.[54]

Women with a molar pregnancy generally present with vaginal bleeding suggestive of a threatened abortion. They may have pelvic pain or pressure. Nausea and vomiting may be present and have been reported in 20% of patients with molar pregnancies. Of these patients, 5% to 10% have signs and symptoms suggestive of preeclampsia. Ultrasound is diagnostic and shows a characteristic snowstorm appearance, with a uterus that is large for gestational age. hCG is always increased, and the level correlates with the size of the mole.

Since the first report of hyperthyroidism with molar pregnancy in 1955,[1] it is now well appreciated that hyperthyroidism frequently complicates this disorder. The exact prevalence of hyperthyroidism with molar pregnancy is unknown, but it has been reported that thyroid function is increased in 20% to 64% of molar pregnancies.[55,56] Thyroid tests show increased free T_4 and free T_3 and low TSH concentrations. The serum T_4/T_3 ratio is higher in thyrotoxic patients with gestational trophoblastic disease compared with patients with Graves' disease.[55] There is decreased TSH response to thyrotropin-releasing hormone (TRH).[57] Thyroid radioiodine uptake is diffusely increased.[58] Thyroid antibodies are negative. There is no opthalmopathy, in contrast with Graves' disease. The thyroid gland is generally not enlarged or minimally enlarged, but is rarely more than twice normal size. There is less increase in TBG concentration in women with trophoblastic tumors compared with normal pregnancy, because these tumors secrete less estrogen than normal placental tissue.[55] It is important to distinguish hyperthyroidism associated with molar pregnancy from Graves' disease, because they are treated very differently.

Women with molar pregnancy may present with varying degrees of hyperthyroidism. Some may have no clinical symptoms, with only minimal or moderate increase in free T_4 and free T_3 levels, others may have hyperthyroid symptoms associated with significantly elevated levels of thyroid hormones, and still others may have severe hyperthyroidism. It has been reported that 5% of molar pregnancies present with clinical symptoms of hyperthyroidism, including tachycardia, heat intolerance, weight loss, tremor, nervousness, and palpitation.[9] Severe cardiac failure resulting in pulmonary edema may occur with molar pregnancy.[8] Variability and lack of symptoms has been suggested to result from the brief duration of increased thyroid function, with insufficient time for thyrotoxic symptoms to develop.[59] Some have proposed that hCG concentrations higher than 200 U/mL need to be present for several weeks to develop clinical hyperthyroidism.[9] Furthermore, a focus on the toxemia associated with the molar pregnancy may obscure the diagnosis of hyperthyroidism. In recent years, the extensive use of ultrasound has resulted in the diagnosis of hydatidiform moles at an earlier stage, when they are smaller and hCG levels are much lower; such patients are not likely to be hyperthyroid.

The hyperthyroidism associated with trophoblastic tumors is suggested to result from the cross-reactivity of hCG at the TSH receptor. The serum concentration of hCG in hydatidiform molar pregnancy may be extraordinarily high, often more than 300 U/mL and almost always higher than 100 U/mL.[7,60] However, some molar pregnancies with very elevated hCG levels are not associated with hyperthyroidism. Thus, it has been proposed that some other factor may be playing a causative role in the hyperthyroidism. hCG isoforms with increased thyrotropic activity have been isolated from sera in molar pregnancies associated with hyperthyroidism. Basic hCG isoforms with less sialic acid have been shown to have a higher ratio of biologic to immunologic activity (see Fig. 16-2)[27] and have been isolated in high concentrations from patients with hydatidiform moles.[25] Nicked hCG isoforms, which also demonstrate more potent thyroid stimulating activity in vitro, have been isolated from patients with trophoblastic tumors.[20] It is important to note that even though desialylated hCG and nicked hCG have increased thyrotropic potential, they have a shorter half-life, because sialic acid protects against hepatic binding and degradation in vivo.[29]

Hydatidiform moles must be treated with surgical evacuation,[61] which should be done as soon as possible. Prognosis is good, with cure rates greater than 95%.[62] Surgical evacuation of the mole cures the hyperthyroidism. After removal of the mole, there is a decline in hCG, T_4, and T_3 concentrations, as well as decrease in thyroid-stimulating activity (Fig. 16-8).[7] Treatment of hyperthyroidism prior to evacuation of the mole may or may not be necessary, depending on the severity of symptoms. β-Adrenergic blocking drugs may be used to treat hyperthyroid symptoms until definitive treatment is undertaken. Antithyroid medications may be necessary, depending on clinical presentation. However, propylthiouracil or methimazole may not be the ideal treatment for patients presenting with severe symptoms because of the lag in therapeutic effect. Treatment with potassium iodide or sodium ipodate results in a rapid decrease in serum T_4 and T_3 levels and may benefit patients with extreme thyrotoxic symptoms. Surgical thyroidectomy is not recommended. Follow-up and monitoring after evacuation of the hydatidiform mole include monitoring of hCG levels to detect remaining molar tissue or development of choriocarcinoma.

Choriocarcinoma

Choriocarcinoma is a malignant germ cell tumor that is very aggressive because of early hematogenous dissemination. Choriocarcinoma has been reported to occur in 1 in 20,000 to 50,000 pregnancies.[63] Half of these cases occur in patients with previous complete hydatidiform moles, and the other cases occur after nonmolar pregnancies (normal gestation, ectopic pregnancy, or abortion). About 3% to 5% of molar pregnancies are complicated by choriocarcinoma.[9] Clinically, women present with vaginal bleeding and weight loss, generally within 1 year of pregnancy. Choriocarcinoma may be confined to the uterus, but in most cases it is widely metastatic to the pelvis, liver, lung, and brain. There may be symptoms of cough, hemoptysis, dyspnea, or pleuritic chest pain associated with lung metastases. Focal neurologic signs or convulsions may be present in the setting of brain metastases. Epigastric and right upper quadrant pain may indicate hepatic metastases.

In men, choriocarcinoma is the most aggressive testicular germ cell tumor, with most cases being widely metastatic at diagnosis. Men may present with a painless testicular mass, gynecomastia caused by elevated estrogen concentration, and other signs and symptoms consistent with metastatic disease to the liver, lung, or brain.

Diagnosis of choriocarcinoma is based on pathology showing sheets of syncytiotrophoblastic

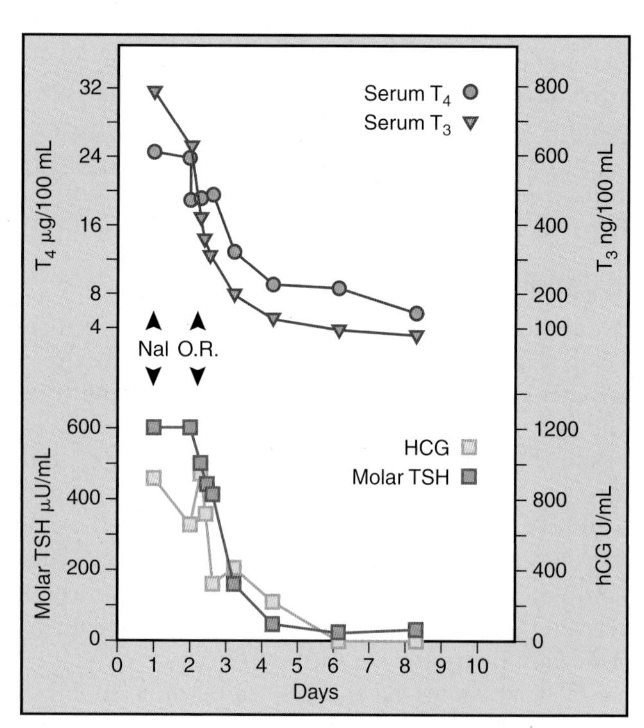

Figure 16–8 Serum thyroxine (T_4), triiodothyronine (T_3), human chorionic gonadotropin (hCG), and molar thyroid-stimulating hormone (TSH) in a patient with hydatidiform mole and hyperthyroidism. After evacuation of the mole, there was a decline in hCG levels, with a parallel decrease in T_4, T_3, and molar TSH. *(Adapted from Higgins HP, Hershman JM, Kenimer JG, et al: The thyrotoxicosis of hydatidiform mole. Ann Intern Med 83:307-311, 1975.)*

and cytotrophoblastic cells, with hemorrhage and necrosis. There may be invasion of blood vessels, because metastasis occurs via hemorrhagic extension. hCG levels are generally substantially elevated, sometimes higher than 1000 U/mL.

Hyperthyroidism has been reported to occur in patients diagnosed with choriocarcinoma, although the exact prevalence is unknown. Weight loss, tachycardia, and anxiety are often present as a consequence of the primary disease, so that hyperthyroidism may be overlooked. In one report of 20 female patients with trophoblastic tumors seen in 1 year, 5 patients (25%) had associated hyperthyroidism, 3 with choriocarcinoma and 2 with hydatidiform mole.[56] The prevalence of basic hCG isoform with less than 3% oligosaccharide side chains isolated from patients with choriocarcinoma[64] is believed to confer a higher thyrotropic potential in these patients; however, hCG isolated from choriocarcinoma in men is mostly the acidic isoform.[65,66]

Treatment of choriocarcinoma requires chemotherapy at a center with expertise in this area. With treatment, survival can reach up to 90% to 95% in women[62] but the prognosis is generally poorer in men, with a 5-year survival of only 35% to 47%.[67] Patients who present with choriocarcinoma and associated hyperthyroidism overall have poorer prognosis because this suggests a larger tumor burden, with metastatic disease associated with very high hCG levels that cause the hyperthyroidism. Curing the choriocarcinoma cures the hyperthyroidism. Control of hyperthyroid symptoms may be achieved with β-adrenergic blocking medication. Antithyroid medication may be necessary, but should be reserved for patients presenting with significant thyrotoxic features. Surgical thyroidectomy is not recommended.

Other Human Chorionic Gonadotropin–Secreting Tumors

Testicular germ cell tumors may secrete high levels of human chorionic gonadotropin. In one study, 15% to 20% of seminomas and 40% to 60% of nonseminomas were associated with abnormal hCG levels.[68] Thyrotoxicosis has been reported in men presenting with widely metastatic germ cell tumors. In a review of 17 men with germ cell tumors and hCG levels higher than 50 U/mL,[69] an associated elevated thyroxine level was noted in 7 patients (41%), with 3 of them having clinical signs and symptoms of hyperthyroidism. The most common and sometimes only suggestion of hyperthyroidism in men with germ cell tumor is an unexplained tachycardia. Most of these men with thyrotoxicosis had a choriocarcinoma, but embryonal, endodermal sinus, and teratomas were other notable histologies. The hCG level was invariably higher in men with hyperthyroidism than in those without and the hCG concentration paralleled the T_4 concentration, suggesting that hCG itself was the thyrotropic modulator. The hCG isoform isolated from testicular germ cell tumor was predominantly acidic.[65,66] Acidic variants have been shown in vitro to have thyrotropic activity[65] and delayed clearance from circulation.[30] Successful treatment of germ cell tumors in men resulted in a decline of hCG level and improvement in symptoms of hyperthyroidism.

Hyperplacentosis

Hyperplacentosis is a rare condition with an increase in placental weight caused by excess trophoblastic activity, leading to a higher hCG concentration compared with normal pregnancy. It has been reported to occur with diabetes, thalassemia, erythroblastosis, and multiple-gestation pregnancies.[70] Symptoms of hyperplacentosis include tachycardia, nausea, vomiting, and heat intolerance, similar to those of hyperthyroidism. There has been one case report of a patient with thyrotoxicosis secondary to hyperplacentosis[70] who required antithyroid drugs. Ultimately hysterotomy was necessary to remove the enlarged placenta, which led to a rapid decline in the hCG level and a parallel decline in T_4 concentration. It is unclear whether there are any specific isoforms of hCG associated with this condition.

Thyroid-Stimulating Hormone Receptor Mutation

A unique mutation in the TSH receptor that confers an increased affinity for hCG has been described in a patient and her mother.[71] Both had pregnancies complicated by transient gestational thyrotoxicosis in the setting of normal hCG levels, and both required antithyroid treatment only during pregnancy. Hyperthyroidism resolved completely postpartum in each case, and there was no evidence of recurrent hyperthyroidism until subsequent pregnancies. Both also had prior pregnancies complicated by nausea and vomiting that resulted in miscarriages.

Evaluation of the TSH receptor from these two patients has revealed a substitution of guanine for adenine at codon 183 within exon 7.[71] As a result, arginine, instead of lysine, was placed at position 183 of the TSH receptor, a substitution in the middle of the extracellular N-terminal domain of the TSH receptor. When the mutant TSH receptor was transfected into COS-7 cells, it showed a high sensitivity to hCG (Fig. 16-9).[71] It is believed that the change from lysine to arginine results in the release of nearby negatively charged glutamate at position 157 from the

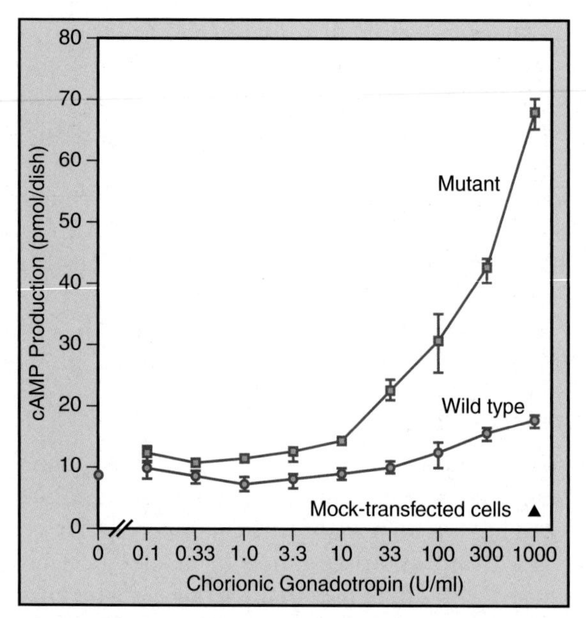

Figure 16–9 Mutant thyroid-stimulating hormone (TSH) receptor shows increased sensitivity to human chorionic gonadotropin (hCG) compared with wild-type. cAMP, cyclic adenosine monophosphate. *(Adapted from Rodien P, Brémont C, Sanson MLR, et al: Familial gestational hyperthyroidism caused by a mutant thyrotropin receptor hypersensitive to human chorionic gonadotropin. N Engl J Med 339:1823-1826, 1998.)*

normal salt bridge, with lysine at position 183.[71] This would allow glutamate to bind with greater affinity to the positively charged hCG and activate the thyroid cells, even when hCG is present at normal gestational concentrations. This increased stability of the hCG interaction at the TSH receptor is believed to be responsible for the hyperthyroidism in these otherwise normal pregnancies.

Subsequent studies of the TSH receptor have shown that substitution of other amino acids (methionine, asparagine, glutamine) for lysine at position 183 also result in similar gain of function at the TSH receptor,[72] suggesting that nature may have strategically placed lysine at this position to prevent overt hyperthyroidism from occurring with all normal pregnancies. No other families with this mutation or similar mutations of the TSH receptor have yet been identified.

References

1. Tisne L, Barzelatto J, Stevenson C: Study of thyroid function during pregnancy and the post partum period with radioactive iodine [in Spanish]. Bol Soc Chil Obstet Ginecol 20:246-251, 1955.
2. Hershman JM: Role of human chorionic gonadotropin as a thyroid stimulator [editorial]. J Clin Endocrinol Metab 74:258-259, 1992.
3. Merz WE: Biosynthesis of human chorionic gonadotropin: A review. Eur J Endocrinol 16:722-725, 1996.
4. Pierce JG, Parson TF: Glycoprotein hormones: Structure and function. Annu Rev Biochem 50:465-495, 1981.
5. Pierce JG. Thyroptropin: Chemistry. In Ingbar SH, Braverman LE (eds): Werner's The Thyroid, 5th ed, Philadelphia, JB Lippincott, 1986, pp 267-318.
6. Nagayama Y, Rapoport B: The thyrotropin receptor and the regulation of thyrocyte function and growth. Endocr Rev 13:596-611, 1992.
7. Higgins HP, Hershman JM, Kenimer JG, et al: The thyrotoxicosis of hydatidiform mole. Ann Intern Med 83:307-311, 1975.
8. Hershman JM, Higgins HP: Hydatidiform mole—a cause of clinical hyperthyroidism. N Engl J Med 284:573-577, 1971.
9. Hershman JM: Physiological and pathological aspects of the effect of human chorionic gonadotropin on the thyroid. Best Pract Res Clin Endocrinol Metab 18:249-265, 2004.
10. Kenimer JG, Hershman JM, Higgins HP: The thyrotropin in hydatidiform moles is human chorionic gonadotropin. J Clin Endocrinol Metab 40:482-491, 1975.
11. Hershman JM, Lee H-Y, Sugawara M, et al: Human chorionic gonadotropin stimulates iodide uptake, adenyalate cyclase, and deoxyribonucleic acid synthesis in cultured rat thyroid cells. J Clin Endocrinol Metab 67:74-79, 1988.
12. Davis RF, Platzer M: hCG-induced TSH receptor activation and growth acceleration in FRTL-5 thyroid cells. Endocrinology 118:2149-2151, 1986.
13. Yoshimura M, Nishikawa M, Horimoto M, et al: Thyroid-stimulating activity of human chorionic gonadotropoin in sera of normal pregnancy women. J Clin Endocrinol Metab 69:891-895, 1989.
14. Yoshikawa N, Nishikawa M, Horimoto M, et al: Human chorionic gonadotropin promotes thyroid growth via thyrotropin receptors in FRTL-5 cells. Endocrinol Jpn 37:639-648, 1990.
15. Yoshimura M, Nishikawa M, Mori Y, et al: Human chorionic gonadotropin induces c-myc mRNA expression via TSH receptor in FRTL-5 rat thyroid cells. Thyroid 2:315-319, 1992.
16. Carayon P, Lefort G, Nisula B: Interaction of human chorionic gonadotropin and human luteinizing hormone with human thyroid membranes. Endocrinology 106:1907-1916, 1980.
17. Kraim Z, Sadeh O, Blithe DL, et al: Human chorionic gonadotropin stimulates thyroid hormone secretion, iodide uptake, organification and adenosine 3′,5′-monophosphate formation in cultured human thyrocytes. J Clin Endocrinol Metab 79:595-599, 1994.
18. Tomer Y, Huber GK, Davies TF: Human chorionic gonadotropin (hCG) interacts directly with recombinant human TSH receptors. J Clin Endocrinol Metab 77:1477-1479, 1992.

19. Yoshimura M, Hershman JM, Pang XP, et al: Activation of the thyrotropin (TSH) receptor by human chorionic gonadotropin and luteinizing hormone in Chinese hamster ovary cells expressing functional human TSH receptors. J Clin Endocrinol Metab 77:1009-1013, 1993.
20. Yoshimura M, Pekary AE, Pang XP, et al: Effect of peptide nicking in the human chorionic gonadotropin beta-subunit on stimulation of recombinant human thyroid-stimulating hormone receptors. Eur J Endocrinol 130:92-96, 1994.
21. Kimura A, Amino N, Tamaki H, et al: Gestational thyrotoxicosis and hyperemesis gravidarum: Possible role of hCG with higher stimulating activity. Clin Endocrinol (Oxf) 38:345-350, 1993.
22. Yomazaki K, Sato K, Shizume K, et al: Potent thyrotropic activity of human chorionic gonadotropin variants in terms of ^{125}I incorporation and de novo synthesized thyroid hormone release in human thyroid follicles. J Clin Endocrinol Metab 80:473-479, 1995.
23. Pekary AE, Jackson IMD, Goodwin TM, et al: Increased in vitro thyrotropic activity in partially sialated human chorionic gonadotropin extracted from hydatidiform moles of patients with hyperthyroidism. J Clin Endocrinol Metab 76:70-74, 1993.
24. Hoermann R, Keutmann HT, Amir SM: Carbohydrate modification transforms human chorionic gonadotropin into a potent stimulator of adenosine 3′,5′-monophosphate and growth responses in FRTL-5 thyroid cells. Endocrinology 128:1129-1135, 1991.
25. Yoshimura M, Pekary AE, Pang XP, et al: Thyrotropic activity of basic isoelectric forms of human chorionic gonadotropin extracted from hydatidiform mole tissues. J Clin Endocrinol Metab 78:862-866, 1994.
26. Hoermann R, Broecker M, Grossmann M, et al: Interaction of human chorionic gonadotropin (hCG) and asialo-hCG with recombinant human thyrotropin receptor. J Clin Endocrin Metabol 78:933-938, 1994.
27. Yoshimura M, Hershman JM: Thyrotropic action of human chorionic gonadotropin. Thyroid 5:425-434, 1995.
28. Cole LA, Kardana A, Park SY, et al: The deactivation of hCG by nicking and dissociation. J Clin Endocrinol Metab 76:704-710, 1997.
29. Hoermann R, Kubota K, Amir SM: Role of subunit sialic acid in hepatic binding, plasma survival rate, and in vivo thyrotropic activity of human chorionic gonadotropin. Thyroid 3:41-47, 1993.
30. Cassels JW Jr, Mann K, Blithe DL, et al: Reduced metabolic clearance of acidic variants of human chorionic gonadotropin from patients with testicular cancer. Cancer 64:2313-2318, 1989.
31. Harada A, Hershman JM, Reed AW, et al: Comparison of thyroid stimulators and thyroid hormone concentrations in the sera of pregnant women. J Clin Endocrinol Metab 48:793-797, 1979.
32. Glinoer D, De Nayer P, Bourdoux P, et al: Regulation of maternal thyroid during pregnancy. J Clin Endocrinol Metab 71:276-287, 1990.
33. Glinoer D, De Nayer R, Robyn C, et al: Serum levels of intact human chorionic gonadotropoin (hCG) and its free alpha and beta subunits, in relation to maternal thyroid simulation during pregnancy. J Endocrinol Invest 16:881-888, 1993.
34. Grün JP, Sylvain M, De Nayer P, Glinoer D: The thyrotropic role of human chorionic gonadotrophin (hCG) in the early stages of twin (versus single) pregnancies. Clin Endocrinol (Oxf) 46:719-725, 1997.
35. Glinoer D: The thyroid in pregnancy: A European perspective. Thyroid Today 18:1-11, 1995.
36. Tamaki H, Itoh E, Kaneda T, et al: Crucial role of serum human chorionic gonadotropin for the aggravation of thyrotoxicosis in early pregnancy in Graves' disease. Thyroid 3:189-193, 1993.
37. Tsuruta E, Tada H, Tamaki H, et al: Pathogenic role of asialo human chorionic gonadotropin in gestational thyrotoxicosis. J Clin Endocrinol Metab 80:350-355, 1995.
38. Talbot JA, Lambert A, Anobile CJ, et al: The nature of human chorionic gonadotrophin glycoforms in gestational thyrotoxicosis. Clin Endocrinol 55:33-39, 2001.
39. Goodwin T, Hershman JM: Hyperthryoidism due to inappropriate production of human chorionic gonadotropin. Clin Obstet Gynecol 40:32-44, 1997.
40. Verberg MF, Gillott DJ, Al-Fardan N, et al: Hyperemesis gravidarum, a literature review. Hum Reprod Update 11:527, 2005.
41. Tsang IS, Katz VL, Wells SD: Maternal and fetal outcomes in hyperemesis gravidarum. Int J Gynaecol Obstet 55:231-235, 1996.
42. Swaminathan R, Chin RK, Lao TTH, et al: Thyroid function in hyperemesis gravidarum. Acta Endocrinol 120:155-160, 1989.
43. Bouillon R, Naesens M, Van Assche FA, et al: Thyroid function in patients with hyperemesis gravidarum. Am J Obstet Gynecol 143:922-926, 1982.
44. Bober SA, McGill AC, Tunbridge WM: Thyroid function in hyperemesis gravidarum. Acta Endrocrinol 111:404-410, 1986.
45. Shulman A, Shapiro MS, Behary C, et al: Abnormal thyroid function in hyperemesis gravidarum. Acta Obstet Gynecol Scand 55:33-37, 1996.
46. Al-Yatama M, Diejomaoh M, Nandakumaran M, et al: Hormone profile of Kuwaiti women with hyperemesis gravidarum. Arch Gynecol Obstet 266:218-222, 2002.
47. Goodwin T, Montoro M, Mestman J, et al: The role of chorionic gonadotropin in transient hyperthyroidism of hyperemesis gravidarum. J Clin Endocrinol Metab 75:1333-1337, 1992.
48. Soules MR, Hughes CL, Garcia JA, et al: Nausea and vomiting in pregnancy: Role of human chorionic gonadotropin and 17-hydroxyprogesterone. Obstet Gynecol 55:696-700, 1980.

49. Depue RH, Bernstein L, Ross RK, et al: Hyperemesis gravidarum in relation to estradiol levels, pregnancy outcome, and other maternal factors: A seroepidemiologic study. Am J Obstet Gynecol 156:1137-1141, 1987.
50. Jordan V, MacDonald J, Crichton S, et al: Acidic isoforms of chorionic gonadotrophin in European and Samoan women are associated with hyperemesis gravidarum and may be thyrotrophic. Clin Endocrinol (Oxf) 50:619-627, 1999.
51. Chihara H, Otsubo Y, Yoneyama Y, et al: Basal metabolic rate in hyperemesis gravidarum: Comparison to normal pregnancy and response to treatment. Am J Obstet Gynecol 188:434-438, 2003.
52. Bashiri A, Neumann L, Maymon E, et al: Hyperemesis gravidarum: Epidemiologic features, complications and outcome. Eur J Obstet Gynecol Reprod Biol 63:135-138, 1995.
53. Palmar JR: Advances in the epidemiology of gestational trophoblastic disease. J Reprod Med 39:155-162, 1994.
54. Fisher RA, Newlands ES: Gestational trophoblastic disease. Molecular and genetic studies. J Reprod Med 43:87-97, 1998.
55. Desai RK, Norman RJ, Jialal I, et al: Spectrum of thryoid function abnormalities in gestational trophoblastic neoplasia. Clin Endocrinol 29:583-592, 1988.
56. Rajatanavin R, Chailurkit LO, Srisupandit S, et al: Trophoblastic hyperthyroidism: Clinical and biochemical features of five cases. Am J Med 85:237-241, 1988.
57. Miyai K, Tanizawa O, Yamamoto T: Pituitary-thyroid function in trophoblastic disease. J Clin Endocrinol Metabol 42:254-259, 1976.
58. Galton VA, Ingbar SH, Jimenez-Fonseca J, et al: Alterations in thyroid hormone economy in patients with hydatidiform mole. J Clin Invest 50:1345-1354, 1971.
59. Nagataki S, Mizuno M, Sakamoto S, et al: Thyroid function in molar pregnancy. J Clin Endocrinol Metab 44:254-263, 1977.
60. Morley JE, Jacobson RJ, Melamed J, et al: Choriocarcinoma as a cause of hyperthyroidism. Am J Med 60:1036-1040, 1976.
61. Committee on Practice Bulletins-Gynecology, American College of Obstetricians and Gynecologists: ACOG Practice Bulletin #53: Diagnosis and treatment of gestational trophoblastic disease. Obstet Gynecol 103:1365-1377, 2004.
62. Fisher PM, Hancock BW: Gestational trophoblastic diseases and their treatment. Cancer Treatment Rev 23:1-16, 1997.
63. Brinton LA, Braken AB, Connelly RR: Choriocarcinoma incidence in the United States. Am J Epidemiol 123:1094-1100, 1986.
64. Mizouchi T, Nishimura R, Derappe C, et al: Structures of the asparagine-linked sugar chains of human chorionic gonadotropin produced in choriocarcinoma. J Biol Chem 258:14126-14129, 1983.
65. Mann K, Schneider N, Hoermann R: Thyrotropic activity of acidic isoelectric variants of human chorionic gonadotropin from trophoblastic tumors. Endocrinology 118:1558-1566, 1986.
66. Cain JH, Pannall PR, Kotasek D, et al: Choriogonadotropin-mediated thyrotoxicosis in a man. Clin Chem 37:1127-1131, 1991.
67. Donovan JF, Williams RD: Tumors of the testis. In Way LW, editor: Current Surgical Diagnosis and Treatment. Norwalk, Conn, Appleton & Lange, 1994, pp 959-962.
68. Bosl GJ, Motzer RJ: Testicular germ cell cancer. N Engl J Med 337:242-253, 1997.
69. Giralt SA, Dexeus F, Amato R, et al: Hyperthyroidism in men with germ cell tumors and high levels of beta-human chorionic gonadotropin. Cancer 69:1286-1290, 1992.
70. Ginsberg J, Lewanczuk RZ, Honore LH: Case history: Hyperplacentosis: A novel cause of hyperthyroidism. Thyroid 11:393-396, 2001.
71. Rodien P, Brémont C, Sanson MLR, et al: Familial gestational hyperthyroidism caused by a mutant thyrotropin receptor hypersensitive to human chorionic gonadotropin. N Engl J Med 339:1823-1826, 1998.
72. Smits G, Govaerts C, Nubourgh I, et al: Lysine 183 and glutamic acid 157 of the TSH receptor: Two interacting residues with a key role in determining specificity toward TSH and human CG. Mol Endocrinol 16:722-725, 2002.

Section B

HYPOFUNCTION

Chapter 17

Chronic Thyroiditis

Suzanne Myers Adler and Kenneth D. Burman

Key Points

- Chronic lymphocytic thyroiditis is the most common cause of primary hypothyroidism.
- Hypotheses for pathogenesis of autoimmunity leading to this disease include so-called molecular mimicry, abnormal expression of major histocompatibility complex class II proteins on thyrocytes, and apoptosis induced by the Fas ligand–Fas system.
- Signs and symptoms such as fatigue, cold intolerance, lethargy, and weight gain reflect the overall slowing of the body's metabolism, and manifestations typically progress to involve multiple organ systems.
- Diagnosis may be based on clinical presentation with elevated serum thyroid-stimulating hormone level, low serum free thyroxine or triiodothyronine level, and increased concentration of antithyroperoxidase antibodies.
- Treatment with exogenous levothyroxine can reverse most hypothyroid manifestations.

Hypothyroidism occurs when there is insufficient production of thyroid hormones by the thyroid gland. Chronic lymphocytic thyroiditis is the most frequent cause of endogenous primary hypothyroidism, followed by hypothyroidism induced by thyroid surgery, radioactive iodine, or medications, topics reviewed elsewhere in this text. Chronic lymphocytic thyroiditis is an autoimmune disease with an underlying disease mechanism that remains unclear with respect to cause and progression. This chapter will review epidemiology, risk factors, and current knowledge regarding the pathogenesis of this disease before reviewing the clinical course, diagnosis, and treatment of chronic lymphocytic thyroiditis.

EPIDEMIOLOGY, RISK FACTORS, AND PATHOGENESIS

Epidemiology

Estimates of the prevalence of hypothyroidism vary among countries because there is no internationally standardized definition of hypothyroidism, and there are likely true differences in the prevalence of hypothyroidism among international populations. The National Health and Nutrition Examination Survey (NHANES) III trial sampled over 17,000 individuals ages 12 years or older who were specifically chosen to represent the U.S. population distribution. It found that the prevalence of hypothyroidism was 4.6%, which included 0.3% clinically significant hypothyroidism (defined as thyroid-stimulating hormone [TSH] > 4.5 mIU/L and thyroxine [T_4] < 57.9 nmol/L) and 4.3% subclinical or mild hypothyroidism (defined as TSH > 4.5 mIU/L and $T_4 \geq 57.9$ nmol/L). Free T_4 measurements were not performed in NHANES III, and it is well known that the presence of increased estrogens can increase thyroid-binding globulin and hence total T_4 concentrations. However, the prevalence of thyroid disease in this population was essentially unchanged when pregnant women and women on estrogen were removed from analysis. The prevalence of hypothyroidism was highest for whites (5.1%) and Hispanic-Americans (4.1%) and lowest for African Americans (1.7%); the prevalence of hypothyroidism in those whose race was not denoted as one of these three groups was approximately that of Hispanic Americans (4.2%). Additional subanalysis revealed that economic status, geographic region, and urban versus rural residence were not significantly associated with an effect on hypothyroidism prevalence. However, there was a marked gender difference, with a hypothyroidism prevalence of 5.8% in females compared with 3.4% in males. In addition, NHANES III found that the prevalence of hypothyroidism significantly increases for females in the 50 to 59 and 60 to 69 year age groups.[1] The Colorado Thyroid Disease Prevalence Study collected data from over 25,000 individuals at a state health fair and determined the prevalence of hypothyroidism to be 4% to 21% in women and 3% to 16% in men, with an overall prevalence of 9.5%. In addition, this study found an increase in hypothyroidism prevalence with age.[2] The Whickam, England study assessed TSH levels and found the prevalence of TSH > 6 mIU/L to be 7.5% of females and 2.8% of males.[3] A follow-up analysis of 12 studies from various countries concluded the prevalence of hypothyroidism to be 5%.[4]

Risk Factors

There are numerous risk factors for chronic autoimmune thyroiditis that have been described in the literature (Table 17-1). Also, a history of thyroid surgery and radioactive iodine treatment are also risk factors for the development of primary thyroid hypofunction. There is a weak association of autoimmune thyroiditis with the human leukocyte antigen (HLA) DR3 and DR5 haplotypes manifesting as hypothyroidism or thyrotoxicosis. Lack of iodine sufficiency deserves specific mention (Fig. 17-1).[5] The World Health Organization (WHO) recommends a daily intake of at least 150 μg of iodine for adults, 200 μg for pregnant women, 90 to 120 μg for children aged 2 to 11 years, and 50 μg for infants younger than 2 years. It is thought that these minimum daily iodine intakes are sufficient to maintain normal thyroid homeostasis, whereas lower intakes may be associated with goiter and hypothyroidism and perhaps thyroid hormone deficiency in infants of mothers with iodine deficiency. Although over the last several decades implementation of public health measures to enhance iodine intake has reduced the worldwide prevalence of iodine deficiency (e.g., iodized salt, iodized oil injections), there is evidence to suggest that dietary iodine intake is now decreasing even in developed countries. In the NHANES I trial (1971-1974), the median urine iodine excretion was 320 μg/day. A follow-up survey showed decreasing urine excretion and, by deduction, intake. The NHANES III (1998-1994) analysis of 20,369 individuals aged 6 to 74 years found that the median urine iodine excretion was 145 μg/day, and a short-term analysis from 2001 to 2002 showed it to be 161 μg/day.[6,7] Because almost all the iodine ingested is excreted in the urine, it is generally thought that the urine iodine measurement accurately reflects intake. In NHANES III, approximately 15% of women of childbearing potential, 7% of pregnant women, and 12% of adults had urine iodine values lower than 50 μg/day. It is not known how consistent daily iodine intake or urine iodine measurements were in these subjects. Although the international promotion of worldwide iodinated salt continues, most iodine intake in most countries is actually derived from ingestion of dairy and flour products.

Table 17–1 Risk Factors for Development or Aggravation of Chronic Thyroiditis

Risk Factors
Prior diagnosis of thyroid disease
History of autoimmune disease
First-degree relative with autoimmune thyroid disease (hyper- or hypofunction)
Age older than 60 years
Female
Perimenopausal or postmenopausal
Pregnant or postpartum woman
Obesity
Presence of thyroid autoantibodies
History of tobacco use
Use of lithium, amiodarone, iodine, kelp, bladder wrack (also called black tang, rockweed, sea wrack, or bugleweed) or soy isoflavone supplements
History of radiation exposure to head, neck, chest
Heavy consumption of raw Brussels sprouts, rutabaga, turnips, kohlrabi, radishes, cauliflower, African cassava, millet, babassu, cabbage, kale, soy protein supplements (e.g., protein powders)
Iodine deficiency

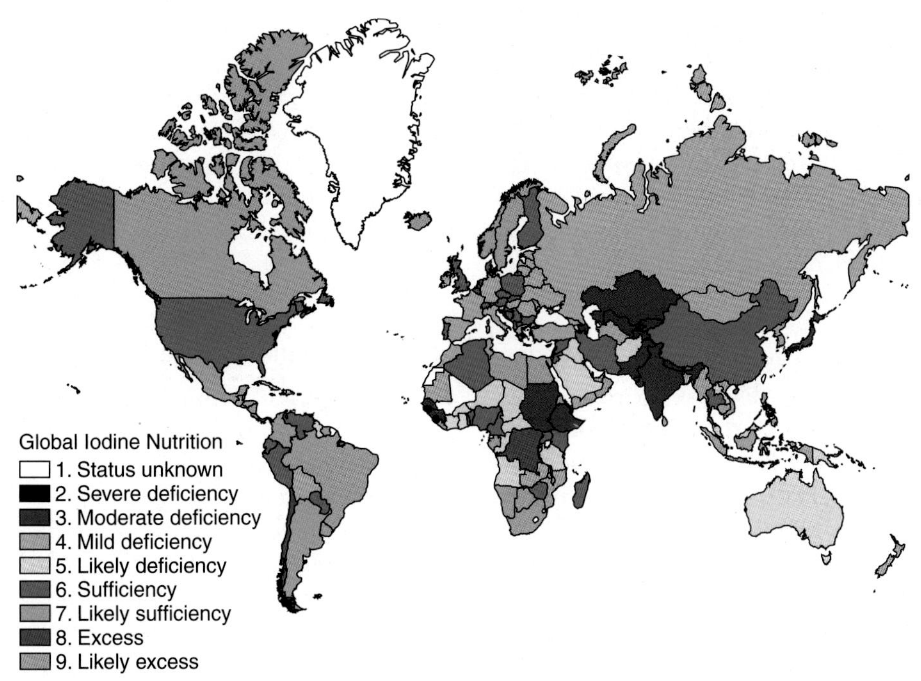

Figure 17–1 Global iodine nutrition. *(From the International Council for the Control of Iodine Deficiency Disorders: Iodine nutrition map. Accessed at http://www.iccidd.org.)*

Pathogenesis

Chronic autoimmune thyroiditis, the most common cause of primary hypothyroidism, is characterized by lymphocytic infiltration of the thyroid gland and by the presence of serum thyroid autoantibodies—namely, anti–thyroid peroxidase (anti-TPO) antibody and antithyroglobulin (anti-TG) antibody. It is believed that this results in thyroid gland destruction. In 1912, Dr. Harkaru Hashimoto first described the clinical entity of struma lymphomatosa, consisting of a goitrous thyroid with histologic features of lymphoid tissue including lymphocytic infiltration, fibrosis, parenchymal atrophy, and eosinophilic changes in acinar cells.[8] The clinical spectrum of chronic autoimmune thyroiditis includes both Hashimoto's thyroiditis, or goitrous autoimmune thyroiditis, and atrophic thyroiditis, which are believed to evolve via the same pathogenic mechanism, although this has not yet been entirely elucidated.

There are several hypotheses that remain under investigation regarding the pathogenesis of chronic lymphocytic thyroiditis. First, the introduction of a foreign protein antigen, such as from a viral or bacterial infection, that is structurally similar to a thyroid protein may induce an autoimmune response that cannot distinguish between the infectious and thyroid proteins, thus attacking both, so-called molecular mimicry. A second hypothesis is based on the observation that thyroid cells in patients with autoimmune thyroid disease express major histocompatibility complex (MHC) class II proteins on their cell surfaces; thyroid cells from healthy individuals do not express MHC-II. MHC-II proteins function to present antigen to helper T cells, and their expression on thyroid follicular cells enables these cells to present intracellular thyroid proteins or foreign proteins to T cells. Evidence suggests that MHC-II expression by thyroid cells is induced by both interferon-gamma and viruses.[9-11] Therefore, interferon-gamma released from activated T cells may induce MHC-II expression in thyroid cells, which in turn may restimulate T cells and propagate the autoimmune process.[12,13] A third hypothesis involves thyroid cell apoptosis directly induced by the Fas ligand–Fas system; Fas normally expressed on lymphoid cells is expressed on follicular cells in autoimmune thyroid glands but is not normally expressed in healthy thyroid glands. Cell death ensues when Fas cross-links with Fas ligand expressed by activated T cells.[14] Interleukin-1 (IL-1) may play an important role because healthy thyroid cells can be induced to express Fas in the presence of IL-1, and there is some support that Fas ligand expressed on thyroid cells may interact with Fas expressed by the same cell to cause self-apoptosis.[15] However, experimentally induced expression of high titers of Fas ligand on thyroid follicular cells in mice has prevented the immune attack of thyroid cells by activated T cells and hence autoimmune thyroiditis.[16] In one small study, more than 38% of those with Hashimoto's thyroiditis were found to have lymphoid cells in the thyroid, with Fas gene mutations, thus further supporting a role of this system in the pathogenesis of autoimmune thyroid disease.[17] Other possible ligands involved in apoptosis of thyroid cells include tumor necrosis factor (TNF)–alpha and TNF-related apoptosis including ligand (TRAIL).[18] Clearly, more investigation is needed to elucidate the pathogenesis of autoimmune thyroid disease further.

These multiple hypotheses all converge on the notion that activated CD4 helper T cells induce cytokine-mediated, cytotoxic, CD8 T-cell direct apoptosis of thyroid cells, predominantly via IL-2, interferon gamma, and TNF-beta. There may also be a more secondary role of anti-TPO and anti-TG antibody-mediated complement fixation and lysis of thyroid cells. However, this process is likely to play a minor role, if any, given that placental transmission of anti-TPO antibodies frequently occurs, and typically does not lead to fetal thyroid gland destruction. In addition, not just thyroid antibody-secreting B cells but thyroid follicular cells themselves may stimulate T-cell activity.[19-22,13] More recent evidence has suggested that those with chronic autoimmune thyroiditis have a reduced percentage of circulating natural killer and CD25+ cells compared with healthy controls, perhaps indicative of some degree of specific peripheral immunodeficiency in those with this disease.[23]

Finally, thyroid-stimulating hormone (TSH)–binding inhibition immunoglobulins (TBII) prevent the binding of TSH to its receptor (TSH-R) and can lead to hypothyroidism. These antibodies are distinct from thyroid-stimulating immunoglobulin (TSI). Whereas TSI binds to the amino terminus of the TSHR extracellular domain (residues 8-165), TBII binds to the carboxyl terminus (residues 270-395), accounting for at least some of the differences in clinical manifestations.[24] However, concentrations of both TBII and TSI may change over time, which can lead to both hypo- and hyperthyroidism in the same individual.[25] The Fas ligand–Fas-mediated apoptosis of thyroid cells described earlier may be inhibited by TSH[26]; TBII prevents the inhibitory action of TSH on this interaction, resulting in thyroid gland destruction.

CLINICAL FEATURES

Chronic autoimmune thyroiditis may present with varying degrees of severity, ranging from asymptomatic goiter to, rarely, myxedema coma. Those with hypothyroidism may present with nonspecific symptoms consistent with the overall slowing of the body's metabolism, including fatigue, cold intolerance, lethargy, and weight gain. However, Hashimoto's thyroiditis and Graves' disease may be considered to be autoimmune diseases of the thyroid on opposite ends of the clinical spectrum. Therefore, an individual patient may exhibit signs of hypothyroidism requiring thyroid hormone replacement but then develop TSH-R stimulating antibodies that may clinically manifest as hyperthyroidism, so-called Hashitoxicosis.[27,28] Here, an overview of hypothyroid symptoms and effects on various organ systems is provided.

Cardiovascular System

Bradycardia is a common manifestation of overt hypothyroidism and, together with decreased myocardial contractility, leads to low cardiac output.[29-36] The ventricular diastolic relaxation phase is decreased, resulting in reduced ventricular filling, further exacerbating cardiac output. Furthermore, because thyroid hormone is known to cause nitric oxide–mediated smooth muscle relaxation, hypothyroidism causes decreased nitric oxide release. This, in conjunction with low cardiac output, may cause up to a 50% increase in systemic vascular resistance, resulting in mild hypertension, typically from diastolic dysfunction. Although edema may be present as a consequence of low cardiac output, clinical congestive heart failure secondary to hypothyroidism is not often seen, and it is uncommon for oxygen delivery to the tissues to be compromised despite low cardiac output, given the overall reduced metabolic rate and hence oxygen demands. Hypothyroidism may also prolong the cardiac action potential and hence the QT interval on electrocardiography, which may rarely lead to torsades de pointes. Pericardial effusions may develop in 3% to 6% of hypothyroid individuals, but these are usually asymptomatic and occur with greater frequency and severity in the myxedematous state. Nonetheless, the possibility of the presence of a clinically significant pericardial effusion should always be considered in the appropriate setting of a patient with hypothyroidism.

Various forms of hyperlipidemia may occur in up to 50% to 90% of hypothyroid individuals. Although elevations in very low-density lipoprotein (VLDL) and triglycerides may occur, increases in serum LDL and total cholesterol are the most common predominant manifestations. LDL cell surface receptors are downregulated in terms of number and potentially of function, and hence LDL catabolism decreases. Increased LDL oxidation may also have an important role in contributing to hyperlipidemia. It remains unclear whether hypothyroidism-induced cardiac changes and related dyslipidemia may predispose certain individuals to coronary artery disease above the risk of the general population. Lipid abnormalities may normalize completely in hypothyroid

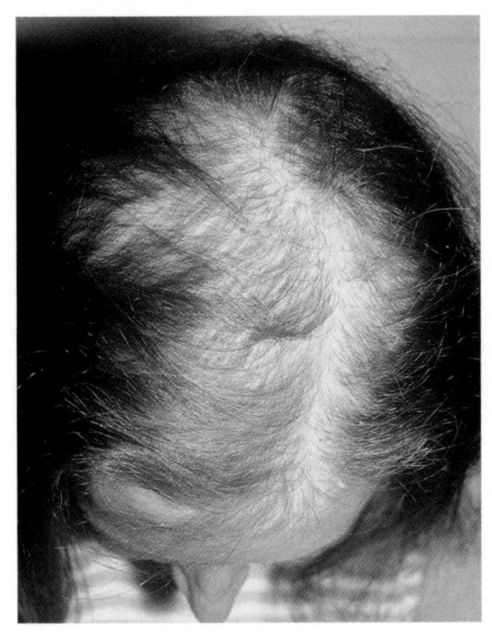

Figure 17–2 Generalized hair thinning, with dry and brittle hair. *(From Burman K, McKinley-Grant L: Dermatologic aspects of thyroid disease. Clin Dermatol 24:250, 2006.)*

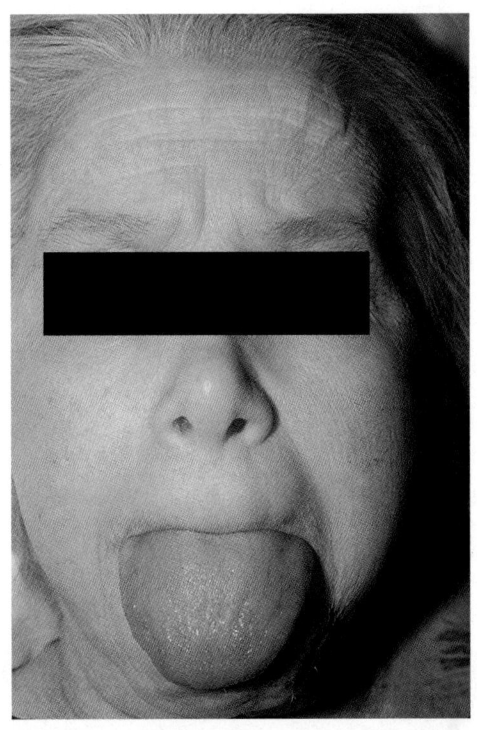

Figure 17–3 Skin pallor, macroglossia, and periorbital edema seen in hypothyroidism. *(From Burman K, McKinley-Grant L: Dermatologic aspects of thyroid disease. Clin Dermatol 24:250, 2006.)*

individuals with thyroid hormone replacement alone. The degree of cholesterol reduction seems proportional to the magnitude of cholesterol elevation above normal, with more dramatic improvements in overall lipid parameters observed in those with higher baseline cholesterol levels. However, selected individuals may need additional therapy with diet modification, exercise, and perhaps lipid-lowering pharmacologic therapy.

Respiratory System

Hypothyroid individuals may present with dyspnea on exertion and decreased exercise tolerance, which likely result from a combination of skeletal muscle weakness and cardiac and respiratory dysfunction.[37-43] The skeletal musculature is adversely affected by hypothyroid-induced myopathy and neuropathy leading to diaphragmatic dysfunction that reverses with the administration of thyroxine. Pulmonary function testing demonstrates a restrictive pattern in hypothyroid patients and administration of thyroxine may reverse pulmonary function abnormalities, particularly in nonobese individuals with a body mass index (BMI) < 30 kg/m^2. There is a reduction in hypoxic and hypercapnic ventilatory drive that correlates with the severity of hypothyroidism, and alveolar hypoventilation is a well-known manifestation of myxedema. Thyroid hormone replacement has been shown to improve hypoxic, but not hypercapnic, ventilatory drive in myxedematous patients. Hypothyroid individuals in rare cases may develop isolated exudative pleural effusions, but these are more often associated with pericardial effusions or ascites. Obstructive sleep apnea is more common in hypothyroid individuals, and evidence suggests an improvement in apneic episodes following levothyroxine replacement.

Dermatologic System

Skin, hair, and nail changes associated with hypothyroidism are nonspecific and may vary, depending on an individual's ethnicity and the extent and duration of hypothyroidism.[44-46] Changes include skin thickening and dryness, thinning and coarsening of the hair (Fig. 17-2), and loss of the lateral aspect of the eyebrows. Livedo reticularis of the extremities, skin pallor, macroglossia, xerosis, and periorbital edema can also occur in more severe hypothyroidism (Fig. 17-3). Those with chronic autoimmune thyroiditis are at increased risk for developing other autoimmune disorders in general, and those of the skin include vitiligo (Fig. 17-4), alopecia areata (Fig. 17-5), pemphigus vulgaris, pemphigus foliaceous, and dermatitis herpetiformis; however, a rigorous analysis of these disease states in autoimmune thyroid disease has not been performed. In addition, because there is overlap between Hashimoto's thyroiditis and Graves' hyperthyroidism, similar skin and ocular findings can occur in both, including pretibial, preradial, or

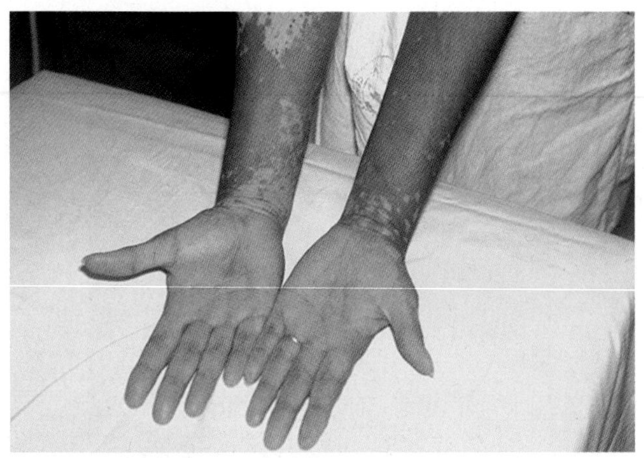

Figure 17–4 Vitiligo, an autoimmune disorder with loss of pigment associated with autoimmune thyroid disease. *(Courtesy of Brian E. Staveley, Department of Biology, Memorial University, Newfoundland and Labrador, Canada.)*

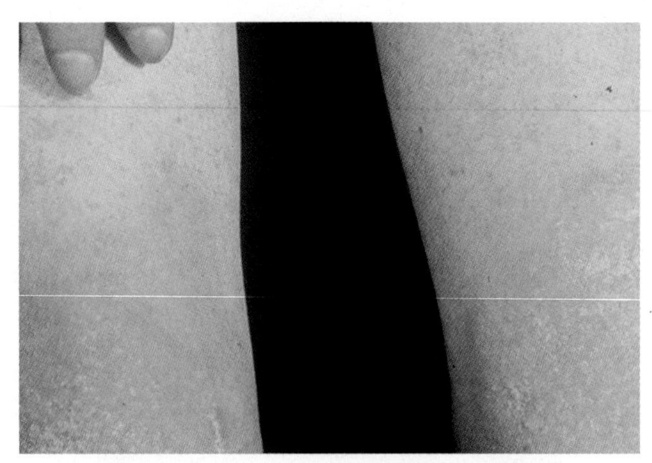

Figure 17–6 Pretibial myxedema, with bilateral erythema and thickening. *(From Burman K, McKinley-Grant L: Dermatologic aspects of thyroid disease. Clin Dermatol 24:248, 2006.)*

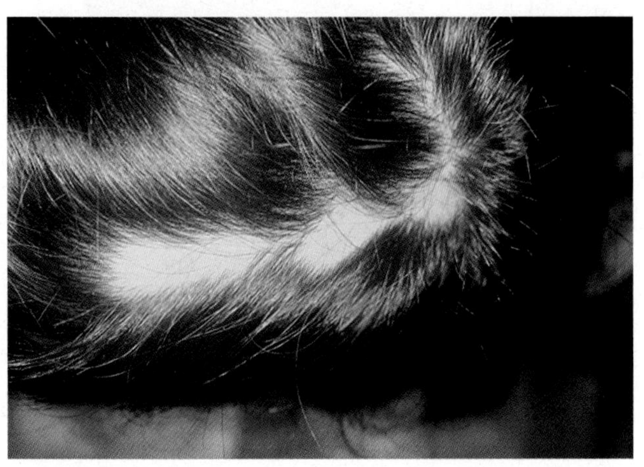

Figure 17–5 Alopecia areata, an autoimmune skin disorder associated with thyroid disease. *(From Burman K, McKinley-Grant L: Dermatologic aspects of thyroid disease. Clin Dermatol 24:251, 2006, with permission)*

scalp myxedema (Fig. 17-6), conjunctivitis, diplopia, enlarged extraocular muscles, and blurred vision.

Gastrointestinal System

Constipation is a frequent symptom of hypothyroidism resulting from decreased gut motility.[47-50] The transit time of food to the colon decreases following thyroid hormone replacement in hypothyroid individuals. In those with preexisting constipation prior to the onset of hypothyroidism, constipation may be exacerbated and, in some cases, can lead to ileus or even intestinal obstruction. In addition, approximately 2% to 4% of those with autoimmune thyroid disease have concomitant celiac sprue, and up to 43% of those with Hashimoto's have immunohistochemical markers (e.g., increased density of gamma-delta T-cell receptors bearing intraepithelial lymphocytes, IL-2 receptors on lamina propria T cells, or HLA-DR molecules on crypt epithelial cells), indicative of the potential to develop celiac disease. In those diagnosed with celiac sprue, seldom does a gluten-free diet reduce the need for thyroid hormone replacement. Up to one third of those with autoimmune thyroid disease may also have atrophic gastritis with detectable antiparietal antibodies, predisposing approximately 10% to 20% of these individuals to pernicious anemia. Given these associations, the possibility of the presence of celiac sprue should be entertained in patients with Hashimoto's thyroiditis even with subtle appropriate signs or symptoms.

Neurologic System

Cognitive dysfunction, including poor concentration, short-term memory impairments, decreased verbal fluency, learning and attention impairments, diminished visuospatial perception, slowed speech, delayed reflexes, and reduced psychomotor speed are associated with hypothyroidism, and may be even more dramatic in the older adult population.[51-57] The magnitude of these defects does not seem to correlate with the degree of TSH elevation. Although depression, mood scores, and verbal memory retrieval may improve following thyroid hormone replacement, many neurocognitive parameters may not normalize after correction of TSH. Carpal tunnel syndrome is an associated diagnosis in approximately 10% of patients with hypothyroidism; symptoms result from accumulation of mucinous material deposited in the carpal tunnel, leading to median nerve impingement. Carpal tunnel syndrome symptoms may develop, even in the euthyroid state, while a patient is taking thyroid hormone replacement. Still others may experience a polyneuropathy thought to be associated with demyelination and axonal degeneration resulting in sensory loss, painful dysesthesias or, most commonly, delayed relaxation phase of the deep tendon reflexes, all of which typically resolve following thyroid hormone replacement. Hashimoto's encephalopathy is a controversial entity characterized by the presence of serum thyroid antibodies—namely, anti-TPO or anti-TG—mental confusion, seizures, or altered consciousness with thyroid function tests consistent with the hypothyroid, euthyroid, or hyperthyroid state. It is thought to result from the autoimmune process itself rather than the clinical manifestations of hypothyroidism, and frequently responds to corticosteroids.

Endocrine System

Multiple endocrinopathies are associated with hypothyroidism.[58] Hyperprolactinemia can occur in the setting of clinical hypothyroidism, probably because of the loss of negative feedback of thyroid hormone on thyrotropin-releasing hormone (TRH), which stimulates the secretion of TSH and prolactin from the anterior pituitary. Many women with hypothyroidism experience menstrual irregularities, including oligomenorrhea or anovulation, with consequential fertility difficulties. Although prolactin levels normalize with replacement of thyroid hormone unless there is a coexistent pituitary abnormality, menstrual irregularities may persist in a subgroup of women. In men, primary hypothyroidism is associated with hypogonadotropic hypogonadism, with low free testosterone levels that can increase to normal following thyroid hormone replacement. Because prolactin levels are not consistently elevated in men with low free testosterone and primary hypothyroidism, decreased responsiveness of luteinizing hormone (LH) to gonadotropin-releasing hormone (GnRH) is thought to cause the findings. Sex hormone–binding globulin (SHBG) concentrations are known to decrease, and therefore may result in low total testosterone levels, but should not affect free testosterone measurements. In addition, chronic autoimmune hypothyroidism is a component of autoimmune polyglandular syndrome type 2, along with type 1 diabetes mellitus and primary adrenal insufficiency.

Renal System

The mechanism whereby hypothyroidism induces hyponatremia is not entirely understood.[59-63] Patients with primary hypothyroidism have impaired free water excretion, which can be reversed by thyroid hormone replacement. Although once thought to be secondary to inappropriately elevated arginine vasopressin (AVP) levels, hypothyroidism-induced hyponatremia is now thought to be mediated by AVP-independent mechanisms. Evidence has suggested appropriately suppressed AVP levels in a population of hyponatremic myxedema patients who demonstrated a degree of impaired urinary dilution during water loading. Decreased renal function and glomerular filtration rate (GFR) may also occur in up to 90% of those with severe hypothyroidism compared with the prior euthyroid state, and creatinine values typically normalize following thyroid hormone replacement to their baseline values. Therefore, the major cause of impaired water excretion in hypothyroidism appears to be an alteration in renal perfusion and GFR secondary to systemic effects of thyroid hormone deficiency on cardiac output and peripheral vascular resistance. Special attention should be given to hypothyroid patients who may be predisposed to develop hyponatremia, such as following excess water intake.

Myxedema Coma

Myxedema coma is an endocrinologic emergency and is the most clinically severe form of hypothyroidism.[64-66] Although it is rarely seen today, myxedema coma still carries a high risk of death unless treated promptly. Signs and symptoms include hypothermia, bradycardia, altered mental status, hypotension, and eventual respiratory failure from hypoventilation and carbon dioxide retention. Mental status abnormalities typically begin with lethargy and confusion, but may also present as memory difficulties and psychosis prior to decompensating to overt coma. Up to 25% of patients may experience seizure activity secondary to hypoglycemia, hyponatremia, or hypoxemia induced by decreased blood flow to the brain. Often, infection is the precipitating factor, but stroke, worsening cardiac status, severe electrolyte abnormalities (e.g., hypoglycemia, hyperkalemia, hyponatremia, hypercalcemia), systemic illness, and medications, including narcotics, sedatives, anesthetics, and hypnotics, have all been known to precede or worsen myxedema coma. During the winter months, older women seem to be at particular risk for developing myxedema coma.

DIAGNOSIS

The diagnosis of hypothyroidism begins with a thorough history and physical examination. Although a TSH determination alone may be adequate for screening the general population without symptoms of thyroid disease, laboratory evaluation for anyone suspected of having hypothyroidism entails determining the serum TSH level and a free thyroxine (FT_4) and total or free triiodothyronine (T_3) level to be able to distinguish between primary and central hypothyroidism. If initial thyroid function studies are abnormal, evaluation of anti-TPO antibodies is warranted. In addition, it is prudent to obtain a baseline comprehensive metabolic panel, complete blood count, and lipid panel, because those with chronic autoimmune thyroiditis are at risk for other autoimmune diseases, electrolyte abnormalities, and dyslipidemia. Some clinicians will also obtain a thyroid ultrasound, in particular if there is a suspicion for thyroid nodules. The ultrasound appearance of the thyroid in chronic autoimmune thyroiditis is heterogeneous, occasionally with pseudonodules. If the serum TSH value is not appropriately elevated when the FT_4 is decreased, consideration of a pituitary or hypothalamic abnormality should be considered and evaluated.

Modest controversy persists regarding the normal reference range of TSH, which is currently 0.4 to 4 mIU/L,[67,68] because some believe that the reference range should be narrowed further to approximately 0.3 to 2.5 mIU/L.[69] The diagnosis of primary hypothyroidism is clear, with an elevated TSH above the reference range in the setting of a free T_4 below the reference range. A normal FT_4 with a slightly elevated TSH is consistent with subclinical hypothyroidism, and individuals should have thyroid function routinely followed as clinically indicated for the development of overt hypothyroidism. The diagnosis of overt hypothyroidism becomes more difficult in the setting of acute illness. In this case, thyroid function tests may be consistent with nonthyroidal illness syndrome, with FT_4 and TSH values that may vary from low to normal and that could even be as high as 15 to 20 mIU/L in the recovery phase of the nonthyroidal illness syndrome.[70] Thus, it might be difficult to discern from true primary thyroid hypofunction.

TREATMENT

Treatment goals in chronic autoimmune thyroiditis are to improve symptoms and normalize thyroid hormone function parameters. Standard treatment for chronic autoimmune thyroiditis and related hypothyroidism involves thyroid hormone replacement with levothyroxine (L-T_4). There has been controversy surrounding replacement with T_4 alone or thyroxine in combination with T_3. However, a meta-analysis of randomized controlled trials published from 1999 to 2005 has concluded that there is no advantage to T_4-T_3 combination therapy for patients with hypothyroidism compared with standard T_4 monotherapy. Furthermore, there was no improvement in quality of life, fatigue, bodily pain, anxiety, depression, attention, concentration, lipids, or weight change.[71] Some have hypothesized that the difference in response to combination therapy may relate to the amount of endogenous thyroid secretory function. Although Hashimoto's patients with some residual thyroid secretory function might not benefit from combination therapy, patients following thyroidectomy who lack residual thyroid secretory capacity might benefit from the addition of T_3 to T_4 replacement.[72] However, the treatment of choice in hypothyroidism, according to most experts, remains L-T_4 monotherapy.

The starting dose of L-T_4 has also been a topic of debate. A prospective randomized trial has found that euthyroidism is achieved more rapidly after initiation of L-T_4 with a full replacement dose compared with a low 25 µg daily starting dose, with a dosage increase every 4 weeks. Furthermore, no cardiac events were documented in individuals in the full replacement or dose titration groups during the 6 months of the study.[73] Therefore, for most patients, therapy can be initiated with a full replacement dose of 1.7 µg/kg body weight, although it is prudent to initiate a lower starting dosage of 25 to 50 µg daily in older patients or those with preexisting cardiac disease. Clinical judgment is needed to select which patients should have L-T_4 therapy started slowly. Following the initiation of therapy, repeat thyroid function studies should be performed and the L-T_4 dose titrated to a TSH level of 0.5 to 2.5 mIU/L.[69] Thyroid function tests should be routinely evaluated after equilibration at 4 to 6 weeks. However, some patients may require closer monitoring and require examinations and laboratory tests more frequently. All patients should be advised to contact health care personnel if they manifest symptoms of chest pain, shortness of breath, or other possibly relevant symptoms (e.g., dizziness). Because L-T_4 is generally not well absorbed, it is prudent to counsel patients to administer this medication at the same time every day, in particular with respect to meals, because absorption is improved in the fasting state. Also, it is important to separate L-T_4 administration from medications known to decrease levothyroxine absorption, such as calcium supplements and antacids (Table 17-2).

The treatment for severe myxedema (or coma) requires prompt administration of thyroid hormone, intensive care monitoring, and supportive care. Intravenous volume repletion is essential, with careful monitoring of serum sodium levels so as not to worsen hyponatremia. Hypertonic 3% saline

Table 17–2 Factors Possibly Leading to Decreased Efficacy of Levothyroxine (L-T_4)

Pregnancy
Malabsorption
Celiac Sprue
Small Bowel Surgery
Nephrotic Syndrome
High-Fiber Diet
Soy Products
Drugs Increasing L-T_4 Clearance
Barbiturates
Carbamazepine
Phenobarbital
Phenytoin
Rifabutin
Rifampin
Drugs Decreasing L-T_4 Absorption
Aluminum hydroxide
Bile acid binding resins
Calcium salts
Cholestyramine
Didanosine
Estrogens
Iron
Kayexalate
Magnesium salts
Proton pump inhibitors
Raloxifene
Sertraline
Simethicone
Sucralfate

should be given when hyponatremia is severe and symptomatic.[59] Vasopressors and ventilatory support are required in most cases. Younger patients may be given an IV L-T_4 loading dose of 300 to 500 μg and older patients may be given a more conservative loading dose of 4 μg/kg body weight to minimize the risks of high-dose thyroid hormone therapy.[64] Following the loading dose, L-T4, 50 to 100 μg, may be given daily. Some also favor coadministering liothyronine (L isomer of T_3), 10 μg every 8 to 12 hours, until the patient stabilizes to account for the decreased rate of extrathyroidal T_4 to T_3 conversion in critically ill hypothyroid patients.[74] In addition, hydrocortisone should be administered in so-called stress doses, given the possibility of concomitant primary or secondary adrenal insufficiency.

CLINICAL COURSE AND PREVENTION

Although many of the detrimental effects of hypothyroidism such as dyslipidemia are reversed with thyroid hormone replacement and TSH normalization, the results of a recent Scottish study have revealed an increased risk of cardiovascular morbidity, but not of all-cause mortality, in those with treated hypothyroidism compared with the general population. Flynn and colleagues[75] evaluated 15,889 primary hypothyroid patients compared with 524,152 patients in the general population and found treated hypothyroid individuals to be at increased risk of diabetes and of morbidity associated with circulatory diseases, ischemic heart disease, and dysrhythmias, even after adjustment for the diagnosis of diabetes. They suggested possible explanations for their findings: (1) thyroid hormone replacement might not completely reverse the pathogenesis of atherosclerosis and/or (2) individuals might not be receiving optimal treatment because their TSH is not at goal or the TSH reference range is not appropriate.[75] It has been estimated that up to 40% of patients on thyroid replacement therapy have TSH values outside the normal reference range.[2] NHANES III found that of those in the studied population on thyroid medication, 15% have biochemical evidence of hypothyroidism and more than 18% have hyperthyroidism, indicating that only 67% of those with thyroid disease are appropriately dosed with thyroid medication.[1] Therefore, reevaluation of the TSH level is important 4 to 6 weeks following any L-T_4 dose adjustment to ensure proper dosing. As a routine, many clinicians recommend yearly evaluation in stable patients.

Association with Thyroid Malignancy

There is a higher incidence of Hashimoto's thyroiditis in those diagnosed with papillary thyroid cancer than in the general population, and meta-analysis has suggested that there may be a survival benefit in papillary thyroid cancer with coexistent Hashimoto's disease.[76] *RET/PTC* rearrangements occur in approximately 20% to 40% of sporadic papillary thyroid cancers.[77,78] *RET/PTC* rearrangements, in particular *RET/PTC1* and *RET/PTC3*, have been reported to occur in high frequency in those with Hashimoto's thyroiditis,[79,80] leading to the hypothesis that there are submicroscopic foci of papillary thyroid cancer in Hashimoto's thyroiditis.[81] However, others argue that the methodologies used leading to such conclusions lend themselves to false-positive results and consequently to the reporting of a higher number of Hashimoto's patients with this gene rearrangement than actually occur.[82] More recent evidence has suggested that *RET/PTC* rearrangements are not frequently present in those with coexistent Hashimoto's thyroiditis and papillary thyroid cancer as compared with those with papillary thyroid cancer not associated with Hashimoto's thyroiditis. This suggests a molecular basis for the association between papillary thyroid cancer and Hashimoto's thyroiditis, independent of the *RET/PTC* rearrangement.[83]

There is an association with Hashimoto's thyroiditis and lymphoma of the thyroid gland, which constitutes approximately 2% of all thyroid malignancies and less than 2.5% of all lymphomas.[84,85] Because Hashimoto's thyroiditis affects mostly women, it is not surprising that most individuals with thyroid lymphoma are also female. Compressive symptoms from a rapidly enlarging thyroid goiter of mass in the thyroid gland are common symptoms on presentation of thyroid lymphoma. One study has documented the prevalence of thyroid lymphoma by histology to be 50% diffuse large B-cell lymphoma (DLCL), 23% mucosa-associated lymphoid tissue (MALT) lymphoma, 12% follicular lymphoma, 7% Hodgkin's disease, 4% small lymphocytic lymphoma, and 4% Burkitt's lymphoma. However, MALT lymphoma is most closely associated with Hashimoto's thyroiditis.[85] Findings on thyroid ultrasound include an asymmetrical pseudocystic pattern in the vast majority of lesions. Cytologic analysis consistent with thyroid lymphoma following fine-needle aspiration reveals an abundance of monomorphic lymphoid cells infiltrating the thyroid tissue.[86] However, there are limitations to cytology as a means of diagnosis. Whereas DLCLs are cytologically more distinguishable, MALT lymphomas may be virtually indistinguishable from cytologic changes related to Hashimoto's thyroiditis itself.[84] MALT lymphomas of the thyroid characteristically demonstrate B-cell follicles and neighboring intraepithelial B cells, also known as lymphoepithelial lesions. Most MALT lymphomas usually originate from tissue that is not normally comprised of lymph tissue (e.g., the stomach), and instead develop in tissue affected by a condition that predisposes that tissue to lymphoid infiltration, such as the thyroid in Hashimoto's thyroiditis.[87] In general, MALT lymphoma occurs in a thyroid gland that has been affected by Hashimoto's thyroiditis for some time, even 20 to 30 years, and has a fairly good prognosis. However, transformation to more aggressive lymphoma subtypes, such as DLCL, carries a much poorer prognosis.

Treatment options vary with the histologic subtype and disease stage. For example, more aggressive, even disseminated, DLCL tumors respond well to an anthracycline-containing multidrug chemotherapy regimen (e.g., CHOP [**c**yclophosphamide, **h**ydroxydaunomycin, **O**ncovin, **p**rednisone] or a related regimen) without surgery, whereas localized MALT tumors have excellent response rates to total thyroidectomy, with the addition of radiation and chemotherapy for more disseminated disease.[85]

Table 17–3 Patients with Inadequately Treated Hypothyroidism (%)

Study, Year	Inadequate Levothyroxine Therapy (High Serum TSH Level)	Excessive Levothyroxine Therapy (Low Serum TSH Level)
Hollowell et al, 2002[1]	15	18
Canaris et al, 2000[2]	18	22
Parle et al, 1993[91]	27	21
Ross et al, 1990[92]	18	14

TSH, thyroid-stimulating hormone.

Newer chemotherapeutic regimens (e.g., EPOCH-R, RICE, and rituximab alone) have not been adequately evaluated in thyroid associated lymphomas, but may also be of benefit.

Pitfalls and Complications: Monitoring Thyroid Function

Many patients with hypothyroidism have inadequately treated disease as reflected by serum TSH levels outside the normal reference range (Table 17-3). A chart review of approximately 400 patients receiving L-T_4 therapy has revealed that within 1 year of follow-up, only 72% of patients after L-T_4 initiation or dose change had their TSH levels monitored every 3 months until normal, and then yearly, and only 61% of those with an abnormal serum TSH level had their L-T_4 dose adjusted.[88] This therefore stresses the importance of not only regular monitoring, but careful attention to L-T_4 dose titration when needed.

Controversies: Subclinical Hypothyroidism

Subclinical hypothyroidism is defined as an elevated level of TSH in the setting of free T_4 and T_3 levels within the normal reference range. NHANES III has found the prevalence of subclinical hypothyroidism with a TSH level > 4.5 mIU/L in the U.S. adult population to be 4.3%,[1] with autoimmune thyroiditis as the most common cause in adults.[89] Although some may experience mild symptoms of overt hypothyroidism, as described earlier, many with subclinical hypothyroidism are asymptomatic. A trial of L-T_4 may be considered in some patients (Table 17-4). However, in one study, 37% of patients with subclinical hypothyroidism were found to normalize their TSH levels without intervention over an average follow-up period of 31.7 months. In this same study, the presence of thyroid antibodies reduced the likelihood of spontaneous TSH normalization

Table 17–4 Recommendations for Management of Subclinical Hypothyroidism

Thyroid-Stimulating Hormone (mIU/L)	Symptomatic?	Recommendations
4.5-10	No	Repeat TSH within 1 month and then every 6 months when asymptomatic.
4.5-10	Yes	Consider trial of thyroid hormone replacement.
>10	—	In most cases, administer thyroid hormone replacement.

because 61.5% of those without antibodies compared with only 30% of those with positive antibodies were found to normalize their TSH levels.[90] Therefore, initiation of therapy in those with subclinical hypothyroidism should be individualized to the specific patient.

References

1. Hollowell J, Staehling N, Flanders W, et al: Serum TSH, T_4, and thyroid antibodies in the United States population (1988 to 1994): National Health and Nutrition Examination Survey (NHANES III). J Clin Endocrinol Metab 87:489-499, 2002.
2. Canaris G, Manowotz N, Mayor G, et al: The Colorado thyroid disease prevalence study. Arch Intern Med 160:526-534, 2000.
3. Tunbridge W, Evered D, Hall R, et al: The spectrum of thyroid disease in a community: The Whickham survey. Clin Endocrinol (Oxf) 7:481-493, 1977.
4. Vanderpump M, Tunbridge W: The epidemiology of thyroid disease. In Braverman L, Utiger R (eds): The Thyroid. Philadelphia, Lippincott-Raven, 1996, pp 474-482.
5. International Council for the Control of Iodine Deficiency Disorders: Iodine nutrition map (http://www.iccidd.org).
6. Hollowell J, Staehling N, Hannon W, et al: Iodine nutrition in the United States. Trends and public health implications: Iodine excretion data from National Health and Nutrition Examination Surveys I and III (1971-1974 and 1988-1994). J Clin Endocrinol Metab 83:3401-3408, 1998.
7. Cooper DS: Regulation of thyroid function: The thyroid and disruption of thyroid function in humans. Presented at the American Thyroid Association Spring Symposium—Thyroid Health and the Environment. Washington, DC, Threats and Effects, March 24, 2006, pp 33-53.
8. Hashimoto H: Zur Kenntniss der lymphomatosen Veranderung der Schilddruse (struma lymphomatosa). Arch Klin Chir 97:219-248, 1912.
9. Khoury E, Pereira L, Greenspan F: Induction of HLA-DR expression on thyroid follicular cells by cytomegalovirus infection in vitro: Evidence for a dual mechanism of induction. Am J Pathol 137:1209-1223, 1991.
10. Neufeld D, Platzer M, Davies TF: Reovirus induction of MHC class II antigen in rat thyroid cells. Endocrinology 124:543-545, 1989.
11. Todd I, Pujol-Borrell R, Hammond L, et al: Interferon-gamma induces HLA-DR expression by thyroid epithelium. Clin Exp Immunol 51:265-273, 1985.
12. Bottazzo G, Pujol-Borrell R, Hanafusa T, et al: Role of aberrant HLA-DR expression an antigen presentation in induction of endocrine autoimmunity. Lancet 2:1115-1119, 1983.
13. Dayan C, Daniels G: Chronic autoimmune thyroiditis. N Engl J Med 335:99-108, 1996.
14. Stassi G, DiLiberto D, Todaro M, et al: Control of target cell survival in thyroid autoimmunity by T helper cytokines via regulation of apoptotic proteins. Nat Immunol 1:483-488, 2000.
15. Giordano C, Stassi G, De Maria R, et al: Potential involvement of Fas and its ligand in the pathogenesis of Hashimoto's thyroiditis. Science 275:960-963, 1997.
16. Batteux F, Lores P, Bucchini D, et al: Transgenic expression of Fas ligand on thyroid follicular cells prevents autoimmune thyroiditis. J Immunol 164:1681-1688, 2000.
17. Dong Z, Takakuwa T, Takayama H, et al: Fas and Fas ligand gene mutations in Hashimoto's thyroiditis. Lab Invest 82:1611-1616, 2002.
18. Stassi G, DeMaria R: Autoimmune thyroid disease: New models of cell death in autoimmunity. Nat Rev Immunol 2:195-204, 2002.
19. Fisfalen M, Palmer E, van Seventer G, et al: Thyrotropin-receptor and thyroid peroxidase-specific T cell clones and their cytokine profile in autoimmune thyroid disease. J Clin Endocrinol Metab 82:3655-3663, 1997.
20. Chiovato L, Bassi P, Santini F, et al: Antibodies producing complement-mediated thyroid cytotoxicity in patients with atrophic or goitrous autoimmune thyroditis. J Clin Endocinol Metab 77:1700-1705, 1993.
21. Khoury E, Hammond L, Bottazzo G, et al: Presence of organ-specific 'microsomal' autoantigen on the surface of human thyroid cells in culture: Its involvement in complement-mediated cytotoxicity. Clin Exp Immunol 45:316-328, 1981.
22. Weetman A, Cohen S, Oleeskky D, et al: Terminal complement complexes and c1/c1 inhibitor complexes in autoimmune thyroid disease. Clin Exp Immunol 77:25-30, 1989.
23. Ciampolillo A, Guastamacchia E, Amati L, et al: Modifications of the immune responsiveness in patients with autoimmune thyroiditis: Evidence for a systemic immune alteration. Curr Pharm Des 24:1946-1950, 2003.

24. Kohn L, Harii N: Thyrotropin receptor autoantibodies: Epitopes, origins and clinical significance. Autoimm 36:331-337, 2003.
25. Takasu N, Yamada T, Takasu M, et al: Disappearance of thyrotropin-blocking antibodies and spontaneous recovery from hypothyroidism in autoimmune thyroiditis. N Engl J Med 326:513-518, 1992.
26. Kawakami A, Eguchi K, Matsuoka N, et al: Thyroid-stimulating hormone inhibits Fas antigen-mediated apoptosis of human thyrocytes in vitro. Endocrinology 137:3163-3169, 1996.
27. Olczak S, McCulloch A, Clark A: Thyrotoxic Graves' disease after primary hypothyroidism. Br Med J 2:666, 1978.
28. Fatourechi V, McConahey W, Woolner L: Hyperthyroidism associated with histologic Hashimoto's thyroiditis. Mayo Clin Proc 46:682-689, 1971.
29. Wieshammer S, Keck F, Waitzinger J, et al: Acute hypothyroidism slows the rate of left ventricular diastolic relaxation. Can J Physiol Pharmacol 67:1007-1010, 1989.
30. Ojamaa K, Klemperer J, Klein I: Acute effects of thyroid hormone on vascular smooth muscle. Thyroid 6:505-512, 1996.
31. Klein I, Ojamaa K: Thyroid hormone and the cardiovascular system. N Engl J Med 344:501-509, 2001.
32. Taddei S, Caraccio N, Virdis A: Impaired endothelium-dependent vasodilatation in subclinical hypothyroidism: Beneficial effect of levothyroxine therapy. J Clin Endocrinol Metab 88:3731-3737, 2003.
33. Fredlund B, Olsson S: Long QT interval and ventricular tachycardia of "torsade de pointe" type in hypothyroidism. Acta Med Scand 213:231-235, 1983.
34. Thompson G, Soutar A, Spengel F, et al: Defects of receptor-mediated low density lipoprotein catabolism in homozygous familial hypercholesterolemia and hypothyroidism in vivo. Proc Natl Acad Sci U S A 78:2591-2595, 1981.
35. Kabadi U, Kumar S: Pericardial effusion in primary hypothyroidism. Am Heart J 120:1393-1395, 1990.
36. Tanis B, Westendorp G, Smelt H: Effect of thyroid substitution on hypercholesterolemia in patients with subclinical hypothyroidism: A reanalysis of intervention studies. Clin Endocrinol (Oxf) 44:643-649, 1996.
37. Zwillich C, Pierson D, Hofeldt F, et al: Ventilatory control in myxedema and hypothyroidism. N Engl J Med 292:662-665, 1975.
38. Sachdev Y, Hall L: Effusions into body cavities in hypothyroidism. Lancet 1:564-566, 1975.
39. Gottehrer A, Roa J, Stanford G, et al: Hypothyroidism and pleural effusions. Chest 98:1130-1132, 1990.
40. Martinez F, Bermudez-Gomez M, Celli B: Hypothyroidism: A reversible cause of diaphragmatic dysfunction. Chest 96:1059-1063, 1989.
41. Sharifi F, Amari A: The effect of levothyroxine on pulmonary function tests of hypothyroid patients. Int J Endocrinol Metab 1:48-51, 2005.
42. Grunstein R, Sullivan C: Sleep apnea and hypothyroidism: Mechanisms and management. Am J Med 85:775-779, 1988.
43. Rajagopal K, Abbrecht P, Derderian S, et al: Obstructive sleep apnea in hypothyroidism. Ann Intern Med 101:491-494, 1984.
44. Burman K, McKinley-Grant L: Dermatologic aspects of thyroid disease. Clin Dermatol 24:247-255, 2006.
45. Jubbour S: Cutaneous manifestations of endocrine disorders: A guide for dermatologists. Am J Clin Dermatol 4:315-331, 2003.
46. Leonhardt J, Heymann W: Thyroid disease and the skin. Dermatol Clin 20:473-481, 2002.
47. Shafer R, Prentiss R, Bond J: Gastrointestinal transit in thyroid disease. Gastroenterology 86:852-855, 1984.
48. Valentino R, Savastano S, Maglio M, et al: Markers of potential celiac disease in patients with Hashimoto's thyroiditis. Eur J Endocrinol 146:479-483, 2002.
49. Collin P, Kaukinen K, Valimaki M, et al: Endocrinological disorders and celiac disease. Endocr Rev 23:464-483, 2002.
50. Centanni M, Marignani M, Gargano L, et al: Atrophic body gastritis in patients with autoimmune thyroid disease: An underdiagnosed association. Arch Int Med 159:1726-1730, 1999.
51. Bono G, Fancellu R, Blandini F, et al: Cognitive and affective status in mild hypothyroidism and interactions with L-thyroxine treatment. Acta Neurol Scand 110:59-66, 2004.
52. Osterweil D, Syndulko K, Cohen S, et al: Cognitive function in non-demented older adults with hypothyroidism. J Am Geriatr Soc 40:325-335, 1992.
53. Wekking E, Appelhof B, Fliers E, et al: Cognitive functioning and well-being in euthyroid patients on thyroxine replacement therapy for primary hypothyroidism. Eur J Endocrinol 153:747-753, 2005.
54. Miller K, Parsons T, Whybrow P, et al: Memory improvement with treatment of hypothyroidism. Int J Neurosci 116:895-906, 2006.
55. Palumbo C, Szabo R, Olmsted S: The effects of hypothyroidism and thyroid replacement on the development of carpal tunnel syndrome. J Hand Surg [Am] 25:734-739, 2000.
56. Duyff R, Van den Bosch J, Laman D, et al: Neuromuscular findings in thyroid dysfunction: A prospective clinical and electrodiagnostic study. J Neurol Neurosurg Psychiatry 68:750-755, 2000.
57. Kececi H, Degirmenci Y: Hormone replacement therapy in hypothyroidism and nerve conduction study. Neurophysiol Clin 36:79-83, 2006.
58. Meikle AW: The interrelationships between thyroid dysfunction and hypogonadism in men and boys. Thyroid 14(Suppl 1):S17-S25, 2004.
59. Adler SM, Verbalis JG: Disorders of body water homeostasis in critical illness. Endocrinol Clin N Am 35:873-894, 2006.
60. Iwaski Y, Oiso Y, Yamauchi K, et al: Osmoregulation of plasma vasopressin in myxedema. J Clin Endocrinol Metab 70:534-539, 1990.

61. Derubertis F Jr, Michelis M, Bloom M, et al: Impaired water excretion in myxedema. Am J Med 51:41-53, 1971.
62. Hanna F, Scanlon M: Hyponatremia, hypothyroidism, and role of arginine-vasopressin. Lancet 350:755-756, 1997.
63. Schmitz P, de Meijer P, Meinders A: Hyponatremia due to hypothyroidism: A pure renal mechanism. Neth J Med 58:143-149, 2001.
64. Wartofsky L: Myxedema coma. Endocrinol Clin N Am 35:687-698, 2006.
65. Sanders V: Neurologic manifestations of myxedema. N Engl J Med 266:547-551, 1962.
66. Westphal S: Unusual presentations of hypothyroidism. Am J Med Sci 314:333-337, 1997.
67. Surks M, Ortiz E, Daniels G, et al: Subclinical thyroid disease: Scientific review and guidelines for diagnosis and management. JAMA 291:228-238, 2004.
68. Gharib H, Tuttle RM, Baskin HJ, et al: Consensus statement: Subclinical thyroid dysfunction: A joint statement on management from the American Association of Clinical Endocrinologists, the American Thyroid Association, and the Endocrine Society. J Clin Endocrinol Metab 90:581-585, 2005.
69. Wartofsky L, Dickey R: The evidence for a narrower thyrotropin reference range is compelling. J Clin Endocrinol Metab 90:5483-5488, 2005.
70. Burman KD, Wartofsky L: Endocrine and metabolic dysfunction syndromes in the critically ill: Thyroid function in the intensive care unit setting. Crit Care Clin 17:43-57, 2001.
71. Grozinsky-Glasberg S, Fraser A, Nahshoni E, et al: Thyroxine-triiodothyronine combination therapy versus thyroxine monotherapy for clinical hypothyroidism: Meta-analysis of randomized controlled trials. J Clin Endocrinol Metab 91:2592-2599, 2006.
72. Bunevicius R, Prange AJ: Mental improvement after replacement therapy with thyroxine plus triiodothyronine: Relationship to cause of hypothyroidism. Int J Neuropsychopharmacol 3:167-174, 2000.
73. Roos A, Linn-Rasker S, van Domburg R, et al: The starting dose of levothyroxine in primary hypothyroidism treatment: Prospective, randomized, double-blind trial. Arch Intern Med 165:1714-1720, 2005.
74. Wartofsky L, Burman KD: Alterations in thyroid function in patients with systemic illness: The euthyroid sick syndrome. Endocr Rev 3:164-217, 1982.
75. Flynn RWV, MacDonald T, Jung R, et al: Mortality and vascular outcomes in patients treated for thyroid dysfunction. J Clin Endocrinol Metab 91:2159-2164, 2006.
76. Singh B, Shaha A, Trivedi H, et al: Coexistent Hashimoto's thyroiditis with papillary thyroid carcinoma: Impact on presentation, management, and outcome. Surgery 126:1070-1076, 1999.
77. Tallini G, Asa SL: RET oncogene activation in papillary thyroid carcinoma. Adv Anat Pathol 8:345-354, 2001.
78. Nikiforov YE. RET/PTC rearrangement in thyroid tumors. Endocr Pathol 13:3-16, 2002.
79. Wirtschafter A, Schmidt R, Rosen D. Expression of the RET/PTC fusion gene as a marker for papillary carcinoma in Hashimoto's thyroiditis. Laryngoscope 107:95-100, 1997.
80. Sheils O, O'Eary J, Uhlmann V, et al: RET/PTC-1 activation in Hashimoto thyroiditis. Int J Surg Pathol 8:185-189, 2000.
81. Arif S, Blanes A, Diaz-Cano S: Hashimoto's thyroiditis shares features with early papillary thyroid carcinoma. Histopathology 41:357-362, 2002.
82. Nikiforov, YE. RET/PTC rearrangement—a link between Hashimoto's thyroiditis and thyroid cancer…or not. J Clin Endocrinol Metab 91:2040-2042, 2006.
83. Nikiforova M, Caudill C, Biddinger P, et al: Prevalence of RET/PTC rearrangements in Hashimoto's thyroiditis and papillary thyroid carcinomas. Int J Surg Pathol 10:15-22, 2002.
84. Sangalli G, Serio G, Zampatti C, et al: Fine needle aspiration cytology of primary lymphoma of the thyroid: A report of 17 cases. Cytopathology 12:257-263, 2001.
85. Thieblemont C, Mayer A, Dumontet C, et al: Primary thyroid lymphoma is a heterogeneous disease. J Clin Endocrinol Metab 87:105-111, 2002.
86. Matsuzuka F, Miyauchi A, Katayama S, et al: Clinical aspects of primary thyroid lymphoma: Diagnosis and treatment based on our experience of 119 cases. Thyroid 3:93-99, 1993.
87. Isaacson P, Spencer J. The biology of low grade MALT lymphoma. J Clin Pathol 48:395-397, 1995.
88. Stelfox H, Ahmed S, Fiskio J, et al: An evaluation of the adequacy of outpatient monitoring of thyroid replacement therapy. J Eval Clin Pract 10:525-530, 2004.
89. Diez JJ: Hypothyroidism in patients older than 55 years: An analysis of the etiology and assessment of the effectiveness of therapy. J Gerontol A Biol Sci Med Sci 57:M315-M320, 2002.
90. Diez JJ, Iglesias P: Spontaneous subclinical hypothyroidism in patients older than 55 years: An analysis of natural course and risk factors for the development of overt thyroid failure. J Clin Endocrinol Metab 89:4890-4897, 2004.
91. Parle J, Franklyn J, Cross K, et al: Thyroxine prescription in the community: Serum thyroid stimulating hormone level assays as an indicator of the undertreatment or overtreatment. Br J Gen Pract 43:107-109, 1993.
92. Ross D, Daniels G, Gouveia D: The use and limitations of a chemiluminescent thyrotropin assay as a single thyroid function test in an outpatient endocrine clinic. J Clin Endocrinol Metab 71:764-769, 1990.

Chapter 18

Central Hypothyroidism

Aniket Sidhaye

Key Points

- Central hypothyroidism is most commonly caused by suprasellar masses.
- Diagnosis is suggested by TSH values that are inappropriate for low thyroxine levels.
- TSH values should not be used to monitor or adjust treatment in central hypothyroidism.
- Adrenal insufficiency may coexist with central hypothyroidism and should be diagnosed and treated before initiating treatment for hypothyroidism.

Central hypothyroidism is defined as pathologically low thyroxine levels caused by decreased secretion of thyroid-stimulating hormone (TSH) or secretion of biologically inactive TSH. Central hypothyroidism (CH) is relatively rare. Indirect estimates based on the prevalence of pituitary tumors have indicated that central hypothyroidism occurs in 0.0002% of the population.[1] Other groups have suggested that the frequency of central hypothyroidism is 0.005%.[2] This is in contrast to a prevalence of 1% to 2% for primary hypothyroidism. Also, in newborns, hypothyroidism caused by pituitary or hypothalamic dysfunction occurs with an incidence of 1 in 25,000 to 100,000 births.[3,4] There is an equal gender distribution. Most commonly, central hypothyroidism is caused by sellar or suprasellar masses that cause a decreased mass of functional thyrotropes or an interruption of the hypothalamic-pituitary portal circulation. Thus, the diagnosis of central hypothyroidism often occurs in the setting of deficiency or excess of other pituitary hormones.[5] Finally, it is important to note that TSH values may be low, normal, or slightly elevated in patients with central hypothyroidism and therefore measurement of TSH value alone cannot be used to diagnose or monitor patients.

PATHOGENESIS

The pathogenesis of central hypothyroidism is caused by decreased secretion of TSH or secretion of biologically inactive TSH. This can occur because of the following:

1. Destruction or compression of existing thyrotropes. This is usually caused by pituitary masses but may also be caused by vascular, infectious, or inflammatory destruction of thyrotrope cells.
2. Deficient or defective secretion of thyrotropin-releasing hormone (TRH). This may be caused by interruption of the hypophyseal portal blood flow to the anterior pituitary or hypothalamic lesions. Theoretically, this is caused by TRH deficiency alone and thus replacement of TRH could result in normal TSH secretion. One study has provided indirect evidence for this concept by correcting hypothyroxinemia with repeated injections of TRH.[6]
3. Congenital defects in thyrotrope development or secretion of biologically active TSH.
4. Functional defects in TSH secretion.

A common finding in central hypothyroidism is disruption of the normal diurnal rhythm of TSH secretion (Fig. 18-1). TSH secretion occurs in a circadian pattern, with a nocturnal surge beginning at about 1900 hours, peaking at about 2400 hours.[7] In central hypothyroidism, this nocturnal surge is absent or blunted in almost all cases. This occurs because of a decrease in the TSH pulse amplitude at night; pulse frequency is preserved.[2] It appears that the nocturnal surge is important because the thyroid is particularly stimulated at night. Based on this, some have suggested that testing for the absence of the nocturnal TSH surge is a sensitive way to identify cases of central hypothyroidism.

Biologically Inactive Thyroid-Stimulating Hormone

The presence of low thyroxine (T_4) levels, in association with normal levels of TSH in patients with known pituitary or hypothalamic disease, had been

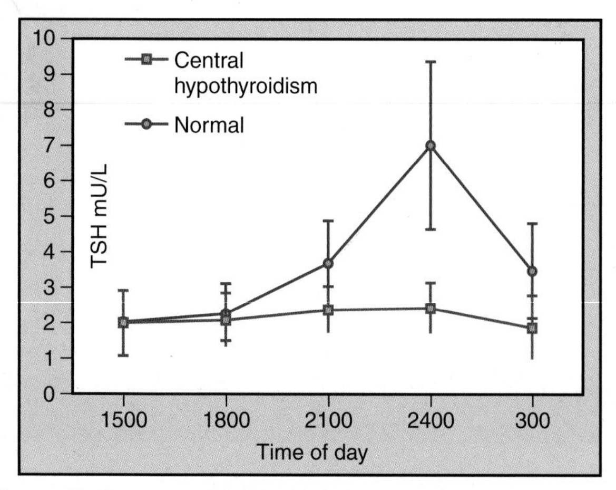

Figure 18–1 Normal individuals have a surge in thyroid-stimulating hormone, peaking at about 2400 hours. In contrast, patients with central hypothyroidism have a blunted nocturnal surge. *(Adapted from Rose SR: Disorders of thyrotropin synthesis, secretion, and function. Curr Opin Pediatr 12:375-381, 2000.)*

recognized in patients not likely to have primary hypothyroidism because of the absence of autoimmunity and an adequate response to exogenous TSH. Furthermore, exogenous TRH produced an appropriate or even exaggerated rise in TSH but with an inadequate increase of triiodothyronine (T_3) levels. Assays for TSH biologic activity, such as Chinese hamster ovary (CHO) cells transfected[8] with TSH receptor or adenylate cyclase activity from FRTL-5 cells,[9] have suggested that the ratio of biologic to immunologic TSH is reduced in some patients with central hypothyroidism. Furthermore, it was shown that chronic oral TRH treatment but not acute IV treatment could restore TSH biologic activity, suggesting a requirement of TRH for full biologic activity of TSH.[10] Subsequently, an abnormal glycosylation pattern in a rat model of central hypothyroidism was shown to be reversed by TRH treatment, with a restoration of normal TSH values.[11] It has now been established that TRH ensures the proper glycosylation of TSH and that there are abnormal glycosylation patterns associated with CH. Investigators have demonstrated abnormal glycosylation patterns, including reduced sialylation of TSH in patients with central, but not primary, hypothyroidism.[12-14] Many studies have documented secretion of bioinactive TSH in central hypothyroidism. Furthermore, this may be a common finding in cases of both pituitary and hypothalamic disease.[13]

CAUSES

There are a number of causes of central hypothyroidism (Table 18-1).

Table 18–1 Etiology of Central Hypothyroidism

Tumors
Pituitary adenomas
Craniopharyngioma
Meningioma
Dysgerminoma
Cysts
Vascular
Postpartum pituitary necrosis (Sheehan's syndrome)
Pituitary infarction (apoplexy)
Infectious
Tuberculosis
Syphilis
Toxoplasmosis
African trypanosomiasis
Abscess
Infiltrative
Sarcoidosis
Histiocytosis
Lymphocytic hypophysitis
Hemochromatosis
Iatrogenic
External-beam radiation
Surgery
Bexarotene
Ribavirin/interferon-α
Trauma
Congenital defects
Combined pituitary hormone deficiency (mutations in *Prop-1*, Pit-1, *Hesx-1*, and other factors)
Isolated thyroid-stimulating hormone (TSH) deficiency (mutations in TSH-β, TRH-receptor)

Pituitary Mass Lesions

Pituitary masses are the most common cause of central hypothyroidism, accounting for almost 75% of hypopituitarism cases in one series.[15] Most often, this is caused by nonfunctioning or functioning adenomas of the pituitary and is often seen in conjunction with other pituitary hormone deficits. The cause of hypothyroidism is likely from compression of nontumorous thyrotropes or interruption of the hypophyseal portal circulation caused by involvement of the stalk from suprasellar extension.[2] Less commonly, pituitary tumor apoplexy has also been associated with hypopituitarism and warrants workup. Interestingly, after surgery for pituitary adenomas, 57% of those who were hypothyroid preoperatively recovered function.[16] A blunted response to TRH preoperatively predicted the inability to recover anterior pituitary function in general. A similar rate of recovery occurs after surgical decompression to treat pituitary tumor apoplexy.[17] However, surgery for larger pituitary tumors is also associated with the development of pituitary deficits postoperatively, with hypothyroidism occurring in about 10% of cases.[2] Metastatic tumors to the hypothalamic-pituitary region can occur with breast, lung, and other cancers.[5] Usually, this is in the setting of advanced disease and the uncommon finding of hypopituitarism is often associated with diabetes insipidus.

Extrasellar Masses

Craniopharyngiomas, especially in younger patients, are frequently associated with central hypothyroidism. TSH deficiency is present in 21% to 42% of cases.[18] In contrast to pituitary adenomas, surgery rarely resolves the hormone deficiency and the 10-year probability of hormone deficiency is high. Meningiomas, cysts, and abscesses are also reported causes of hypopituitarism.[2]

Congenital Defects

Combined pituitary hormone deficiency (CPHD) is a syndrome of deficient secretion of the anterior pituitary hormones prolactin (PRL), growth hormone (GH), and TSH. Research into the stages of pituitary development has revealed a cascade of transcription factors that control when and how the different anterior pituitary cell lineages develop. Molecular defects have been identified in many of these transcription factors:

1. Pit-1, the pituitary-specific transcription factor (or Pou1f1), is expressed relatively late in the pituitary development cascade and its expression is preserved throughout life. Whereas GH and PRL deficiencies are present early in life, TSH deficiency may present later in childhood. The first described mutations were homozygous nonsense mutations[19] or acted as dominant negatives.[20]
2. *Prop-1* is believed to be required for Pit-1 expression and does not persist into adulthood. Mutations in *Prop-1* are associated with GH, TSH, PRL, and gonadotropin deficiencies. Deficiency of GH, TSH, and PRL is milder for mutations in *Prop-1* than in *Pit-1* mutations. Although most patients present with early-onset growth hormone deficiency, TSH deficiency is variable and may not be present at birth. Hypogonadism is also variable in onset and severity. Finally, there is an evolving cortisol deficiency with age, but the cause of this adrenocorticotropic hormone (ACTH) deficiency is unknown.[21,22] In some series of CPHD, mutations in *Prop-1* appear to be the most common cause of sporadic and familial CPHD.[23]
3. *HESX1* is a member of the paired-like class of homeobox genes and is one of the earliest markers of the murine pituitary primordium. It acts as a transcriptional repressor but its downstream targets are unknown. In humans, mutations in *HESX-1* were first identified in association with septo-optic dysplasia.[24]
4. *PITX2* heterozygous mutations are associated with Rieger's syndrome, characterized mainly by defects in the anterior chamber of the eye and by tooth malformations in humans.[25]
5. *Lhx3* and *Lhx4* belong to the LIM family of homeobox genes that are expressed early in Rathke's pouch and into adulthood. Lhx3 is believed to act synergistically with Pou1f1 to activate TSH beta (TSH-β) and PRL promoters. Mutations in humans are identified and have hormone deficiencies similar to patients with *PROP-1* mutations (i.e., GH, TSH, and PRL, in addition to gonadotropin deficiency) but also have a short, rigid cervical spine, with limited head rotation.[26] There is one report of an *Lhx4* mutation associated with a poorly formed sella turcica, ectopic posterior pituitary, absent infundibulum, and pointed cerebellar tonsils.[27]

Investigation into familial cases of central hypothyroidism has revealed mutations in the TSH-β subunit gene. Mutations near the NH_2 terminus have been identified that result in an altered TSH-β subunit unable to bind the alpha subunit.[28,29] The mutations are in the so-called CAGYC region, which is conserved in the beta subunit glycoproteins. The mutations resulted in an arginine substitution for glycine. Patients were described as homozygous for the mutation. Another group has identified three patients in two related Greek families with nonsense mutations in exon 2, giving rise to a truncated peptide including only the first 11 amino acids of the TSH-β peptide.[30] In all these cases, TSH was undetectable. Similar other mutations have been reported (*E12X, G29R, Q49X*, a splice site mutation at exon 2, and 114 X).[31,32] In another report, two related Brazilian families with central hypothyroidism were determined to have a detectable but biologically inactive form of TSH based on in vitro and in vivo studies.[33] The mutation was in a critical carboxy terminal cysteine residue (C105V) in the TSH-β subunit gene. Crystallographic studies of the chorionic gonadotropin have suggested that cysteine residues C19 and C105 in the TSH-β subunit form the buckle of a seat belt that surrounds the alpha subunit and maintains bioactivity of the hormone. Some have suggested that codon 105 represents a "hot spot" for mutation, although a founder effect cannot be ruled out.[31]

Finally, a defective TRH-receptor was identified in a single patient with isolated central hypothyroidism. Defects in the TRH receptor were suspected when the patient did not show expected changes in TSH and prolactin after the administration of TRH. The patient was found to be compound heterozygous for mutations in the TRH receptor. The mutations were in the 5′ region of the gene and the mutated receptors did not bind TRH.[34]

Infiltrative Diseases

Sarcoidosis of the central nervous system occurs in approximately 5% of sarcoid cases.[35] Of these, hypopituitarism is seen in 10%, usually with profound endocrine dysfunction. TSH deficiency occurs in about 50% of cases.[35] However, sarcoidosis can also present as isolated involvement of the central nervous system (CNS) without pituitary dysfunction. On imaging, it may present as a sellar or suprasellar mass or as a cystic sellar mass. More suggestive findings on magnetic resonance imaging (MRI) include thickening of the central portion of the pituitary stock and loss of the posterior pituitary bright spot.

Langerhans cell histiocytosis (LCH) is a multisystem disorder with a propensity for hypothalamic-pituitary involvement. The most common endocrine disorder is diabetes insipidus, which occurs in about 50% of cases of multisystem LCH. Central hypothyroidism occurs in about 10% to 15% of cases and can occur after many years of disease.[36,37]

Lymphocytic hypophysitis (LH) is an infiltrative disease of the pituitary of unknown, although likely, autoimmune cause. Endocrine dysfunction can be seen in approximately 80% of cases, with an interesting predilection for thyrotropes and corticotropes.[38] Hypothyroidism can occur in 50% of cases of LH. Imaging often shows an enlarged pituitary with a symmetrical shape, homogeneous gadolinium enhancement, a relatively low signal on T1-weighted images and high signal on T2-weighted images, serving to distinguish LH from a pituitary adenoma. The frequent co-occurrence of LH with Hashimoto's thyroiditis, type 1 diabetes mellitus (DM), Addison's disease, and pernicious anemia has led it to be considered as part of the autoimmune polyglandular syndrome type 1.[39]

Hereditary hemochromatosis is caused by increased absorption of dietary iron, leading to parenchymal iron overload. Deposition of iron in the anterior pituitary usually causes hypogonadotropic hypogonadism.[40] TSH deficiency can occur, is rare, and can be resolved with iron depletion treatment.[41] In thalassemia patients who receive multiple transfusions, pituitary iron deposition may occur. Furthermore, thyroid dysfunction is observed, but it appears that this is not commonly caused by central hypothyroidism.[42]

Infectious Disorders

Tuberculosis, toxoplasmosis, African trypanosomiasis, and syphilis have been associated with central hypothyroidism in association with pituitary disease.[2]

Iatrogenic Factors

If the hypothalamic-pituitary axis falls within the field of external radiation, hypopituitarism may ensue. This has long been recognized for patients receiving radiation therapy for primary brain tumors,[43,44] total body irradiation for other illnesses, and, importantly, in children undergoing cranial irradiation for prophylaxis in acute lymphoblastic leukemia. Furthermore, the incidence appears to be dose-related, with doses of more than 30 Gy associated with a 90% incidence of hypopituitarism at 10 years.[45] Although it is generally believed that GH is affected earlier and more commonly, one study has suggested that 50% of patients receiving cranial irradiation developed central hypothyroidism.[44] In addition, longer term follow-up studies of survivors of childhood cancers have suggested that central hypothyroidism occurs in 65% of patients after brain or nasopharyngeal tumors, in 35% after bone marrow transplantation, and in 15% after leukemia.[46]

Rexinoids have been shown to decrease TSH. Specifically, bexarotene, a selective retinoid X receptor (RXR)–α agonist, was found to suppress TSH in most patients being treated for cutaneous T-cell lymphoma, and many of these patients had hypothyroidism.[47] Subsequently, it was shown that bexarotene can suppress TSH, even in healthy subjects.[48] It is believed that this is caused by a direct effect of RXR-α on the TSH-β promoter and is reversible.

There is also a report of ribavirin and interferon alpha treatment of hepatitis C being associated with central hypothyroidism and hypophysitis that is apparently different from the autoimmune thyroid disease seen with interferon alpha treatment.[49]

Trauma

Hypopituitarism can occur following head trauma. Although gonadotropin deficiency is the most common finding, central hypothyroidism occurs in approximately 50% of post-traumatic hypopituitarism.[50] Some studies have suggested that in cases of unexplained central hypothyroidism, a history of head trauma should be sought. Furthermore, the incidence of hypothyroidism following head trauma may be underappreciated.[51] In addition, patients with poor outcomes had lower thyroid hormone values in the first days following injury as compared with those patients who recovered well.[52]

Functional Defects in Thyroid-Stimulating Hormone Secretion

There are several clinical scenarios associated with functional defects in TSH secretion. In most cases, this defect need not be treated, because there is no hypothyroidism per se.

After withdrawal of suppressive T_4 therapy for nontoxic goiter or after treatment of hyperthyroidism with radioiodine, antithyroid agents, or surgery, the serum TSH level may remain low for approximately 25 days.[53] During this period, if thyroid hormone replacement is not initiated, then T_4 values could fall to below normal. Thus, a low TSH and low free T_4 may incorrectly suggest central hypothyroidism without knowledge of the patient's history. Similarly, during recovery from the thyrotoxic phase of subacute thyroiditis, TSH levels may remain low even as the T_4 values become normal or even low during the recovery period.

Nonthyroidal illness is characterized by a low T_4 associated with a low TSH.[54] One reason for this may be the induction of type II deiodinase,[55] which is present in hypothalamic and pituitary cells and thus plays an important role in feedback regulation of TSH. Others have noted a defective nocturnal surge in different types of nonthyroidal illness.[56] Increases in interleukin 6 (IL-6) have also been noted, but whether this is part of the pathogenesis of nonthyroidal illness is unknown.[57,58] During nonthyroidal illness, however, most patients have a normal response to TRH and biologic activity of the TSH is normal or even increased. Specific illnesses with thyroid hormone values resembling those of CH are decompensated diabetes, chronic renal failure, burn, and post–bone marrow transplantation.[2] Interestingly, after glycemic control has been restored, nocturnal TSH surge normalizes but only in patients with residual C-peptide secretion.[59]

Functional central hypothyroidism can be seen in Cushing's syndrome or prolonged glucocorticoid therapy.[60] In Cushing's syndrome, the nocturnal TSH surge is absent and there may be a decreased response of TSH to TRH.[61]

GH decreases thyroid function by central and peripheral mechanisms. GH decreases the TSH nocturnal surge and its secretory response to TRH, probably because of stimulation of hypothalamic somatostatin. Furthermore, it increases the metabolism of T_4 to T_3.[62] There is an interaction between T_4 and GH. Both primary and central hypothyroidism can impair endogenous GH secretion and it is recommended that in children with suspected GH deficiency, euthyroidism be verified before provocative testing or treatment with recombinant GH is started. Most studies have suggested that treatment of adult growth hormone deficiency patients with recombinant human GH is associated with a reduction in T_4, increase in T3, and no change in TSH.[63,64] Two studies have suggested that 36% to 47% of patients become hypothyroid within 3 to 6 months after initiation of GH treatment[64] and are less likely to show improvement in quality of life.[65] GH has central and peripheral effects on thyroid function, as noted. In cases in which there is underlying pituitary pathology, CH may be masked[65] by growth hormone deficiency.

Anorexia nervosa is associated with a low T_3 and normal TSH peak after TRH, but a delayed return to baseline.[66]

Similarly, depression is also associated with functional disorders of TSH secretion. A blunted response of TSH to TRH may be seen in up to 25% of patients with depression,[67] and others have noted that a decreased nocturnal TSH surge may be more common than absent TRH responses.[68] It is not generally thought that this merits treatment.

Aging is associated with a small but progressive decrease in TSH as well as a blunted response of TSH to TRH.[69,70]

CLINICAL FEATURES

The patient with central hypothyroidism can present with a variable manifestations, depending on the severity and duration of hypothyroidism, the nature of the underlying illness, and the number and degree of other pituitary hormones affected. Features related to hypothyroidism, such as cold intolerance, fatigue, slowed speech, weight gain, constipation, and loss of mental acuity, are similar to what is seen in primary hypothyroidism, although generally they are thought to be less severe. Onset in childhood may be characterized by delay in sexual maturation and/or bone development in addition to growth failure. Isolated hypothyroidism caused by inherited defects presents as dwarfism or cretinism. On physical examination, bradycardia, hypothermia, and delay in the relaxation phase of deep tendon reflexes can been seen. Because of the strong likelihood of associated deficiencies in other pituitary hormones, the skin may not be coarse and dry but only pale and cool. Instead of periorbital or peripheral edema, there may be fine, dry wrinkling of the skin. Thinning of hair and lateral eyebrows and loss of pubic, axillary, or facial hair is more pronounced than in primary hypothyroidism.

Because central hypothyroidism often occurs in the setting of other pituitary hormone deficiencies, these symptoms may predominate. Gonadotropin and growth hormone deficiency often precede thyrotropin deficiency. In children, this manifests as growth failure and delayed sexual maturation. In adults, there may be no symptoms related to growth hormone deficiency. Gonadotropin deficiency in adults may present with decreased pubic and axillary hair. In men, there is decreased libido, impotence, thinning of the beard, and testicular atrophy and in women there is infertility and amenorrhea. Corticotropin deficiency generally occurs after the development of thyrotropin deficiency and thus patients may complain of nausea, abdominal discomfort, and lassitude. Postural hypotension and depigmented areas of the skin may also be noted. Hypoglycemia can occur with adrenal insufficiency and decreased insulin requirements in a diabetic patient with growth hormone deficiency. It is important to recognize the possibility of concomitant adrenal insufficiency because there is a risk for life-threatening adrenal crisis in the setting of infection, trauma, or surgery.

If the cause of central hypothyroidism is related to a sellar or suprasellar mass, the patient's presentation may be dominated by symptoms and signs related to mass effect. Thus, headache and visual loss may be the presenting signs of a nonfunctioning tumor extending out of the sella. Similarly, in the setting of a pituitary tumor associated with hormone oversecretion, the patient is likely to present with symptoms related to this problem rather than hypothyroidism. Thus, female patients may present with amenorrhea and galactorrhea in the setting of a prolactinoma. Men may only note decreased libido and impotence. GH- and ACTH-secreting tumors are less common but, in these cases, acromegaly and Cushing's syndrome, respectively, will be the presenting findings. Craniopharyngiomas may also cause diabetes insipidus and growth failure in children and hypogonadism in adults. Other diseases in which diabetes insipidus is common include sarcoidosis and histiocytosis X because of hypothalamic or posterior pituitary involvement. Another interesting feature of hypothalamic lesions is the possibility of meningeal signs early in the course of disease. Finally, because appetite- and temperature-regulating centers are present in the hypothalamus, obesity and abnormal temperature regulation can occur with hypothalamic lesions.

Other causes often have unique clinical scenarios. Thus, severe headache is a prominent feature of pituitary apoplexy as well as sudden visual loss and involvement of the third and fifth cranial nerves. Postpartum pituitary necrosis often occurs in the setting of a complicated delivery involving hemorrhage and shock, followed by deficient lactation and delay in resumption of menses.

DIAGNOSIS

Laboratory Studies

THYROID-STIMULATING HORMONE AND FREE THYROXINE

Since the development of ultrasensitive TSH assays, the diagnosis of central hypothyroidism can be confirmed by the presence of low free thyroxine levels in the presence of low, inappropriately normal, or even mildly elevated TSH. Even prior to the availability of sensitive TSH assays, one study showed that 35% of patients had undetectable serum TSH, 41% had normal TSH, and 25% had elevated TSH.[71] Despite normal or elevated TSH levels, it is believed that these TSH molecules are bioinactive.

Measurement of total or free T_3 levels is generally not useful because they are frequently in the normal range. One prospective study has noted that free T_3 levels are within normal range in approximately 25% of patients with low free T_4 whereas total T_4 and T_3 values are normal in an even higher percentage of cases.[72] TSH values in patients with pituitary and hypothalamic disease exhibit considerable overlap and thus the TSH value alone cannot distinguish the site of pathology.

LOSS OF NOCTURNAL THYROID-STIMULATING HORMONE SURGE

As noted, TSH secretion occurs in a diurnal rhythm, with a surge in the late evening hours that is under hypothalamic control. Some investigators have suggested that serum TSH samples obtained between 2300 hours and 0200 hours every 30 minutes can document reliably the absence of this nocturnal surge and is a sensitive measure of central hypothyroidism.[46]

THYROTROPIN-RELEASING HORMONE STIMULATION TESTING

The rationale behind using TRH stimulation testing is to identify the site of pathology. That is, based on the control mechanism for TSH, it was anticipated that patients with pituitary disease would have an absent or blunted TSH response to TRH and patients with hypothalamic disease would have a preserved response. In normal individuals, after IV administration of TRH (5 μg/kg), TSH values generally peak in 30 minutes and return to basal levels in 120 minutes.[73] Patients with pituitary or hypothalamic disease exhibit a different pattern. In these cases, after TRH administration, there is a delayed rise in TSH, often followed by a sustained increase. Maximal TSH response may be blunted or even absent. This is more often seen in patients with pituitary disease, although patients with hypothalamic disease and no apparent pituitary involvement may also have this finding. Lastly, a normal or exaggerated rise in what is likely bioinactive TSH occurs occasionally after TRH administration in patients with hypothalamic disease and central hypothyroidism.[74] However, occasional patients with only pituitary pathology exhibit similar responses. For example, in one study, the plasma TSH response to TRH was absent in 13.5%, impaired in 16.8%, normal in 47.2%, and exaggerated in 22.5% of cases, with delayed and/or prolonged pattern of response in 65% of cases.[71] Thus, TRH testing alone cannot reliably distinguish between hypothalamic or pituitary causes of central hypothyroidism. For this reason, it is important to examine the complete clinical picture along with the thyroid function tests to determine the site of the lesion causing hypothyroidism. Furthermore, although a nocturnal TSH surge is common in pediatric patients with central hypothyroidism, a TRH test may still be unrevealing.[75,76]

However, in newborns, TRH testing may have a role in distinguishing central hypothyroidism from mild primary hypothyroidism or other conditions associated with a low T_4 and normal TSH levels, such as TBG deficiency, euthyroid sick syndrome, and hypothyroxinemia of prematurity.[77] A recent study has characterized the neonatal response to TRH stimulation in a small cohort of patients with persistently low T_4 and normal TSH values, identified initially only by newborn screening.[78] In such patients, who can be diagnostically challenging because of the absence of other features suggesting hypopituitarism, such as hypoglycemia or midline defects, the TRH stimulation test may be useful. Newborns with confirmed pituitary dysmorphology had a higher peak TSH, with persistent TSH elevation, although such a response is expected in primary hypothyroidism as well. A second group had absent or diminished response to TSH, showed male predominance, and had a lower incidence of multiple hormone deficiency. Given the importance of instituting proper replacement therapy, this test maybe a diagnostically useful tool if further studies confirm its applicability.

Imaging Studies

Computed tomography (CT) and MRI are sensitive techniques to identify hypothalamic and pituitary lesions. Imaging characteristics may help determine the cause. For example, calcifications and cysts may suggest craniopharyngioma. Loss of a bright spot in the posterior pituitary or thickening of the infundibulum may suggest an infiltrative process, such as sarcoidosis. As noted, lymphocytic hypophysitis has specific features that help distinguish it from a pituitary adenoma, which may be important, given the difference in clinical course.

TREATMENT

The goal of treatment is euthyroidism. Central hypothyroidism is treated in a similar manner as primary hypothyroidism, with levothyroxine (L-T_4) in dosages of 1.4 to 1.6 μg/kg/day. However, in patients who may be at risk from overtreatment, such as older adults or patients with existing cardiovascular disease, treatment is begun at dosages of 0.3 to 0.7 μg/kg of L-T_4 and adjusted every 3 to 4 weeks. In infants or children, the dose of L-T_4 required may be higher because of the potential of greater risk of underreplacement as a result of increased T_4 clearance. The consequence of undertreatment in this setting is mental retardation and delay of physical growth, so it is important to provide adequate treatment from the outset. However, to monitor treatment, TSH is not useful and should not be measured. Clinical assessment must be combined with measurements of free T_4 and free T_3. There is evidence to suggest that free T_3 values can be a more sensitive measure of overtreatment whereas free T_4 may disclose undertreatment.[72]

Patients with hypopituitarism have decreased quality of life, despite replacement hormonal therapy.[15] The TSH level is not useful for monitoring, so treatment of central hypothyroidism is more challenging because the "target" for free T_4 values in this setting is not well established. For example, one study of pituitary deficiency found lower free T_4 values in patients compared with the free T_4 values of healthy controls. Some have suggested that free T_4 in the middle of the normal range indicates appropriate dosage whereas others have suggested the upper third of the normal range as the correct target. However, the detriment of overtreatment cannot be overlooked; it includes decreased bone mineral density and susceptibility to atrial fibrillation in those older than 60 years.[79] Finally, growth hormone deficiency is common in patients with central hypothyroidism and is associated with reduced conversion of T_4 to T_3. Thus the free T_4 level may not reflect adequate tissue levels of T_3. A recent study has compared empirical T_4 treatment, which resulted in an average dose of 1.1 μg/kg body weight, with a body weight–adapted T_4 treatment, in which T_4 was dosed at 1.6 μg/kg body weight. The latter treatment resulted in improved clinical signs and symptoms of hypothyroidism and parameters, such as lipid levels, muscle enzymes, and body weight.[80] Another nonrandomized study has found that aiming treatment for a normal free T_3 and free T_4 concentrations led to subtle hypothyroidism.[72] In addition, patients with central hypothyroidism may need higher doses of levothyroxine than patients with primary hypothyroidism. One study examined clinically euthyroid patients with free T_4 in the upper half of the normal range and found that patient with central hypothyroidism received more exogenous T_4 (1.9 μg/kg/day) than patients with primary hypothyroidism from autoimmune thyroiditis or radioiodine treatment (1.6 μg/kg/day).[81] In this study, the authors noted lower TSH values in central versus primary hypothyroidism and suggested that even small amounts of TSH maybe biologically important.

Finally, it is important to evaluate for adrenal insufficiency prior to initiating treatment with T_4. T_4 accelerates the metabolism of cortisol. Therefore, if T_4 treatment is initiated in the setting of untreated adrenal insufficiency, a life-threatening adrenal crisis may be precipitated.

References

1. Hershman J: Hypothalamic and pituitary hypothyroidism. In Bastenie TA, Bonnyns M, Vanhaelst L (eds): Progress in the Diagnosis and Treatment of Hypothyroid Conditions. Amsterdam, Excerpta Medica, 1980, p 40.
2. Martino E, Bartalena L, Pinchera A: Central hypothyroidism. In Braverman LE, Utiger RD (eds): Werner and Ingbar's The Thyroid: A Fundamental and Clinical Text, 8th ed. Philadelphia, Lippincott, Williams & Wilkins, 2000, pp 762-773.
3. Hanna CE, Krainz PL, Skeels MR, et al: Detection of congenital hypopituitary hypothyroidism: Ten-year experience in the Northwest Regional Screening Program. J Pediatr 109:959-964,1986.
4. Fisher DA, Klein AH: Thyroid development and disorders of thyroid function in the newborn. N Engl J Med 304:702-712, 1981.
5. Samuels MH, Ridgway EC: Central hypothyroidism. Endocrinol Metab Clin North Am 21:903-919, 1992.
6. Van den Berghe G, de Zeghe F, Baxter RC, et al: Neuroendocrinology of prolonged critical illness: Effects of exogenous thyrotropin-releasing hormone and its combination with growth hormone secretagogues. J Clin Endocrinol Metab 83:309-319, 1998.
7. Rose SR: Disorders of thyrotropin synthesis, secretion, and function. Curr Opin Pediatr 12:375-381, 2000.
8. Persani L, Tonacchera M, Beck-Peccoz P, et al: Measurement of cAMP accumulation in Chinese hamster ovary cells transfected with the recombinant human TSH receptor (CHO-R): A new bioassay for human thyrotropin. J Endocrinol Invest 16:511-519, 1993.
9. Beck-Peccoz P, Persani L: Variable biological activity of thyroid-stimulating hormone. Eur J Endocrinol 131:331-340, 1994.
10. Beck-Peccoz P, Amr S, Menezes-Ferreira, et al: Decreased receptor binding of biologically inactive thyrotropin in central hypothyroidism. Effect of treatment with thyrotropin-releasing hormone. N Engl J Med 312:1085-1090, 1985.
11. Taylor T, Weintraub BD: Altered thyrotropin (TSH) carbohydrate structures in hypothalamic hypothyroidism created by paraventricular nuclear lesions are corrected by in vivo TSH-releasing hormone administration. Endocrinology 125:2198-2203, 1989.
12. Miura Y, Perkel VS, Papenberg KA, et al: Concanavalin-A, lentil, and ricin lectin affinity binding characteristics of human thyrotropin: Differences in the sialylation of thyrotropin in sera of euthyroid, primary, and central hypothyroid patients. J Clin Endocrinol Metab 69:985-995, 1989.
13. Persani L, Ferretti E, Borgato S, et al: Circulating thyrotropin bioactivity in sporadic central hypothyroidism. J Clin Endocrinol Metab 85:3631-3635, 2000.
14. Oliveira JH, Persani L, Beck-Peccoz P, Abucham J: Investigating the paradox of hypothyroidism and increased serum thyrotropin (TSH) levels in Sheehan's syndrome: Characterization of TSH carbohydrate content and bioactivity. J Clin Endocrinol Metab 86:1694-1699, 2001.
15. Bates AS, Van't Hoff W, Jones PJ, Clayton RN: The effect of hypopituitarism on life expectancy. J Clin Endocrinol Metab 81:1169-1172, 1996.
16. Arafah BM: Reversible hypopituitarism in patients with large nonfunctioning pituitary adenomas. J Clin Endocrinol Metab 62:1173-1179, 1986.
17. Arafah BM, Harrington JF, Madhoun ZT, Selman WR: Improvement of pituitary function after surgical decompression for pituitary tumor apoplexy. J Clin Endocrinol Metab 71:323-328, 1990.
18. Karavitaki N, Cudlip S, Adams CB, Wass JA: Craniopharyngiomas. Endocr Rev 27:371-397, 2006.
19. Tatsumi K, Miyai K, Notomi T, et al: Cretinism with combined hormone deficiency caused by a mutation in the PIT1 gene. Nat Genet 1:56-58, 1992.
20. Radovick S, Nation M, Du Y, et al: A mutation in the POU-homeodomain of Pit-1 responsible for combined pituitary hormone deficiency. Science 257:1115-1118, 1992.

21. Agarwal G, Bhatia V, Cook S, Thomas PQ: Adrenocorticotropin deficiency in combined pituitary hormone deficiency patients homozygous for a novel PROP1 deletion. J Clin Endocrinol Metab 85:4556-4561, 2000.
22. Mendonca BB, Osorio MG, Latronico AC, et al: Longitudinal hormonal and pituitary imaging changes in two females with combined pituitary hormone deficiency caused by deletion of A301,G302 in the PROP1 gene. J Clin Endocrinol Metab 84:942-945, 1999.
23. Deladöey J, Fluck C, Buyukgebiz A, et al: "Hot spot" in the PROP1 gene responsible for combined pituitary hormone deficiency. J Clin Endocrinol Metab 84:1645-1650, 1999.
24. Dattani MT, Martinez-Barbera JP, Thomas PQ, et al: Mutations in the homeobox gene HESX1/Hesx1 associated with septo-optic dysplasia in human and mouse. Nat Genet 19:125-133, 1998.
25. Dattani MT: Growth hormone deficiency and combined pituitary hormone deficiency: Does the genotype matter? Clin Endocrinol (Oxf) 63:121-130, 2005.
26. Netchine I, Sobrier ML, Krude H, et al: Mutations in LHX3 result in a new syndrome revealed by combined pituitary hormone deficiency. Nat Genet 25:182-186, 2000.
27. Machinis K, Pantel J, Netchine I, et al: Syndromic short stature in patients with a germline mutation in the LIM homeobox LHX4. Am J Hum Genet 69:961-968, 2001.
28. Hayashizaki Y, Hiraoka Y, Endo Y, et al: Thyroid-stimulating hormone (TSH) deficiency caused by a single base substitution in the CAGYC region of the beta-subunit. EMBO J 8:2291-2296, 1989.
29. Hayashizaki Y, Hiraoka Y, Tatsumi K, et al: Deoxyribonucleic acid analyses of five families with familial inherited thyroid stimulating hormone deficiency. J Clin Endocrinol Metab 71:792-796, 1990.
30. Dacou-Voutetakis C, Feltquate DM, Drakopoulou M, et al: Familial hypothyroidism caused by a nonsense mutation in the thyroid-stimulating hormone beta-subunit gene. Am J Hum Genet 46:988-993, 1990.
31. Deladöey J, Vuissoz JM, Domene HM, et al: Congenital secondary hypothyroidism caused by a mutation C105Vfs114X thyrotropin-beta mutation: Genetic study of five unrelated families from Switzerland and Argentina. Thyroid 13:553-559, 2003.
32. Borck G, Topaloglu AK, Korsch E, et al: Four new cases of congenital secondary hypothyroidism caused by a splice site mutation in the thyrotropin-beta gene: Phenotypic variability and founder effect. J Clin Endocrinol Metab 89:4136-4141, 2004.
33. Medeiros-Neto G, Herodotou DT, Rajan S, et al: A circulating, biologically inactive thyrotropin caused by a mutation in the beta subunit gene. J Clin Invest 97:1250-1256, 1996.
34. Collu R, Tang J, Castagné J, et al: A novel mechanism for isolated central hypothyroidism: Inactivating mutations in the thyrotropin-releasing hormone receptor gene. J Clin Endocrinol Metab 82:1561-1565, 1997.
35. Freda PU, Silverberg SJ, Post KD, Wardlaw SL: Hypothalamic-pituitary sarcoidosis. Trends Endocrinol Metab 3:321-325, 1992.
36. Nanduri VR, Bareille P, Pritchard J, Stanhope R: Growth and endocrine disorders in multisystem Langerhans' cell histiocytosis. Clin Endocrinol (Oxf) 53:509-515, 2000.
37. Kaltsas GA, Powles TB, Evanson J, et al: Hypothalamo-pituitary abnormalities in adult patients with langerhans cell histiocytosis: Clinical, endocrinological, and radiological features and response to treatment. J Clin Endocrinol Metab 85:1370-1376, 2000.
38. Powrie JK, Powell M, Ayers AB, et al: Lymphocytic adenohypophysitis: Magnetic resonance imaging features of two new cases and a review of the literature. Clin Endocrinol (Oxf) 42:315-322, 1995.
39. Molitch ME, Gillam MP: Lymphocytic hypophysitis. Horm Res 68(Suppl 5):145-150, 2007.
40. McDermott JH, Walsh CH: Hypogonadism in hereditary hemochromatosis. J Clin Endocrinol Metab 90:2451-2455, 2005.
41. Hudec M, Grigerova M, Walsh CH: Secondary hypothyroidism in hereditary hemochromatosis: Recovery after iron depletion. Thyroid 18:255-257, 2008.
42. Zervas A, Katopodi A, Protonotariou A, et al: Assessment of thyroid function in two hundred patients with beta-thalassemia major. Thyroid 12:151-154, 2002.
43. Harrop JS, Davies TJ, Capra LG, Marks V: Hypothalamic-pituitary function following successful treatment of intracranial tumours. Clin Endocrinol (Oxf) 5:313-321, 1976.
44. Constine LS, Woolf PD, Cann D, et al: Hypothalamic-pituitary dysfunction after radiation for brain tumors. N Engl J Med 328:87-94, 1993.
45. Littley MD, Shalet SM, Beardwell CG, et al: Radiation-induced hypopituitarism is dose-dependent. Clin Endocrinol (Oxf) 31:363-373, 1989.
46. Rose SR, Lusti RH, Pitukcheewanont P, et al: Diagnosis of hidden central hypothyroidism in survivors of childhood cancer. J Clin Endocrinol Metab 84:4472-4479, 1999.
47. Sherman SI, Gopal J, Haugen BR, et al: Central hypothyroidism associated with retinoid X receptor-selective ligands. N Engl J Med 340:1075-1079, 1999.
48. Golden WM, Webe KB, Hernandez TL, et al: Single-dose rexinoid rapidly and specifically suppresses serum thyrotropin in normal subjects. J Clin Endocrinol Metab 92:124-130, 2007.
49. Ridruejo E, Christensen AF, Mando OG: Central hypothyroidism and hypophysitis during treatment of chronic hepatitis C with pegylated interferon alpha and ribavirin. Eur J Gastroenterol Hepatol 18:693-694, 2006.
50. Benvenga S, Campenni A, Ruggeri RM, Trimarchi FJ: Clinical review 113: Hypopituitarism secondary to head trauma. J Clin Endocrinol Metab 85:1353-1361, 2000.

51. Benvenga S, Vigo T, Ruggeri RM, et al: Severe head trauma in patients with unexplained central hypothyroidism. Am J Med 116:767-771, 2004.
52. Woolf PD, Lee LA, Hamill RW, McDonald JV: Thyroid test abnormalities in traumatic brain injury: Correlation with neurologic impairment and sympathetic nervous system activation. Am J Med 84:201-208, 1988.
53. Uy HL, Reasner CA, Samuels MH: Pattern of recovery of the hypothalamic-pituitary-thyroid axis following radioactive iodine therapy in patients with Graves' disease. Am J Med 99:173-179, 1995.
54. Wehmann RE, Gregerman RI, Burns WH, et al: Suppression of thyrotropin in the low-thyroxine state of severe nonthyroidal illness. N Engl J Med 312:546-552, 1985.
55. Fekete C, Gereben B, Doleschall M, et al: Lipopolysaccharide induces type 2 iodothyronine deiodinase in the mediobasal hypothalamus: Implications for the nonthyroidal illness syndrome. Endocrinology 145:1649-1655, 2004.
56. Adriaanse R, Romijn JA, Brabant G, et al: Pulsatile thyrotropin secretion in nonthyroidal illness. J Clin Endocrinol Metab 77:1313-1317, 1993.
57. Davies PH, Black EG, Sheppard MC, Franklyn JA: Relation between serum interleukin-6 and thyroid hormone concentrations in 270 hospital in-patients with non-thyroidal illness. Clin Endocrinol (Oxf) 44:199-205, 1996.
58. Bartalena L, Grasso L, Brogioni S, Martino E: Interleukin 6 effects on the pituitary-thyroid axis in the rat. Eur J Endocrinol 131:302-306, 1994.
59. Coiro V, Volpi R, Marchesi C, et al: Influence of residual C-peptide secretion on nocturnal serum TSH peak in well-controlled diabetic patients. Clin Endocrinol (Oxf) 47:305-310, 1997.
60. Samuels MH, Luther M, Henry P, Ridgway EC: Effects of hydrocortisone on pulsatile pituitary glycoprotein secretion. J Clin Endocrinol Metab 78:211-215, 1994.
61. Duick DS, Wahner HW: Thyroid axis in patients with Cushing's syndrome. Arch Intern Med 139:767-772, 1979.
62. Laron Z: Interactions between the thyroid hormones and the hormones of the growth hormone axis. Pediatr Endocrinol Rev 1(Suppl 2):244-249, 2003.
63. Jørgensen JO, Moller J, Laursen T, et al: Growth hormone administration stimulates energy expenditure and extrathyroidal conversion of thyroxine to triiodothyronine in a dose-dependent manner and suppresses circadian thyrotrophin levels: Studies in GH-deficient adults. Clin Endocrinol (Oxf) 41: 609-614, 1994.
64. Porretti S, Giavoli C, Ronchi C, et al: Recombinant human GH replacement therapy and thyroid function in a large group of adult GH-deficient patients: When does L-T(4) therapy become mandatory? J Clin Endocrinol Metab 87:2042-2045, 2002.
65. Agha A, Walker D, Perry L, et al: Unmasking of central hypothyroidism following growth hormone replacement in adult hypopituitary patients. Clin Endocrinol (Oxf) 66:72-77, 2007.
66. Croxson MS, Ibbertson HK: Low serum triiodothyronine (T_3) and hypothyroidism in anorexia nervosa. J Clin Endocrinol Metab 44:167-174, 1977.
67. Hein MD, Jackson IM: Review: Thyroid function in psychiatric illness. Gen Hosp Psychiatry 12:232-244, 1990.
68. Bartalena L, Placidi GF, Martino E, et al: Nocturnal serum thyrotropin (TSH) surge and the TSH response to TSH-releasing hormone: Dissociated behavior in untreated depressives. J Clin Endocrinol Metab 71:650-655, 1990.
69. Sell MA, Schott M, Tharandt L, et al: Functional central hypothyroidism in the elderly. Aging Clin Exp Res 20:207-210, 2008.
70. Mariotti S, Barbesino G, Caturegli P, et al: Complex alteration of thyroid function in healthy centenarians. J Clin Endocrinol Metab 77:1130-1134, 1993.
71. Faglia G, Bitensky L, Pinchera A, et al: Thyrotropin secretion in patients with central hypothyroidism: Evidence for reduced biological activity of immunoreactive thyrotropin. J Clin Endocrinol Metab 48:989-998, 1979.
72. Ferretti E, Persani L, Jaffrain-Rea ML, et al: Evaluation of the adequacy of levothyroxine replacement therapy in patients with central hypothyroidism.J Clin Endocrinol Metab 84:924-929, 1999.
73. Snyder PJ, Utiger RD: Response to thyrotropin-releasing hormone (TRH) in normal man. J Clin Endocrinol Metab 34:380-385, 1972.
74. Faglia G, Beck-Peccoz P, Ferrari C, et al: Plasma thyrotropin response to thyrotropin-releasing hormone in patients with pituitary and hypothalamic disorders. J Clin Endocrinol Metab 37:595-601, 1973.
75. Caron PJ, Nieman LK, Rose SR, Nisula BC: Deficient nocturnal surge of thyrotropin in central hypothyroidism. J Clin Endocrinol Metab 62:960-964, 1986.
76. Rose SR, Manasco PK, Pearce S, Nisula BC: Hypothyroidism and deficiency of the nocturnal thyrotropin surge in children with hypothalamic-pituitary disorders. J Clin Endocrinol Metab 70:1750-1755, 1990.
77. Divall SA, Wondisford FE: TRH testing in its infancy. J Clin Endocrinol Metab 93:378-379, 2008.
78. van Tijn DA, de Vijlder JJ, Vulsma T: Role of the thyrotropin-releasing hormone stimulation test in diagnosis of congenital central hypothyroidism in infants. J Clin Endocrinol Metab 93:410-419, 2008.
79. Sawin CT, Geller A, Wolf PA, et al: Low serum thyrotropin concentrations as a risk factor for atrial fibrillation in older persons. N Engl J Med 331: 1249-1252, 1994.

80. Slawik M, Klawitter B, Meiser E, et al: Thyroid hormone replacement for central hypothyroidism: A randomized controlled trial comparing two doses of thyroxine (T_4) with a combination of T_4 and triiodothyronine. J Clin Endocrinol Metab 92:4115-4122, 2007.

81. Gordon MB, Gordon MS: Variations in adequate levothyroxine replacement therapy in patients with different causes of hypothyroidism. Endocr Pract 5:233-238, 1999.

PART IV

Conditions with Variable Effects

Chapter 19

Pregnancy

Neil Tran and Gregory Brent

Key Points

- Maternal hypothyroidism is associated with an increased risk of adverse outcomes for the mother and fetus.
- Women with known hypothyroidism should have thyroxine dosage adjustment prior to pregnancy, targeting serum thyroid-stimulating hormone level in the low-normal range.
- Women at increased risk for thyroid disease should be identified for testing (e.g., those with personal or family history of thyroid disease, those with other autoimmune disorders, such as type 1 diabetes mellitus).
- Hyperthyroidism in the first trimester of pregnancy can be difficult to diagnose; must be distinguished from gestational transient thyrotoxicosis caused by elevated human chorionic gonadotropin.
- Treatment goal of hyperthyroidism in pregnancy is to maintain maternal free thyroxine concentration in the upper normal range (using lowest possible dose of antithyroid drug).

Pregnancy is associated with changes in thyroid physiology that ensure an optimal thyroid environment for fetal growth and development.[1] The net effect of these changes is a requirement for increased maternal thyroid hormone production. Successful adaptation to these pregnancy-related changes requires a normally functioning thyroid gland and adequate iodine intake. The presence of thyroid disease or iodine deficiency impairs the ability of the thyroid to compensate for pregnancy. In areas of iodine insufficiency, or in women with antithyroid antibodies, adaptation to these changes are associated with an increase in serum thyroid-stimulating hormone (TSH) and, in some cases, an increase in the size of the thyroid gland and serum thyroglobulin. The management of preexisting thyroid disease is influenced by pregnancy. Thyroid disease may first be diagnosed during pregnancy or in the postpartum period. Most women who are on exogenous thyroid hormone replacement will require an increase in their levothyroxine dose during pregnancy. Treatment of hyperthyroidism in pregnancy must be carefully adjusted to adequately treat the mother, but avoid excessive antithyroid treatment that might lead to fetal thyroid hormone deficiency and impaired neurologic development.

THYROID PHYSIOLOGY IN PREGNANCY

The earliest factor influencing thyroid physiology in pregnancy is the estrogen-induced increase in the concentration of circulating thyroxine-binding globulin (TBG).[1] This occurs primarily because of altered glycosylation of TBG induced by estrogen, which reduces clearance and prolongs the circulating half-life. This change is so strongly associated with a viable pregnancy that a fall in serum TBG concentration in the first trimester is associated with impending miscarriage. Because of the increase in the level of TBG, there is an increase in the serum concentration of total thyroxine (T_4) and triiodothyronine (T_3), but the free fraction remains in the normal range.

Another important early influence on thyroid function is placental human chorionic gonadotropin (hCG), which is a weak TSH receptor agonist.[2] Chorionic gonadotropin and TSH share a common alpha subunit and the unique beta subunits have significant homology. The chorionic gonadotropin luteinizing hormone and TSH receptors also share a significant amount of structural similarity. The increased levels of hCG in the first half of pregnancy directly stimulate the TSH receptor and increase thyroid hormone production, and the transient increase in free thyroxine level results in a reduced, and sometimes suppressed, serum TSH. Transient TSH suppression in the first trimester is seen in as many as 10% to 15% of women and is a reflection of direct thyroidal stimulation caused by high levels of hCG. Clinical thyrotoxicosis from an extreme excess of hCG is seen in molar pregnancy and trophoblastic disease. Pregnant women with multiple gestations, a condition associated with higher serum levels of hCG, have a lower TSH compared with women with singleton pregnancies.

An additional factor influencing thyroid hormone levels in pregnancy is altered thyroid hormone volume of distribution and metabolism.[1] Placental 5-deiodinase type 3 (D3) activity is increased as pregnancy progresses. This leads to increased conversion of T_4 to the inactive metabolic product of T_3, reverse T_3. D3 is also expressed in the uterus. Although the role of placental and uterine D3 expression is not known, it may function to increase the supply of iodine to the fetus for thyroid hormone synthesis, as well as protect the developing fetus from excess maternal serum T_4 concentrations.

The increase in thyroid hormone production during pregnancy leads to an increased iodine requirement.[1] Pregnancy is normally associated with an increased glomerular filtration rate, which increases the renal excretion of iodine. During this time of increased iodine requirement, there is also increased urinary iodine loss. Markers of insufficient iodine intake include the presence of maternal goiter, increased serum TSH, increased serum thyroglobulin, and fetal or neonatal goiter, all of which are corrected with iodine supplementation. Current guidelines recommend an iodine intake of 220 μg/day of iodine during pregnancy and lactation, to be met by dietary intake and a supplement of 150 μg/day.[3]

The prevalence of TSH suppression varies, depending on the stage of pregnancy. A transient subnormal serum TSH is seen in as many as 18% of women in the first trimester, 10% in the second trimester, and 5% in the third trimester.[1] This corresponds to the highest serum hCG in the first trimester and subsequent reduction through the later stages of pregnancy. The mean TSH is significantly lower in the first trimester of pregnancy compared with nonpregnant controls, and a trimester-specific reference range should be used (Fig. 19-1).[4] Free T_4 measurements by the analog method, used in essentially all automated laboratory platforms, are normal in early pregnancy. In the third trimester, however, results in normal pregnancy are typically in the lower normal or subnormal reference range developed for nonpregnant women. The extent of subnormal free T_4 measurement varies among the different assays and is likely related to the changes in thyroid hormone binding protein, rather than a true reduction in free hormone concentration. Direct measurement of the free fraction of T_4 by the equilibrium dialysis technique can be performed and is usually normal. Hyperemesis gravidarum is associated with a more pronounced elevation in hCG and, in more severe

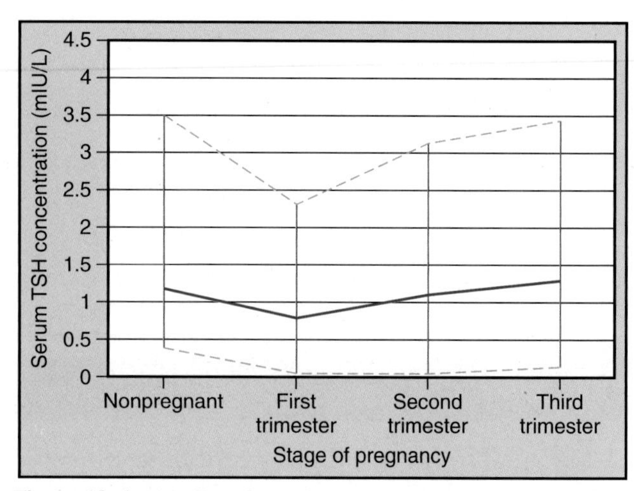

Figure 19–1 Median thyroid-stimulating hormone (TSH) level (solid line) and 95% confidence interval (dashed line) in nonpregnant women and at each trimester of pregnancy *(Adapted from Panesar NS, Li CY, Rogers MS: Reference intervals for thyroid hormones in pregnant Chinese women. Ann Clin Biochem 38:329-332, 2001.)*

cases, a suppressed TSH and elevated serum free T_4.[2] The TSH and T_4 levels generally normalize by the second trimester, unlike Graves' disease, in which the TSH and T_4 are persistently abnormal, and the serum T_3 is also often elevated.

In the first trimester, the fetus depends entirely on transplacental passage of maternal thyroid hormone.[1] Fetal thyroid hormone production begins around the 12th to 14th week of gestation and is under control of the pituitary around the 20th week. As a result, maternal euthyroxinemia, especially during early gestation, may be especially important for normal fetal neurologic development. The hCG-induced increase in serum T_4 in early pregnancy may be adaptive to supply thyroid hormone to the developing fetus. Normal maternal thyroid hormone levels likely play a role throughout pregnancy for normal brain and somatic development, even when the fetal thyroid gland is functioning, as well as acting on the placenta. Preterm infants have transient hypothyroxinemia, which is associated with impaired neurologic development.[5]

Pregnancy-associated thyroid abnormalities represent a spectrum of disorders, including subclinical hypothyroidism, overt hypothyroidism, autoimmune thyroiditis, goiter formation, and hyperthyroidism. A description of these conditions and an approach to clinical management will be presented.

HYPOTHYROIDISM IN PREGNANCY

The early diagnosis and effective management of hypothyroidism in pregnancy is essential to optimize the outcome for both the mother and her fetus.[6]

Women with preexisting hypothyroidism, as well as those first diagnosed with hypothyroidism during pregnancy, must be monitored carefully to ensure adequate thyroid hormone therapy and reduce the risks of adverse outcomes (Table 19-1). The approach to diagnosis, treatment, and monitoring will be described.

Table 19–1 Adverse Pregnancy Outcomes Associated with Maternal Overt and Subclinical Hypothyroidism

Maternal Outcome	Fetal Outcome
Spontaneous abortion	Fetal distress
Pregnancy-induced hypertension	Breech delivery
Placental abruption	Low birth weight
Preterm delivery	Perinatal death
	Impaired neuropsychological development

Epidemiology

Overt hypothyroidism, defined as an elevated serum TSH and reduced serum free T_4 concentration, occurs in approximately 0.2% of all pregnancies.[7] Subclinical hypothyroidism, defined as a normal range free T_4 and elevated serum TSH, is much more common, found in 2% to 5% of pregnancies, depending on the TSH reference range used. A number of studies have shown that the upper limit of the TSH reference range in the first trimester of pregnancy is lower than for nonpregnant women, likely because of suppression caused by an hCG-stimulated increase in thyroid hormone production; it is in the range of 2.5 mIU/L (see Fig. 19-1).[2,4]

Risk Factors

A number of factors increase the possibility of abnormal thyroid function in pregnant women.[8] Identification of any of these factors or conditions should prompt measurement of thyroid function. Women with type 1 diabetes mellitus have an especially high incidence of positive thyroid peroxidase (TPO) antibodies and thyroid disease, as high as 20% in some series.

Risk factors include the following:

- Iodine insufficiency or deficiency (most common cause worldwide of maternal thyroid deficiency)
- Personal history of goiter, radioiodine ablation, or thyroidectomy
- Use of thyroid hormone therapy
- Treatment with antithyroid drugs
- Personal or family history of autoimmune thyroid disease
- Personal history of diabetes mellitus type 1 or other autoimmune endocrine disease (e.g., primary autoimmune adrenal destruction)
- History of postpartum thyroiditis (following delivery or miscarriage)
- Personal history of autoimmune disease (e.g., rheumatoid arthritis, lupus)

Pathogenesis

The most common cause of primary hypothyroidism (subclinical or overt) in pregnant or nonpregnant women is chronic lymphocytic thyroiditis (Hashimoto's disease). Hashimoto's thyroiditis is characterized by lymphocytic thyroidal infiltration and destruction of thyroid tissue mediated by anti-TPO antibodies. Several studies have shown that pregnant women with positive TPO antibodies have a higher serum TSH throughout pregnancy compared with TPO-negative women.[1] This is true even when women with an abnormally high serum TSH are excluded from the analysis. Some TPO-positive women with a normal range TSH show reduced thyroid volume by ultrasound, likely because of thyroid atrophy. In addition to thyroid autoimmunity, other factors associated with reduced thyroidal reserve in pregnancy include previous thyroid surgery, radioiodine treatment, and external radiation.

In the first trimester of pregnancy, women with positive anti-TPO antibodies and a normal range serum TSH have a two- to fourfold increase in miscarriage rates.[9] Similarly, a higher incidence of recurrent abortion is associated with thyroid antibody positivity. Although essentially all studies to date have demonstrated a strong link between thyroid antibodies and spontaneous loss of pregnancy, a clear mechanism of how thyroid autoimmunity leads to termination of pregnancy has not been established. Thyroid autoantibodies may be a marker of overall increased autoimmunity, leading to a higher level of autoantibodies that directly result in miscarriage. Another possible mechanism is a direct effect of thyroid autoantibodies on fetal loss, which is supported by observations from several mouse models of autoimmune thyroid disease. In these models, elevation of thyroid autoantibodies is directly linked to embryonic loss during pregnancy. Alternatively, women with positive thyroid antibodies may have subtle thyroid dysfunction that worsens during early gestation. This mild reduction in maternal serum thyroxine concentration results in a suboptimal thyroid environment in early pregnancy, and may lead to miscarriage. If maternal thyroid status is the key

Table 19–2 Recommended Daily Iodine Requirements for Pregnant Women

Organization	Recommended Amount (μg/day)
American Thyroid Association (ATA)	220*
Institute of Medicine	220 (lactation, 290)
World Health Organization (WHO)	200

*ATA recommends a supplement of 150 μg/day to reach this total daily amount.

factor, then intervention with thyroxine replacement should reduce the miscarriage rate. Others have suggested that antibody-positive women have reduced fertility and tend to become pregnant at an older age, which is itself a risk factor for fetal demise.

The other major cause of thyroid hypofunction during pregnancy, and the most common cause of compromised thyroid function worldwide, is iodine insufficiency or deficiency.[1,3] The clinical presentation varies depending on the severity and duration of iodine restriction. The National Health and Nutrition Examination Survey (NHANES), performed regularly in a representative sample of the U.S. population, has shown that dietary iodine intake has fallen significantly over the past 20 years. Preliminary analysis of the most recent survey, however, indicates that iodine intake has stabilized, with the mean iodine intake remaining in the range of 150 μg/day.[10] This is sufficient iodine intake for a woman who is not pregnant, but the recommended intake of iodine during pregnancy and lactation is in the range of 200 to 220 μg/day (Table 19-2). A survey measuring urinary iodine in pregnant women in Boston has shown that the mean of the lowest quintile was 52 μg/L liter of urine collected, indicating a significant fraction of women with an estimated intake of less than 100 μg/day.[11] An effect of iodine intake on thyroid hormone levels is consistently detected with an iodine intake of 50 μg/day or less, and can occur at an iodine intake less than 100 μg/day.[1] The content of iodine in various brands of bread, cows' milk, and infant formula was measured and found to be highly variable, often not matching the amount stated on the label.[12] Only about one third of prenatal vitamin preparations contain iodine, and most do not contain the recommended amount of iodine supplement for pregnancy.[13] These findings emphasize the importance of public awareness of iodine nutrition and the need for supplementation during pregnancy. Because of the difficulty in timely identification and iodine repletion in pregnant women, another recommended approach to ensure iodine sufficiency in pregnancy is to increase iodine nutrition in the general population by a higher level of iodine supplementation in salt and flour.

Secondary hypothyroidism occurs as a result of pituitary insufficiency. The characteristic laboratory test profile is a reduced serum free T_4 and an inappropriately normal range or low serum TSH. Because of the long half-life of T_4 (7 days), the serum T_4 may be normal in the setting of acute pituitary insufficiency. Pituitary insufficiency can have various causes, including pituitary tumors, such as prolactinomas, lymphocytic hypophysitis, and pituitary ischemia and necrosis in the postpartum period (Sheehan's syndrome). These conditions are rare and usually, but not always, have manifestations in addition to hypothyroidism, which should raise suspicion of an underlying pituitary disorder. In women of reproductive age, the most common manifestation of pituitary insufficiency is irregular or absent menstrual periods, or difficulty lactating in the postpartum period.

Overall, reduced thyroidal reserve, regardless of the cause, predisposes the expectant mother to thyroid insufficiency. The thyroid gland is unable to compensate for the increased thyroid hormone requirement that results from the normal physiologic changes accompanying pregnancy.

Clinical Features

Overt hypothyroidism can present with fatigue, constipation, cold intolerance, and muscle cramps. Other symptoms include insomnia, weight gain, hair loss, voice changes, and reduced ability to concentrate.[6] Signs of hypothyroidism include periorbital edema, macroglossia, bradycardia, dry skin, and a delayed relaxation phase of deep tendon reflexes. A goiter can be seen in patients with chronic autoimmune thyroiditis or those with iodine deficiency.

Most patients with hypothyroidism, however, are asymptomatic. Even when patients become symptomatic, their signs and symptoms are usually subtle and nonspecific, and may be mistaken for changes that are part of normal pregnancy. Therefore, it is important to make an early diagnosis of hypothyroidism. Clinicians should have a low threshold for testing thyroid function in pregnancy, especially in those women with risk factors.

Diagnosis

The most important test used to evaluate maternal thyroid function, as in the nonpregnant state, is determination of the serum TSH level. It is important, however, to recognize that there are physiologic changes occurring during pregnancy that influence interpretation of the TSH. A subnormal TSH level can be seen in normal pregnancy, most commonly during the first trimester (up to 15% of pregnant women). The upper limit of the reference range in the first trimester is lower than in nonpregnant women (see Fig. 19-1). A serum TSH in the high-normal TSH range, above 2.5 to 3 μU/mL, may indicate thyroid hypofunction. Most consider a TSH level above 2.5 mIU/L in the first trimester as an indication of thyroid dysfunction.[4] Some have suggested that even in the nonpregnant state, a TSH level in the 2.5- to 4.5 mIU/L range reflects early thyroid dysfunction. There are dynamic changes in serum TSH that occur throughout pregnancy and indicate the need for gestational age-specific TSH reference ranges. A study of more than 13,000 pregnancies has identified differences in the TSH reference ranges for each trimester, as well as lower TSH levels in twin compared with singleton pregnancies, likely because of the higher levels of hCG with multiple gestation.[14]

Measurement of FT_4 by the analog method, the most commonly used assay, may not accurately reflect free T_4 levels in pregnancy because of the increase in TBG concentration.[15] In most assays, especially during the third trimester, the results of the free T_4 analog assay underestimate the true free T_4 in pregnancy. In contrast to TSH, there are currently no gestational age-specific reference ranges for free T_4. Alternatively, measurement of total T_4, adjusting the reference range for the elevated level of TBG, may serve as a more accurate estimate of free T_4. A reference range for total T_4 can be approximated by multiplying the usual nonpregnant reference limits by 1.5—that is, in a typical assay reference range of 5 to 12 μg/dL, a level below 7.5 μg/dL would be considered maternal hypothyroxinemia.[15]

When hypothyroidism is first diagnosed during pregnancy, measurement of the TPO antibody may assist in establishing an autoimmune cause of hypothyroidism and help predict the risk of developing long-term hypothyroidism.

A subgroup of pregnant women with isolated hypothyroxinemia, normal TSH but FT_4 levels in the lowest tenth percentile, has been identified in studies from Europe.[16] These changes may be in part related to the lower iodine intake in those countries studied. This maternal thyroid function test profile of a normal TSH and a low free T_4 in early gestation, has been associated with adverse developmental outcomes in the offspring, if the free T_4 does not normalize in later stages of pregnancy.[16]

Treatment

Hypothyroid women of reproductive age should have their thyroxine replacement optimized prior to conception. Optimization should include sufficient thyroxine to target a serum TSH in the low-normal range (0.5 to 2.0 mIU/L). If hypothyroidism is first diagnosed during pregnancy, early institution of levothyroxine supplementation is important. The fetal thyroid gland does not function until late in the first trimester and any thyroid requirement for early fetal brain development depends exclusively on a maternal source of thyroid hormone.[17]

The recommended dosage for treatment of overt hypothyroidism is levothyroxine, 1.6 to 1.8 μg/kg/day, although the dose is typically 25% to 50% higher in pregnancy. TSH should be monitored at intervals of 4 weeks, a shorter time than the typical 6- to 8-week intervals outside of pregnancy, until the TSH is normalized. The levothyroxine dosage is usually adjusted in 25-μg increments.

The potential for other medications or food to reduce thyroxine absorption should be considered. Pregnancy may be the first time that a women takes calcium, iron supplements, or soy milk products, all of which have the potential to reduce thyroxine absorption.[6] It is recommended that the patient take thyroid hormone on an empty stomach. Otherwise, levothyroxine administration should be separated by 4 hours or more from anything that might interfere with absorption. Another factor that should be considered in levothyroxine therapy is the bioequivalence among the different available formulations. The variation in bioavailable hormone may be clinically important for some women, and a consistent levothyroxine formulation should be used during pregnancy.

The goal of treatment is to maintain the serum TSH in the lower half of the reference range, between 0.5 and 2.0 mIU/L.[6] The resulting free T_4 concentration is generally in the upper half of the normal range. It is relevant to note that a change in TSH may lag behind a dose change for up to 6 weeks, because of the 7- to 10-day half-life of levothyroxine. Although it is usually recommended to wait 6 to 8 weeks to determine the full effect of changes on levothyroxine dosage, one can obtain thyroid function testing in 3 to 4 weeks to ensure that the TSH and free T_4 levels are improving and moving toward their targets. The consequences of even short-term insufficient treatment during early treatment can be significant.

Table 19–3 Pregnancy Outcomes with Maternal Hypothyroidism

Study	Patients (N)	Obstetrical Outcome	
Abalovich et al[20]		Abortion	Term delivery
	Hypo adequate L-T_4 (27)	0%	93%
	Hypo inadequate L-T_4 (24)	67%	21%
Tan et al[21]		Placental abruption	Placenta previa
	Euthyroid (20,499)	1.9%	1.0%
	Hypothyroid on L-T_4 (419)	1.2%	0.7%
Casey et al[22]		Placental abruption	Preterm delivery
	Euthyroid (20,499)	0.3%	2.5%
	SCH (404)	1%	4%
Negro et al[23]	Euthyroid +/– TPO	Miscarriage	Preterm delivery
	TPO+/L-T_4– (58)	13.8%	22.4%
	TPO+/L-T_4+ (57)	3.5%	7%
	TPO–/L-T_4– (869)	2.4%	8.2%

Adequate L-T_4, adequate levothyroxine treatment (TSH < 4 mIU/L); hypo, hypothyroidism; inadequate L-T_4, inadequate levothyroxine treatment (TSH > 4 mIU/L); L-T_4–, L-T_4–negative; L-T_4+, L-T_4–positive; SCH, subclinical hypothyroidism; TPO+, thyroid peroxidase–positive; TPO–, TPO-negative; TSH, thyroid-stimulating hormone.

In women with known hypothyroidism, a serum TSH level should be determined as soon as pregnancy is confirmed. At least 50% of women with hypothyroidism will require an increase in their usual thyroxine replacement dose during pregnancy.[6,18] The timing and magnitude of dose change, however, varies depending on the cause of maternal hypothyroidism and the prepregnancy dose. Essentially, all athyreotic patients will require an increase in thyroxine dose. The need for an increased dose in women with autoimmune hypothyroidism will vary depending on the stage and severity of the underlying thyroid disease. A prospective study of a cohort of hypothyroid women has attempted to define the timing and degree of increase of levothyroxine requirements in pregnancy.[19] Levothyroxine dosage needed to be increased as early as week 5, reaching a plateau at the 16th to 20th week of gestation. A 47% increase in dose, compared with the prepregnancy level, was required to normalize the serum TSH level. The median time for the first increase in thyroxine dose was at the eighth week of gestation. The authors recommended that women who have a prior diagnosis of hypothyroidism should increase their levothyroxine dose as soon as pregnancy is confirmed, taking two additional doses per week. Others, however, caution that the levothyroxine dose should not be changed until an abnormal TSH is demonstrated by thyroid function testing. For those women whose dosage remains unchanged, thyroid function testing can be carried out once every trimester. Overreplacement with levothyroxine may also produce adverse effects on pregnancy outcome (see later), so it is important to monitor therapy carefully.

Following delivery, levothyroxine dosage should be immediately reduced to the prepregnancy level, and a TSH level measured at 6 to 8 weeks postpartum. Breast-feeding is not contraindicated while the mother is on levothyroxine.

Clinical Course

MATERNAL OUTCOME

Most studies evaluating pregnancy outcome in hypothyroid mothers have been retrospective. It is difficult in this type of study to identify an appropriate control group and accurately account for the influence of other co-morbidities and prenatal care. Previous studies have shown a range of adverse outcomes in pregnancies associated with both overt and subclinical hypothyroidism (Table 19-3).[1,6] A common feature of almost all studies has been that hypothyroid mothers treated with levothyroxine sufficient to achieve a normal serum TSH do not have any associated adverse outcomes. Because thyroid autoantibodies are still present in these women, this finding suggests that the autoantibodies are not directly involved in mediating the adverse outcomes associated with hypothyroidism and pregnancy. It is more likely that the low maternal thyroxine levels mediate the adverse effects.

Table 19–4 Fetal Outcomes with Maternal Hypothyroidism

Study	Test	Outcomes in Each Group (N)		
Haddow et al[25]		Euthyroid (124)	Children of untreated SCH mothers (48)	Children of treated SCH mothers (14)
	IQ	107	100	111
Pop et al[16]		Euthyroid (57) (1 year/2 year)	Maternal low FT_4 1 year old (58)	Maternal low FT_4 2 year old (58)
	Bayley Mental Score	105/106	95	98
	Bayley Motor Score	99/102	91	92

FT_4, free thyroxine; IQ, intelligence quotient; SCH, subclinical hypothyroidism.

The impact of levothyroxine therapy on pregnancy outcomes was investigated in a study of 150 pregnancies in women with primary hypothyroidism.[20] One third of these pregnancies occurred when the mother was hypothyroid. Women on adequate thyroxine therapy, defined as a TSH level less than 4 mIU/L, were compared with those who were inadequately treated and had an elevated TSH. Inadequately treated women had a marked increase in spontaneous abortions and only a small fraction, approximately 20%, had full-term deliveries. Women on adequate levothyroxine therapy had adverse outcomes comparable to those seen in euthyroid pregnant women. A similar rate of adverse outcomes was seen in women with overt and subclinical hypothyroidism.

Similar outcomes were seen in a study of more than 20,000 pregnant women comparing obstetric outcomes in euthyroid mothers compared with those with treated hypothyroidism.[21] The prevalence of hypothyroidism, diagnosed before or early in pregnancy, was 2% in this study. There was a higher incidence of hypothyroidism among white women and those with advanced maternal age, at least 35 years old. The levothyroxine dose was adjusted every 6 to 8 weeks to maintain a TSH level less than 2.5 mIU/L. Women with treated hypothyroidism did not have a significant difference in their mode of delivery or rate of complications, or in maternal, fetal, or neonatal outcomes.

A large prospective study of over 15,000 pregnant women at Parkland Hospital in Dallas has identified a subset of about 400 women with untreated subclinical hypothyroidism.[22] These women were not treated with levothyroxine and were assessed for adverse outcomes in mother and fetus. In the women with subclinical hypothyroidism, there was a threefold higher incidence of placental abruption and a twofold higher incidence of preterm delivery at or before the 34th week of gestation. Infants of these mothers had more adverse outcomes associated with preterm delivery, including respiratory distress syndrome and prolonged stay in the intensive care unit. These associations were determined after adjustments for maternal age, race, and placental abruption.

The first reported prospective randomized levothyroxine treatment study of hypothyroidism in pregnancy used a cohort of almost 1000 pregnant women.[22] Women with normal TSH and free T_4 concentrations, were separated into those with and without TPO antibodies. Women with positive TPO antibodies were randomized to a levothyroxine treatment or a no-treatment control group. The women with positive TPO antibodies had a higher TSH and graded doses of levothyroxine were given based on the initial TSH. Untreated women with positive antibodies developed higher TSH and lower FT_4 levels during pregnancy, compared with levothyroxine-treated women with positive antibodies. Untreated women with positive TPO antibodies had an increased rate of miscarriage and preterm delivery. The TPO antibody-positive women treated with levothyroxine, however, had a level of miscarriage and preterm delivery the same as those women without TPO antibodies. These findings strongly suggest that thyroxine therapy is beneficial for pregnancy outcomes, even in mild or subclinical hypothyroidism.

FETAL OUTCOME

Maternal hypothyroidism is associated with impaired neurologic development in the offspring (Table 19-4).[24] Some of the developmental abnormalities may be a consequence of premature birth. Subtle but selective cognitive deficits and mild reduction in performance score on global intelligence were seen in 5-year old children born to mothers with mild hypothyroidism, a serum TSH level ranging from 5 to 7 mIU/L. These findings suggest that maternal thyroid hormone supply may be important to the fetus for development of specific brain areas.

A retrospective study has identified 62 women who had subclinical hypothyroidism during pregnancy with an elevated TSH (mean TSH, 13 mU/L), but normal free T_4.[25] More than 75% of these women had positive thyroid antibodies. Their offspring were all delivered at full term and all had normal thyroid function at birth. The women with abnormal serum TSH were matched with controls for maternal age, maternal years of education, child's gender, and age (mean age, 8 years). Children whose mothers were hypothyroid had a reduction in intellectual performance of 7 IQ points compared with the offspring of euthyroid mothers. There was also a significant increase in the fraction of children with an IQ score less than 85 who were born to hypothyroid mothers as compared with matched control children. There was no adverse outcome on intellectual function in mothers who were hypothyroid but on adequate treatment with levothyroxine.

Isolated maternal hypothyroxinemia, early in pregnancy, may also be associated with abnormal fetal development. A prospective 3-year study has found that the presence of isolated maternal hypothyroxinemia, defined as a free T_4 below the 10th percentile in the first trimester (12th week) with a normal TSH, was associated with delayed mental and psychomotor function in the offspring.[16] This delay was seen in children tested at 1 and again at 2 years of age. In contrast, children born to mothers whose early hypothyroxinemia was normalized at the 24th to 32nd week of gestation scored similarly to their control counterparts, whose mothers had free T_4 levels in the 50th to 90th percentile. In the control group, scores were not affected by the decline of maternal free T_4 at later stages of pregnancy. This observation indicates the importance of attaining an adequate level of thyroid hormone in early gestation, although the relative importance of FT_4 and TSH in early pregnancy is not known.

Prevention

Based on the robust body of evidence supporting the impact of thyroid dysfunction on maternal and fetal outcome, counseling prior to a planned pregnancy is important.[6] Both the patient and her health care provider need to be aware of the expected increase in levothyroxine dosage compared with the prepregnancy level. Smoking and use of other chemicals or medications known to interfere with thyroid hormone synthesis and absorption should also be avoided. The American Thyroid Association (ATA) recommends iodine supplementation of 150 μg/day during pregnancy and lactation, which could be included in prenatal vitamins.[3] The ATA has also called for systematic monitoring of iodine nutrition in pregnant women to ensure adequate intake.

Pitfalls and Complications

- Contribution of smoking to fetal and neonatal iodine deficiency
- Impact of reduced dietary iodine supply on pregnancy and fetal development
- Adjustment of levothyroxine dose during pregnancy and the postpartum period

Early development of the human brain and neurologic system depends on the action of the thyroid hormone.[24] Thyroid hormone synthesis, in turn, is dependent on an adequate iodine supply. Iodine supply throughout fetal development is derived exclusively from maternal sources. After parturition, the neonate continues to use iodine to synthesize thyroid hormone actively, which is used for development, growth, and metabolism. Breast milk is the sole source of iodine in the breast-feeding infant.

The mammary gland concentrates iodine via the same sodium iodide symporter protein expressed in the thyroid gland. The function of this transporter is compromised in the presence of several chemical compounds, including thiocyanate and perchlorate. Maternal smoking during breast-feeding reduces breast milk iodine.[26] Smoking mothers, compared with nonsmokers, have reduced iodine content in breast milk and their infants have lower urinary iodine. Thiocyanate, a byproduct of tobacco smoking, competes with iodine for transport by the sodium iodide symporter and results in less iodine in breast milk. The inhibitory effect of thiocyanate is especially significant in the setting of insufficient iodine intake.

Another environmental toxicant that has been implicated in thyroid dysfunction is perchlorate, a chemical used as a propellant in fireworks and rocket fuel.[27] Ammonium perchlorate has been detected in water, vegetables, cows' milk, and breast milk. Perchlorate inhibits iodine uptake into the thyroid by competitive inhibition of the sodium iodide symporter. At very high levels, this can result in reduced thyroid hormone production. Perchlorate may also block iodine transport in the fetal thyroid gland, resulting in reduced fetal thyroid hormone production. A recent study has shown that perchlorate might influence thyroid function in women with a low iodine intake (less than 100 μg/L), but not in men or women with adequate iodine intake.[28]

The dose of levothyroxine in hypothyroid women should be returned to the prepregnancy level immediately following parturition. In women first diagnosed with hypothyroidism during pregnancy, thyroid function tests in the postpartum period should be followed closely to adjust the levothyroxine dose.

Controversies

- Mechanism whereby maternal hypothyroidism leads to adverse outcome(s)
- Reversibility of developmental abnormalities caused by maternal thyroid hormone deficiency during pregnancy
- Optimal timing, preferred thyroid tests, and threshold for initiation of treatment as they relate to hypothyroidism in pregnancy
- Effects of subclinical hypothyroidism on pregnancy outcomes and whether treatment is beneficial
- Effects of isolated maternal hypothyroxinemia (with normal serum TSH) on pregnancy outcomes
- Effects of overreplacement with thyroid hormone on pregnancy
- Value of universal screening for thyroid disease in pregnancy

It is not established how thyroid hormone deficiency results in adverse gestational outcomes, although placental effects of thyroid hormone may be especially important. In addition, the impact of the severity and duration of maternal hypothyroidism on maternal and fetal outcomes needs to be investigated further.

Although it is uniformly accepted that thyroid hormone is important for fetal brain development, the relative influence of maternal and fetal thyroid hormone production is not established. It is likely that there are key time periods for thyroid hormone actions in brain development. The apparently normal brain function in children with congenital hypothyroidism diagnosed and treated soon after birth indicates that most effects of thyroid hormone deficiency are reversible. Detailed neurocognitive studies in these children, however, have shown some subtle defects that reflect deficits in specific brain areas. These areas may reflect thyroid hormone targets, with many related to sensory integration at critical developmental stages.[29]

The optimal timing for thyroid testing during the course of pregnancy and the threshold of TSH for initiation of thyroid hormone therapy remain unclear.[6] Whether the best screening test is determination of the TSH or FT_4 level, or both, is not established. Thyroid autoimmunity may have an independent role in mediating adverse outcomes. Thyroid autoantibody testing may be important to identify those at risk for abnormal thyroid function during pregnancy and in the postpartum period.

Treatment of subclinical hypothyroidism during pregnancy appears to improve the pregnancy outcome, specifically reducing miscarriage rate and preterm delivery. These adverse outcomes associated with hypothyroidism are seen only in women who have not had adequate replacement of thyroid hormone. A recent prospective, randomized, controlled trial has shown that thyroid hormone replacement prevents the increased miscarriage rate and preterm delivery associated with even a mild degree of maternal subclinical hypothyroidism.[23] The impact of thyroid hormone replacement in this trial on mothers with positive TPO antibodies and normal range serum TSH suggests a link between adverse outcome and mild subclinical hypothyroidism.

The impact of an isolated low free T_4 level on pregnancy is not established.[30] A prospective study followed maternal thyroid function at 12th and 32nd weeks' gestation and then determined their offspring's neurodevelopmental score. Infants born to mothers who had low free T_4 in early gestation were six times more likely to have impaired psychomotor development. It is important that the method of free T_4 measurement, and the influence of pregnancy on the determination, be standardized for these studies.

The effect(s) of levothyroxine overreplacement in pregnancy on the mother and her fetus are less well characterized. Moderately high maternal thyroxine levels in pregnant women treated for hyperthyroidism are associated with a better fetal outcome compared with women treated for normal or low serum T_4 levels. An increase in fetal loss associated with excess thyroid hormone exposure, however, has been reported in women with very high serum T_4 concentration caused by thyroid hormone resistance when the fetus is not thyroid hormone–resistant.[31] It is likely that placental D3, which inactivates T_4 and T_3, may protect the fetus from moderately high maternal thyroid hormone levels, but at higher levels adverse actions are seen. Very high maternal T_4 levels can produce adverse effects on the thyroid hormone–sensitive infant.

Universal screening for thyroid dysfunction in pregnancy is not yet recommended, but a case-finding approach using TSH screening in those at increased risk (e.g., a personal history of thyroid or autoimmune disease, or family history of thyroid disorder) can be used.[32] This approach, however, may miss as many as one third of pregnant women with hypothyroidism. Physicians and other health care providers need to be aware of potential challenges associated with thyroid function screening and intervention during pregnancy. The correct thyroid tests to carry out, the timing of testing, and indications for intervention are not established. The results of several prospective randomized studies of levothyroxine treatment of mild hypothyroidism in pregnancy currently in progress will guide the approach to diagnosis and treatment.[32]

Comprehensive evidenced-based clinical guidelines for the management of thyroid disease in pregnancy have recently been published.[33] These were developed by The Endocrine Society with contributions from an international panel and have been endorsed by the major endocrine societies in the United States. These guidelines should contribute to a more uniform approach to diagnosis and treatment.

HYPERTHYROIDISM IN PREGNANCY

Hyperthyroidism is challenging to diagnose and treat during pregnancy and, if not properly managed, is associated with adverse outcomes for mother and fetus.

Epidemiology

Overt hyperthyroidism is reported in about 0.2% to 0.4% of all pregnancies. Subclinical hyperthyroidism is present in 1.7% of pregnancies, with a higher incidence in African American and parous women.[13]

Risk Factors

- Personal or family history of autoimmune thyroid disease
- Personal of family history of other autoimmune diseases, especially type 1 diabetes mellitus
- History of Graves' disease in remission after medical and/or ablative therapy
- Symptoms suggestive of thyroid overactivity
- Presence of goiter

Pathogenesis

The most common cause of overt hyperthyroidism during pregnancy is Graves' disease.[13] In addition, gestational transient thyrotoxicosis, toxic multinodular goiter, autonomous thyroid adenoma, and thyroiditis can all occur during pregnancy.

In Graves' disease, thyroid-stimulating immunoglobulins (TSIs) bind to TSH receptors on the thyroid gland and mimic the action of TSH. This results in increased production and secretion of thyroid hormone. The degree of hyperthyroidism or thyrotoxicosis generally, but not always, diminishes throughout pregnancy because immunosuppression increases in the second and third trimesters. The activity of Graves' disease can be followed by measuring the serum levels of thyroid-stimulating antibodies as well as following thyroid hormone levels and TSH.

Gestational transient thyrotoxicosis (GTT) is caused by direct stimulation of the TSH receptors by high concentrations of hCG.[2] This syndrome occurs most commonly during the first half of pregnancy or in conditions associated with a high level of hCG, such as a molar or twin pregnancy. GTT is associated with a higher amplitude and longer duration of hCG elevation superimposed on underlying thyroid abnormalities, such as micronodular or enlarged thyroid gland. GTT is associated with hyperemesis gravidarum. This condition is usually self-limited and improves in the second trimester. Antithyroid drug treatment does not alter the course of the condition. It could lead to severe dehydration and metabolic disturbances, requiring hospitalization. There appears to be a relationship among the magnitude of hCG elevation, severity of vomiting, and suppression of TSH.[36]

Clinical Features

As in the case of gestational hypothyroidism, hyperthyroidism in pregnancy is not easily diagnosed clinically, because the signs and symptoms overlap with findings in normal pregnancy. Typical symptoms of hyperthyroidism include weight loss or failure to gain weight with progression of pregnancy, excessive sweating, heat intolerance, palpitations, and hyperdefecation. Signs include opthalmopathy, tachycardia, and widened pulse pressure. In many women with hyperthyroidism, there may be no clear symptoms or signs indicating the diagnosis.

Although thyroid storm is rare in pregnancy, it represents a life-threatening condition. Clinically, patient may have fever, tachycardia, dehydration, altered mental status, nausea, vomiting, and/or diarrhea.

Hyperemesis gravidarum occurs more commonly than hyperthyroidism in pregnancy. In such cases, there are usually no or mild signs or symptoms of hyperthyroidism. Biochemical abnormalities (i.e., suppressed TSH and elevated T_4) usually resolve in the early part of the second trimester (15th to 18th week of gestation). Hyperemesis gravidarum rarely has typical manifestations of hyperthyroidism.

Diagnosis

Overt hyperthyroidism is confirmed by thyroid function test measurements, with findings of a suppressed TSH and elevated free T_4 and T_3 levels in the mother. Use of the nonpregnant range for free T_4 is acceptable early in pregnancy. Thyroid-stimulating antibody titers can be helpful to make a diagnosis if the thyroid function test changes are not clear. TSI levels can also be used to track the response to therapy, and very high levels are associated with an increased risk of neonatal hyperthyroidism. A diagnostic radioiodine uptake scan, the gold standard for diagnosing hyperthyroidism, cannot be performed in pregnancy because of radiation exposure to the fetus from the excreted isotope and the potential for concentration of isotope in the fetal thyroid gland.

Assessment of the fetal thyroid gland by ultrasound may be used as an adjunct diagnostic tool in the management of maternal Graves' disease during pregnancy.[37] An enlarged fetal thyroid can reflect an effect of excess antithyroid drug treatment to the mother or neonatal Graves' disease. Cardiac echocardiography may reveal a hypertrophic heart. Fetal thyroid function can be assessed from cord blood or amniotic fluid sampling, but this is rarely necessary.

It is important to differentiate thyrotoxicosis secondary to Graves' disease from gestational transient thyrotoxicosis, because each condition has a different course and management. The free T_3 level is usually elevated in Graves' disease but not gestational thyrotoxicosis. Elevated serum levels of TSI are found only in Graves' disease.

Treatment

Although milder forms of hyperthyroidism are generally well tolerated, more severe forms of hyperthyroidism require treatment. The primary treatment for hyperthyroidism in pregnancy is antithyroid drugs (ATDs).[38,39] A surgical thyroidectomy is considered when very high doses or ATDs are required, or when the patient experiences significant ATD-associated complications. The use of therapeutic radioactive iodine for thyroid ablation is absolutely contraindicated in pregnancy.

The antithyroid drugs propylthiouracil (PTU) and methimazole (MMI) have both been used in pregnant thyrotoxic patients. There has been no clinical trial to date comparing these two medications. PTU, however, is the preferred drug in North America because it is thought to cross the placenta less than MMI. Recent studies, however, do not support this view. MMI, but not PTU, has been associated with congenital anomalies, including aplasia cutis and choanal atresia.[38] Both PTU and MMI are in the U.S. Food and Drug Administration (FDA) category D because of the potential risk of fetal hypothyroidism. They are, however, considered to be safe for breast-feeding women and their infants. Side effects from the thionamide ATDs include agranulocytosis, hepatitis, and vasculitis.

Adrenergic blockers may be used to treat hyperthyroidism in pregnancy, but pose the potential risks of intrauterine growth retardation and neonatal respiratory distress, as well as hypothermia, bradycardia, and hypoglycemia in the postnatal period. Thyroid function testing should be performed at least every 4 to 6 weeks to observe the effect of treatment, and more often in women with active disease. It is especially important to avoid overtreatment of maternal hyperthyroidism, which can lead to maternal or fetal hypothyroidism.

The goal of medical treatment is to maintain the serum free T_4 concentration in the upper third of the normal nonpregnant range while using the lowest possible dosage of ATDs.[38] This is generally associated with a serum TSH level suppressed below normal. A midnormal range TSH usually represents an excessive ATD dose and an elevated TSH definitely indicates excessive ATD. An upper normal or modestly elevated level of maternal free T_4 has been shown to be associated with a fetal free T_4 in the midnormal range, therefore minimizing the risk of fetal hypothyroidism.[40] Alternatively, one can use the total T_4 level targeted at 1.5 times the normal nonpregnant range. Fetal hypothyroidism can impair neurologic development and can be associated with a significant goiter.

Surgery, if necessary, is best performed during the second trimester. The risk of miscarriage is high if thyroid surgery is performed prior to the 16th week of gestation. Premature delivery is a risk of surgery when the woman is more than 26 weeks pregnant. The preoperative use of β-adrenergic blockade and iodide is indicated to minimize the risk of thyroid storm. Surgery is only recommended when very high doses of ATD are required or severe side effects, such as agranulocytosis or hepatic inflammation, prevent the continued use of ATDs.

The treatment of thyroid storm requires supportive measures and removal of precipitating factor(s). The initial treatment is high-dose PTU, up to 1 g, followed by continuous administration of PTU in 200-mg doses at intervals of 4 hours. Because no parenteral form is available, this can be given by nasogastric tube. Once adequate doses of PTU have been given to block thyroid hormone synthesis, iodine is given to prevent thyroidal release of T_3 and T_4. Depending on the fetal stage, administration of iodine to the mother can also block thyroid hormone production and release in the fetus, so caution must be exercised, especially with prolonged treatment. In addition, dexamethasone has been used to block peripheral conversion of T_4 to T_3. Tachycardia can be managed short-term by the use of a β-adrenergic receptor blocking agent.

Table 19–5 Adverse Pregnancy Outcomes Associated with Maternal Hyperthyroidism

Maternal	Fetal
Preeclampsia	Craniosynostosis
Congestive heart failure	Goiter
Preterm delivery	Tachycardia
Thyrotoxicosis (thyroid storm in extreme cases)	Intrauterine growth retardation
	Low birth weight
	Fetal hydrops
	Fetal death

Clinical Course

MATERNAL OUTCOME

Overt maternal hyperthyroidism has been linked to a higher incidence of adverse maternal outcomes (Table 19-5). The evidence in this area, however, is more limited than studies of the effects of maternal hypothyroidism on pregnancy outcome. Some but not all studies have shown an increased incidence of miscarriages with maternal hyperthyroidism.[13]

In contrast to subclinical hypothyroidism, maternal subclinical hyperthyroidism has not been associated with pregnancy complications or perinatal morbidity when compared with normal subjects.[34]

FETAL OUTCOME

There is limited evidence on the influence of maternal hyperthyroidism on fetal outcomes (see Table 19-5). A study of mothers affected by resistance to thyroid hormone has shown that very high maternal thyroid hormone levels are associated with an increased incidence of miscarriage and low birth weight when the fetus does not have resistance to thyroid hormone.[31] If the fetus also had thyroid resistance, no adverse effect of maternal hyperthyroxinemia was seen. Although these findings in patients with thyroid resistance may not be transferable to pregnant women without thyroid resistance, they do suggest that very high maternal thyroid hormone levels can exert a direct effect on the fetus and placenta. This effect is evidenced by the increased incidence of miscarriages and low birth weight. Another reported complication of maternal hyperthyroidism is neonatal central hypothyroidism, which can be permanent.

Transient congenital hyperthyroidism is seen in about 1% of infants of mothers with Graves' disease.[38] This occurs because of transfer of TSIs from mother to fetus, which is usually associated with high titers of TSI in the mother during pregnancy. Elevated levels of TSI can persist in women with Graves' disease, even after thyroidectomy or radioiodine ablation prior to pregnancy. It is important to consider the possibility of neonatal Graves' disease, even if the mother has previously had definitive ablative treatment for Graves' disease. Fetal hypothyroidism and goiter can occur because of excessive thionamide usage in the mother during pregnancy.

Prevention

Hyperthyroidism is not preventable, but early diagnosis and treatment can minimize the associated maternal and fetal complications during pregnancy. It is important to inquire about family or personal history of prior thyroid disease or autoimmune disorders, along with careful attention to signs and symptoms suggestive of hyperthyroidism. Because of the unreliability of symptoms and signs in pregnancy, there should be a low threshold to perform thyroid function testing.

Pitfalls and Complications

- Risk of fetal and neonatal hyperthyroidism and hypothyroidism in maternal Graves' disease
- Use of antithyroid drugs for Graves' disease during pregnancy
- Monitoring of ATD therapy during the postpartum and the impact on breast feeding
- Neonatal Graves' disease

Close titration of antithyroid drug should be guided by the maternal total T_4 (with adjusted normal range) or free T_4 level, measured at 2-to 6-week intervals. Because Graves' disease tends to improve as pregnancy progresses, drug dose reduction or even withdrawal is encouraged whenever possible, usually after the 4th to 6th month of gestation. In contrast to the usual goal of a normal range serum TSH, the target is an upper normal to slightly elevated free T_4 level, which is often associated with a persistently suppressed serum TSH. An elevated TSH always indicates ATD overtreatment.

Close follow-up in the first postpartum year is important because of a high risk of exacerbation of Graves' disease. There is also an increased incidence of Graves' disease first diagnosed during the postpartum period.[38] Although thionamides are transferred to a small extent into breast milk, their use is not contraindicated during breast-feeding. If the mother requires antithyroid drugs while breast-feeding, however, it is recommended that as low a dose as possible be used. Some experts recommend periodic monitoring of the child's thyroid function if the mother is taking ATDs,[41] although most recommend this only when the ATD doses are high. PTU has greater protein binding compared with MMI, and is probably less likely to be transferred in breast milk.

Neonatal Graves' disease is uncommon, seen in only about 1% of offspring of mothers with Graves' disease during pregnancy. The risk is increased in mothers with more severe Graves' disease—evidenced by a greater magnitude of thyroid function test elevation and goiter—and higher levels of TSIs during the second trimester.

Controversies

- Impact and treatment of subclinical hyperthyroidism
- Optimal thyroid function target in treatment of maternal hyperthyroidism

Universal screening of thyroid function, especially in the first trimester, would identify a number of women with a suppressed TSH level. There is no evidence from a recent study of a cohort of mothers with suppressed TSH and normal free thyroxine levels of any adverse outcome.[34] There may be a protective effect of subclinical hyperthyroidism to reduce the incidence of hypertension in this subset of pregnant women. There is no clear indication of when women with a suppressed TSH should be treated. The correlation of these thyroid function test abnormalities in pregnancy with postpartum thyroid disease, and the appropriate follow-up, has not been established.

The high serum T_4 levels in women with resistance to thyroid hormone, approximately twofold above normal, were found to be harmful to the fetuses, which did not have resistance to thyroid hormone.[31] The usual target of serum T_4, in the upper part or slightly above normal range, protects the fetus from hypothyroidism and is unlikely to cause the adverse effects seen in the infants of mothers with resistance to thyroid hormone. The optimal maternal T_4 level, however, is unknown.

OTHER CONDITIONS

Thyroid Nodule in Pregnancy

Pregnancy does not appear to influence the natural history of thyroid carcinoma or thyroid nodules significantly.[33] The high levels of hCG in pregnancy might promote thyroid cancer growth by weak stimulation of the TSH receptor, but this effect does not seem to be clinically relevant. Thyroid nodules detected during pregnancy should be evaluated with diagnostic fine-needle aspiration if the nodule(s) meets one or more of the following criteria:

- Rapid enlargement or causing compressive symptoms
- Size larger than 1 to 1.5 cm
- Ultrasound characteristics suspicious for malignancy
- Presence of cervical lymphadenopathy

If there is evidence of thyroid carcinoma by cytology, surgery can be considered during the second trimester, although radioiodine cannot be given until after delivery. If the nodule is stable in size or if the diagnosis is made in the second half of pregnancy, surgery is usually delayed until after delivery, unless compressive symptoms in the neck are present. Postoperative management should include thyroid hormone suppression therapy. Breast-feeding is not influenced by the mother taking thyroid hormone replacement. Radioiodine, however, is concentrated in breast milk and breast-feeding can usually not be continued if therapeutic radioiodine at the doses required for thyroid cancer is planned. There are strategies to pump and discard contaminated breast milk in the post-treatment period. The long half-life of ^{131}I and the persistent activity of the sodium iodide symporter in the breast for weeks after breast-feeding is stopped, however, makes this difficult to accomplish safely.

A woman of childbearing age can have ^{131}I ablation treatment for thyroid cancer without necessarily affecting her fertility following treatment. However, it is usually recommended that she wait at least 6 to 12 months following radioactive iodine treatment before attempting conception. It is also important that any decision about an additional pregnancy take into account the nature and likely course of the thyroid cancer, especially the need for additional radioiodine scans or treatments.

Postpartum Thyroiditis

Postpartum thyroiditis is a form of painless subacute thyroiditis that occurs in 5% to 10% of women in the postpartum period and can also occur following miscarriage.[42] It can present as only hyperthyroidism, only hypothyroidism, or go through both phases. The first phase is usually a hyperthyroid phase, which occurs 1 to 3 months after delivery and lasts approximately 1 month. The thyroid is inflamed and thyroid hormone stores are released. The second phase is a hypothyroid phase, which occur 3 to 5 months postpartum and can lasts up to 9 months, although it is usually shorter. During the hypothyroid phase, levothyroxine replacement can be given if the patient has symptoms or persistent and significant elevation of serum TSH levels. Levothyroxine therapy does not seem to influence the duration of the hypothyroidism. Most patients return to the euthyroid state within 12 months. One study has reported that as many as 50% of women with positive TPO antibodies during pregnancy developed postpartum thyroid dysfunction. Furthermore, 25% of women in this high risk group went on to have overt thyroid failure within 1 year.[43] Others have shown that 30% to 50% of patients with postpartum thyroiditis develop hypothyroidism within 5 years.

A decision analysis model has supported the cost-effectiveness of measuring thyroid TPO antibodies during prenatal screening for postpartum thyroiditis. Despite having several limitations, this study argued for TSH being a cost-effective screening test in the general obstetric population.[44] This would also identify women at increased risk for hypothyroidism during pregnancy.

References

1. Glinoer D: The regulation of thyroid function in pregnancy: Pathways of endocrine adaptation from physiology to pathology. Endocr Rev 18:404-433, 1997.
2. Hershman JM: Human chorionic gonadotropin and the thyroid: Hyperemesis gravidarium and trophoblastic tumors. Thyroid 9:653-657, 1999.
3. Becker DV, Braverman LE, Delange F, et al: Iodine supplementation for pregnancy and lactation—United States and Canada: Recommendations of the American Thyroid Association. Thyroid 16: 949-951, 2006.
4. Panesar NS, Li CY, Rogers MS: Reference intervals for thyroid hormones in pregnant Chinese women. Ann Clin Biochem 38:329-332, 2001.
5. Reuss ML, Paneth N, Pinto-Martin JA, et al: The relation of transient hypothyroxinemia in preterm infants to neurologic development at two years of age. N Engl J Med 334:821-827, 1996.
6. Brent GA: Maternal hypothyroidism: Recognition and management. Thyroid 9:661-665, 1999.
7. Casey BM: Subclinical hypothyroidism and pregnancy. Obstet Gynecol Surv 61:415-420, 2006.
8. Vaidya B, Anthony S, Bilous M, et al: Detection of thyroid dysfunction in early pregnancy: Universal screening or targeted high-risk case finding? J Clin Endocrinol Metab 92:203-207, 2007.
9. Stagnaro-Green A, Glinoer D: Thyroid autoimmunity and the risk of miscarriage. Best Pract Res Clin Endocrinol Metab 18:167-181, 2004.
10. Caldwell KL, Jones R, Hollowell JG: Urinary iodine concentration: United States National Health and Nutrition Examination Survey 2001-2002. Thyroid 15:692-699, 2005.
11. Pearce EN, Bazrafshan HR, He X, et al: Dietary iodine in pregnant women from the Boston, Massachusetts area [letter]. Thyroid 14:327-328, 2004.
12. Pearce EN, Pino S, He X, et al: Sources of dietary iodine: Bread, cows' milk, and infant formula in the Boston area. J Clin Endocrinol Metab 89: 3421-3424, 2004.
13. Lee SL, Roper J: Inadequate iodine supplementation in American multivitamins. Endocr Pract 10(Suppl1):46-52, 2004.
14. Dashe JS, Casey BM, Wells CE, et al: Thyroid-stimulating hormone in singleton and twin pregnancy: Importance of gestational age-specific reference ranges. Obstet Gynecol 106:753-757, 2005.
15. Mandel SJ, Spencer CA, Hollowell JG: Are detection and treatment of thyroid insufficiency in pregnancy feasible? Thyroid 15:44-53, 2005.
16. Pop VJ, Brouwers EP, Vader HL, et al: Maternal hypothyroxinaemia during early pregnancy and subsequent child development: A 3-year follow-up study. Clin Endocrinol 59:282-288, 2003.
17. Vulsma T, Gons M, de Vijlder J: Maternal-fetal transfer of thyroxine in congenital hypothyroidism because of a total organification defect of thyroid agenesis. N Engl J Med 321:13-16, 1989.
18. Mandel SG, Larsen PR, Seely EW, et al: Increased need for thyroxine during pregnancy in women with primary hypothyroidism. N Engl J Med 323: 91-96, 1990.
19. Alexander EK, Marqusee E, Lawrence J, et al: Timing and magnitude of increases in levothyroxine requirements during pregnancy in women with hypothyroidism. N Engl J Med 351:241-249, 2004.
20. Abalovich M, Gutierrez S, Alcaraz G, et al: Overt and subclinical hypothyroidism complicating pregnancy. Thyroid 12:63-68, 2002.
21. Tan TO, Cheng YW, Caughey AB: Are women who are treated for hypothyroidism at risk for pregnancy complications? Am J Obstet Gynecol 194:e1-3, 2006.
22. Casey BM, Dashe JS, Wells CE, et al: Subclinical hypothyroidism and pregnancy outcomes. Obstet Gynecol 105:239-245, 2005.
23. Negro R, Formoso G, Mangieri T, et al: Levothyroxine treatment in euthyroid pregnant women with autoimmune thyroid disease: Effects on obstetrical complications. J Clin Endocrinol Metab 9: 2587-2591, 2006.
24. Williams GR: Neurodevelopmental and neurophysiological actions of thyroid hormone. J Neuroendocrinol 20:784-794, 2008.
25. Haddow JE, Palomaki GE, Allan WC, et al: Maternal thyroid deficiency during pregnancy and subsequent neuropsychological development of the child. N Engl J Med 341:549-555, 1999.
26. Laurberg P, Nohr S, Pedersen KM, et al: Iodine nutrition in breast-fed infants is impaired by maternal smoking. J Clin Endocrinol Metab 89:181-187, 2004.
27. Hershman JM: Perchlorate and thyroid function: What are the environmental issues? Thyroid 15: 427-431, 2005.
28. Blount BC, Pirkle JL, Osterloh JD, et al: Urinary perchlorate and thyroid hormone levels in adolescent and adult men and women living in the United States. Envir Health Perspect 114:1865-1871, 2006.

29. Rovet JF: Congenital hypothyroidism: Long-term outcome. Thyroid 9:741-748, 1999.
30. Pop VJ, Vulsma T: Maternal hypothyroxinemia during (early) gestation. Lancet 365:1604-1606, 2005.
31. Anselmo J, Cao D, Karrison T, et al: Fetal loss associated with excess thyroid hormone exposure. JAMA 292:691-695, 2004.
32. Brent GA: Diagnosing thyroid dysfunction in pregnant women: Is case finding enough [editorial]? J Clin Endocrinol Metab 91:39-41, 2007.
33. Abalovich M, Amino N, Barbour LA, et al: Management of thyroid dysfunction during pregnancy and postpartum: An Endocrine Society clinical practice guideline. J Clin Endocrinol Metab 92:S1-S47, 2007.
34. Casey BM, Dashe JS, Wells CE, et al: Subclinical hyperthyroidism and pregnancy outcomes. Obstet Gynecol 107:337-341, 2006.
35. Glinoer D: Thyroid hyperfunction during pregnancy. Thyroid 8:859-864, 1998.
36. Goodwin TM, Montoro M, Mestman JH: Transient hyperthyroidism and hyperemesis gravidarum: Clinical aspects. Am J Obstet Gynecol 167:648-652, 1992.
37. Luton D, Le Gac I, Vuillard E, et al: Management of Graves' disease during pregnancy: The key role of fetal thyroid gland monitoring. J Clin Endocrinol Metab 90:6093-6098, 2005.
38. Chan GW, Mandel SJ: Therapy insight: Management of Graves' disease during pregnancy. Nat Clin Pract Endocrinol Metab 3:470-478, 2007.
39. Brent GA: Graves' disease. N Engl J Med 358: 2594-2605, 2008.
40. Momotani N, Noh J, Oyanagi H, et al: Antithyroid drug therapy for Graves' disease during pregnancy. N Engl J Med 315:24-28, 1986.
41. Vanderpump MP, Ahlquist JA, Franklyn JA, et al: Consensus statement for good practice and audit measures in the management of hypothyroidism and hyperthyroidism. British Med J 313:539-544, 1996.
42. Stagnaro-Green A: Clinical review 152: Postpartum thyroiditis. J Clin Endocrinol Metab 87:4042-4047, 2002.
43. Premawardhana LD, Parkes AB, Ammari F, et al: Postpartum thyroiditis and long-term thyroid status: Prognostic influence of thyroid peroxidase antibodies and ultrasound echogenicity. J Clin Endocrinol Metab 85:71-75, 2000.
44. Bonds DE, Freeberg KA: Cost-effectiveness of prenatal screening for postpartum thyroiditis. J Wom Health Gender-Based Med 10:649-658, 2001.

Chapter 20

Nonthyroidal Illness Syndrome

Ronald J. Koenig

The nonthyroidal illness syndrome (NTIS), also called the sick euthyroid syndrome, is the state of a low serum triiodothyronine (T_3) level associated with illness in the absence of intrinsic disease of the hypothalamic-pituitary-thyroid axis.[1,2] Additional thyroid function test abnormalities may occur. NTIS occurs with essentially all acute and chronic diseases. The magnitude of thyroid function test abnormalities correlates with the severity of illness, and the test abnormalities resolve on recovery from the illness. NTIS may have evolved as a means to conserve energy in times of severe stress.

THYROID FUNCTION ABNORMALITIES IN NONTHYROIDAL ILLNESS SYNDROME

Triiodothyronine

In its mildest form, NTIS is associated with a low serum T_3 level without other thyroid function test abnormalities. The free T_3 has generally,[3-8] although not universally,[9] been reported as low. The temporal relationship between the onset of illness and the decrease in T_3 usually is not known because of the lack of appropriate stored sera, but this issue has been addressed in specific cases. During coronary artery bypass surgery, the total T_3 reaches a nadir (approximately 50% decrease) 30 minutes after the onset of cardiopulmonary bypass, and even shows a 5% to 10% decrease 30 minutes after induction of anesthesia.[10,11] Fasting also is associated with NTIS. An approximately 20% decrease in total T_3 is detected by 24 hours of fasting, although values decline further with continued fasting.[12] Interestingly, subjects who consumed a calorie-restricted diet with adequate nutrients over a period of years also demonstrated an approximately 20% reduction in total T_3, and the free T_3 is low in at least those with the lowest total T_3 values.[13]

Thyroxine

The serum total thyroxine (T_4) level is normal in mild cases of NTIS but falls below normal in proportion to the severity of illness, reaching values below 2 μg/dL in the most severely ill patients.[14-17] The free T_4 has been difficult to measure in NTIS and has been the subject of much controversy. Different commercial free T_4 assays can produce disparate results when analyzing sera from patients with NTIS.[18-20] Equilibrium dialysis is problematic not only because of its technically challenging nature, but also because even small amounts of heparin administered to patients can generate sufficient free fatty acids during the dialysis to displace T_4 from thyroxine binding globulin (TBG) and thus artifactually elevate the free T_4.[21] Ultrafiltration has yielded variable results, but usually returns low values for free T_4 in the most severe cases.[3] Because no methodology has been rigorously demonstrated to measure free T_4 in NTIS accurately, it is not possible to say with certainty whether the free T_4 is low in cases with low total T_4 levels. However, numerous reports have shown that patients with very low total T_4 values also have low measured free T_4 levels, but this finding is not universal.

Thyroxine-Binding Globulin

The time honored T_3 resin uptake test often yields high values in NTIS,[22] consistent with a low level of thyroxine-binding globulin (TBG). In the setting of sepsis,[23] and probably also cardiopulmonary bypass,[24] TBG is subject to cleavage by inflammatory proteases such as elastase, resulting in a reduction of thyroid hormone–binding capacity and affinity for thyroxine.[25] TBG cleavage may partially account for the fall in total T_3 during cardiopulmonary bypass, and may help explain why the total T_4 often decreases to a greater extent than the free T_4 in severe NTIS.

3,3′,5′-Triiodothyronine (Reverse Triiodothyronine)

3,3′,5′-Triiodothyronine (reverse T_3, rT_3) is an inactive metabolite of T_4 that results from inner ring deiodination (see later). The serum level of rT_3 is often elevated in NTIS, but this finding is not universal, especially when the T_4 level is very low.[22]

In practice, measurement of the serum rT_3 concentration rarely is helpful in the evaluation of patients with the NTIS.

Thyrotropin (Thyroid-Stimulating Hormone)

The thyroid-stimulating hormone (TSH) level is normal in mild cases of NTIS, but drops below normal in more severe illness. However, it is unusual for the TSH level to fall below approximately 0.01 to 0.05 mIU/L because of NTIS.[26] In contrast, patients with clinically apparent thyrotoxicosis usually have TSH values below this level. TSH normally is secreted in a pulsatile manner and has a circadian rhythm characterized by a small nocturnal surge; both of these characteristics are blunted in patients with NTIS.[27-29] The TSH response to thyrotropin-releasing hormone (TRH) injection often is blunted in NTIS.[9,30] In addition, circulating TSH in NTIS has altered glycosylation (reduced binding to concanavalin A) and reduced bioactivity.[31] Similar reductions in TSH bioactivity and concanavalin A binding are seen in patients with central hypothyroidism,[32] probably because TRH is required to stimulate the full glycosylation of TSH. The findings in NTIS suggest that this condition also is associated with diminished TRH secretion (see later).

The TSH level rises during the recovery phase of nonthyroidal illness and, in some patients, can reach values mildly above the assay reference range (Fig. 20-1).[33,34] Typically, the TSH does not rise above 10 mIU/L, but on rare occasions can transiently reach values of about 20 mIU/L. This elevated TSH can persist for a few weeks, but then returns to normal as the serum T_3 and T_4 levels normalize. Frequent sampling in patients recovering from severe NTIS with low T_4 levels has demonstrated that the rise in TSH precedes the rise in T_4 by 5 to 14 hours (Fig. 20-2).[34]

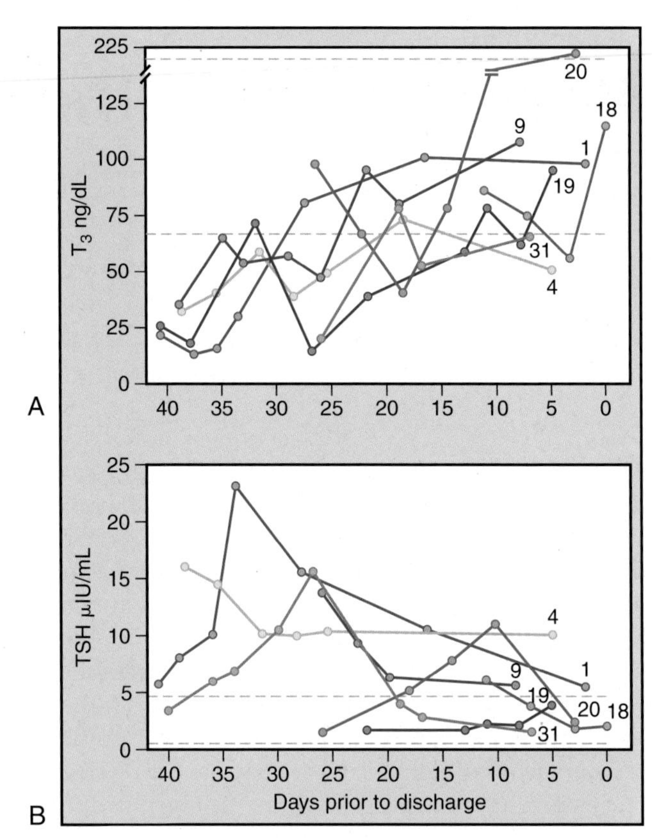

Figure 20–1 Elevation of TSH during the recovery phase of nonthyroidal illness syndrome (NTIS). The figure shows triiodothyronine (T_3) and thyroid-stimulating hormone (TSH) concentrations in hospitalized patients with NTIS who were eventually discharged. Patients are identified by case number. The broken lines indicate ±2 SD of the mean value in the normal subjects. *(Adapted from Bacci V, Schussler GC, Kaplan TB: The relationship between serum triiodothyronine, thyrotropin during systemic illness. J Clin Endocrinol Metab 54:1229-1235, 1982.)*

Clinical Situations with Variations in Laboratory Findings

In patients with AIDS, the TBG often is elevated and the rT_3 level tends to be low. The T_3 can remain normal until late in the disease, and it has been hypothesized that this may contribute to AIDS-associated weight loss.[35] The atypical aspects of NTIS in AIDS may be a consequence of associated hepatitis with increased TBG release and of immune dysfunction.

Patients with chronic renal failure[36] tend to have normal levels of rT_3 and TBG. The remainder of the thyroid function test results resemble those in typical NTIS. The levels of total T_4 and T_3 decrease in proportion to the degree of renal failure, perhaps in part caused by inhibitors of hormone binding to TBG present in uremic plasma. The free T_4 generally is measured as normal, the free T_3 is typically low, and the TSH is usually normal, although low values and minimally elevated values also have been reported.

Determining Whether Patients with Nonthyroidal Illness Syndrome Are Hypothyroid

The low serum total and free T_3 values that characterize NTIS suggest the presence of hypothyroidism, but it is difficult to prove or disprove this conclusion rigorously. The clinical examination generally is unhelpful in that patients are by definition very ill, and hence signs or symptoms consistent with hypothyroidism could simply reflect the underlying nonthyroidal illness. Measurements of the expression of T_3 target genes are difficult to interpret in that many other factors that can be altered in NTIS (e.g., nutrition, cytokines) also influence the expression of such genes. Additional observations, however, are consistent with

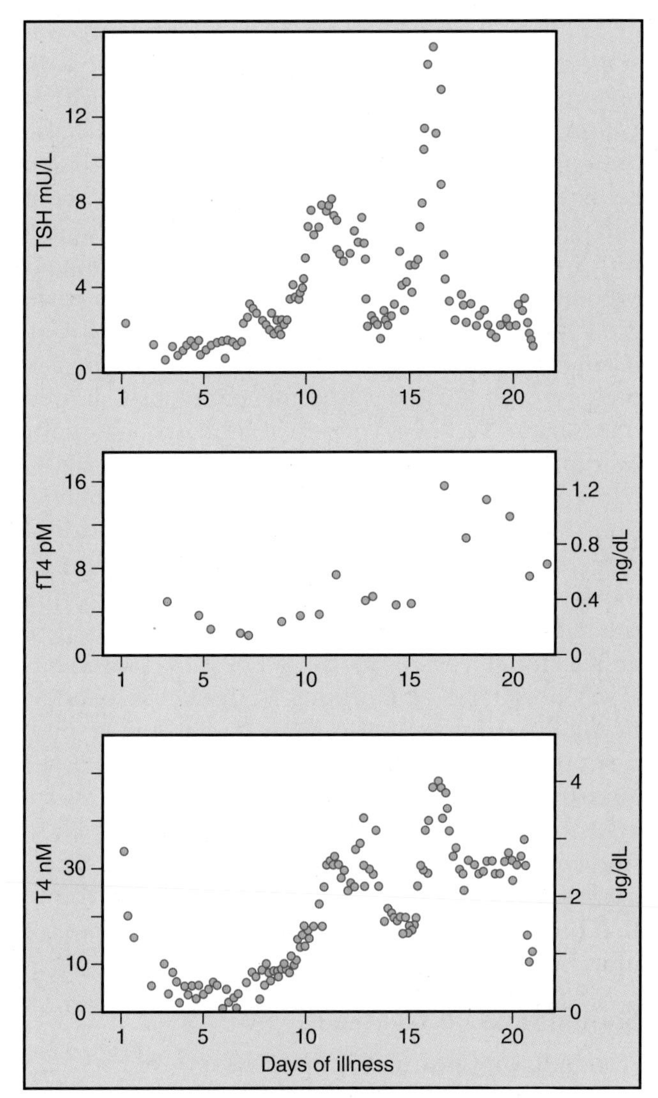

Figure 20–2 The relationship between thyroid-stimulating hormone (TSH) and thyroxine (T_4) during the recovery phase of the NTIS. The figure shows serum TSH, free T_4 (fT_4), and total T_4 concentrations during 22 days of illness in a patient with 70% burns from whom an average of five serum samples per day were obtained. A close relationship is found between changes in TSH, fT_4, and total T_4 levels. *(Adapted from Hamblin PS, Dyer SA, Mohr VS, et al: Relationship between thyrotropin, thyroxine changes during recovery from severe hypothyroxinemia of critical illness. J Clin Endocrinol Metab 62:717-722, 1986.)*

the hypothesis that patients with NTIS are hypothyroid. A study of autopsy specimens from 12 subjects dying with NTIS versus 10 subjects dying suddenly of trauma has demonstrated decreased concentrations of T_3 in the cerebral cortex, hypothalamus, pituitary, liver, kidney, and lung of NTIS patients.[37] A study of 79 patients who died while in intensive care has shown that the level of serum T_3 correlates highly with the levels of T_3 in liver and skeletal muscle—that is, a low serum T_3 predicted low tissue T_3.[38] A caveat, however, is that it is not known whether decreased tissue total T_3 signifies decreased tissue free (biologically available) T_3. The fact that the serum TSH level rises, sometimes above the reference range, during the recovery phase of NTIS suggests that the body is recovering from central hypothyroidism that was secondary to the illness.

DIFFERENTIAL DIAGNOSIS

Primary Hypothyroidism

It usually is not difficult to distinguish nonthyroidal illness from primary hypothyroidism, because the TSH level is normal or low in the former and elevated in the latter. In addition, T_4 falls earlier and to a greater extent than T_3 in primary hypothyroidism, but the opposite is found in NTIS. It is conceivable that a patient with mild primary hypothyroidism might have the TSH level fall from just above the reference range to within the reference range with concomitant NTIS. Although it would be difficult to exclude such an occurrence during the illness, it seems unlikely that this mild untreated primary hypothyroidism would be of substantial clinical importance. Patients with more significant primary hypothyroidism still manifest an elevated TSH level during nonthyroidal illness, although the magnitude of elevation may be diminished.

If the TSH is first measured when the clinical situation is improving, it can be impossible to distinguish primary hypothyroidism from the recovery phase of the NTIS, because the TSH may rise above the reference range during this period of time. A prior history of primary hypothyroidism, the presence of antithyroid peroxidase or antithyroglobulin antibodies, or a TSH level above approximately 15 to 20 mIU/L would suggest that the elevated TSH during recovery from nonthyroidal illness may reflect true primary hypothyroidism. The only way to be certain is to reassess thyroid function in several weeks. If clinically indicated, the patient could be treated with levothyroxine and reassessed subsequently by halving the dose or discontinuing the replacement and then measuring TSH.

Central Hypothyroidism

Distinguishing NTIS from "true" central hypothyroidism caused by pituitary or hypothalamic disease can be difficult or impossible. Fortunately, true central hypothyroidism is uncommon, and most cases are associated with previously known pituitary or hypothalamic disease or predisposing conditions. Because gonadotropic dysfunction usually precedes thyrotropic dysfunction, normal gonadal axis function (indicated by a normal testosterone level in a man, elevated luteinizing hormone and follicle-stimulating hormone levels in a postmenopausal woman, or regular menses in a reproductive age woman) argues against true central hypothyroidism. Unfortunately, however, severe illness often causes a functional suppression of the hypothalamic-pituitary-gonadal axis analogous to NTIS,[39] and therefore laboratory findings consistent with central hypogonadism cannot be interpreted as evidence for structural disease causing true central hypothyroidism. In situations in which true central hypothyroidism is a serious consideration that cannot be rigorously excluded, it may be appropriate to treat the patient with levothyroxine, or perhaps even levothyroxine plus liothyronine (triiodothyronine) because of the blockade of T_4 to T_3 conversion associated with NTIS (see later). It is important to exclude cortisol deficiency in patients with central hypothyroidism or provide glucocorticoid replacement.

Dopamine

Special mention should be made of patients treated with dopamine, which is a potent inhibitor of TSH secretion. For this reason, TSH levels measured during dopamine therapy cannot be interpreted as reflecting normal feedback mechanisms or the adequacy of circulating thyroid hormone levels. A study of intensive care unit (ICU) patients who had received dopamine (5 μg/kg/min IV) for 83 to 296 hours demonstrated a sharp rise in TSH beginning 20 minutes after dopamine withdrawal, achieving a mean TSH of 7.5 mIU/L (range, 0.74 to 22.4) 2 hours after withdrawal with increments in serum T_4 of 57% and T_3 of 82% within 24 hours.[40] In that same report, the effects of a brief (15- to 21-hour) dopamine infusion (5 μg/kg/min IV) were evaluated in a separate group of ICU patients using a randomized crossover design. The TSH level was low in all patients during dopamine infusion. An increase in TSH was detectable 20 minutes after dopamine withdrawal, with peak values of 1.7 to 5.5 mIU/L 3 hours after withdrawal. However, there was no significant decrease in serum T_4 or T_3 at the end of this infusion. Overall, the data indicate that prolonged dopamine therapy can cause central hypothyroidism. However, most patients do not receive dopamine for sufficient time for this to be of concern.

PROGNOSTIC FACTORS

Severity of Nonthyroidal Illness Syndrome Predicts Mortality

The severity of NTIS has been shown to be a strong predictor of mortality in a wide variety of clinical conditions. For example, in 113 patients admitted to an ICU, the best prediction of mortality was achieved by combining the APACHE II score with measurements of total T_3 and TSH obtained within 1 hour of ICU admission.[41] For every 10-ng/dL decrement in T_3, the odds of dying in the ICU increased by 49% after accounting for the APACHE II score and TSH level. In a study of 573 patients hospitalized for cardiac disease, free T_3 was the strongest predictor of mortality over the subsequent year, even stronger than dyslipidemia, age, and left ventricular ejection fraction.[5] A separate study of 281 patients with dilated cardiomyopathy also showed that serum T_3 was an independent risk factor for mortality over the subsequent year.[7] A study of 100 patients who underwent bone marrow transplantation showed that a high rT_3/T_3 ratio (indicative of more severe NTIS) 1 month post transplantation was an independent predictor of mortality during the subsequent year.[42] In 451 patients admitted to an ICU for at least 5 days, a high rT_3/T_3 ratio on day 1 was predictive of mortality.[43] Among 32 patients hospitalized for acute or acute on chronic respiratory failure, a low free T_3 (measured within 1 day of admission) was the only factor significantly associated with an increased risk of mortality.[6] Finally, a study of 200 hemodialysis patients followed prospectively for an average of 42 months has also found that the free T_3 level is an independent predictor of mortality.[8]

Should NTIS Be Treated?

It is commonly postulated that NTIS evolved because tissue hypothyroidism would conserve energy in times of illness or injury. This would imply that NTIS is an adaptive response to severe illness, or at least that it has been such a response. However, in the modern era of ICU medicine, might NTIS be maladaptive? The strong correlation between the severity of NTIS and risk of mortality raises the question of whether NTIS itself contributes to poor clinical outcome or is simply a marker of poor prognosis. An often asked question is whether NTIS should ever be treated. If yes, then which patients and which type of treatment? These important questions can be answered only by randomized clinical studies with adequate statistical power. Sufficient data do not exist to provide definitive answers. Thus, the standard of care, perhaps reflecting a "do no harm" philosophy, has been not to treat the NTIS. However, encouraging data, at least in some clinical settings, have indicated that further research is needed to resolve this issue better. The current literature on clinical trials of thyroid hormone therapy in NTIS is reviewed here.

CLINICAL TRIALS OF THYROID HORMONE THERAPY

A number of clinical trials of thyroid hormone therapy in patients with NTIS have been undertaken. In one study, 28 men who suffered severe burns were randomly assigned to treatment with placebo or triiodothyronine (200 μg/day in four divided doses) until their wounds healed.[44] Four of 14 patients in each group died, so there was no effect of T_3 therapy on survival. In a separate study, 23 ICU patients with total T_4 levels < 5 μg/dL were randomized to a control group or therapy with levothyroxine, 1.5 μg/kg/day, for 2 weeks.[45] The mortality rates were 75% in the control group and 73% in the levothyroxine-treated group, so again there was no benefit to therapy. However, these were small clinical studies with correspondingly small statistical power to detect real effects.

Several larger studies have evaluated the effects of triiodothyronine therapy in patients undergoing cardiac surgery, with the overall results suggesting beneficial effects. In one such study, 142 patients were randomized prior to coronary artery bypass surgery to receive triiodothyronine or dextrose postoperatively.[11] The treated group received 0.8 μg/kg T_3 IV at the time of removal of the aortic cross clamp, followed by an IV infusion of 0.113 μg/kg/hr for 6 hours and then a 3-hour taper. T_3 therapy increased cardiac output and lowered systemic vascular resistance but did not affect the need for inotropic or vasodilator drugs, the duration of postoperative mechanical ventilation, the length of ICU or hospital stay, or perioperative morbidity or mortality. A subsequent analysis has revealed that the T_3-treated patients had an approximately 50% reduction in the incidence of atrial fibrillation, with fewer required cardioversions and fewer patients being anticoagulated.[46] A separate double-blind study randomized 170 coronary artery bypass graft patients to receive placebo or T_3 starting at the time of removal of the aortic cross clamp, and found that the T_3-treated patients had better postoperative ventricular function, less need for inotropic agents and mechanical devices, and a lower incidence of myocardial ischemia.[47] Another double-blind study randomized coronary artery bypass graft patients to receive placebo, glucose-insulin-potassium, T_3, or glucose-insulin-potassium plus T_3.[48] Compared with placebo, all three treatment groups showed improved hemodynamic performance and reduced serum cardiac troponin I levels, but the combination therapy was not superior to glucose-insulin-potassium alone or T_3 alone.

Because premature infants have very low serum T_3 and T_4 levels that correlate with poor outcome, a randomized controlled trial of levothyroxine supplementation was conducted in 200 infants born at less than 30 weeks' gestational age.[49] The treatment group received T_4 at 8 μg/kg birth weight/day for the first 6 weeks of life. Upon follow up at a mean age of 10.5 years, the T_4 treated group demonstrated better school outcome in those born at <27 weeks' gestation and better motor outcome in those born at <28 weeks' gestation, but the T_4 treated subjects fared worse than those born at 29 weeks' gestation. These authors also reported similar findings at age 5.5 years.

Mechanisms Underlying Nonthyroidal Illness Syndrome: Data from Human Studies

When reviewing data that address the mechanisms underlying the NTIS, it is important to recognize that there may be differences between acute versus chronic illness, as well as differences among types of illnesses. Nevertheless, many of the underlying mechanisms are likely to be generally applicable.

Patients Receiving Levothyroxine Replacement

Wadwekar and Kabadi[50] studied six subjects who were receiving chronic levothyroxine therapy for hypothyroidism, with normal outpatient TSH levels, who were admitted to an ICU for acute illnesses. All six continued to receive their usual doses of levothyroxine during hospitalization. Despite this, during the first 2 hospital days all subjects demonstrated typical laboratory changes of NTIS, with decreased levels of T_4 and T_3, elevated rT_3, and borderline low TSH. The patients recovered and their TSH levels rose to slightly above the reference range on hospital day 7, with all test results normalizing after discharge. The fact that these changes were observed in subjects receiving exogenous levothyroxine suggests that the changes of NTIS are secondary to alterations in thyroid hormone metabolism, rather than thyroid gland secretion.

Thyroid Hormone Kinetic Studies in Intensive Care Unit Patients

Kinetic studies were performed following the injection of radiolabeled T_4, T_3, or rT_3 into severely ill patients with NTIS and total T_4 levels < 3 μg/dL.[51] In these patients, the total T_3 levels were decreased to 22% of normal and the free T_3 levels were reduced to 49% of normal. This quantitative discrepancy was at least in part accounted for decreased serum protein binding, which also resulted in an increased metabolic clearance rate. The T_3 production rate was only 27% of normal, and this appeared to result from decreased peripheral T_4 to T_3 conversion (5′ deiodination).

Although the total T_4 levels were low, the free T_4 levels (by equilibrium dialysis) were generally in the lower portion of the normal range, as were the T_4 production rates. Binding of T_4 to serum proteins was decreased and the metabolic clearance rate was increased. Although these patients had elevated rT_3 levels, the rT_3 production rate was normal. However, the metabolic clearance rate of rT_3 was decreased, consistent with impaired rT_3 deiodination.

Hypothalamic Thyrotropin-Releasing Hormone Expression in Postmortem Specimens

Fliers and colleagues[52] performed in situ hybridization for TRH mRNA in paraventricular nuclei (PVN) of hypothalami from a series of patients who had died acutely without developing NTIS, or who had died with NTIS because of severe protracted illness. The amount of TRH mRNA correlated with the serum T_3 level; that is, patients with the most severe NTIS had the lowest expression of TRH (Fig. 20-3). In a separate study, when patients who had been critically ill for several weeks were given TRH infusions for 21 hours, the serum T_4 level rose by 44% and the T_3 by 116%.[28] These data suggest that decreased TRH secretion (functional tertiary hypothyroidism) is an important component of NTIS. Although this may appear to conflict with previous studies, suggesting that NTIS results from alterations in thyroid hormone metabolism, the difference may relate to the duration of illness, with hypothalamic TRH deficiency playing more of a role in chronic NTIS. Even if decreased TRH does not cause the low serum T_3 level, the failure of TRH to increase likely is important in sustaining the low T_3.

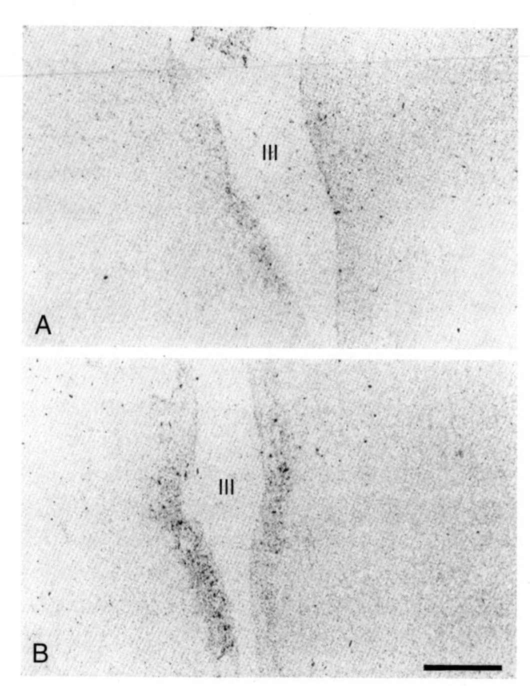

Figure 20–3 Decreased expression of thyrotropin-releasing hormone (TRH) in the paraventricular nucleus (PVN) of the hypothalamus in a patient who died with nonthyroidal illness syndrome (NTIS). The figure demonstrates in situ hybridizations of TRH mRNA from two subjects, showing the PVN along the wall of the third ventricle. **A,** Low-intensity hybridization signal in the PVN of a subject whose premortem serum thyroid hormone concentrations showed NTIS. **B,** High-intensity hybridization signal in the PVN of a subject who had a normal serum concentration of triiodothyronine who died from cardiac arrest. Scale bar represents 2 mm. III, third ventricle. *(From Fliers E, Guldenaar SE, Wiersinga WM, et al: Decreased hypothalamic thyrotropin-releasing hormone gene expression in patients with nonthyroidal illness. J Clin Endocrinol Metab 82:4032-4036, 1997.)*

The mechanism underlying the decrease in PVN TRH is not known. Perhaps illness-related factors override the normal negative feedback relationship between T_3 and TRH, or perhaps there actually is increased T_3 in the PVN (despite decreased serum T_3), with normal feedback suppression of TRH. However, as noted earlier, the tissue T_3 concentration was decreased in the hypothalami and pituitaries from patients who had died with severe NTIS, compared with patients who had died suddenly from trauma.[37] This result argues for true tissue hypothyroidism and hence inappropriately low TRH expression. A caveat is that the total tissue T_3 level may not reflect the free hormone concentration in the PVN. Animal studies (see later) suggest that the concentration of T_3 in the PVN may not be low in NTIS.

Deiodinase Expression in Liver and Skeletal Muscle

There are three enzymes capable of removing iodide from thyroid hormones. Types 1 and 2 deiodinase (D1, D2) have outer ring (5′) deiodinase activity and therefore convert T_4 to T_3, whereas D3 is an inner ring deiodinase that inactivates T_4 to rT_3 and T_3 to 3,3′-diiodothyronine (T_2). The relative importance of D1 and D2 as contributors to circulating T_3 in humans is controversial. Liver is the major source of D1, and the importance of this enzyme is suggested by the fact that a polymorphism in the human *DIO1* gene correlates with the serum free T_4/free T_3 ratio.[53] Skeletal muscle contains extremely low levels of D2, but because the mass of skeletal muscle is large, it is possible that this D2 also contributes significantly to the serum T_3. Without knowing the true relative contributions of D1 and D2 in normal physiology, it is difficult to evaluate the significance of changes associated with NTIS. Nevertheless, measurements of peripheral organ deiodinase levels are of great interest, given the data supporting an important role for abnormalities in thyroid hormone metabolism in the NTIS. In one study, liver and skeletal muscle biopsies were taken within minutes after death from approximately 65 ICU patients and then assayed for deiodinase enzyme activity.[54] The patients with the most severe NTIS, as judged by low ratios of serum T_3/rT_3, had the lowest liver D1 activity. D1 appeared to be downregulated especially in patients who died from cardiovascular collapse or multiple organ failure and sepsis. These data are consistent with decreased hepatic D1 contributing to the low T_3 level in NTIS. Surprisingly, most of the liver and muscle biopsies had measurable D3 activity, even though D3 normally is not expressed in these organs. Because D3 inactivates T_4 and T_3, this result also potentially implicates the induction of D3 in the cause of the low T_3 state.

In principle, the low T_3 state also could be caused by decreased D2, because D1 and D2 both convert T_4 to T_3. However, skeletal muscle D2 enzyme activity was not found to be decreased in NTIS patients versus control subjects.[55,56]

The elevated rT_3 that accompanies NTIS could be secondary to the decrease in D1 (D1 is the major pathway for rT_3 clearance) or the induction of D3 (D3 converts T_4 to rT_3). However, as noted, radiolabeled rT_3 kinetic studies in ICU patients implicate impaired rT_3 clearance rather than increased production in the NTIS.[51]

Thyroid Hormone Transporters

Whether specific cell surface transporters are necessary for T_4 and T_3 to gain entry into cells has long been debated. This issue has recently been resolved, at least for some organs, by the discovery that the monocarboxylate transporter 8 gene (*MCT8*) encodes a thyroid hormone transporter[57] and that patients with *MCT8* mutations have abnormal thyroid function test results and neurologic abnormalities that might be explained by neuronal thyroid hormone deficiency.[58,59] By analogy, T_4 or T_3 entry into cells might be diminished in NTIS if MCT8 or another transporter is downregulated in key organs, contributing to the phenotype of this condition. MCT8 is, in fact, expressed in TRH neurons of the PVN.[60] However, in patients who died with NTIS, skeletal muscle or liver MCT8 expression did not correlate with the ratio of serum-to-tissue T_3 (or T_4) concentrations,[38] suggesting that decreased liver and skeletal muscle thyroid hormone concentrations are not accounted for by decreased MCT8 expression. However, it is possible that the decreased expression or function of currently unidentified T_3 transporters contributes to low tissue T_3 concentrations in the NTIS.

Cytokine Levels

Increased cytokine levels may underlie the changes in thyroid hormone economy in NTIS, in part because cytokines are induced in almost all illnesses and NTIS occurs under similar conditions. In a study of 140 consecutive internal medicine hospital admissions, the serum interleukin 6 (IL-6) level correlated inversely with the serum T_3 level ($r = -0.56$).[61] Furthermore, infusion of IL-6 into healthy subjects resulted in decreased levels of TSH and T_3 and elevation of rT_3.[62,63] These data are consistent with the hypothesis that increased IL-6, at least in part, causes the thyroid function test abnormalities in NTIS.

Administration of endotoxin to healthy subjects results in decreases in serum T_4, T_3, and TSH and an increase in rT_3, similar to changes observed in NTIS. These endotoxin-induced changes were not prevented by co-infusion of an IL-1 receptor antagonist,[64] and serum IL-1 levels do not correlate well with the severity of NTIS.[65] The findings with tumor necrosis factor (TNF) have been similar. Administration of recombinant TNF to healthy subjects induces changes typical of NTIS, including decreases in T_3 and TSH and an increase in rT_3.[66] However, neutralization of TNF by administration of a recombinant TNF receptor–immunoglobulin G (IgG) fusion protein did not prevent the endotoxin-induced changes in serum thyroid hormone levels,[67] and serum TNFα levels do not correlate well with the magnitude of thyroid hormone changes in NTIS patients.[68] These findings suggest that IL-1 and TNF are not essential to the development of NTIS, although they do not exclude the possibility that IL-1 and TNF are two of many cytokines (or other factors) that contribute to the NTIS.

Leptin

Data from rodent studies (see later) have indicated that leptin positively regulates the hypothalamic-pituitary-thyroid axis. Because circulating leptin levels decrease in starvation, leptin deficiency might be implicated in some patients with NTIS. For example, four patients who consumed a hypocaloric diet for more than 2 weeks to achieve 10% weight loss had significant decreases (within the normal ranges) in serum T_4 and T_3 levels, and these changes were reversed by leptin administration.[69] Leptin administration to women with hypothalamic amenorrhea (secondary to strenuous exercise or low weight) increased the free T_3 from low normal to midnormal.[70] A study of three obese children with genetic deficiencies of leptin demonstrated that they had normal levels of free T_4, free T_3, and TSH, but that leptin replacement therapy still increased the free T_4 level in all three and the free T_3 in two.[71] Conversely, even though a 72-hour fast resulted in decreases in circulating leptin and T_3 and an increase in rT_3, leptin administration did not reverse the changes in T_3 and rT_3.[72] These findings suggest that diminished leptin might partially account for the decreased TRH secretion and changes in circulating thyroid hormones in NTIS patients, presuming that such patients are undernourished for a sufficiently long period. However, even critically ill patients generally receive nutritional supplementation and hence are not starved. A study of 8 critically ill patients with NTIS showed that their leptin levels were normal or elevated, not low.[73] In contrast, a subset of elderly subjects with NTIS was found to have decreased leptin levels, which correlated with a low body mass index.[74] The authors did not test whether leptin administration would increase the serum T_3, but it is possible that leptin deficiency contributes to NTIS in chronically undernourished subjects.

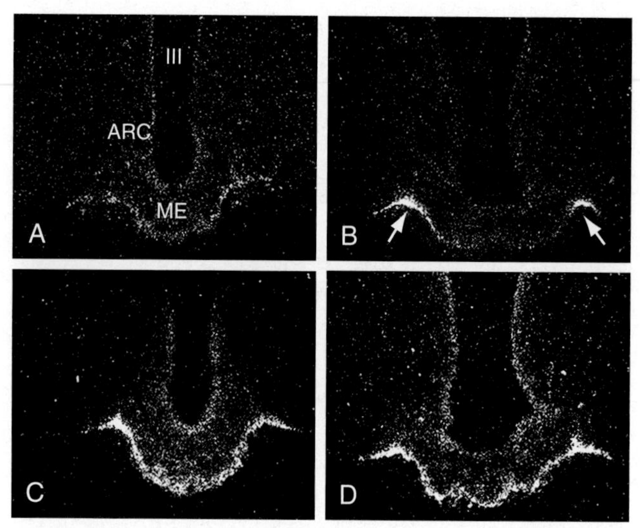

Figure 20–4 Endotoxin induces type 2 deiodinase (D2) expression in the mediobasal hypothalamus of rats. Rats were injected with lipopolysaccharide (LPS) or saline and were sacrificed 12 hours later. Low-power dark field micrographs from two rostrocaudal levels of the median eminence (ME) are shown, illustrating the effect of LPS treatment on D2 mRNA expression as assessed by in situ hybridization. **A, B,** Controls. **C, D,** LPS-treated animals. Silver grains denoting D2 mRNA are accumulated along the wall of the third ventricle (III) in tanycytes, which send processes to the tuberoinfundibular sulci (arrows) and the external zone of the ME. After LPS administration, the density of silver grains denoting tanycyte D2 mRNA is markedly increased. ARC, arcuate. *(From Fekete C, Gereben B, Doleschall M, et al: Lipopolysaccharide induces type 2 iodothyronine deiodinase in the mediobasal hypothalamus: Implications for the nonthyroidal illness syndrome. Endocrinology 145:1649-1655, 2004.)*

Mechanisms Underlying Nonthyroidal Illness Syndrome: Data from Animal and In Vitro Studies

Interleukin 6 in Mouse Models

The role of IL-6 in NTIS was assessed by inducing illness in wild-type versus IL-6 null mice in three different ways; administration of endotoxin (lipopolysaccharide [LPS]), infection with *Listeria monocytogenes*, or turpentine injection into the hind limbs to induce sterile inflammation.[75] In each case, the decrease in serum T_3 was smaller in the knockout mice, implying that induction of IL-6 is partially responsible for the low T_3 state in these animal models.

Hypothalamic-Pituitary Regulation in Animal Models

Administration of LPS to rats reduces the serum T_3 and also decreases expression of TRH mRNA in the PVN of the hypothalamus and TSHβ mRNA in the anterior pituitary. Serum glucocorticoid levels are induced in stress, including in this animal model, and therefore might contribute to the TRH-TSH axis suppression in NTIS. However, adrenalectomized, corticosterone-replaced rats also develop decreased TRH and TSHβ mRNA following LPS administration,[76] indicating that stress-induced increases in steroid levels are not required for this NTIS response.

Type 2 deiodinase is expressed in specialized cells of the mediobasal hypothalamus called tanycytes that line the third ventricle and that may function to supply T_3 to the TRH neurons in the PVN.[77] Interestingly, the administration of LPS to rats acutely induces tanycyte D2 (Fig. 20-4), an effect mediated, at least in part, by activation of nuclear factor–kappa B (NF-κB).[78] This local D2 induction may result in the delivery of excess T_3 to the PVN and/or anterior pituitary, essentially creating tissue-specific thyrotoxicosis and suppressing the TRH-TSH axis, despite a decreased serum T_3 level. LPS administration to mice also decreases TSHβ mRNA,[79] which might occur because of diminished TRH, which could further contribute to axis suppression. However, this tissue-specific thyrotoxicosis hypothesis needs to be resolved with the finding of decreased hypothalamic and pituitary T_3 levels in patients dying with NTIS.[37]

As noted, leptin has important regulatory effects on TRH expression in rodents. Fasted rats have low serum T_4 and T_3 levels and decreased expression of TRH mRNA in the PVN of the hypothalamus; all these changes were reversed with leptin administration.[80] The serum TSH also is decreased in fasted rats and leptin administration also prevents this decrease.[81]

Hepatic Type 1 Deiodinase in Animal Models

Mice given LPS develop NTIS, which is associated with decreased hepatic D1 mRNA and enzyme activity.[82] However, in contrast to the data from patients who succumbed to critical illness, D3 activity is not induced in the livers of these mice.

Type 1 deiodinase, which probably is the major source of peripheral T_4 to T_3 conversion in rat, is induced at the transcriptional level by T_3. Exposure of primary cultures of rat hepatocytes to IL-1 or IL-6 has little effect on D1 expression when the culture media lack T_3, but these cytokines block the T_3 induction of D1 mRNA and enzyme activity.[83,84] This cytokine effect is prevented by forced expression of the thyroid hormone receptor coactivator, steroid receptor coactivator-1 (SRC-1, NCoA-1). If these results apply in vivo, cytokines would decrease D1 expression from a euthyroid level to a hypothyroid level; this would result in decreased T_3 production, which would further decrease D1 in a self-reinforcing loop. To test this hypothesis, mice were injected with a control adenovirus or an adenovirus that expresses SRC-1, which efficiently expresses in liver. The mice then were treated with LPS to induce NTIS. It was found that pretreatment with the SRC-1 adenovirus prevents the LPS-induced decrease in hepatic D1, and also prevents the fall in serum T_3 that characterizes NTIS.[84] The results imply that, in this model of NTIS, inhibition of hepatic D1 plays a key role in the decreased serum T_3, and the syndrome can be overcome by forced expression of SRC-1.

In separate studies, exposure of HepG2 hepatoma cells to IL-1 also was found to decrease D1 mRNA, with activation of both AP-1 and NF-KB being involved in this process.[85] Exposure of HepG2 hepatoma cells to TNF-α also impaired T3 induction of D1, and this effect was dependent on NF-KB.[86]

Hepatic Nuclear Receptors in Mouse Models

Additional mechanisms may underlie the decreased T_3-dependent expression of hepatic D1 in NTIS. Mice treated with LPS have decreased expression of liver thyroid hormone receptors and their heterodimerization partner, retinoid X receptor alpha (RXRα).[87] Furthermore, LPS administration to mice caused a redistribution of hepatic RXRα from the nucleus to the cytoplasm,[88] and IL-1 treatment of HepG2 cells had the same effect.[89] The movement of RXRα from the nucleus could contribute to the decreased ability of T_3 to induce D1.

Induction of Type 3 Deiodinase at Sites of Inflammation and Local Nonthyroidal Illness Syndrome

As noted, the induction of liver and skeletal muscle D3 in NTIS patients was unexpected and suggested the catabolism of T_3 as a contributing factor to the low T_3 state. This phenomenon also has been observed in rodents, where it has been studied in some detail. The injection of turpentine into the hind limbs of mice induces sterile inflammation, which was associated with the local induction of D3.[82] In this model, the D3-containing cells appeared to be the infiltrating polymorphonuclear leukocytes, rather than the myocytes.

Type 3 deiodinase also was induced in the hearts of rats subjected to myocardial infarction.[90] In another model of heart disease, rats were subjected to pulmonary hypertension, resulting in right ventricular hypertrophy and congestive heart failure.[91] Type 3 deiodinase was induced in the right ventricle, associated with decreased expression of a thyroid hormone–responsive reporter gene, suggesting that D3 is inducing functionally significant local hypothyroidism. These changes were not observed in the left ventricle, demonstrating that the response was specific to the diseased tissue. These results suggest that the induction of D3 at sites of inflammation and disease may induce local hypothyroidism (local NTIS) that may be important in disease pathology, perhaps independent of any effects on circulating T_3 levels.

Peripheral Organ Type 2 Deiodinase

Human studies discussed earlier indicate that skeletal muscle D2 does not decrease in NTIS, and hence the low T_3 state is not likely explained by decreased D2. Potential changes in skeletal muscle D2 in NTIS cannot readily be modeled in rats or mice because these animals do not express D2 in muscle. Cell culture studies have demonstrated that D2 expression is regulated primarily at the protein level by ubiquitination and proteasome-mediated degradation,[92] which can be rescued by deubiquitination.[93] If the net ubiquitination of D2 is increased by nonthyroidal illness, the result would be a rapid decline in D2-dependent T_3 production and hence potentially a fall in serum T_3. Thus, it remains possible that changes in D2 levels in unidentified organs may contribute to the low T_3 state of nonthyroidal illness.

FUTURE CONSIDERATIONS

A number of important questions can be resolved only with further studies, including the following:

- What is the mechanism(s) underlying the low TRH and TSH state despite a low serum T_3 level? Induction of tanycyte D2, with resulting local thyrotoxicosis, is attractive as a contributing factor, but further evidence is needed.
- Are there other tissues in which the local thyroid hormone status is not reflected by the serum values, and what are the physiologic consequences of this?
- What are the relative contributions of decreased D1 and increased D3 (and perhaps, decreased D2 in unknown organs) to the decrease in serum T_3? Multiple mechanisms probably underlie

these changes, but which are most important? What are the roles of cytokines or other factors in establishing these changes?

- Do other abnormalities make important contributions to NTIS, such as decreased expression or activity of thyroid hormone transporters which could limit the access of circulating T_3 to target cells?

The ultimate question is whether NTIS should ever be treated and, if so, how? A better understanding of its mechanisms of action will help resolve this issue. For example, if the low T_3 state reflects a functional deficiency in coactivators such as SRC-1, as is suggested by mouse data,[84] perhaps therapies directed at this underlying deficiency would be more appropriate than treatment with T_3.

References

1. Carter JN, Eastman CJ, Corcoran JM, et al: Effect of severe, chronic illness on thyroid function. Lancet 2:971-974, 1974.
2. Bermudez F, Surks MI, Oppenheimer JH: High incidence of decreased serum triiodothyronine concentration in patients with nonthyroidal disease. J Clin Endocrinol Metab 41:27-40, 1975.
3. Wang YS, Hershman JM, Pekary AE: Improved ultrafiltration method for simultaneous measurement of free thyroxine, free triiodothyronine in serum. Clin Chem 31:517-522, 1985.
4. Chopra IJ, Taing P, Mikus L: Direct determination of free triiodothyronine (T3) in undiluted serum by equilibrium dialysis/radioimmunoassay (RIA). Thyroid 6:255-259, 1996.
5. Iervasi G, Pingitore A, Landi P, et al: Low- T3 syndrome: A strong prognostic predictor of death in patients with heart disease. Circulation 107:708-713, 2003.
6. Scoscia E, Baglioni S, Eslami A, et al: Low triiodothyronine (T3) state: A predictor of outcome in respiratory failure? Results of a clinical pilot study. Eur J Endocrinol 151:557-560, 2004.
7. Pingitore A, Landi P, Taddei MC, et al: Triiodothyronine levels for risk stratification of patients with chronic heart failure. Am J Med 118:132-136, 2005.
8. Zoccali C, Mallamaci F, Tripepi G, et al: Low triiodothyronine, survival in end-stage renal disease. Kidney Int 70:523-528, 2006.
9. Faber J, Kirkegaard C, Rasmussen B, et al: Pituitary-thyroid axis in critical illness. J Clin Endocrinol Metab 65:315-320, 1987.
10. Chu SH, Huang TS, Hsu RB, et al: Thyroid hormone changes after cardiovascular surgery: Clinical implications. Ann Thorac Surg 52:791-796, 1991.
11. Klemperer JD, Klein I, Gomez M, et al: Thyroid hormone treatment after coronary-artery bypass surgery. N Engl J Med 333:1522-1527, 1995.
12. Merimee TJ, Fineberg ES: Starvation-induced alterations of circulating thyroid hormone concentrations in man. Metabolism 25:79-83, 1976.
13. Fontana L, Klein S, Holloszy JO, et al: Effect of long-term calorie restriction with adequate protein and micronutrients on thyroid hormones. J Clin Endocrinol Metab 91:3232-3235, 2006.
14. McLarty DG, Ratcliffe WA, McColl K, et al: Letter: Thyroid-hormone levels and prognosis in patients with serious non-thyroidal illness. Lancet 2:275-276, 1975.
15. Slag MF, Morley JE, Elson MK, et al: Hypothyroxinemia in critically ill patients as a predictor of high mortality. JAMA 245:43-45, 1981.
16. Kaptein EM, Weiner JM, Robinson WJ, et al: Relationship of altered thyroid hormone indices to survival in nonthyroidal illnesses. Clin Endocrinol (Oxf) 16:565-574, 1982.
17. Kantor MJ, Leef KH, Bartoshesky L, et al: Admission thyroid evaluation in very-low-birth-weight infants: Association with death and severe intraventricular hemorrhage. Thyroid 13:965-969, 2003.
18. Kaptein EM, MacIntyre SS, Weiner JM, et al: Free thyroxine estimates in nonthyroidal illness: Comparison of eight methods. J Clin Endocrinol Metab 52:1073-1077, 1981.
19. Melmed S, Geola FL, Reed AW, et al: A comparison of methods for assessing thyroid function in nonthyroidal illness. J Clin Endocrinol Metab 54:300-306, 1982.
20. Wong TK, Pekary AE, Hoo GS, et al: Comparison of methods for measuring free thyroxinE in nonthyroidal illness. Clin Chem 38:720-724, 1992.
21. Jaume JC, Mendel CM, Frost PH, et al: Extremely low doses of heparin release lipase activity into the plasma and can thereby cause artifactual elevations in the serum-free thyroxine concentration as measured by equilibrium dialysis. Thyroid 6:79-83, 1996.
22. Kaptein EM, Grieb DA, Spencer CA, et al: Thyroxine metabolism in the low thyroxine state of critical nonthyroidal illnesses. J Clin Endocrinol Metab 53:764-771, 1981.
23. Jirasakuldech B, Schussler GC, Yap MG, et al: A characteristic serpin cleavage product of thyroxine-binding globulin appears in sepsis sera. J Clin Endocrinol Metab 85:3996-3999, 2000.
24. Afandi B, Schussler GC, Arafeh AH, et al: Selective consumption of thyroxine-binding globulin during cardiac bypass surgery. Metabolism 49:270-274, 2000.
25. Janssen OE, Golcher HM, Grasberger H, et al: Characterization of T_4-binding globulin cleaved by human leukocyte elastase. J Clin Endocrinol Metab 87:1217-1222, 2002.
26. Spencer CA, LoPresti JS, Patel A, et al: Applications of a new chemiluminometric thyrotropin assay to subnormal measurement. J Clin Endocrinol Metab 70:453-460, 1990.

27. Romijn JA, Wiersinga WM: Decreased nocturnal surge of thyrotropin in nonthyroidal illness. J Clin Endocrinol Metab 70:35-42, 1990.
28. Van den Berghe G, de Zegher F, Baxter RC, et al: Neuroendocrinology of prolonged critical illness: Effects of exogenous thyrotropin-releasing hormone, its combination with growth hormone secretagogues. J Clin Endocrinol Metab 83:309-319, 1998.
29. Van den Berghe G, de Zegher F, Veldhuis JD, et al: Thyrotrophin, prolactin release in prolonged critical illness: Dynamics of spontaneous secretion and effects of growth hormone-secretagogues. Clin Endocrinol (Oxf) 47:599-612, 1997.
30. Vierhapper H, Laggner A, Waldhausl W, et al: Impaired secretion of TSH in critically ill patients with 'low T4-syndrome.' Acta Endocrinol (Copenh) 101:542-549, 1982.
31. Lee HY, Suhl J, Pekary AE, et al: Secretion of thyrotropin with reduced concanavalin-A–binding activity in patients with severe nonthyroid illness. J Clin Endocrinol Metab 65:942-945, 1987.
32. Beck-Peccoz P, Amr S, Menezes-Ferreira MM, et al: Decreased receptor binding of biologically inactive thyrotropin in central hypothyroidism. Effect of treatment with thyrotropin-releasing hormone. N Engl J Med 312:1085-1090, 1985.
33. Bacci V, Schussler GC, Kaplan TB: The relationship between serum triiodothyronine, thyrotropin during systemic illness. J Clin Endocrinol Metab 54:1229-1235, 1982.
34. Hamblin PS, Dyer SA, Mohr VS, et al: Relationship between thyrotropin and thyroxine changes during recovery from severe hypothyroxinemia of critical illness. J Clin Endocrinol Metab 62: 717-722, 1986.
35. LoPresti JS, Fried JC, Spencer CA, et al: Unique alterations of thyroid hormone indices in the acquired immunodeficiency syndrome (AIDS). Ann Intern Med 110:970-975, 1989.
36. Wartofsky L, Burman KD: Alterations in thyroid function in patients with systemic illness: The "euthyroid sick syndrome." Endocr Rev 3:164-217, 1982.
37. Arem R, Wiener GJ, Kaplan SG, et al: Reduced tissue thyroid hormone levels in fatal illness. Metabolism 42:1102-1108, 1993.
38. Peeters RP, van der Geyten S, Wouters PJ, et al: Tissue thyroid hormone levels in critical illness. J Clin Endocrinol Metab 90:6498-6507, 2005.
39. Spratt DI, Cox P, Orav J, et al: Reproductive axis suppression in acute illness is related to disease severity. J Clin Endocrinol Metab 76:1548-1554, 1993.
40. Van den Berghe G, de Zegher F, Lauwers P: Dopamine and the sick euthyroid syndrome in critical illness. Clin Endocrinol (Oxf) 41:731-737, 1994.
41. Chinga-Alayo E, Villena J, Evans AT, et al: Thyroid hormone levels improve the prediction of mortality among patients admitted to the intensive care unit. Intensive Care Med 31:1356-1361, 2005.
42. Schulte C, Reinhardt W, Beelen D, et al: Low T3-syndrome and nutritional status as prognostic factors in patients undergoing bone marrow transplantation. Bone Marrow Transplant 22:1171-1178, 1998.
43. Peeters RP, Wouters PJ, van Toor H, et al: Serum 3,3′,5′-triiodothyronine (rT3) and 3,5,3′-triiodothyronine/r T3 are prognostic markers in critically ill patients and are associated with postmortem tissue deiodinase activities. J Clin Endocrinol Metab 90:4559-4565, 2005.
44. Becker RA, Vaughan GM, Ziegler MG, et al: Hypermetabolic low triiodothyronine syndrome of burn injury. Crit Care Med 10:870-875, 1982.
45. Brent GA, Hershman JM: Thyroxine therapy in patients with severe nonthyroidal illnesses and low serum thyroxine concentration. J Clin Endocrinol Metab 63:1-8, 1986.
46. Klemperer JD, Klein IL, Ojamaa K, et al: Triiodothyronine therapy lowers the incidence of atrial fibrillation after cardiac operations. Ann Thorac Surg 61:1323-1327, discussion 1328-1329, 1996.
47. Mullis-Jansson SL, Argenziano M, Corwin S, et al: A randomized double-blind study of the effect of triiodothyronine on cardiac function and morbidity after coronary bypass surgery. J Thorac Cardiovasc Surg 117:1128-1134, 1999.
48. Ranasinghe AM, Quinn DW, Pagano D, et al: Glucose-insulin-potassium and triiodothyronine individually improve hemodynamic performance and are associated with reduced troponin I release after on-pump coronary artery bypass grafting. Circulation 114:I245-I250, 2006.
49. van Wassenaer AG, Westera J, Houtzager BA, et al: Ten-year follow-up of children born at <30 weeks' gestational age supplemented with thyroxine in the neonatal period in a randomized, controlled trial. Pediatrics 116:e613-618, 2005.
50. Wadwekar D, Kabadi UM: Thyroid hormone indices during illness in six hypothyroid subjects rendered euthyroid with levothyroxine therapy. Exp Clin Endocrinol Diabetes 112:373-377, 2004.
51. Kaptein EM, Robinson WJ, Grieb DA, et al: Peripheral serum thyroxine, triiodothyronine and reverse triiodothyronine kinetics in the low thyroxine state of acute nonthyroidal illnesses. A noncompartmental analysis. J Clin Invest 69:526-535, 1982.
52. Fliers E, Guldenaar SE, Wiersinga WM, et al: Decreased hypothalamic thyrotropin-releasing hormone gene expression in patients with nonthyroidal illness. J Clin Endocrinol Metab 82:4032-4036, 1997.
53. Panicker V, Cluett C, Shields B, et al: A common variation in deiodinase 1 gene *DIO1* is associated with the relative levels of free thyroxine and triiodothyronine. J Clin Endocrinol Metab 93:3075-3081, 2008.
54. Peeters RP, Wouters PJ, Kaptein E, et al: Reduced activation and increased inactivation of thyroid hormone in tissues of critically ill patients. J Clin Endocrinol Metab 88:3202-3211, 2003.

55. Mebis L, Langouche L, Visser TJ, et al: The type II iodothyronine deiodinase is up-regulated in skeletal muscle during prolonged critical illness. J Clin Endocrinol Metab 92:3330-3333, 2007.
56. Rodriguez-Perez A, Palos-Paz F, Kaptein E, et al: Identification of molecular mechanisms related to nonthyroidal illness syndrome in skeletal muscle and adipose tissue from patients with septic shock. Clin Endocrinol (Oxf) 68:821-827, 2008.
57. Friesema EC, Ganguly S, Abdalla A, et al: Identification of monocarboxylate transporter 8 as a specific thyroid hormone transporter. J Biol Chem 278:40128-40135, 2003.
58. Friesema EC, Grueters A, Biebermann H, et al: Association between mutations in a thyroid hormone transporter and severe X-linked psychomotor retardation. Lancet 364:1435-1437, 2004.
59. Dumitrescu AM, Liao XH, Best TB, et al: A novel syndrome combining thyroid and neurological abnormalities is associated with mutations in a monocarboxylate transporter gene. Am J Hum Genet 74:168-175, 2004.
60. Alkemade A, Friesema EC, Unmehopa UA, et al: Neuroanatomical pathways for thyroid hormone feedback in the human hypothalamus. J Clin Endocrinol Metab 90:4322-4334, 2005.
61. Boelen A, Platvoet-Ter Schiphorst MC, Wiersinga WM: Association between serum interleukin-6 and serum 3,5,3′-triiodothyronine in nonthyroidal illness. J Clin Endocrinol Metab 77:1695-1699, 1993.
62. Stouthard JM, van der Poll T, Endert E, et al: Effects of acute and chronic interleukin-6 administration on thyroid hormone metabolism in humans. J Clin Endocrinol Metab 79:1342-1346, 1994.
63. Torpy DJ, Tsigos C, Lotsikas AJ, et al: Acute and delayed effects of a single-dose injection of interleukin-6 on thyroid function in healthy humans. Metabolism 47:1289-1293, 1998.
64. van der Poll T, Van Zee KJ, Endert E, et al: Interleukin-1 receptor blockade does not affect endotoxin-induced changes in plasma thyroid hormone and thyrotropin concentrations in man. J Clin Endocrinol Metab 80:1341-1346, 1995.
65. Damas P, Reuter A, Gysen P, et al: Tumor necrosis factor and interleukin-1 serum levels during severe sepsis in humans. Crit Care Med 17:975-978, 1989.
66. van der Poll T, Romijn JA, Wiersinga WM, et al: Tumor necrosis factor: A putative mediator of the sick euthyroid syndrome in man. J Clin Endocrinol Metab 71:1567-1572, 1990.
67. van der Poll T, Endert E, Coyle SM, et al: Neutralization of TNF does not influence endotoxin-induced changes in thyroid hormone metabolism in humans. Am J Physiol 276:R357-362, 1999.
68. Chopra IJ, Sakane S, Teco GN: A study of the serum concentration of tumor necrosis factor-alpha in thyroidal and nonthyroidal illnesses. J Clin Endocrinol Metab 72:1113-1116, 1991.
69. Rosenbaum M, Murphy EM, Heymsfield SB, et al: Low-dose leptin administration reverses effects of sustained weight-reduction on energy expenditure and circulating concentrations of thyroid hormones. J Clin Endocrinol Metab 87:2391-2394, 2002.
70. Welt CK, Chan JL, Bullen J, et al: Recombinant human leptin in women with hypothalamic amenorrhea. N Engl J Med 351:987-997, 2004.
71. Farooqi IS, Matarese G, Lord GM, et al: Beneficial effects of leptin on obesity, T cell hyporesponsiveness, and neuroendocrine/metabolic dysfunction of human congenital leptin deficiency. J Clin Invest 110:1093-1103, 2002.
72. Chan JL, Heist K, DePaoli AM, et al: The role of falling leptin levels in the neuroendocrine, metabolic adaptation to short-term starvation in healthy men. J Clin Invest 111:1409-1421, 2003.
73. Bornstein SR, Torpy DJ, Chrousos GP, et al: Leptin levels are elevated despite low thyroid hormone levels in the "euthyroid sick" syndrome. J Clin Endocrinol Metab 82:4278-4279, 1997.
74. Corsonello A, Buemi M, Artemisia A, et al: Plasma leptin concentrations in relation to sick euthyroid syndrome in elderly patients with nonthyroidal illnesses. Gerontology 46:64-70, 2000.
75. Boelen A, Maas MA, Lowik CW, et al: Induced illness in interleukin-6 (IL-6) knock-out mice: A causal role of IL-6 in the development of the low 3,5,3′-triiodothyronine syndrome. Endocrinology 137:5250-5254, 1996.
76. Kondo K, Harbuz MS, Levy A, et al: Inhibition of the hypothalamic-pituitary-thyroid axis in response to lipopolysaccharide is independent of changes in circulating corticosteroids. Neuroimmunomodulation 4:188-194, 1997.
77. Tu HM, Kim SW, Salvatore D, et al: Regional distribution of type 2 thyroxine deiodinase messenger ribonucleic acid in rat hypothalamus and pituitary and its regulation by thyroid hormone. Endocrinology 138:3359-3368, 1997.
78. Fekete C, Gereben B, Doleschall M, et al: Lipopolysaccharide induces type 2 iodothyronine deiodinase in the mediobasal hypothalamus: Implications for the nonthyroidal illness syndrome. Endocrinology 145:1649-1655, 2004.
79. Boelen A, Kwakkel J, Thijssen-Timmer DC, et al: Simultaneous changes in central, peripheral components of the hypothalamus-pituitary-thyroid axis in lipopolysaccharide-induced acute illness in mice. J Endocrinol 182:315-323, 2004.
80. Legradi G, Emerson CH, Ahima RS, et al: Leptin prevents fasting-induced suppression of prothyrotropin-releasing hormone messenger ribonucleic acid in neurons of the hypothalamic paraventricular nucleus. Endocrinology 138:2569-2576, 1997.
81. Seoane LM, Carro E, Tovar S, et al: Regulation of in vivo TSH secretion by leptin. Regul Pept 92:25-29, 2000.

82. Boelen A, Kwakkel J, Alkemade A, et al: Induction of type 3 deiodinase activity in inflammatory cells of mice with chronic local inflammation. Endocrinology 146:5128-5134, 2005.
83. Yu J, Koenig RJ: Regulation of hepatocyte thyroxine 5′-deiodinase by T3 and nuclear receptor coactivators as a model of the sick euthyroid syndrome. J Biol Chem 275:38296-38301, 2000.
84. Yu J, Koenig RJ: Induction of type 1 iodothyronine deiodinase to prevent the nonthyroidal illness syndrome in mice. Endocrinology 147:3580-3585, 2006.
85. Kwakkel J, Wiersinga WM, Boelen A: Differential involvement of nuclear factor-κB, activator protein-1 pathways in the interleukin-1β-mediated decrease of deiodinase type 1 and thyroid hormone receptor β1 mRNA. J Endocrinol 189:37-44, 2006.
86. Nagaya T, Fujieda M, Otsuka G, et al: A potential role of activated NF-κB in the pathogenesis of euthyroid sick syndrome. J Clin Invest 106:393-402, 2000.
87. Beigneux AP, Moser AH, Shigenaga JK, et al: Sick euthyroid syndrome is associated with decreased TR expression and DNA binding in mouse liver. Am J Physiol Endocrinol Metab 284:E228-E236, 2003.
88. Ghose R, Zimmerman TL, Thevananther S, et al: Endotoxin leads to rapid subcellular re-localization of hepatic RXRα: A novel mechanism for reduced hepatic gene expression in inflammation. Nucl Recept 2:4, 2004.
89. Zimmerman TL, Thevananther S, Ghose R, et al: Nuclear export of retinoid X receptor α in response to interleukin-1β–mediated cell signaling: Roles for JNK, SER260. J Biol Chem 281:15434-15440, 2006.
90. Olivares EL, Marassi MP, Fortunato RS, et al: Thyroid function disturbance and type 3 iodothyronine deiodinase induction after myocardial infarction in rats—a time course study. Endocrinology 148:4786-4792, 2007.
91. Simonides WS, Mulcahey MA, Redout EM, et al: Hypoxia-inducible factor induces local thyroid hormone inactivation during hypoxic-ischemic disease in rats. J Clin Invest 118:975-983, 2008.
92. Gereben B, Goncalves C, Harney JW, et al: Selective proteolysis of human type 2 deiodinase: A novel ubiquitin-proteasomal mediated mechanism for regulation of hormone activation. Mol Endocrinol 14:1697-1708, 2000.
93. Curcio-Morelli C, Zavacki AM, Christofollete M, et al: Deubiquitination of type 2 iodothyronine deiodinase by von Hippel-Lindau protein–interacting deubiquitinating enzymes regulates thyroid hormone activation. J Clin Invest 112:189-196, 2003.

Chapter 21

Syndromes of Resistance to Thyroid Hormone

Roy E. Weiss and Samuel Refetoff

Key Points

- Syndromes of resistance to thyroid hormone are a heterogeneous group of disorders.
- RTH is mostly caused by mutations in the thyroid hormone receptor β gene.
- Diagnosis is based on persistent elevations of serum free thyroxine and often triiodothyronine levels in absence of thyroid-stimulating hormone (thyrotropin) suppression.
- The key clinical feature is goiter, followed by palpitations and attention-deficit/hyperactivity disorder.
- The best treatment is to ensure that inadvertent thyroid gland ablation or surgical removal is not done.

Resistance to thyroid hormone (RTH), a syndrome of reduced end-organ responsiveness to thyroid hormone (TH), was described in 1967.[1] Various mechanisms to explain the syndrome were postulated, including defects in TH transport, metabolism, and action.[2] Subsequent to the identification of TH receptor (TR) β gene mutations,[3,4] the term *RTH* became synonymous with defects of the TR.[5] The recent discoveries of genetic defects that reduce the effectiveness of TH through altered cell membrane transport (see Chapter 22) and metabolism[6] have broadened the definition of TH insensitivity to encompass all defects that can interfere with the biologic activity of a chemically intact hormone secreted in normal amounts. In this chapter, use of the acronym RTH is limited to the syndrome produced by reduced intracellular action of the active TH, triiodothyronine (T_3).

Expression of TH effects requires the presence of sufficient amount of the active hormone T_3 within the cell. Rapid nongenomic action is exerted at the level of the plasma membrane and cytoplasm.[7] However, the principal, best-studied, and characterized effect requires the translocation of the hormone into the nucleus, where it interacts with TRs to activate or repress transcription of specific target genes. These genes contain nucleotide sequences at or near their promoter regions (TH response elements, or TREs) recognized by TRs for binding. In the absence of TH, TRs associate with other molecules, most notably the coregulator retinoid X receptor (RXR), and corepressors. These complexes have silencing effect on genes positively regulated by TH. The latter undergo conformational changes initiated by T_3 binding, which in turn trigger a chain of processes including release of the corepressor and recruitment of coactivators and a large number of other proteins. In positively controlled genes, this results in making the DNA more accessible for transcription.[8]

The cardinal features of RTH are elevated serum levels of free thyroxine (T_4) and often free T_3, normal or slightly increased serum thyrotropin (TSH), and absence of typical symptoms and metabolic consequences of TH excess.[5,9] Theoretically, interference at any step in the pathway following hormonogenesis that leads to hormone action would result in resistance. Whereas those caused by defective transport into the cell, subsequent metabolism, and action at the TR have been identified, defects in cytosolic action, translocation into the nucleus, and cofactors interacting with the TR remain to be elucidated (Fig. 21-1). If the defect responsible for TH action were restricted to specific organs or tissues, then the particular tissue would be hypothyroid relative to unaffected tissues, despite normal TH levels. More commonly, the hyposensitivity of the pituitary to TH produces an increase in TSH secretion, causing an increase in the circulating levels of TH

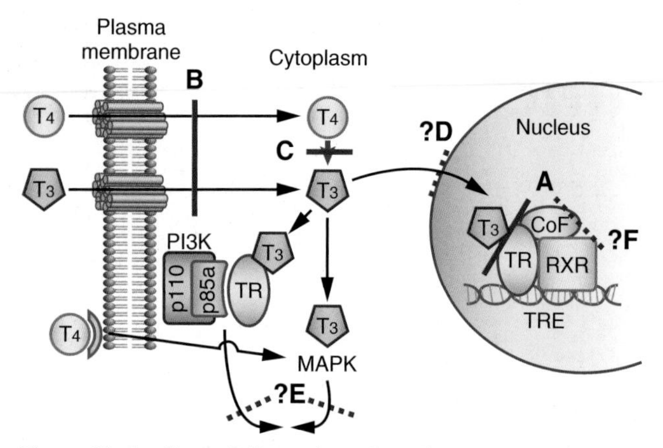

Figure 21–1 Sites of disruption of posthormonogenesis pathways involved in thyroid hormone (TH) activity. The most common cause of resistance to thyroid hormone (RTH), as described in this chapter, is impaired action of the TH receptor **(A).** However, a defect in transport of TH into the cell **(B)** as seen in *MCT8* mutations (see Chapter 22) or a defect in the conversion of thyroxine (T_4) to triiodothyronine (T_3), as seen in *SECISBP2* mutations,[6] can occur **(C).** Although possible but not yet described, impaired T_3 and TR translocation to the nucleus **(D)** or defects in nongenomic pathways of TH action **(E)** can by hypothesized. In addition, a defective cofactor interaction with thyroid hormone receptor (TR) **(F)** may also be responsible for non–thyroid hormone receptor resistance to thyroid hormone.

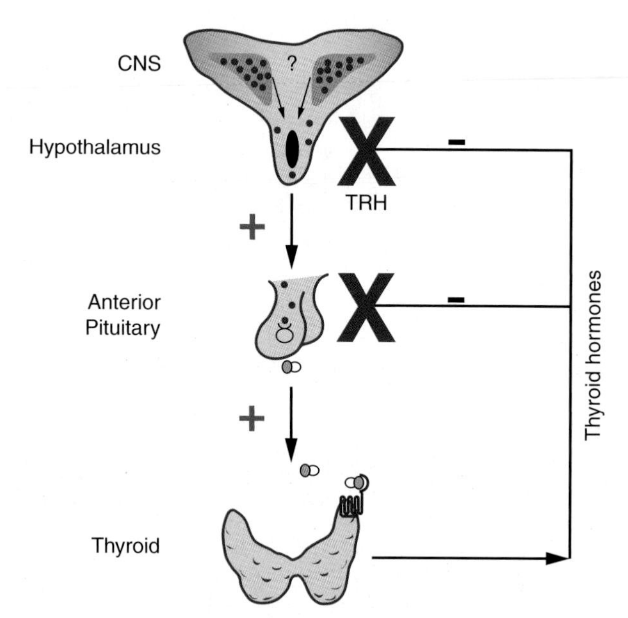

Figure 21–2 Regulation of thyroid hormone synthesis and secretion by the hypothalamus and pituitary. In resistance to thyroid hormone (RTH) syndrome, impaired feedback of thyroid hormone to the thyrotropes in the anterior pituitary and thyrotropin-releasing hormone (TRH) neurons in the hypothalamus result in increased stimulation of the thyroid gland to produce excess amounts of triiodothyronine and thyroxine. CNS, central nervous system. ***(Courtesy of Dr. Fredric Wondisford.)***

(Fig. 21-2). This provides compensation to tissues that are equally resistant whereas other tissues, such as the heart, which are primarily dependent on the TRα isoform, manifest signs of TH hormone excess.

The two TRs encoded by different genes, TRα and TRβ, are of similar structure.[10] They are members of the nuclear receptor superfamily that include, among others, receptors for vitamin D, glucocorticoids, mineralocorticoids sex hormones, retinoic acid, retinoid X (RXR), and the peroxisome proliferator-activated receptor (PPAR).[11-15] Defects in all these receptors produce syndromes reflecting the resulting reduced sensitivity to the cognate hormone.[16-21] The lack of other mechanisms causing resistance in hormones other than the thyroid likely reflects our inability to predict the clinical consequences resulting from transport and activation defects for most hormones. In the case of RTH, 85% of affected individuals have a mutation of the *TRβ* gene. The other 15% are presumed to have defects in cofactors or coregulators involved in the mediation of TH action at the nuclear level, although their precise nature remains unknown.[22-24]

Careful clinical evaluation of subjects with RTH-like syndromes can be helpful in determining the site of the defect (see later). For example, administration of incremental doses of T_3 and T_4 can identify a defect in iodothyronine metabolism when T_3 but not T_4 appropriately suppresses the serum TSH.[6] RTH, in contrast, will show resistance to the suppressive effects of both iodothyronines. Proper interpretation of seemingly paradoxical thyroid function tests is necessary for appropriate diagnosis. The purpose of this chapter is to present the methods available for diagnosis of RTH and suggest options for management of this condition.

EPIDEMIOLOGY, RISK FACTORS, PATHOGENESIS

The precise incidence of RTH is not known because it is usually not detected by routine neonatal screening for hypothyroidism, using blood spot TSH determination. A limited screen for high T_4 values found a prevalence of 1 in 40,000 life births.[25] Equal number of males and females are affected, although the prevalence of RTH without TR mutations is more common in females.[26]

In most cases, RTH is caused by mutations in the *TRβ* gene, located on chromosome 3. Mutations have been found in the carboxyl terminus of the TRβ covering the ligand-binding domain and adjacent hinge domain of the TRβ protein (Fig. 21-3).[27-29] They are contained within three clusters rich in CG hot spots, separated by areas devoid of mutations (cold regions). The latter are located

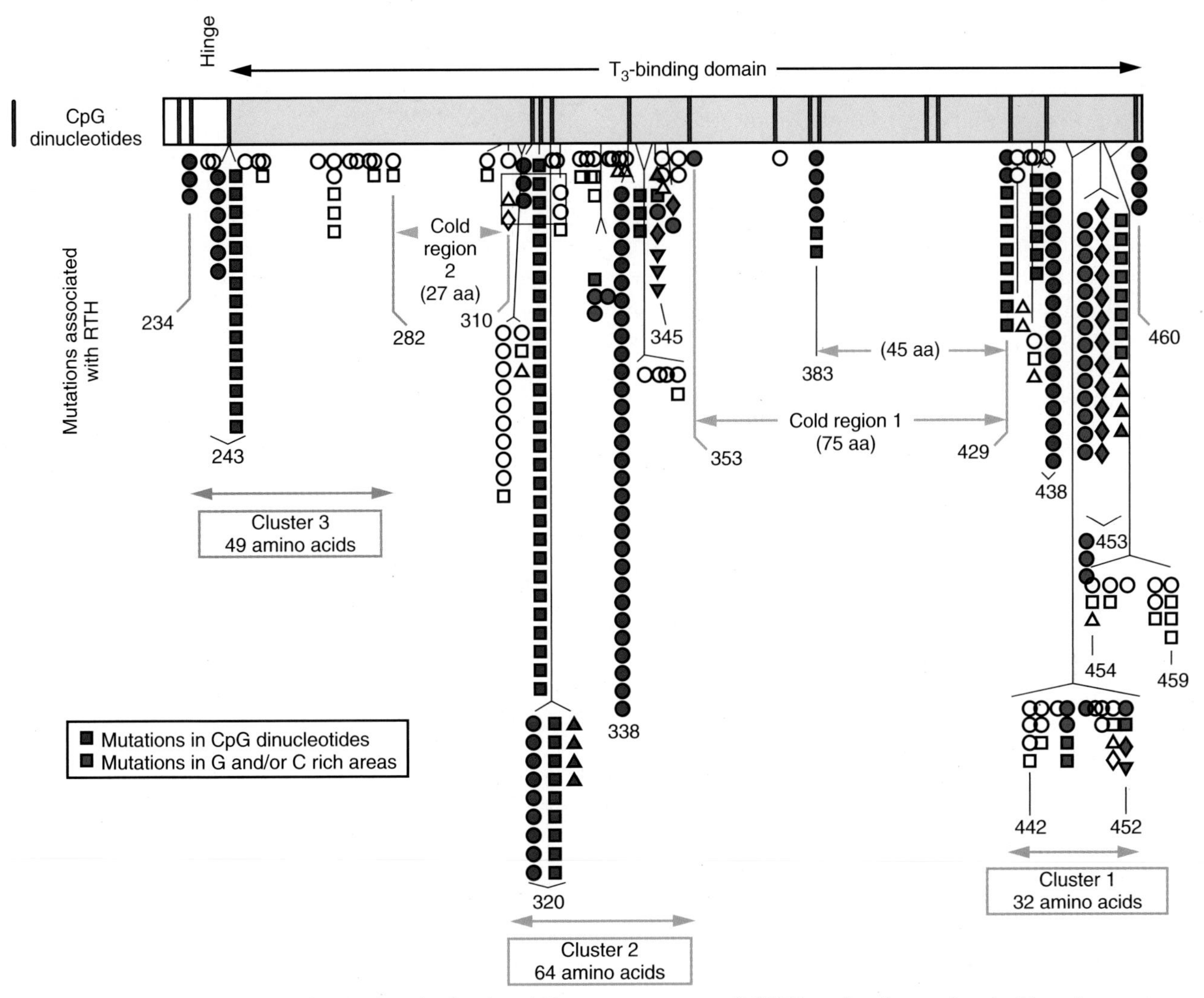

Figure 21–3 Location of natural mutations in the thyroid hormone receptor β (TRβ) molecule associated with resistance to thyroid hormone (RTH). The triiodothyronine (T_3)–binding domain and distal end of the hinge region, which contain the three mutation clusters, are expanded and show the positions of CpG dinucleotide mutational hot spots in the corresponding TRβ gene. The location of the 121 different mutations detected in 299 unrelated families are each indicated by a symbol. Identical mutations in members of unrelated families are represented by the same shading pattern of vertically placed symbols. Cold regions are areas devoid of mutations associated with RTH. *(Adapted from Refetoff S: Defects of Thyroid Hormone Transport in Serum, 2007. Available at http://www.thyroidmanager.org/Chapter16/16c-frame.htm.)*

between codons 282 and 310 and, with the exception of 383, codons 353 and 429. No mutation has been reported upstream of codon 234. Because cold regions are not devoid of hot spots, the lack of mutations reflects the observation that mutations in the second cold region do not impair TR function and therefore are not expected to produce a phenotype.[30]

TRβ gene defects have been identified in 344 families, comprising 124 distinct mutations. We have found mutations in 148 families (a partial listing is available online at http://www.receptors.org/cgi-bin/nrmd/nrmd.py). Although mostly missense mutations, nucleotide deletion and insertions producing frame shifts have created nonsense proteins with two additional amino acids in five cases. In four cases, single nucleotide deletions have produced truncated receptors. In only one family, complete *TRβ* gene deletion resulted in recessively inherited RTH.[31] The following mutations have been identified in more than 10 unrelated families, often the consequence of de novo mutations: *R243Q* (15 families); *A317T* (29 families); *R338W* (30 families); *R438H* (17 families); *P453T* (17 families); and *P453S* (12 families). Of these frequently observed mutations, all are in CG hot spots or long stretches of Cs (see Fig. 21-3).

The mutant TRβ molecules have reduced affinity for T_3[27,28] or impaired interaction with one of the cofactors involved in the mediation of thyroid hormone action.[28,32-34] Because TR mutants are still able to bind to TREs on DNA and dimerize with normal TRs or the RXR partner, they interfere with the function of the normal TRs, explaining the dominant mode of inheritance. Therefore, it is not surprising that in the single family reported with a deletion of all coding sequences of the *TRβ* gene, only homozygotes manifested the phenotype of RTH.[31]

A family with two de novo *TRβ* gene mutations occurring in the same nucleotide has been reported.[35] The proposita with apparent de novo missense mutation (GTG to GGG) in codon 458 of the *TRβ* gene *(V458G)* transmitted this mutation to her affected son. The mutant allele underwent another de novo mutation that was transferred to her affected daughter as GAG *(V458E)*. This apparent attempt of repair is more likely the result of the creation of a mutagenic three-guanine sequence by the first mutation.

No mutations in the *TRα* gene have been identified so far in humans. Based on observations in transgenic mice (see later, "Animal Models"), a putative *TRα* gene mutation should not cause RTH.

Non–Thyroid Hormone Receptor Resistance to Thyroid Hormone

In 1996, we reported a family in which RTH manifested in the absence of *TRβ* gene mutation and a *TRβ* gene transcript of normal size and abundance.[24] Nevertheless, fibroblasts were resistant to the in vitro effect of TH. Recombinant wild-type (WT) TRβ interacted aberrantly with nuclear extracts of fibroblasts from affected individuals of the family but not from normal individuals or subjects with complete *TRβ* gene deletion, and far-Western analysis has revealed an additional 84-kD band. More families with non-TR RTH were subsequently reported.[22,36-38] We have identified non-TR RTH in 27 out of 175 families with RTH studied. Similarly, glucocorticoid and androgen resistance have now been described in the absence of mutations in the respective receptors,[39,40] as well as partial resistance to several steroid hormones in the same subjects.[41] It should be noted that mosaicism should be considered in any subject with phenotypic RTH in whom no mutation can be demonstrated in a particular cell lineage.[42]

Animal Models

The generation of mice with *TRβ* deletion (knockout [KO]) and with mutations (knock-in [KI]) replicating those observed in humans have been important in understanding TR function and the pathophysiology of RTH. Similar manipulations of the *TRα* gene have allowed the prediction of a putative phenotype for corresponding human gene abnormalities.[43]

TRβ Gene Manipulation

TRβ KO mice manifest all the features of humans with *TRβ* gene deletion. Heterozygotes are normal and homozygotes have the typical thyroid function test abnormalities as well as sensorineural deafness and monochromatic vision.[44] Thus, deaf mutism and color blindness in humans can be fully explained by the TRβ deficiency.[1] *TRβ* KO mice have increased heart rate that can be corrected with reduction of the TH level. This finding, together with the lower heart rate in *TRα1* KO mice,[43] supports the concept that TH affects heart rate through TRα1, and explains the tachycardia observed in some patients with RTH.

TRβ KI mice, produced according to human *TRβ* gene mutations, are true models of the dominantly inherited form of RTH. Heterozygous KI mice manifest many of the abnormalities observed in humans. In addition, homozygotes develop metastatic thyroid cancer.[45]

TRα Gene Manipulation

TRα gene deletions, total or only α*1*, do not produce important alterations in thyroid function.[46] Several human mutations occurring in the *TRβ* gene[47-49] were targeted in homologous regions of the *TRα* gene of the mouse. The resulting phenotypes were variable but had no resemblance to RTH. The heterozygotes showed severe postnatal development and growth retardation, as well as increased body fat and insulin resistance. Decreased heart rate and reduced fertility were also observed. All *TRα* KIs were lethal in the homozygous state, in agreement with the noxious effect of unliganded TRα1.

Combined *TRα* and *TRβ* Gene Deletions

Deletion of both α and β TRs is compatible with life.[50,51] This contrasts with the complete TH deficiency as in the athyreotic *Pax8* KO mouse that, if untreated, dies prior to weaning. Removal of the TRα gene rescues the *Pax8* KO mice from death.[52] Deletion of the *TRα1* gene also prevents the development of cerebellar abnormalities during TH deprivation.[53] Although the unliganded TRα is not required for the upregulation of TSH, it allows TH-mediated suppression in the absence of TRβ.

Cofactor and Coregulator Deletion

Mice deficient in the coactivator SRC-1 have resistance to TH in addition to sex hormones.[54] Mice deficient in RXRγ, the dimerization partner of TR, are also mildly resistant to TH.[55]

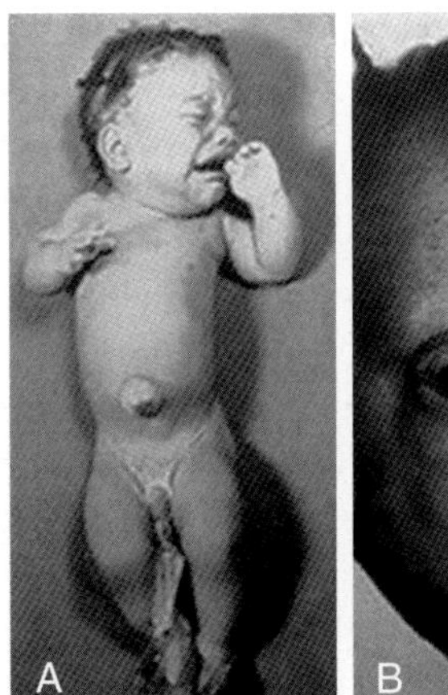

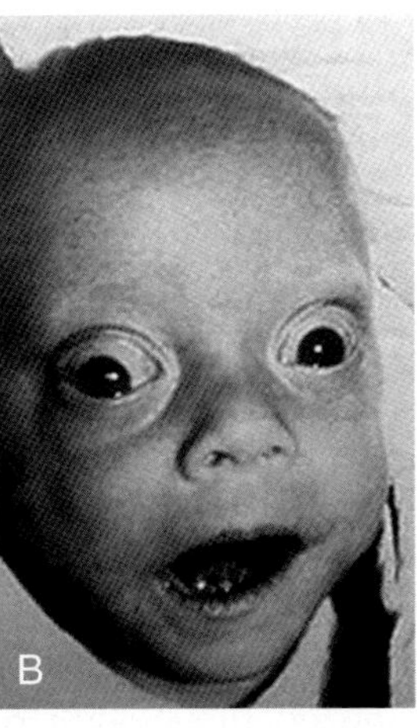

Figure 21–4 Two children with resistance to thyroid hormone (RTH) syndrome showing clinical manifestations at the extremes of the spectrum. **A,** 1-month old infant homozygous for a single amino acid (Thr 337) deletion in the *TRβ* gene showing emaciation and a stare caused by lid retraction or hydrocephalus, giving the appearance of thyrotoxicosis. **B,** 7-month old infant with typical cretinoid and hypothyroid appearance, including narrow forehead, pug nose, large tongue, thin extremities, pot belly, and umbilical hernia. *(**A** from Ono S, Schwartz ID, Mueller OT, et al: Homozygosity for a dominant negative thyroid hormone receptor gene responsible for generalized resistance to thyroid hormone. J Clin Endocrinol Metab 73:990-994, 1991; **B** from Refetoff S, Weiss RE, Usala SJ: The syndromes of resistance to thyroid hormone. Endocr Rev 14:348-399, 1993.)*

Table 21–1 Clinical Features: Frequency of Symptoms and Signs

Findings	Frequency (%)
Thyroid gland	Goiter (66-95)
Heart	Tachycardia (33-75)
Nervous system	Emotional disturbances (60) Hyperkinetic behavior (33-68) Attention-deficit/hyperactivity disorder (40-60) Learning disability (30) Mental retardation, IQ < 70 (4-16) Hearing loss, sensorineural (10-22)
Growth and development	Short stature, less than 5th percentile (18-25) Delayed bone age > 2 SD (29-47) Low body mass index (in children) (33)
Recurrent ear and throat infections	Viral (55)

IQ, intellectual quotient.

(Data from Refetoff S, Weiss RE, Usala SJ: The syndromes of resistance to thyroid hormone. Endocr Rev 14:348-399, 1993; Beck-Peccoz P, Chatterjee VK: The variable clinical phenotype in thyroid hormone resistance syndrome. Thyroid 4:225-232, 1994; and Brucker-Davis F, Skarulis MC, Grace MB, et al: Genetic and clinical features of 42 kindreds with resistance to thyroid hormone. The National Institutes of Health Prospective Study. Ann Intern Med 123:572-583, 1995.)

CLINICAL FEATURES

Presenting Complaints

RTH lacks specific clinical manifestations. When present, they are variable and signs of TH deficiency and excess often coexist.[5,56] Investigation may be initiated when hypothyroidism is suspected in a child with short stature, learning disability, or mental retardation. In contrast, thyrotoxicosis may be the reason for investigation in a hyperactive youngster or an adult with tachycardia. The detection of a goiter has been also a reason for thyroid testing in children and adults. Formerly, the diagnosis was often missed because of failure to recognize the normal or elevated TSH, leading to treatment aimed at normalizing the elevated TH levels. In such patients, symptoms of fatigue, somnolence, depression, and weight gain associated with bradycardia have ensued. More dramatic is the growth retardation resulting from treatment of children with antithyroid drugs. This has been less common in the last decade with wider recognition of RTH.

Although most patients with RTH are clinically euthyroid, presentation can range from a stare suggestive of exophthalmos to hypotonia, umbilical hernia, and cretinoid facies (Fig. 21-4). Symptoms and sign and their frequency are shown in Table 21-1.

Thyroid Gland

Goiter is by far the most common abnormality. In several studies, its prevalence has been reported to range from 66% to 95%. Large goiters are, however, rare.[5] One severely affected RTH newborn presented with tracheal compression and respiratory difficulty[57] and one subject had esophageal constriction secondary to a goiter.[58]

Growth and Development

Failure to thrive and growth delay are not uncommon. However, this rarely results in short stature. More often, children have delay in bone age and low body mass index. Permanent short stature is associated mental retardation (IQ < 70).

Psychological Profile

Emotional disturbances are found in two thirds of subjects with RTH. Most common is the occurrence of attention-deficit/hyperactivity disorder (ADHD), identified in 40% to 60% of cases. Although ADHD is common in individuals with RTH, the latter is rarely found in subjects with the primary diagnosis of ADHD. It is of note that children with combined RTH with ADHD have a lower IQ than those with ADHD only.[59] Learning disabilities alone or in combination with ADHD pose significant problems in school, and many children requiring special classes and treatment with methylphenidate.

Heart

Tachycardia has been reported in 33% to 75% of cases. Together with hyperactivity, it is a common finding suggestive of thyrotoxicosis. It is the consequence of TH excess acting on the heart that expresses the mutant *TRβ* at a very low level. The resulting symptom of palpitations prompts 25% of adults with RTH to seek medical advice.

Ears

Deafness is rare and has been reported only in three affected members of one family homozygous for *TRβ* gene deletion.[31] On the other hand, mild hearing impairment as result of recurrent ear infections has been reported 50% of cases.[60]

Osteoporosis

Bone is a TRα–dependent tissue.[61,62] Subjects with RTH have increased bone marker turnover[63] and therefore are at risk for decreased bone mineral density.

Miscellaneous Findings

Various physical findings that cannot be explained on the basis of TH deprivation or excess have been noted. These include major or minor somatic defects, such as winged scapulae, vertebral anomalies, pigeon breast, prominent pectoralis, birdlike facies, scaphocephaly, short fourth metacarpals, and craniosynostosis as well as Besnier's prurigo, ectodermal dysplasia, and congenital ichthyosis. Bull's eye–type macular atrophy, resulting in color blindness, is on the other hand caused by TR deletion, as in mice.[64] The following conditions have been reported in individuals with RTH: enuresis, schizophrenia, recurrent pneumonia, seizures, rheumatic fever, empty sella, medullary cystic disease of the kidney, types 1 and 2 diabetes mellitus, migraine, and proptosis.[5]

Concurrent Thyroid Disease

Clinically challenging is the diagnosis of RTH when it occurs in combination with other thyroid conditions that independently alter TH concentrations. RTH has been reported with concurrent autoimmune hypothyroidism[65-67] and in a patient with thyroid dysgenesis.[68] The resulting limited thyroidal reserve prevents full compensation, and subjects present with very high TSH levels, despite normal TH concentrations. *TRβ* gene sequencing is important in confirming the diagnosis of RTH in such cases. We have found autoimmune hyperthyroidism in two individuals with RTH (unpublished findings).

Fertility and Pregnancy

An accurate evaluation of fertility and pregnancy outcome in RTH had been difficult to obtain until the discovery of a large Azorean kindred harboring the TRβ mutation *R343Q*.[69,70] A three- to fourfold increase in the rate of miscarriages was observed in affected women as compared with that in spouses of affected fathers or unaffected first-degree relatives. Fertility was not impaired in affected couples, regardless of whether women or men harbored the mutant *TRβ* gene. The difference in genotype frequency in the progeny of affected mothers (20 affected vs. 11 unaffected offspring), combined with a significantly higher miscarriage rate, suggests that these women tend to lose more normal than affected fetuses. This was not found in the progeny of affected fathers, whose spouses had almost equal number of affected and unaffected offspring (15 and 12, respectively). Because the mothers with RTH were not thyrotoxic and had no thyroid autoantibodies, it may be concluded that miscarriages were the consequence of the fetal exposure to the high levels of TH. This is supported by the improved survival of the affected fetuses for whom high TH levels were physiologic, as in their affected mothers. Contrary to findings in uncontrolled maternal hyperthyroidism, women with RTH have no increased frequency of premature labor, preeclampsia, stillbirths, or perinatal loss.

Unaffected infants born to affected mothers have a significantly lower weight at birth than their affected siblings. This suggests that the high maternal TH level was able to induce a catabolic state during fetal life, similar to what happens in children and adults with uncontrolled hyperthyroidism. That these infants were thyrotoxic is supported by their suppressed blood TSH level at birth (Fig. 21-5).

DIAGNOSIS

Baseline Thyroid Function Tests

RTH should be considered in subjects with elevated TH levels and nonsuppressed TSH values (Fig. 21-6). The differential diagnosis of euthyroid hyperthyroxinemia includes transport defects as well as T_4 to T_3 conversion defects. The presence of a goiter with elevation of free T_4 and, in most cases, free T_3 concentration with normal or elevated TSH levels is diagnostic of RTH. The presence of autoantibodies raises the suspicion that circulating substances may

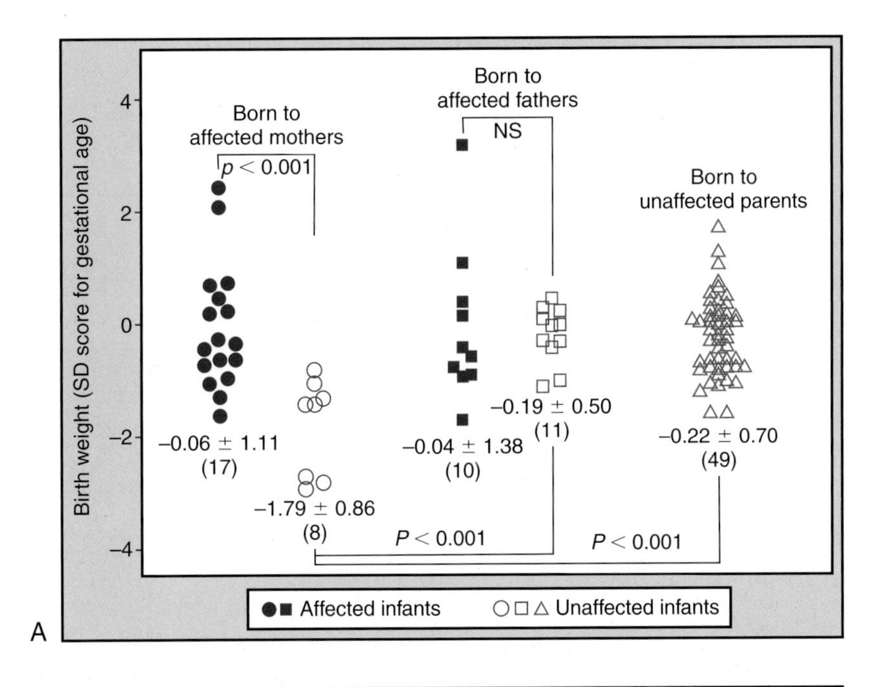

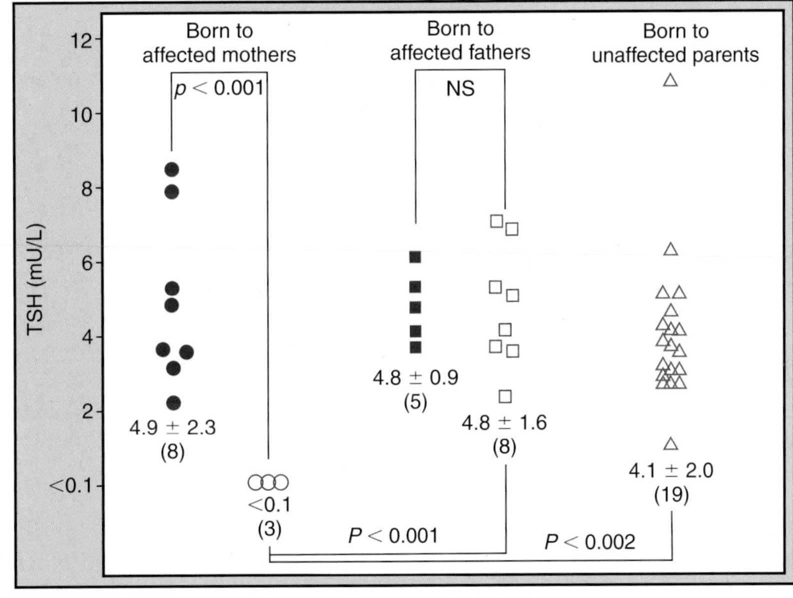

Figure 21–5 **A,** Birth weights in the different groups according to genotype. Data are expressed as mean SD score for gestational age using a chart obtained for singleton infants born to the Portuguese population and adjusted for the sex of the infant. A highly significant reduction in birth weight was found only in unaffected infants born to affected mothers. In additions, 3 of the infants in this group are of low birth weight, according to World Health Organization criteria. **B,** Neonatal blood TSH concentrations in the different groups and according to genotype. Only unaffected infants botn to RTH mothers had undetectable blood TSH values. *(Adapted from Anselmo J, Cao D, Karrison T, et al: Fetal loss associated with excess thyroid hormone exposure. JAMA 292:691-695, 2004.)*

interfere with measurement of THs or, more rarely, of TSH. Exclusion of such antibodies by direct testing or confirmation using different assays is advisable. Reverse T_3 (rT_3) concentrations are also high and the levels of thyroglobulin (TG) reflect the degree of serum TSH elevation. Thyroidal radioiodide uptake is increased and ultrasound of the thyroid gland demonstrates the presence of gland enlargement, diffuse or multinodular. The finding of goiter in the presence of normal serum TSH levels is explained by the increase of TSH bioactivity in RTH.[71]

Distinction between RTH and a TSH-secreting pituitary adenoma (TSH-oma) can be challenging. No single test is conclusive and diagnosis of RTH must rest on a combination of tests and observations: (1) absence of an elevated serum concentration of the alpha pituitary glycoprotein subunit; (2) stimulation of TSH following the administration of TSH-releasing hormone (TRH);

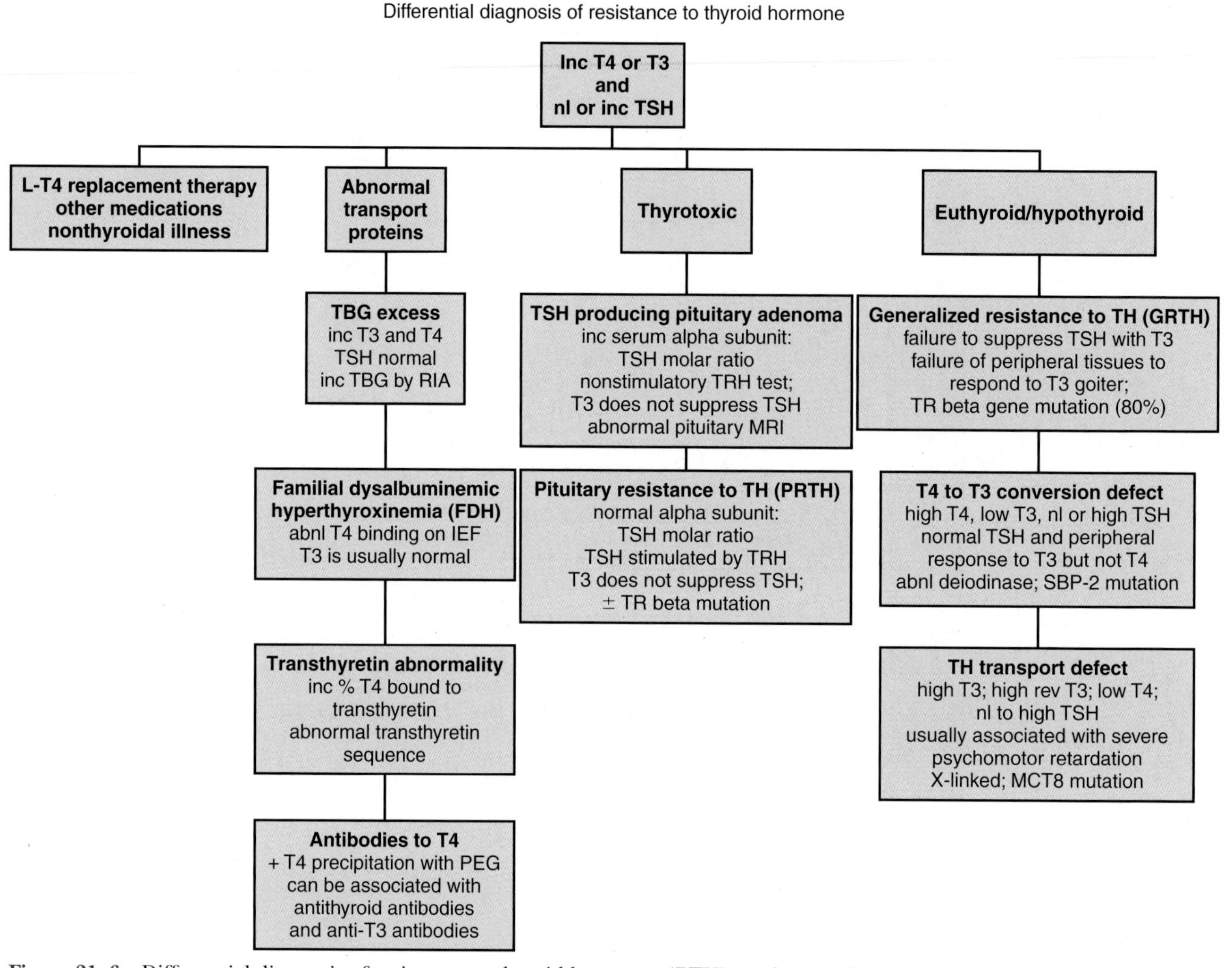

Figure 21–6 Differential diagnosis of resistance to thyroid hormone (RTH) syndrome. IEF, isoelectric focusing; L-T_4, levothyroxine; PEG, polyethylene glycol; RIA, radioimmunoassay; T_3, triiodothyronine; T_4, thyroxine; TBG, thyroxine-binding globulin; TH, thyroid hormone; TR, thyroid hormone receptor; TSH, thyroid-stimulating hormone.

(3) presence of thyroid test abnormalities compatible with RTH in other family members; (4) absence of elevated serum sex hormone–binding globulin (SHBG) concentration, reflecting a euthyroid state; and (5) ability to suppress serum TSH with supraphysiologic doses of levotriiodothyronine (L-T_3).

Thyrotropin-Releasing Hormone Stimulation Test

The TRH stimulation test measures the increase in TSH in serum in response to the administration of synthetic TRH. The magnitude of the response is modulated by the thyrotropic suppressibility by TH and is inversely proportional to the concentration of free TH in serum. The response is exquisitely sensitive to minor changes in the level of circulating TH, which may not be detected by direct measurement. The main use of the test is for the differential diagnosis of inappropriate TSH secretion, in particular when a TSH-oma is suspected. TSH is usually not stimulated by TRH in TSH-omas.[72,73]

The standard test uses a single TRH dose of 200 μg/1.73 m^2 body surface area, given by rapid intravenous injection. Serum is collected before the test, at 15 minutes, and then at 30-minute intervals over a period of 120 to 180 minutes. Many clinicians obtain blood for TSH measurements before and a single postinjection sample at 15, 20, or 30 minutes. Normal peak TSH response is at 15 to 40 minutes (i.e., on average, or five times the basal level). The decline is more gradual, with a return of serum TSH to the preinjection level by 3 to 4 hours.[74] Determination of TSH before and 30 minutes after the injection of TRH provides information concerning the presence or absence of TSH responsiveness but cannot detect delayed or prolonged responses. At the time

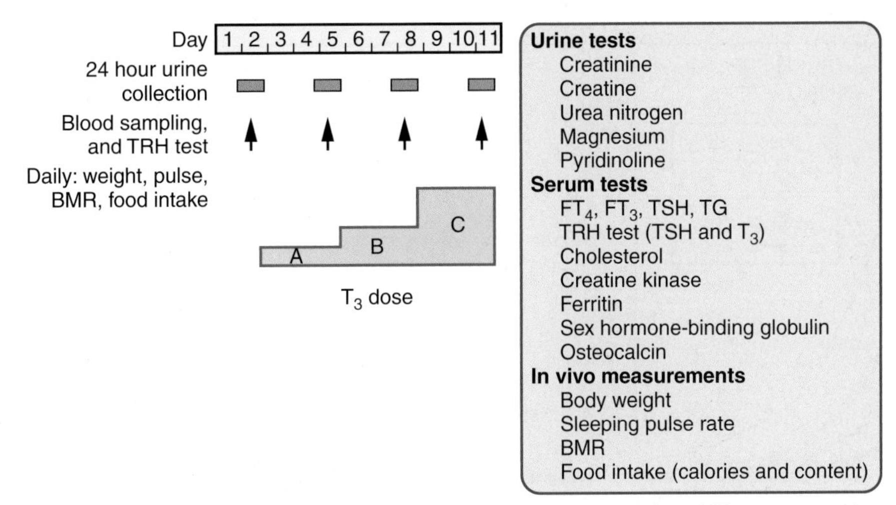

Figure 21–7 Schematic representation of a protocol for the in vivo assessment of thyroid hormone action used at the University of Chicago. It is used to establish the diagnosis of resistance to thyroid hormone (RTH) syndrome. See text for details. BMR, basal metabolic rate; FT_4, free thyroxine; T_3, triiodothyronine; TG, thyroglobulin; TRH, thyrotropin-releasing hormone; TSH, thyroid-stimulating hormone.

of this writing, TRH is not available here but can be obtained for use in the United States (from Ferring Arzneimittel, GmbH, Kiel, Germany) after submitting an investigational new drug (IND) application from the U.S. Food and Drug Administration (FDA).

Levotriiodothyronine Suppression Test

The measurement of responses to the administration of incremental doses of TH is the best method to assess the presence and magnitude of the hormonal resistance and obtain a clinical diagnosis of RTH. The rational for the use of L-T_3 rather than L-T_4 is its direct effect on tissues, independent of variations in T_4 metabolism. The rapid onset of L-T_4 action reduces the period of hormone administration and the shorter half-life of this hormone decreases the duration of symptoms that may arise in hormonally responsive subjects. The protocol is outlined in Figure 21-7 and a detailed description has been published.[5] It involves the administration of three incremental doses of L-T_3, each for 3 days. Amounts range from just below to three times above replacement. Hospitalization for 11 days is required for the detailed study, which includes measurement of sleeping pulse, basal metabolic rate (BMR), and calorie balance, for which food intake is controlled and urinary nitrogen excretion is measured.

Dosages of L-T_3 for adults are 50, 100, and 200 μg/day, each given for three consecutive days in a split dose every 12 hours, a total of six doses per increment. Corresponding doses for children, adjusted for size and age to obtain similar serum levels of T_3, are available.[5] A TRH test is performed at baseline and at the time of the administration of the last L-T_3 dose of each increment. Blood samples drawn over 180 minutes are used to measure the TSH and prolactin responses, as well as the nadir and peak of serum T_3 levels achieved with each incremental dose. Measurements of TG and T_4 assess the magnitude of thyroid gland suppression, whereas those of serum cholesterol, creatine kinase, ferritin, SHBG, and osteocalcin (OC) assess the responses of peripheral tissues to the hormone. Figure 21-8 shows typical results obtained in a normal subject as compared with those of subjects with RTH and with and without TRβ gene mutations.

Color Flow Doppler Sonography

Recently, the use of color flow Doppler sonography of the thyroid gland has been shown to distinguish between patients with TSH-omas and those with RTH.[75] The test is performed during the course of L-T_3 suppression according to the schedule described earlier. The increased pattern and peak systolic velocity normalized in 8 of 10 patients with RTH, but not in any of the 8 patients with a TSH-oma.

Prenatal Diagnosis

Although prenatal diagnosis of RTH based on genetic testing of amniotic fluid has not been reported, we have successfully identified the genotype of fetuses carried by women with RTH who were known to have *TRβ* gene mutations.

TREATMENT

There is no available treatment to correct the specific defect. Current treatments are aimed at alleviating symptoms when present. Most important is not to treat asymptomatic fully compensated individuals

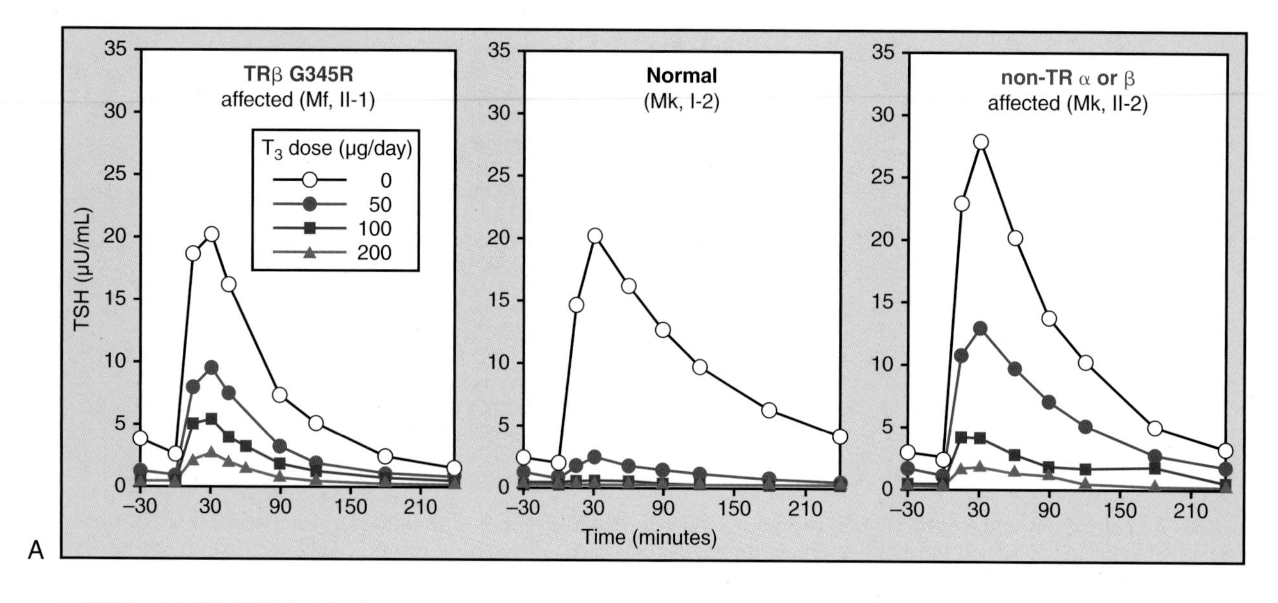

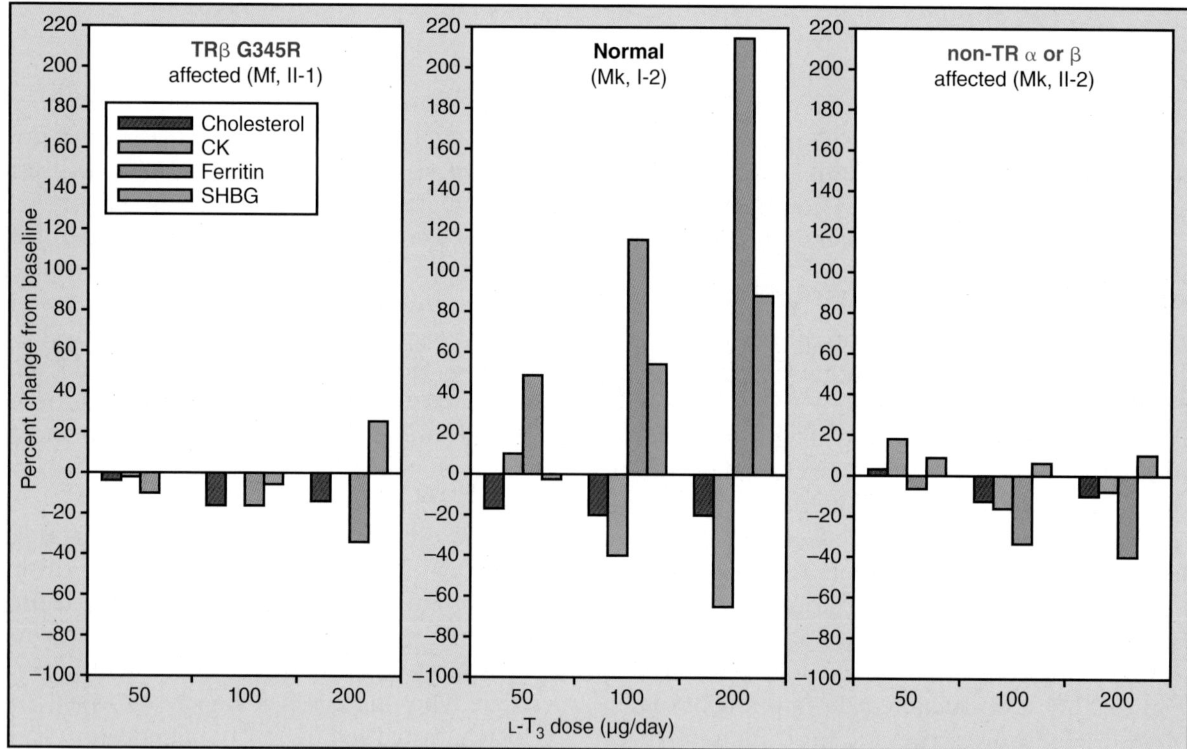

Figure 21–8 **A,** Thyrotropic responses to thyrotropin-releasing hormone (TRH) stimulation at baseline and after the administration of graded doses of levotriiodothyronine (L-T_3). The hormone was given in three incremental doses, each for 3 days, as depicted in Figure 21-7. Results are shown for patients with resistance to thyroid hormone (RTH) syndrome in the presence (left) or absence (right) of a thyroid receptor β (TRβ) gene mutation, together with the unaffected mother of the patient with non-TR RTH (center). **B,** Responses of peripheral tissues to the administration of L-T_3 in the presence or absence of mutations in the TRβ gene. The hormone was given as described in Figure 21-7. Note the stimulation of ferritin and sex hormone–binding globulin (SHBG) and the suppression of cholesterol and creatine kinase (CK) in the normal subject. Responses in affected subjects, with or without a TRβ gene mutation, were blunted or paradoxical. TSH, thyroid-stimulating hormone. *(Adapted from Refetoff S: Defects of Thyroid Hormone Transport in Serum, 2007. Available at http://www.thyroidmanager.org/Chapter16/16c-frame.htm.)*

with the sole purpose of correcting the laboratory test abnormalities. Prior ablative treatment, resulting from misdiagnosis, requires the administration of TH often in supraphysiologic doses.

When Not to Treat

There is no reason to treat subjects with elevated levels of TH appropriate for the degree of both thyrotropic and peripheral tissue resistance. Although the theoretical probability of developing thyrotropic adenomas caused by a long-standing increase in thyrotropic activity has been suggested, only one case of a pituitary adenoma in a subject with RTH has been reported.[76] In mouse models of RTH, pituitary pathology consists of thyrotropic hyperplasia only, particularly in homozygotes, which rarely occurs in humans. Using the same logic, the thyroid gland, which is under increased stimulation by TSH, may also be prone to tumor development, but there is no increased incidence of thyroid cancer in RTH and goiters are rarely obstructive. A mouse model homozygous for a mutation in the *TRβ* gene will develop papillary thyroid cancer,[45] but the relevance in humans is unknown. Therefore, the mainstay for the management of RTH patients who are asymptomatic is to recognize the correct diagnosis and avoid antithyroid treatment.

Real and Apparent Thyroid Hormone Deficiency

Intervention is recommended in patients who present with objective findings of TH deprivation, usually because of treatment aimed to decrease the circulating TH level. If the consequence is reversible, such as antithyroid drugs, treatment should be discontinued. In the case of prior ablative treatment (surgery or radioiodide), judicious administration of supraphysiologic doses of TH are usually required. The dose of TH needs to be titrated in an incremental manner to normalize the serum TSH concentration. Dosages of L-T_4 as high as 500 to 1000 μg/day may be necessary to obtain the desired TH effect. Tachycardia should not be a contraindication for T_4 treatment because it can be managed with atenolol (see later). Most difficult is the treatment of children with apparent hypothyroidism manifesting as growth retardation with delayed bone age and failure to thrive. A guide for TH dosage in such children is growth, bone maturation, and mental development. In addition, it is suggested that BMR, nitrogen balance, and serum SHBG be monitored at each dose increment.

Apparent Thyroid Hormone Excess

The most common symptom suggestive of hyperthyroidism is sinus tachycardia, present in about 50% of patients with RTH. When symptomatic, or limiting exercise tolerance, treatment with a beta-adrenergic blocking agent is effective. Some beta blockers, such as propanolol (Inderal), have an added effect of inhibiting conversion of T_4 to T_3, which is not desirable in RTH. We prefer to use atenolol, which does not have this added effect of depriving the TH-resistant cells of TH. More generalized symptoms of hyperthyroidism, including tremor, heat intolerance, sweating, and agitation, may also benefit from treatment with atenolol. However, this may not be effective in extreme cases. Two other approaches have been used but experience is limited; these are reduction of TSH secretion and blocking the action of TH.

Reduction of Thyroid-Stimulating Hormone Secretion

Agents in this category include glucocorticoids, somatostatin, and dopaminergic drugs. Although effective at reducing the TSH concentration, glucocorticoids have unacceptable side effects and therefore are not clinically useful. Dopaminergic agents such as bromocriptine or pergolide can reduce the TSH concentration but lose their effectiveness when used for a prolonged period. In addition, patients may not tolerate the gastrointestinal side effects.[58,77-79] The somatostatin analogue SMS201-995 was studied in three patients with RTH and found to have a weaker and more transient effect when compared with that in patients with TSH-omas.[80]

Goiter

Thyroid gland enlargement is usually modest, but large goiters occasionally occur. Surgical treatment is not effective in the long term because goiters are notorious for their recurrence, and contrary to autoimmune thyroid disease, there is no underlying destructive process. Thus, it is more effective to inhibit thyroid gland growth by suppression of TSH. The latter has been achieved by treating with a single large dose of L-T_3 given every second day (Fig. 21-9). The high levels of serum T_3 produced a few hours after ingestion of the hormone are effective in suppressing TSH but do not persist, so symptoms of TH excess do not develop.[81]

Reduction Thyroid Hormone Action Using Analogues

Triiodothyroacetic acid (TRIAC) is a TH analogue with low hormonal potency but high affinity for the TR[82] and very rapid turnover, requiring the use of doses more than 1000-fold those of L-T_3. In vitro studies have shown that the binding affinity of TRIAC is almost three times that of T_3 for normal TRβ and similar to T_3 for TRα1.[83] TRIAC was also more potent than T_3 in the transactivation of some

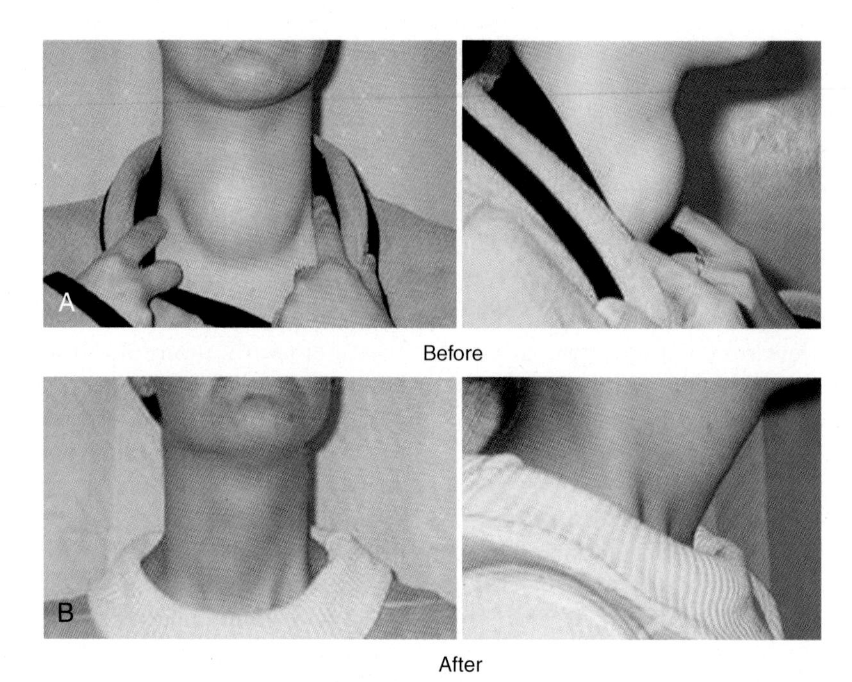

Figure 21–9 Goiter in a patient with resistance to thyroid hormone (RTH) syndrome. **A,** Patient's neck just before beginning of treatment. Although doses of 150 μg of levotriiodothyronine (L-T_3) every other day for 11 months resulted in a decrease in thyroid-stimulating hormone (TSH) level from 1.1 to 0.24 mU/L, there was no decrease in the size of the goiter. **B,** However, treatment with 250 μg L-T_3 every other day for 7 months resulted in disappearance of the goiter and serum TSH levels below 0.08 mU/L, associated with a modest increase in body weight and no symptoms of thyroid hormone excess. *(From Anselmo J, Refetoff S: Regression of a large goiter in a patient with resistance to thyroid hormone by every other day treatment with triiodothyronine. Thyroid 14:71-74, 2004.)*

mutant TRβs, suggesting that TRIAC may overcome a dominant negative effect of these mutant TRβs.[83] Long-term studies on the effect of TRIAC have been reported in several subjects with RTH.[77,79,80,84-91] Although a significant reduction in the basal and TRH-stimulated TSH levels, as well as in serum free T_4 and T_3 levels, were observed in most cases, there was no appreciable change in parameters that measure TH action. This inhibition of TSH secretion without peripheral tissue metabolic effects was seen with TRIAC in normal and hypothyroid patients.[86] In two children, TRIAC produced normal growth and bone maturation.[87,89] In several subjects, there was no change in thyroid function after discontinuing TRIAC, questioning the specificity of the observed effect. Most investigators who used TRIAC reported receiving the drug from Laboratories ANA (Neuilly-sur-Seine, France). It is not available in the United States.

Dextrothyroxine (D-T_4) had been thought to be useful in reducing plasma cholesterol without producing adverse thyromimetic effects[92] in some subjects but not in others.[93,94] Investigators have tried to treat RTH with D-T_4 in an effort to decrease TSH levels.[95-97] Several patients with RTH of various severity have received 2 to 8 mg of D-T_4 daily.[96-99] Clinical changes were minimal and often not supported by objective findings. Given that most preparations contain small amounts of L-T_4, 2% to 3% of the levo substance could fully account for the thyromimetic effect.[95] In most cases, D-T_4 (Dynothel, 2-mg tablet) was obtained from Henning (Berlin).

Treatment of Children and Infants

Infants may be found to have RTH by early testing because of a known affected sibling or parent or, more rarely, because routine neonatal testing revealed an elevated T_4 level and a nonsuppressed TSH. Treatment of these infants is controversial, especially when asymptomatic, because there have been no long-term outcome studies. In general, we tend to treat infants and children with L-T_4 only if any of the following are present: (1) marked elevation of TSH; (2) history of adverse symptoms in other affected family members, such as mental retardation; (3) evidence of failure to thrive; (4) growth retardation; or (5) developmental delays.

There are no guidelines for the treatment of fetuses. Based on the study described earlier,[69] it seems reasonable to reduce the hormone level in a mother with RTH who carries a normal fetus. Although subjects with RTH born to normal mothers, as compared with RTH mothers, had childhood short stature,[60] it is unclear whether treatment with TH during pregnancy would be beneficial in such circumstances.

CLINICAL COURSE AND PREVENTION

There is no evidence to suggest that RTH has an effect on the life span. The few reported infant deaths were from unrelated causes. Only in one subject was RTH thought to have contributed to his demise. This individual,[100] with a homozygous *TRβ* gene mutation and resting heart rate of 190 beats/min, died from a cardiac shock complicating staphylococcal septicemia. Several others with RTH have died from a presumably unrelated illness, the nature of which is unknown, and no information is available from postmortem examinations.

In humans,[101] as in mice[102] with RTH, the serum levels of T_4 and T_3 decline with age, suggesting that the severity of the resistance may improve with time. However, this could represent an exaggerated trend that occurs in normal individuals as well.[101]

PITFALLS, COMPLICATIONS, AND CONTROVERSIES

Correct Diagnosis

A common pitfall in RTH is the failure to make the correct diagnosis. With increased awareness of the syndrome and its inclusion in standard textbooks, ablative therapy is used less frequently. However, clinical and laboratory diagnosis by standard tests is more difficult in patients on TH replacement because of prior surgery or radioiodide treatment. This is particularly important for patients who require higher than the usual replacement doses of TH. In such cases, it is imperative to document carefully that there is a reduced sensitivity to administered TH, to perform genetic testing, and to determine that there are other family members with an RTH phenotype.

Presumed Peripheral Tissue Resistance to Thyroid Hormone Versus Thyroid Hormone Habituation

A common referral to physicians with expertise in RTH is the apparent requirement of high doses of TH, despite TSH suppression. Such individuals are presumed to have selective peripheral tissue resistance to thyroid hormone (PTRTH). Usually, these patients have elevated serum T_4 and T_3 levels with suppressed TSH but the patient continues to feel hypothyroid. Although theoretically possible, this condition has not been convincingly shown to exist. It is acquired and not associated with demonstrable receptor defects. A typical presentation is that of a patient who has undergone thyroid ablation or had a history of mild hyperthyrotropinemia, is dissatisfied with their energy level or weight, and attributes it to insufficient TH replacement. Patients have often tried different TH preparations including L-T_3 and desiccated thyroid. In patients on high doses of L-T_4, the serum rT_3 concentration is disproportionately high relative to T_3. This shunting of T_4 metabolism to produce an inactive hormone explains the scarcity of signs of TH excess. These patients present a challenge to physicians to determine the cause for their complaints and prevent overmedication with TH.

Controversies in Resistance to Thyroid Hormone Syndrome

These include the following:

1. Determination of the cause for the heterogenous phenotype of subjects with identical mutations across and within the same family
2. Development of treatment to revert the dominant negative effect of the receptor and thus cure RTH
3. Management of maternal and fetal TH levels during gestation
4. Cause of non-TR RTH
5. Identification of humans with TRα mutations

References

1. Refetoff S, DeWind LT, DeGroot LJ: Familial syndrome combining deaf-mutism, stuppled epiphyses, goiter and abnormally high PBI: Possible target organ refractoriness to thyroid hormone. J Clin Endocrinol Metab 27:279-294, 1967.
2. Refetoff S, DeGroot LJ, Benard B, DeWind LT: Studies of a sibship with apparent hereditary resistance to the intracellular action of thyroid hormone. Metabolism 21:723-756, 1972.
3. Sakurai A, Takeda K, Ain K, et al: Generalized resistance to thyroid hormone associated with a mutation in the ligand-binding domain of the human thyroid hormone receptor beta. Proc Natl Acad Sci U S A 86:8977-8981, 1989.
4. Usala SJ, Tennyson GE, Bale AE, et al: A base mutation of the C-erbA beta thyroid hormone receptor in a kindred with generalized thyroid hormone resistance. Molecular heterogeneity in two other kindreds. J Clin Invest 85:93-100, 1990.
5. Refetoff S, Weiss RE, Usala SJ: The syndromes of resistance to thyroid hormone. Endocr Rev 14:348-399, 1993.
6. Dumitrescu AM, Liao XH, Abdullah MS, et al: Mutations in SECISBP2 result in abnormal thyroid hormone metabolism. Nat Genet 37:1247-1252, 2005.
7. Bassett JH, Harvey CB, Williams GR: Mechanisms of thyroid hormone receptor–specific nuclear and extra nuclear actions. Mol Cell Endocrinol 213: 1-11, 2003.

8. Fondell JD, Guermah M, Malik S, Roeder RG: Thyroid hormone receptor-associated proteins and general positive cofactors mediate thyroid hormone receptor function in the absence of the TATA box-binding protein-associated factors of TFIID. Proc Natl Acad Sci U S A 96:1959-1964, 1999.
9. Refetoff S, Weiss RE, Usala SJ, Hayashi Y: The syndromes of resistance to thyroid hormone: Update 1994. In Braverman LE, Refetoff S (eds): Endocrine Reviews Monographs. Bethesda, Md, The Endocrine Society, 1994, pp 336-343, 1994.
10. Flamant F, Gauthier K, Samarut J: Thyroid hormones signaling is getting more complex: STORMs are coming. Mol Endocrinol 21:321-333, 2007.
11. Evans RM: The steroid and thyroid hormone receptor superfamily. Science 240:889-895, 1988.
12. Gurnell M, Chatterjee VK: Nuclear receptors in disease: Thyroid receptor beta, peroxisome proliferator–activated receptor gamma and orphan receptors. Essays Biochem 40:169-189, 2004.
13. Kliewer SA, Umesono K, Mangelsdorf DJ, Evans RM: Retinoid X receptor interacts with nuclear receptors in retinoic acid, thyroid hormone and vitamin D_3 signalling. Nature 355:446-449, 1992.
14. Lazar MA: Thyroid hormone receptors: Multiple forms, multiple possibilities. Endocr Rev 14:184-193, 1993.
15. Mangelsdorf DJ, Evans RM: The RXR heterodimers and orphan receptors. Cell 83:841-850, 1995.
16. Arai K, Chrousos GP: Syndromes of glucocorticoid and mineralocorticoid resistance. Steroids 60:173-179, 1995.
17. Bouillon R, Verstuyf A, Mathieu C, et al: Vitamin D resistance. Best Pract Res 20:627-645, 2006.
18. Hughes MR, Malloy PJ, Kieback DG, et al: Point mutations in the human vitamin D receptor gene associated with hypocalcemic rickets. Science 242:1702-1705, 1988.
19. Quigley CA, De Bellis A, Marschke KB, et al: Androgen receptor defects: Histological, clinical, and molecular perspectives. Endocr Rev 16:271-321, 1995.
20. Smith EP, Boyd J, Frank GR, et al: Estrogen resistance caused by a mutation in the estrogen-receptor gene in a man. N Engl J Med 331:1056-1061, 1994.
21. van Rossum EF, Lamberts SW: Glucocorticoid resistance syndrome: A diagnostic and therapeutic approach. Best Pract Res 20:611-626, 2006.
22. Pohlenz J, Weiss RE, Macchia PE, et al: Five new families with resistance to thyroid hormone not caused by mutations in the thyroid hormone receptor β gene. J Clin Endocrinol Metab 84:3919-3928, 1999.
23. Reutrakul S, Sadow PM, Pannain S, et al: Search for abnormalities of nuclear corepressors, coactivators, and a coregulator in families with resistance to thyroid hormone without mutations in thyroid hormone receptor beta or alpha genes. J Clin Endocrinol Metab 85:3609-3617, 2000.
24. Weiss RE, Hayashi Y, Nagaya T, et al: Dominant inheritance of resistance to thyroid hormone not linked to defects in the thyroid hormone receptors alpha or beta genes may be due to a defective co-factor. J Clin Endocrinol Metab 81:4196-4203, 1996.
25. Lafranchi SH, Snyder DB, Sesser DE, et al: Follow-up of newborns with elevated screening T4 concentrations. J Pediatr 143:296-301, 2003.
26. Sadow PM, Reutrakul S, Weiss RE, Refetoff S: Resistance to thyroid hormone in the absence of mutations in the thyroid hormone receptor genes. Curr Opinion Endocrinol Diabetes 7:253-259, 2000.
27. Adams M, Matthews C, Collingwood TN, et al: Genetic analysis of 29 kindreds with generalized and pituitary resistance to thyroid hormone: Identification of thirteen novel mutations in the thyroid hormone receptor β gene. J Clin Invest 94:506-515, 1994.
28. Collingwood TN, Wagner R, Matthews CH, et al: A role for helix 3 of the TRβ ligand-binding domain in coactivator recruitment identified by characterization of a third cluster of mutations in resistance to thyroid hormone. EMBO J 17:4760-4770, 1998.
29. Weiss RE, Weinberg M, Refetoff S: Identical mutations in unrelated families with generalized resistance to thyroid hormone occur in cytosine-guanine-rich areas of the thyroid hormone receptor beta gene. Analysis of 15 families. J Clin Invest 91:2408-2415
30. Hayashi Y, Sunthornthepvarakul T, Refetoff S: Mutations of CpG dinucleotides located in the triiodothyronine (T_3)-binding domain of the thyroid hormone receptor (TR) beta gene that appears to be devoid of natural mutations may not be detected because they are unlikely to produce the clinical phenotype of resistance to thyroid hormone. J Clin Invest 94:607-615, 1994.
31. Takeda K, Sakurai A, DeGroot LJ, Refetoff S: Recessive inheritance of thyroid hormone resistance caused by complete deletion of the protein-coding region of the thyroid hormone receptor-β gene. J Clin Endocrinol Metab 74:49-55, 1992.
32. Liu Y, Takeshita A, Misiti S, et al: Lack of coactivator interaction can be a mechanism for dominant negative activity by mutant thyroid hormone receptors. Endocrinology 139:4197-4204, 1998.
33. Safer JD, Cohen RN, Hollenberg AN, Wondisford FE: Defective release of corepressor by hinge mutants of the thyroid hormone receptor found in patients with resistance to thyroid hormone. J Biol Chem 273:30175-30182, 1998.
34. Yoh SM, Chatterjee VKK, Privalsky ML: Thyroid hormone resistance syndrome manifests as an aberrant interaction between mutant T_3 receptor and transcriptional corepressor. Mol Endocrinol 11:470-480, 1997.
35. Lado-Abeal J, Dumitrescu AM, Liao XH, et al: A de novo mutation in an already mutant nucleotide of the thyroid hormone receptor beta gene perpetuates resistance to thyroid hormone. J Clin Endocrinol Metab 90:1760-1767, 2005.

36. Bottcher Y, Paufler T, Stehr T, et al: Thyroid hormone resistance without mutations in thyroid hormone receptor beta. Med Sci Monit 13:CS67-CS77, 2007.
37. McDermott JH, Agha A, McMahon M, et al: A case of resistance to thyroid hormone without mutation in the thyroid hormone receptor beta. Ir J Med Sci 174:60-64, 2005.
38. Vlaeminck-Guillem V, Margotat A, et al: Resistance to thyroid hormone in a family with no TRβ gene anomaly: Pathogenic hypotheses. Ann Endocrinol (Paris) 61:194-199, 2000.
39. Adachi M, Takayanagi R, Tomura A, et al: Androgen-insensitivity syndrome as a possible coactivator disease. N Engl J Med 343:856-862, 2000.
40. Huizenga NA, de Lange P, Koper JW, et al: Five patients with biochemical and/or clinical generalized glucocorticoid resistance without alterations in the glucocorticoid receptor gene. J Clin Endocrinol Metab 85:2076-2081, 2000.
41. New MI, Nimkarn S, Brandon DD, et al: Resistance to several steroids in two sisters. J Clin Endocrinol Metab 84:4454-4464, 1999.
42. Mamanasiri S, Yesil S, Dumitrescu AM, et al: Mosaicism of a thyroid hormone receptor-beta gene mutation in resistance to thyroid hormone. J Clin Endocrinol Metab 91:3471-3477, 2006.
43. Flamant F, Samarut J: Thyroid hormone receptors: Lessons from knockout and knock-in mutant mice. Trends Endocrinol Metab 14:85-90, 2003.
44. Jones I, Srinivas M, Ng L, Forrest D: The thyroid hormone receptor beta gene: Structure and functions in the brain and sensory systems. Thyroid 13:1057-1068, 2003.
45. Suzuki H, Willingham MC, Cheng SY: Mice with a mutation in the thyroid hormone receptor beta gene spontaneously develop thyroid carcinoma: A mouse model of thyroid carcinogenesis. Thyroid 12:963-969, 2002.
46. Macchia PE, Takeuchi Y, Kawai T, et al: Increased sensitivity to thyroid hormone in mice with complete deficiency of thyroid hormone receptor alpha. Proc Natl Acad Sci U S A 98:349-354, 2001.
47. Kaneshige M, Suzuki H, Kaneshige K, et al: A targeted dominant negative mutation of the thyroid hormone alpha 1 receptor causes increased mortality, infertility, and dwarfism in mice. Proc Natl Acad Sci U S A 98:15095-15100, 2001.
48. Liu YY, Schultz JJ, Brent GA: A thyroid hormone receptor alpha gene mutation (P398H) is associated with visceral adiposity and impaired catecholamine-stimulated lipolysis in mice. J Biol Chem 278:38913-38920, 2003.
49. Tinnikov A, Nordstrom K, Thoren P, et al: Retardation of post-natal development caused by a negatively acting thyroid hormone receptor alpha1. EMBO J 21:5079-5087, 2002.
50. Gauthier K, Chassande O, Plateroti M, et al: Different functions for the thyroid hormone receptors TRalpha and TRbeta in the control of thyroid hormone production and post-natal development. EMBO J 18:623-631, 1999.
51. Gothe S, Wang Z, Ng L, et al: Mice devoid of all known thyroid hormone receptors are viable but exhibit disorders of the pituitary-thyroid axis, growth, and bone maturation. Genes Dev 13: 1329-1341, 1999.
52. Flamant F, Poguet AL, Plateroti M, et al: Congenital hypothyroid Pax8$^{-/-}$ mutant mice can be rescued by inactivating the TRalpha gene. Mol Endocrinol 16:24-32, 2002.
53. Morte B, Manzano J, Scanlan T, et al: Deletion of the thyroid hormone receptor alpha 1 prevents the structural alterations of the cerebellum induced by hypothyroidism. Proc Natl Acad Sci U S A 99:3985-3989, 2002.
54. Weiss RE, Xu J, Ning G, et al: Mice deficient in the steroid receptor co-activator 1 (SRC-1) are resistant to thyroid hormone. EMBO J 18:1900-1904, 1999.
55. Brown NS, Smart A, Sharma V, et al: Thyroid hormone resistance and increased metabolic rate in the RXR-gamma-deficient mouse. J Clin Invest 106:73-79, 2000.
56. Beck-Peccoz P, Chatterjee VK: The variable clinical phenotype in thyroid hormone resistance syndrome. Thyroid 4:225-232, 1994.
57. Wu SY, Cohen RN, Simsek E, et al: A novel thyroid hormone receptor-beta mutation that fails to bind nuclear receptor corepressor in a patient as an apparent cause of severe, predominantly pituitary resistance to thyroid hormone. J Clin Endocrinol Metab 91:1887-1895, 2006.
58. Sasaki J, Tada T, Saito K, Kurihara H: [A case report of Refetoff's syndrome]. Nippon Naika Gakkai Zasshi 65:1286-1293, 1989.
59. Weiss RE, Stein MA, Refetoff S: Behavioral effects of liothyronine (L-T_3) in children with attention deficit hyperactivity disorder in the presence and absence of resistance to thyroid hormone. Thyroid 7:389-393, 1997.
60. Brucker-Davis F, Skarulis MC, Grace MB, et al: Genetic and clinical features of 42 kindreds with resistance to thyroid hormone. The National Institutes of Health Prospective Study. Ann Intern Med 123:572-583, 1995.
61. Bassett JH, O'Shea PJ, Sriskantharajah S, et al: Thyroid hormone excess rather than thyrotropin deficiency induces osteoporosis in hyperthyroidism. Mol Endocrinol 21:1095-1107, 2007.
62. O'Shea PJ, Bassett JH, Cheng SY, Williams GR: Characterization of skeletal phenotypes of TRalpha1 and TRbeta mutant mice: Implications for tissue thyroid status and T_3 target gene expression. Nucl Recept Signal 4:e011, 2006.
63. Persani L, Preziati D, Matthews CH, et al: Serum levels of carboxyterminal cross-linked telopeptide of type I collagen (ICTP) in the differential diagnosis of the syndromes of inappropriate secretion of TSH. Clin Endocrinol 47:207-214, 1997.
64. Ng L, Hurley JB, Dierks B, et al: A thyroid hormone receptor that is required for the development of green cone photoreceptors. Nat Genet 27:94-98, 2001.

65. Aksoy DY, Gurlek A, Ringkananont U, et al: Resistance to thyroid hormone associated with autoimmune thyroid disease in a Turkish family. J Endocrinol Invest 28:379-383, 2005.
66. Fukata S, Brent GA, Sugawara M: Resistance to thyroid hormone in Hashimoto's thyroiditis. N Engl J Med 352:517-518, 2005.
67. Sato H, Sakai H: A family showing resistance to thyroid hormone associated with chronic thyroiditis and its clinical features: A case report. Endocr J 53:421-425, 2006.
68. Grasberger H, Ringkananont U, Croxson M, Refetoff S: Resistance to thyroid hormone in a patient with thyroid dysgenesis. Thyroid 15:730-733, 2005.
69. Anselmo J, Cao D, Karrison T, et al: Fetal loss associated with excess thyroid hormone exposure. JAMA 292:691-695, 2004.
70. Anselmo J, César R: Resistance to thyroid hormone: Report of 2 kindreds with 35 patients. Endocr Pract 4:368-374, 1998.
71. Persani L, Asteria C, Tonacchera M, et al: Evidence for the secretion of thyrotropin with enhanced bioactivity in syndromes of thyroid hormone resistance. J Clin Endocrinol Metab 78:1034-1039, 1994.
72. Beck-Peccoz P, Brucker-Davis F, et al: Thyrotropin-secreting pituitary tumors. Endocr Rev 17:610-638, 1996.
73. Beckers A, Abs R, Mahler C, Vandalem JL, et al: Thyrotropin-secreting pituitary adenomas: Report of seven cases. J Clin Endocrinol Metab 72:477-483, 1991.
74. Haigler ED Jr, Hershman JM, Pittman JA Jr: Response to orally administered synthetic thyrotropin-releasing hormone in man. J Clin Endocrinol Metab 35:631-635, 1972.
75. Bogazzi F, Manetti L, Tomisti L, et al: Thyroid color flow doppler sonography: An adjunctive tool for differentiating patients with inappropriate thyrotropin (TSH) secretion due to TSH-secreting pituitary adenoma or resistance to thyroid hormone. Thyroid 16:989-995, 2006.
76. Safer JD, Colan SD, Fraser LM, Wondisford FE: A pituitary tumor in a patient with thyroid hormone resistance: A diagnostic dilemma. Thyroid 11:281-291, 2001.
77. Beck-Peccoz P, Piscitelli G, Cattaneo MG, Faglia G: Successful treatment of hyperthyroidism due to nonneoplastic pituitary TSH hypersecretion with 3,5,3′-triiodothyroacetic acid (TRIAC). J Endocrinol Invest 6:217-223, 1983.
78. Dorey F, Strauch G, Gayno JP: Thyrotoxicosis due to pituitary resistance to thyroid hormones. Successful control with D thyroxine: A study in three patients. Clin Endocrinol 32:221-228, 1990.
79. Dulgeroff AJ, Geffner ME, Koyal SN, et al: Bromocriptine and Triac therapy for hyperthyroidism due to pituitary resistance to thyroid hormone. J Clin Endocrinol Metab 75:1071-1075, 1992.
80. Beck-Peccoz P, Mariotti S, Guillausseau PJ, et al: Treatment of hyperthyroidism due to inappropriate secretion of thyrotropin with the somatostatin analog SMS 201-995. J Clin Endocrinol Metab 68:208-214, 1989.
81. Anselmo J, Refetoff S: Regression of a large goiter in a patient with resistance to thyroid hormone by every other day treatment with triiodothyronine. Thyroid 14:71-74, 2004.
82. Koerner D, Surks MI, Oppenheimer JH: In vitro demonstration of specific triiodothyronine binding sites in rat liver nuclei. J Clin Endocrinol Metab 38:706-709, 1974.
83. Takeda T, Suzuki S, Liu RT, DeGroot LJ: Triiodothyroacetic acid has unique potential for therapy of resistance to thyroid hormone. J Clin Endocrinol Metab 80:2033-2040, 1995.
84. Salmela PI, Wide L, Juustila H, Ruokonen A: Effects of thyroid hormones (T_4, T_3), bromocriptine and Triac on inappropriate TSH hypersecretion. Clin Endocrinol 28:497-507, 1988.
85. Lind P, Eber O: [Treatment of inappropriate TSH secretion with Triac]. Acta Med Austriaca 13:13-16, 1986.
86. Medeiros-Neto G, Kallas WG, Knobel M, et al: Triac (3,5,3′-triiodothyroacetic acid) partially inhibits the thyrotropin response to synthetic thyrotropin-releasing hormone in normal and thyroidectomized hypothyroid patients. J Clin Endocrinol Metab 50:223-225, 1980.
87. Darendeliler F, Bas F: Successful therapy with 3,5,3′-triiodothyroacetic acid (TRIAC) in pituitary resistance to thyroid hormone. J Pediatr Endocrinol Metab 10:535-538, 1997.
88. Kunitake JM, Hartman N, Henson LC, et al: 3,5,3′-triiodothyroacetic acid therapy for thyroid hormone resistance. J Clin Endocrinol Metab 69:461-466, 1989.
89. Radetti G, Persani L, Molinaro G, et al: Clinical and hormonal outcome after two years of triiodothyroacetic acid treatment in a child with thyroid hormone resistance. Thyroid 7:775-778, 1997.
90. Rivolta CM, Mallea Gil MS, Ballarino C, et al: A novel 1297-1304delGCCTGCCA mutation in the exon 10 of the thyroid hormone receptor beta gene causes resistance to thyroid hormone. Mol Diagn 8:163-169, 2004.
91. Torre P, Bertoli M, Di Giovanni S, et al: Endocrine and neuropsychological assessment in a child with a novel mutation of thyroid hormone receptor: Response to 12-month triiodothyroacetic acid (TRIAC) therapy. J Endocrinol Invest 28:657-662, 2005.
92. Schneeberg NG, Herman E, Menduke H, Altschuler NK: Reduction of serum cholesterol by sodium dextrothyroxine in euthyroid subjects. Ann Intern Med 56:265-275, 1962.
93. Bantle JP, Hunninghake DB, Frantz ID, et al: Comparison of effectiveness of thyrotropin-suppressive doses of D- and L-thyroxine in treatment of hypercholesterolemia. Am J Med 77:475-481, 1984.

94. Gorman CA, Jiang NS, Ellefson RD, Elveback LR: Comparative effectiveness of dextrothyroxine and levothyroxine in correcting hypothyroidism and lowering blood lipid levels in hypothyroid patients. J Clin Endocrinol Metab 49:1-7, 1979.
95. Hamon P, Bovier-Lapierre M, Robert M, et al: Hyperthyroidism due to selective pituitary resistance to thyroid hormones in a 15-month old boy: Efficacy of d-thyroxine therapy. J Clin Endocrinol Metab 67:1089-1093, 1988.
96. Pohlenz J, Knöbl D: Treatment of pituitary resistance to thyroid hormone (PRTH) in an 8-year-old boy. Acta Paediatr 85:387-390, 1996.
97. Schwartz ID, Bercu BB: Dextrothyroxine in the treatment of generalized thyroid hormone resistance in a boy homozygous for a defect in the T_3 receptor. Thyroid 2:15-19, 1992.
98. Sarkissian G, Dace A, Mesmacque A, et al: A novel resistance to thyroid hormone associated with a new mutation (T329N) in the thyroid hormone receptor beta gene. Thyroid 9:165-171, 1999.
99. Usala SJ, Menke JB, Watson TL, et al: A homozygous deletion in the c-erbA beta thyroid hormone receptor gene in a patient with generalized thyroid hormone resistance: Isolation and characterization of the mutant receptor. Mol Endocrinol 5:327-335, 1991.
100. Ono S, Schwartz ID, Mueller OT, et al: Homozygosity for a dominant negative thyroid hormone receptor gene responsible for generalized resistance to thyroid hormone. J Clin Endocrinol Metab 73:990-994, 1991.
101. Pohlenz J, Manders L, Sadow PM, et al: A novel point mutation in cluster 3 of the thyroid hormone receptor beta gene (P247L) causing mild resistance to thyroid hormone. Thyroid 9:1195-1203, 1999.
102. Weiss RE, Chassande O, Koo EK, et al: Thyroid function and effect of aging in combined hetero/homozygous mice deficient in thyroid hormone receptors alpha and beta genes. J Endocrinol 172:177-185, 2002.

Chapter 22

Cell Transport Defects

Alexandra M. Dumitrescu and Samuel Refetoff

Key Points

- Monocarboxylate transporter 8 (MCT8; also known as SLC16A2 and XPCT) is a specific thyroid hormone cell membrane transporter located on the X chromosome.
- *MCT8* gene defect should be suspected when truncal hypotonia and limb spasticity are accompanied by high serum triiodothyronine and low thyroxine and low reverse triiodothyronine concentrations.
- Neurologic manifestations cannot be explained by thyroid function test abnormalities; observed phenotype is different from that of global thyroid hormone deficiency or excess.
- Treatment with physiologic doses of levothyroxine could not correct the phenotype in several patients; efficacy of treatment during pregnancy and use of higher levothyroxine doses and thyroid hormone analogues will have to be tested.
- *Mct8* knockout mice replicate the characteristic thyroid human phenotype.

The effects of thyroid hormone (TH) are dependent on the quantity of the hormone that reaches peripheral tissues, its intracellular availability, and the presence of unaltered TH receptors (TRs). Until recently it was believed that TH enters the cells passively. However, the characterization of several classes of TH membrane transporters with different kinetics and substrate preferences that actively transport TH across cell membranes has changed this paradigm. These proteins belong to different families of solute carriers, organic anion transporters (OATPs), amino acids, and monocarboxylate transporters.[1-5] Their characteristics in terms of tissue distribution and kinetics, as well as binding of other possible ligands, provide them with potentially distinctive roles in the fine tuning of organ-specific TH availability.[6]

Once it is intracellular, the hormone precursor thyroxine (T_4) is activated by removal of the outer ring iodine (5′-deiodination) to form triiodothyronine (T_3) or T_4 and T_3 are inactivated by inner ring 5-deiodination to form reverse T_3 (rT_3) and diiodothyronine (T_2), respectively. The activating deiodinases are D1 and D2, whereas the inactivating enzyme is D3 and, to a lesser extent, D1 (Fig. 22-1). Their presence in changing concentrations in various cell types allows an additional level of local regulation of hormone supply.[7] Finally, the presence and abundance of TRs, through which TH action is mediated, determine the type and degree of hormonal response.[8]

For many years after the identification of TH membrane transporters, their physiologic role remained elusive because no genetic defects were known in humans or animals, and the consequence of a putative defect was unknown. In particular, a defect in liver-specific transporter 1 (LST1) was considered as a possible cause of resistance to TH (RTH). Linkage analysis in several families with RTH has excluded LST1 involvement.[9] However, the recent identification of patients with mutations in the X-linked TH transporter, monocarboxylate transporter 8 (MCT8),[10-16] has revealed the role played by one such transmembrane carrier in the intracellular availability of TH.

Being an X-linked disease, hemizygous males are affected but carrier females are clinically normal. The phenotype of patients with *MCT8* gene mutations has two components: (1) thyroid function test (TFT) abnormalities that include high T_3, low T_4, low rT_3, and slightly elevated TSH concentrations (Fig. 22-2) found in males and to a lesser degree in carrier females and (2) severe motor and developmental delay, gait disturbance, dystonia, and poor head control, found only in males. These neuropsychiatric manifestations have not been previously described in the context of abnormal thyroid function and cannot

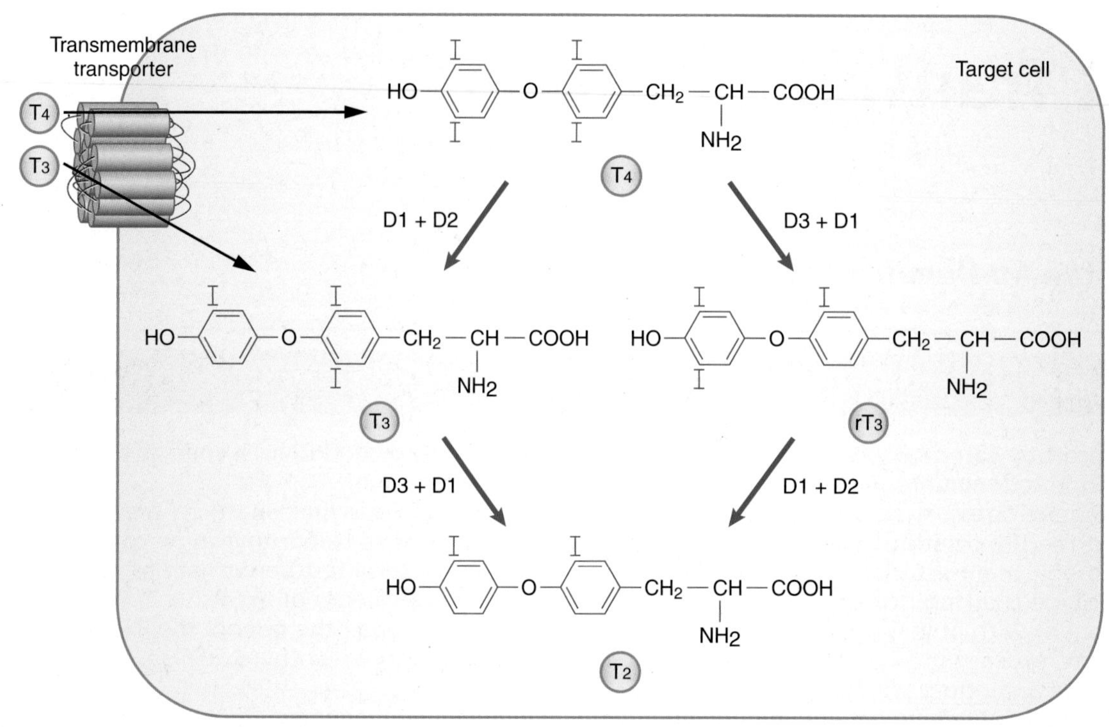

Figure 22–1 Regulation of intracellular thyroid hormone (TH) bioactivity. TH, thyroxine (T_4), and triiodothyronine (T_3), are actively transported across the cell membrane. T_4, the main hormonal precursor secreted by the thyroid gland, undergoes intracellular stepwise deiodination. 5′-deiodination through D1 and D2 activates T_4 by converting it to T_3, whereas 5-deiodination by D3 converts T_4 to the inactive rT_3. T_3 is inactivated by D3 and, to a lesser extent, D1. T_2, diiodothyronine.

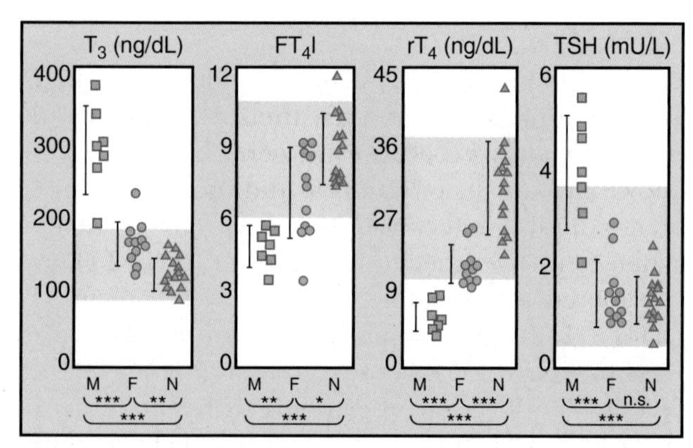

Figure 22–2 Thyroid function test results from six families studied at the University of Chicago. Shown are resuts from 7 affected males (M), 11 carrier females (F), and 15 unaffected family members (N). The shaded areas depict the normal range for the corresponding test. Bars represent 2 SD. FT_4, free thyroxine; rT_3, reverse triiodothyronine; T_3, triiodothyronine; TSH, thyroid-stimulating hormone; *, $P < .05$; **, $P < .01$, ***, $P < .001$.

be explained by the current knowledge and observed TFT result. This is the first genetic defect of a TH transporter and understanding the underlying mechanisms responsible for the phenotype manifested by patients with MCT8 defect will provide new insights into thyroid physiology.

EPIDEMIOLOGY, CAUSE, AND PATHOGENESIS

The *MCT8* gene was first cloned during the physical characterization of the Xq13.2 region known to contain the X inactivation center.[17] It has six exons and a very long (more than 100 kb) first intron. It belongs to a family of genes officially named *SLC16*, the products of which catalyze proton-linked transport of monocarboxylates, such as lactate, pyruvate, and ketone bodies. The deduced products of the *MCT8 (SLC16A2)* gene are proteins of 613 and 539 amino acids (translated from two in-frame start sites) containing 12 transmembrane domains with both amino and carboxyl termini located within the cell.[18] In 2003, Friesema and colleagues[2] demonstrated that the rat homologue was a specific transporter of TH into cells.

A form of mental retardation associated with motor abnormalities was described in 1944[19] and subsequently named the Allan-Herndon-Dudley (A-H-D) syndrome. This condition was further mapped to a locus on chromosome X, Xq13-q21[20] and Xq12-q13.[21] In 2004, two laboratories identified, independently, mutations in the *MCT8* gene in seven unrelated families, in which males presented with high serum T_3, low T_4, and low rT_3 concentrations, together with psychomotor abnormalities reminiscent of the A-H-D syndrome.[10,11] In 2005, it was shown that families

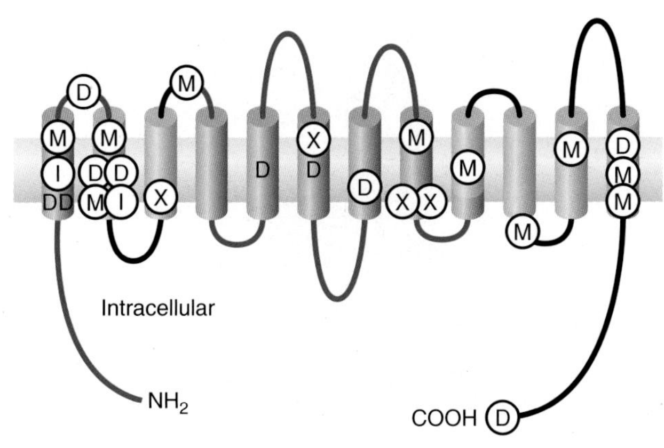

Figure 22–3 Schematic representation of *MCT8* gene mutations in 26 families by type and location. D, deletion; M, missense; X, nonsense; I, insertion.

previously identified as suffering from the A-H-D syndrome, including the first family reported in 1944, harbored mutations in the *MCT8* gene and had high serum T_3 levels.[12]

We know of 26 families with *MCT8* gene mutations.[14,22] The mutations are distributed throughout the coding region of the gene (Fig. 22-3). Single amino acid substitutions causing missense mutations were found in 10 families and in four families they resulted in nonsense mutations. Single amino acid deletions or insertions were reported in two families each. One or two nucleotide deletions or insertions produced two stop codons and, in one case, a 64–amino acid extension of the carboxyl terminus of the MCT8 molecule. Deletions of 10 nucleotides or more were reported in four families, and an intronic mutation, affecting the splice site, in one. It is of note that two mutations, F229Δ and S448X, occurred in two unrelated families each.

The identification of 26 families with a *MCT8* defect in less than 3 years indicates that this syndrome is more common than initially suspected. From a population genetics point of view, the spontaneous *MCT8* mutations could have been maintained in the population because carrier females are asymptomatic, thus preventing any negative selection to take place. Currently, penetrance is thought to be complete. Ethnic origins reported to date include German, Greek, American Indian, English, Irish, French, Japanese, Hispanic, Brazilian, Argentinean, Chilean, Mexican, and Dutch.

Genotype and Phenotype Correlation

Given the variability in the severity of the disease, correlations between phenotypes and genotypes were sought. A comparison of the clinical picture in the families with identical mutations would have been helpful in determining whether such correlations exist. Unfortunately, detailed clinical information in one of each of the two families is not available. However, early deaths were reported in the two families with a truncated MCT8 molecule *(S448X)*. In one family, two affected males died at ages 13 and 39 years and, in the other, deaths occurred at 20, 22, and 30 years. Early death also was reported in subjects harboring the following mutations: P537L, 404 frameshift 416X, F229Δ, S194F, and 612 frameshift with 64–amino acid carboxyl terminal extension. The cause of death in 4 of 14 patients was aspiration pneumonia. Prediction of outcome based on the genotype would help in the care of patients and in genetic counseling.

Functional analysis, in terms of cellular T_3 uptake, of 12 different mutations,[22] revealed no activity in four mutations, two missense (471 and 512) and two nonsense mutations (R245X and 448X). In three mutations (F229Δ, insertion Ile189, and 224), uptake was from 2.4% to 5%. In the remaining five mutations, T_3 uptake ranged from 8.6% to 33% that of the wild-type MCT8; all five were missense mutations (S194F, V235M, R271H, L434W, and L598P).

Using available clinical, chemical, and in vitro information, there is no clear relation between the degree of impairment of T_3 transport by the mutant MCT8 molecules and the level of serum T_3. This is probably because of the important role played by the underlying perturbations in the metabolism of iodothyronines in the production of T_3, as demonstrated in the *Mct8* knockout mice.[23] Furthermore, except for early death, no other clinical consequence appears to correlate significantly with the degree of functional or physical disruption of the MCT8 molecule. Genetic factors, variability of tissue expression of *MCT8*, and other iodothyronine cell membrane transporters could be at the basis of this lack of phenotype or genotype correlation. However, the possibility that MCT8 is involved in the transport of other ligands has not been excluded.

Mouse Model of the Disease

To understand the mechanism underlying the phenotype of MCT8 deficiency better, mice lacking functional Mct8 were created by homologous recombination.[23] These mice replicate the characteristic thyroid phenotype observed in humans: high serum T_3 and low T_4 and rT_3 compared with wild-type (WT) male littermates.[23] Thus, *Mct8* knockout (KO) mice are a good model for the study of the pathophysiology underlying the thyroid phenotype.

Studies of *Mct8* KO[23] have provided much needed insights into the mechanisms responsible for the thyroid phenotype.[24] Measurements of tissue T_3

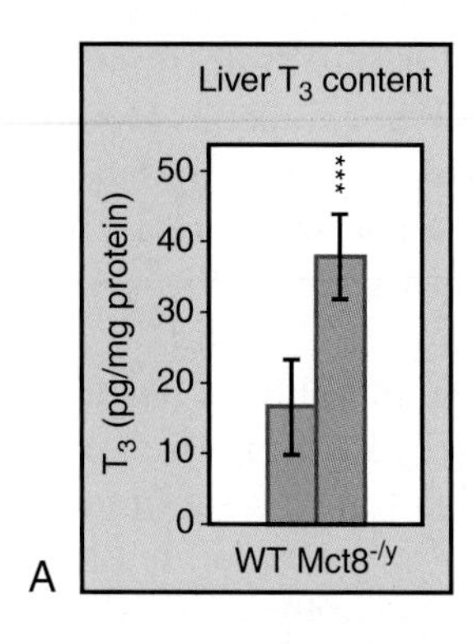

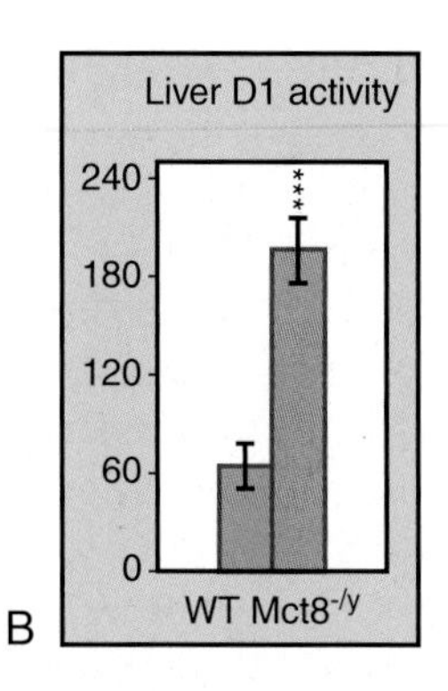

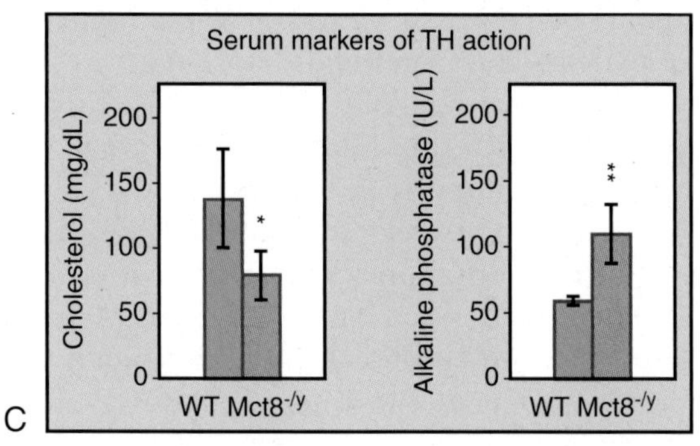

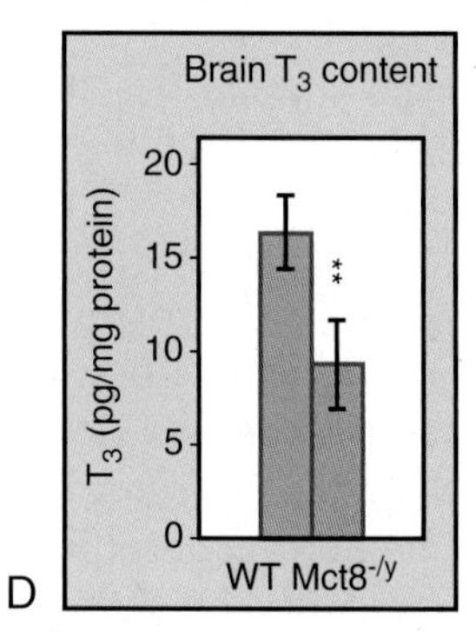

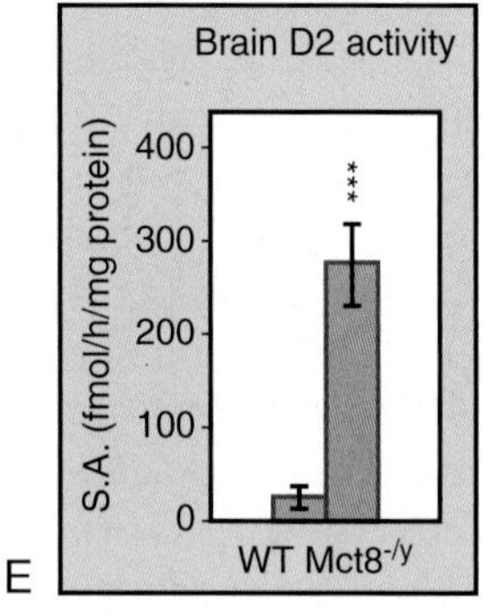

Figure 22–4 Consequences of Mct8 deficiency. **A,** Liver T_3 content. **B,** Liver deiodinase 1 enzymatic activity. **C,** Serum cholesterol and alkaline phosphatase levels. **D,** Brain T_3 content. **E,** Brain deiodinase 2 enzymatic activity. Bars represent mean ± SD. *Mct8*$^{-/y}$, male *Mct8* knockout mice; S.A., specific activity; T_3, triiodothyronine; WT, male wild-type mice; *, $P < .05$; **, $P < .01$; ***, $P < .001$.

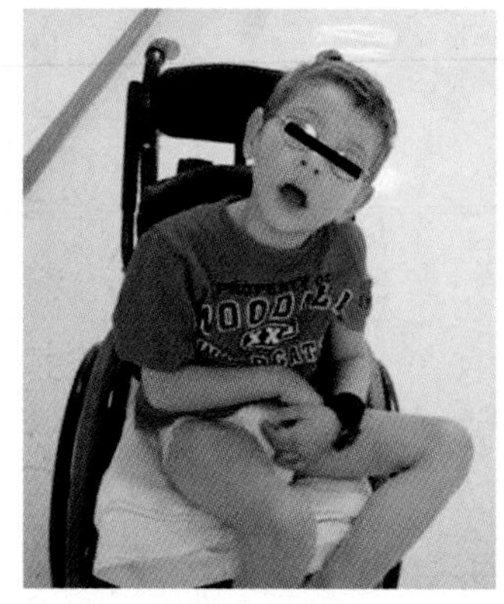

Figure 22–5 This photograph shows a 5-year old with *MCT8* gene mutation. The child cannot talk, walk, or feed himself. He has spastic quadriplegia and has to be propped up and supported in a sitting position.

content demonstrated that the high circulating T_3 levels are differentially available to tissues, depending on the redundancy in TH transmembrane transporters. Tissues that express others transporters in addition to Mct8, such as the liver,[25] manifest hormonal responses that reflect the circulating T_3 levels and are thus thyrotoxic in Mct8-deficient mice (Fig. 22-4A). The baseline hepatic thyrotoxicosis in *Mct8* KO mice results in increased D1 enzymatic activity (see Fig. 22-4B), decreased serum cholesterol, and increased alkaline phosphatase (see Fig. 22-4C). In contrast, tissues with limited redundancy in cellular TH transporters, such as the brain,[25] have decreased T_3 content in *Mct8* KO mice (see Fig. 22-4D). As a consequence, the local D2 enzymatic activity is increased (see Fig. 22-4E). The role of D2 is to maintain local levels of T_3 in the context of TH deficiency and its activity is post-translational, regulated by TH availability.[7]

The findings of coexistent TH excess and deficiency in *Mct8* KO mice can explain, in part, the mechanisms responsible for the pattern of thyroid tests observed in MCT8 deficiency.[23] The increased D1 and D2 activity, stimulated by opposite states of intracellular TH availability, has an additive consumptive effect on T_4 levels and results in increased T_3 generation. The impaired T_3 uptake in the brain makes the circulating T_3 less available for deiodination by D3. The increased liver D1 enzymatic activity also stimulates the metabolism of rT_3. In addition, these tissue-specific differences in intracellular TH content and consecutive changes in TH metabolism are responsible for the unusual clinical presentation of this defect compared with global TH deficiency.

CLINICAL FEATURES

Male patients who are found to have *MCT8* mutations are referred for medical investigation during infancy or early childhood because of neurodevelopmental abnormalities. They present with hypotonia, motor delay, feeding problems, inability to walk, and no speech development (Fig. 22-5). The clinical presentation of more than 100 male patients with *MCT8* gene mutations known to date is similar, with consistent TFT abnormalities (see earlier) and severe psychomotor retardation. Review of these families indicates that parents were not consanguineous and gestation and delivery were normal. Infants are normal in length, weight, and head circumference.

They do not show typical signs of hypothyroidism, such as prolonged neonatal jaundice, macroglossia, umbilical hernia, or signs of hyperthyroidism, increased heart rate, and premature closure of the fontanelles. An early sign of the defect, manifesting in the first few weeks of life, was hypotonia and feeding difficulties.

With advancing age, weight gain lagged behind normal and microcephaly became apparent, whereas linear growth proceeded normally. Although truncal hypotonia persisted, there was progressive development of limb rigidity leading to spastic quadriplegia, often with joint contractures. In these patients, muscle mass is diminished, with generalized muscle weakness, often with myopathic facies but characteristic poor head control, originally described as limber neck.[19] Purposeless movements in the form of choreoathetosis and characteristic paroxysms of kinesigenic dyskinesias are common. These are typically triggered by somatosensory stimuli, such as changing of clothes or lifting the child. The attacks consist of extension of the body, opening of the mouth, and stretching or flexing of the limbs lasting less than minutes.[26] In addition to these nonepileptic events, true seizures can also occur. Reflexes are usually brisk, clonus is often present, but nystagmus and extension plantar responses are less common. Most affected children are never able to sit by themselves or walk; those that manage to do so lose this ability with time, indicating progressive deterioration.

Cognitive impairment is severe. Individuals never develop speech or, at the most, acquire the ability to emit garbled sounds. Their behavior tends to be passive with little evidence of aggressiveness and they appear to respond to their surroundings by a social smile. Although brain MRI scans are often normal, atrophy of the cerebrum, thalamus, and basal ganglia have been reported, probably reflecting dysmyelination.[14,15] Female carries do not manifest any of these psychomotor abnormalities, but intellectual delay and frank mental retardation have been described.[10,16]

DIAGNOSIS

Most characteristic, if not pathognomonic, is the high serum T_3 and low rT_3 concentrations. Although T_4 is reduced in most cases and is usually the first thyroid abnormality identified during neonatal screening, T_4 has been normal in some individuals.[13] TSH levels are normal or slightly elevated, rarely above 6 mU/L. Heterozygous female carriers have serum TH concentrations intermediate between affected males and unaffected family members (see Fig. 22-2). However, they lack the typical psychomotor abnormalities always found in affected males.

Current diagnostic criteria include the characteristic thyroid abnormalities accompanied by truncal hypotonia, limb spasticity, poor head control, motor delays, and absent speech. The definitive diagnosis is made by the identification of mutations in the *MCT8* gene. Our experience has been that the TFT results are specifically associated with MCT8 defect. Sequencing of the *MCT8* gene in males with similar neuropsychiatric manifestations but who do not present the pathognomonic TFT abnormalities has yielded negative results.

The TFT pattern, with high T_3, low T_4, and low rT_3 levels, although characteristic of MCT8 deficiency, could be the consequence of other defects causing TH metabolic abnormalities. However, no genetic defects in deiodinases have so far been identified in humans. All three deiodinase genes were initial candidate genes in MCT8 and other defects with abnormal ratios of active and inactive TH.[27] They were eventually excluded by sequence and linkage analysis. Studies of *Mct8* KO mice have demonstrated secondary defects in TH metabolism caused by the tissue-specific TH availability and by the intrinsic complex regulation of deiodinases. The high serum T_3 levels with normal or slightly elevated TSH is compatible with RTH, but the low T_4 and low rT_3 levels exclude this diagnosis.

Serum transport defects have normal free TH levels, whereas in *MCT8* defects total and free levels are proportionally abnormal. In iodine deficiency, normal T_3 levels may be found in the context of low T_4, but treatments with iodine or T_4 would normalize the TFT abnormalities.

CLINICAL COURSE, PREVENTION, AND TREATMENT

The natural course of the disease caused by *MCT8* gene mutations is characterized by the profound motor impairment and absent speech development. Almost all affected males become wheelchair-bound in adult life. Although some achieve delayed and unsteady independent ambulation, they are dependent on their family's care or are institutionalized. In some families, there is early death; the cause is usually aspiration pneumonia. There are also reports of patients living longer than 70 years.

Finding treatment options for patients with *MCT8* gene mutations is challenging. Detection of elevated TSH by neonatal screening has prompted levothyroxine (L-T_4) treatment in several patients but physiological doses were not able to improve the outcome, because the cellular uptake of TH is impaired in MCT8-dependent tissues. Administration of pharmacologic doses of L-T_4during pregnancy and the efficacy of several TH analogues to bypass the molecular defect by using alternative transporters have therapeutic potential and are being tested in Mct8-deficient mice.

Prenatal testing and genetic counseling of carrier females can prevent the transmission of this defect to male offspring.

PITFALLS, COMPLICATIONS, AND CONTROVERSIES

Diagnostic Pitfalls

1. Because neonatal screening for hypothyroidism is based on the detection of elevated blood TSH and/or low T_4 levels, affected newborns are likely to be missed until suspected on the basis of neurodevelopmental findings.
2. Carrier females are asymptomatic, so the presence of abnormality is not suspected and thus is not sought until the birth of the first affected male.

Complications

1. Aspiration pneumonia
2. Seizures

Although not a constant feature of the syndrome, those with seizures could be refractory to standard anticonvulsants.

Controversies and Uncertainties

1. There is a debate as to whether the severe neuropsychiatric manifestations are caused by the abnormalities in TH transport or whether MCT8 is required for the transport of an important, but yet unidentified, substance.
2. Is the brain damage already present in the embryo or does it develop after birth? This is of great importance in planning therapy.
3. What is the sequence of events that leads to the development of the various thyroid test abnormalities? Does low T_4 precede the elevated T_3 level, and are TFT abnormalities always present at birth?

References

1. Abe T, Suzuki T, Unno M, et al: Thyroid hormone transporters: Recent advances. Trends Endocrinol Metab 13:215-220, 2002.
2. Friesema EC, Ganguly S, Abdalla A, et al: Identification of monocarboxylate transporter 8 as a specific thyroid hormone transporter. J Biol Chem 278:40128-40135, 2003.
3. Pizzagalli F, Hagenbuch B, Stieger B, et al: Identification of a novel human organic anion transporting polypeptide as a high affinity thyroxine transporter. Mol Endocrinol 16:2283-2296, 2002.
4. Hagenbuch B, Dawson P: The sodium bile salt cotransport family SLC10. Pflugers Arch 447:566-570, 2004.
5. Chairoungdua A, Kanai Y, Matsuo H, et al: Identification and characterization of a novel member of the heterodimeric amino acid transporter family presumed to be associated with an unknown heavy chain. J Biol Chem 276:49390-49399, 2001.
6. Friesema EC, Jansen J, Milici C, Visser TJ: Thyroid hormone transporters. Vitam Horm 70:137-167, 2005.
7. Bianco AC, Salvatore D, Gereben B, et al: Biochemistry, cellular and molecular biology, and physiological roles of the iodothyronine selenodeiodinases. Endocr Rev 23:38-89, 2002.
8. Yen PM, Ando S, Feng X, et al: Thyroid hormone action at the cellular, genomic and target gene levels. Mol Cell Endocrinol 246:121-127, 2006.
9. Refetoff S SP, Reutrakul S, Dennis K, et al: Resistance to thyroid hormone in the absence of mutations in the thyroid hormone receptor genes. In Beck-Peccoz P (ed): Syndromes of Hormone Resistance on the Hypothalamic-Pituitary-Thyroid Axis. Boston, Kluwer Academic Publishers, 2004, pp 89-107.
10. Dumitrescu AM, Liao XH, Best TB, et al: A novel syndrome combining thyroid and neurological abnormalities is associated with mutations in a monocarboxylate transporter gene. Am J Hum Genet 74:168-175, 2004.
11. Friesema EC, Grueters A, Biebermann H, et al: Association between mutations in a thyroid hormone transporter and severe X-linked psychomotor retardation. Lancet 364:1435-1437, 2004.
12. Schwartz CE, May MM, Carpenter NJ, et al: Allan-Herndon-Dudley syndrome and the monocarboxylate transporter 8 (MCT8) gene. Am J Hum Genet 77:41-53, 2005.
13. Maranduba CM, Friesema EC, Kok F, et al: Decreased cellular uptake and metabolism in Allan-Herndon-Dudley syndrome (AHDS) due to a novel mutation in the MCT8 thyroid hormone transporter. J Med Genet 43:457-460, 2006.
14. Kakinuma H, Itoh M, Takahashi H: A novel mutation in the monocarboxylate transporter 8 gene in a boy with putamen lesions and low free T_4 levels in cerebrospinal fluid. J Pediatr 147:552-554, 2005.
15. Holden KR, Zuniga OF, May MM, et al: X-linked MCT8 gene mutations: Characterization of the pediatric neurologic phenotype. J Child Neurol 20:852-857, 2005.
16. Herzovich V, Vaiani E, Marino R, et al: Unexpected peripheral markers of thyroid function in a patient with a novel mutation of the MCT8 thyroid hormone transporter gene. Horm Res 67:1-6, 2006.

17. Lafreniere RG, Carrel L, Willard HF: A novel transmembrane transporter encoded by the XPCT gene in Xq13.2. Hum Mol Genet 3:1133-1139, 1994.
18. Halestrap AP, Meredith D: The SLC16 gene family-from monocarboxylate transporters (MCTs) to aromatic amino acid transporters and beyond. Pflugers Arch 447:619-628, 2004.
19. Allan W, Herndon CN, Dudley FC: Some examples of the inheritance of mental deficiency: Apparently sex-linked idiocy and microcephaly. Am J Ment Defic 48:325-334, 1944.
20. Bialer MG, Lawrence L, Stevenson RE, et al: Allan-Herndon-Dudley syndrome: Clinical and linkage studies on a second family. Am J Med Genet 43: 491-497, 1992.
21. Zorick TS, Kleimann S, Sertie A, et al: Fine mapping and clinical reevaluation of a Brazilian pedigree with a severe form of X-linked mental retardation associated with other neurological dysfunction. Am J Med Genet A 127:321-323, 2004.
22. Friesema EC, Jansen J, Heuer H, et al: Mechanisms of disease: Psychomotor retardation and high T3 levels caused by mutations in monocarboxylate transporter 8. Nat Clin Pract Endocrinol Metab 2:512-523, 2006.
23. Dumitrescu AM, Liao XH, Weiss RE, et al: Tissue-specific thyroid hormone deprivation and excess in monocarboxylate transporter (mct) 8-deficient mice. Endocrinology 147:4036-4043, 2006.
24. Bernal J: Role of monocarboxylate anion transporter 8 (MCT8) in thyroid hormone transport: Answers from mice. Endocrinology 147:4034-4035, 2006.
25. Jansen J, Friesema EC, Milici C, Visser TJ: Thyroid hormone transporters in health and disease. Thyroid 15:757-768, 2005.
26. Brockmann K, Dumitrescu AM, Best TT, et al: X-linked paroxysmal dyskinesia and severe global retardation caused by defective MCT8 gene. J Neurol 252:663-666, 2005.
27. Dumitrescu AM, Liao XH, Abdullah MS, et al: Mutations in SECISBP2 result in abnormal thyroid hormone metabolism. Nat Genet 37:1247-1252, 2005.

Chapter 23

Drugs

Ronald N. Cohen

Key Points

- Certain drugs affect the pituitary and its ability to produce thyrotropin.
- Other medications cause frank thyroid dysfunction or lead to altered thyroid autoimmunity.
- Additional physiologic consequences of medications involve alterations in thyroid hormone-binding proteins, deiodinase enzymes, and regulation of thyroid hormone metabolism.
- Certain drugs decrease levothyroxine absorption from the gastrointestinal tract.
- Knowledge of these medications is vital to the appropriate interpretation of thyroid function tests.

The correct interpretation of thyrotropin (TSH) and thyroid hormone (TH) levels is vital for the proper evaluation of thyroid function. However, various medications interfere with these and other thyroid function tests (TFTs). Some drugs lead to thyroid dysfunction, whereas others merely complicate the analysis of TFT results. Knowledge of these effects allows for the correct interpretation of such tests and thus limits inappropriate treatment. In this chapter, we will review medications that have the following effects: (1) disrupt the pituitary regulation of the thyroid gland; (2) alter thyroid gland function itself; (3) interfere with generation of the active form of the thyroid hormone, triiodothyronine (T_3); (4) alter thyroid hormone-binding protein levels and/or function; and (5) impair thyroid hormone absorption from the gastrointestinal tract. An understanding of medications and their effects on thyroid hormone physiology is necessary for the proper diagnosis and treatment of patients with thyroid dysfunction.

DRUGS THAT AFFECT THYROTROPE FUNCTION IN THE PITUITARY

The TSH-producing cell in the anterior pituitary is called the thyrotrope (or thyrotroph). TSH itself is composed of two subunits, both of which are synthesized by the thyrotrope. The alpha subunit is common to TSH, follicle-stimulating hormone (FSH), luteinizing hormone (LH), and human chorionic gonadotropin (hCG). The beta subunit is specific to TSH. A number of medications act on the thyrotrope to decrease TSH synthesis and/or secretion. The effects of these medications must be distinguished from other causes of secondary hypothyroidism. To understand how drugs affect TSH levels, it is important to review the regulation of TSH (Figs. 23-1 and 23-2). The major positive regulator of TSH secretion is the hypothalamic hormone thyrotropin-releasing hormone (TRH). TRH stimulates TSH synthesis, increases TSH secretion, and enhances TSH bioactivity via its effect on TSH glycosylation. The major negative regulator of TSH is thyroid hormone through a classic negative feedback loop. However, a number of other factors also modulate TSH secretion, including the hypothalamic hormones dopamine and somatostatin and the adrenal hormone cortisol. Drugs that modulate and/or mimic these hormones alter TSH levels.

Glucocorticoids bind the glucocorticoid receptor (GR) to modulate gene transcription, either positively or negatively. Glucocorticoids repress transcription of both TSH subunits.[1,2] However, the exact mechanisms underlying GR modulation of TSH subunit gene synthesis by the thyrotrope remain unclear. It is not yet known whether some of these effects are mediated via other pituitary cell types.[3] Glucocorticoids also decrease the TSH pulse amplitude, suggesting an effect also on the TRH neuron.[4]

Glucocorticoid deficiency is associated with increased TSH levels,[5] and studies of patients with Addison's disease have shown that replacement doses of hydrocortisone decrease TSH levels.[6] In contrast, when glucocorticoids are used clinically at pharmacologic doses, TSH levels decrease. Glucocorticoid treatment can occasionally be confused with primary

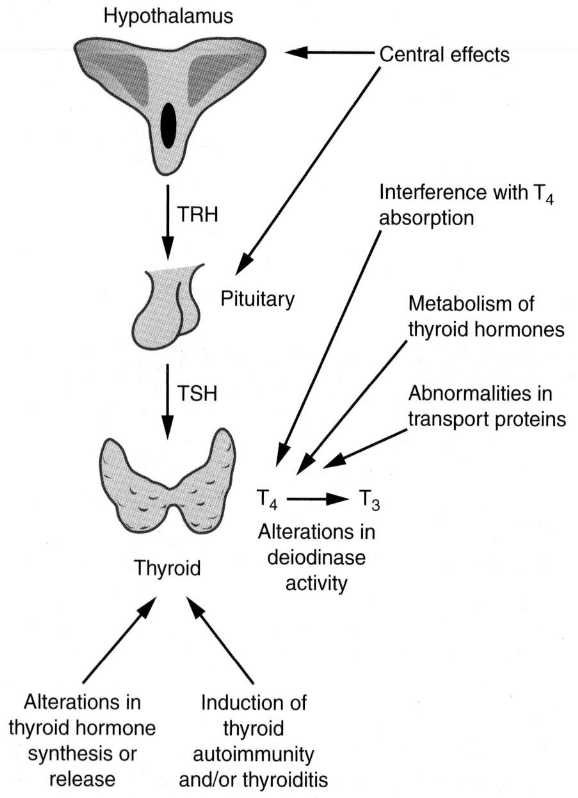

Figure 23–1 Methods whereby alteration can cause thyroid dysfunction or interfere with the interpretation of thyroid function tests. The hypothalamic-pituitary-thyroid axis is shown, along with different ways that medications interfere with thyroid function tests. Medications can affect the axis centrally or cause abnormalities in the thyroid gland. In addition, medications can alter thyroid hormone metabolism, protein binding, and/or absorption. T_3, triiodothyronine; T_4, thyroxine; TRH, thyrotropin-releasing hormone; TSH, thyroid-stimulating hormone.

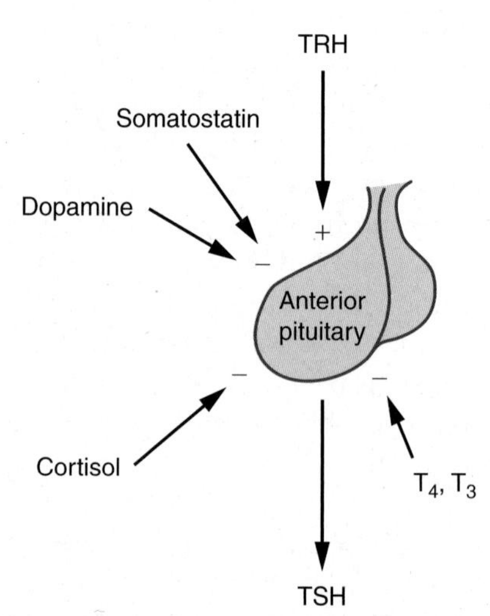

Figure 23–2 Medications can interfere with thyrotrope function. The major positive and negative regulators of thyroid-stimulating hormone (TSH) synthesis and/or secretion are shown. Medications that enhance or interfere with these pathways can change TSH levels and potentially lead to thyroid dysfunction. T_3, triiodothyronine; T_4, thyroxine; TRH, thyrotropin-releasing hormone

Table 23–1 Medications that Affect Pituitary or Thyroid Function

Affect Pituitary Regulation of Thyroid-Stimulating Hormone Secretion
Hydrocortisone
Dopamine
Somatostatin analogues
Bexarotene
Possibly others (e.g., dobutamine)

hyperthyroidism if only the TSH level is measured. In contrast to primary hyperthyroidism, however, TSH levels are not generally fully suppressed during glucocorticoid treatment, so highly sensitive TSH assays often can distinguish between these two situations. Glucocorticoid effects can also be difficult to distinguish from secondary hypothyroidism or severe nonthyroidal illness (NTI), also called sick euthyroid syndrome. Measurement of the reverse T_3 (rT_3) level, which is often elevated in NTI, can sometimes be helpful in this latter situation. Glucocorticoids have a variety of additional effects on thyroid hormone physiology (Table 23-1). They block conversion of thyroxine (T_4) to T_3,[7] decrease thyroxine-binding globulin (TBG) levels,[8] and increase renal iodine clearance. These effects will be discussed later in the appropriate sections.

As noted, TRH is not the only hypothalamic hormone that regulates TSH secretion. Somatostatin and dopamine are other factors important in this process. These agents and/or their analogues are used clinically, so their effects on TSH physiology must be considered. Somatostatin is produced in the brain and elsewhere and binds five subtypes of somatostatin receptors to mediates its effects. Somatostatin analogues are used clinically for the treatment of acromegaly and other disorders.[9] Somatostatin analogues decrease TSH levels but do not usually lead to hypothyroidism on their own. Because of their effects on the thyrotrope, somatostatin analogues are sometimes used to treat patients with TSH-secreting adenomas.[10] In contrast, dopamine is best recognized as the key negative regulator of prolactin secretion. Dopamine also decreases TSH synthesis[11] and secretion.[12] Dopamine antagonists (e.g., metoclopramide) transiently increase TSH levels.[13,14] Dopamine is used clinically in intensive care unit patients with hypotension, particularly in patients with septic shock. Thus, the effects of dopamine need to be differentiated from those of NTI, as well as glucocorticoids. It should be noted that the dopamine agonists bromocriptine and cabergoline

Table 23–2 Medications that Target the Thyroid Gland or Stimulate Thyroid Autoimmunity

Iodine-containing medications
Amiodarone
Iodinated contrast agents
Others
Thionamides
Propylthiouracil
Methimazole
Carbimazole
Perchlorate
Immunomodulatory agents
Interferons
Interleukin-2
Lithium
Sunitinib
Aminoglutethimide

do not seem to have as profound effects on TSH values[15,16] as dopamine itself. Although dopamine clearly has important effects on TSH physiology, the effects of another inotropic agent, dobutamine, is less clear. One study has suggested that dobutamine at high doses decreases TSH secretion, although levels did not fall to below normal.[17]

A novel chemotherapeutic agent, bexarotene, has dramatic effects on TSH levels. Bexarotene is used in the treatment of cutaneous T-cell lymphoma and functions as an agonist for the retinoid X receptor (RXR). RXR is a nuclear receptor that is structurally related to the thyroid hormone receptor (TR).[18] Bexarotene decreases TSH levels, which return to normal after its discontinuation.[19,20] The mechanisms underlying these effects are incompletely understood. Whereas bexarotene has been shown to repress TSH synthesis, one study also suggested that it decreases TSH release.[21] Bexarotene is the first in a class of RXR agonists, termed *rexinoids*, that may have widespread effects.[22]

Other medications that have been implicated in decreased TSH secretion include cimetidine,[23] morphine,[24] and metformin.[25] It is currently unclear how important these effects are clinically.

DRUGS THAT CAUSE HYPOTHYROIDISM OR HYPERTHYROIDISM

Various drugs directly affect the thyroid gland itself and/or modulate thyroid autoimmunity (Table 23-2). These effects should always be considered in patients diagnosed with thyroid dysfunction. In certain cases, stopping the offending medication can return thyroid status to normal, but in other cases, thyroid dysfunction persists. In this section, we will not discuss thionamides such as methimazole and propylthiouracil because they are included elsewhere in this text.

Iodine-Containing Compounds

Iodination of tyrosine residues in thyroglobulin is a key step in thyroid hormone biosynthesis. In one sense, therefore, it is not surprising that excess iodine can lead to increased thyroid hormone production. However, there are mechanisms to control thyroid hormone overproduction in these situations. Therefore, it is important to review the body's response to increased levels of iodine. Iodine is present in a number of medications, including amiodarone (see later), potassium iodide (SSKI), Lugol's solution, CT scan contrast agents, vitamins, and topical antiseptics.[26]

When iodine is in excess, the thyroid gland compensates by inhibiting its organification,[27] a process that has been termed the *Wolff-Chaikoff effect.* Thus, hyperthyroidism does not generally occur after an iodine load in normal individuals. Iodine-induced hyperthyroidism usually occurs in the setting of underlying thyroid nodularity.[28] This is likely caused by the presence of nodules with some degree of autonomous function. These nodules synthesize additional thyroid hormone when exposed to an iodine load. However, patients with other forms of goiter, patients with underlying Graves' disease, and even patients without evidence of thyroid dysfunction[26] can occasionally develop iodine-induced hyperthyroidism.

There is also an escape from the Wolff-Chaik off effect, after which thyroid hormone synthesis resumes. This appears to be caused by decreased transport of iodide across the thyroid follicular cell basolateral membrane resulting from decreased expression of the sodium iodide symporter.[29] Certain patients, however, develop frank hypothyroidism after exposure to large doses of iodine, in part because of the inability to escape from the Wolff-Chaikoff effect. As with iodine-induced hyperthyroidism (see earlier), these patients often have underlying thyroid disorders. Patients with underlying autoimmune thyroid disease, particularly Hashimoto's thyroiditis or treated Graves' disease, are prone to develop iodine-induced hypothyroidism, although normal individuals can develop hypothyroidism if large doses are ingested.[30]

Immunomodulatory Medications

Certain immunomodulatory drugs affect thyroid function by inducing or exacerbating thyroid autoimmunity. Interferon alfa (IFNα)[31] has been implicated in a destructive thyroiditis-like syndrome. It may be more apt to lead to thyroid dysfunction when used in the treatment of hepatitis C.[32] The thyroiditis associated with IFNα is painless, and the 24-hour uptake measurements taken during the thyrotoxic phase are characteristically low. As with other forms of thyroiditis, patients can also develop hypothyroidism. The incidence of thyroid dysfunction during therapy with interferon is variable, but the presence of preexisting antithyroid antibodies is a significant risk factor.[33] In addition to a transient destructive thyroiditis, interferon therapy has also been implicated in the development of Graves' disease, as well permanent hypothyroidism.[33] Interestingly, the development of hypothyroidism may be greater in interferon-treated patients also receiving ribavirin.[34]

Treatment with interleukin-2 (IL-2) can lead to the induction of a thyroiditis and development of thyroid autoimmunity.[35-37] Recently, denileukin, a fusion protein consisting of diphtheria toxin and a portion of IL-2, was also implicated as a cause of thyroiditis.[38] It is likely that novel immunomodulatory agents will also cause similar syndromes.

Lithium

Lithium is commonly used for the treatment of bipolar disorder. It has been known for many years that lithium has complex affects on thyroid function. Lithium treatment can result in goiter[39] and its major effect on the thyroid appears to occur via the inhibition of thyroid hormone release.[40] The mechanisms whereby lithium inhibits thyroid hormone secretion remain unclear, but therapy results in hypothyroidism in up to 20% of treated patients.[41] Hypothyroidism in lithium-treated patients is more common in women than men, and the prevalence increases with age.[42] Patients with preexisting thyroid autoimmunity are more likely to develop lithium-induced hypothyroidism.[43] Lithium may be able to induce thyroid autoimmunity in patients without evidence of thyroid autoantibodies at baseline.[44] Lithium can cause goiter, even in the absence of frank hypothyroidism. One study has suggested that up to 50% of lithium-treated patients may develop goiter, which is more common in smokers than nonsmokers.[45]

In contrast to hypothyroidism, lithium-induced hyperthyroidism is uncommon. Various forms of thyrotoxicosis have been identified in lithium-treated patients.[46] Certain studies have suggested that lithium may in particular cause a destructive thyroiditis.[47,48] Because of its effects on thyroid hormone and iodine release, lithium is sometimes used as an adjunctive therapy in the treatment of hyperthyroidism[49] and thyroid cancer.[50]

Amiodarone

Amiodarone also has complex effects on thyroid hormone physiology (see Table 23-2). A number of excellent reviews on amiodarone effects on thyroid physiology have been published.[51-53] Thus, we will focus mostly on amiodarone effects on TFTs and the development of thyroid dysfunction. Amiodarone contains a significant fraction of iodine, about 75 mg of iodine/200-mg tablet. Elevated levels of iodine mediate many of the effects of amiodarone on thyroid physiology. However, amiodarone has other important actions, including effects on deiodinase activity, thyroid hormone action, and the induction of thyroid cellular damage.

One of the first effects on thyroid homeostatis in amiodarone-treated patients is a block in T_4 to T_3 conversion.[54] Interestingly, in euthyroid patients acutely given intravenous amiodarone, the first alteration seen clinically was actually an increase in TSH levels.[55] Total T_3 levels declined throughout this study, reverse T_3 (rT_3) levels increased, and total and free T_4 levels increased. These effects may all be mediated through the inhibition of types 1 and 2 deiodinase enzymes. There is also evidence that amiodarone or its metabolites interfere with T_3 binding to the thyroid hormone receptor.[56] Thus, in the weeks after initiation of amiodarone therapy, TSH levels may transiently increase. However, during chronic ingestion of amiodarone, TSH levels generally normalize, but thyroid hormone levels in amiodarone-treated patients are different from those in untreated controls. In general, serum total and free T_4 levels are upper normal or mildly elevated, whereas serum T_3 levels are frequently in the low-normal range.[57] In contrast, rT_3 levels are increased or high normal. In the setting of normal TSH levels, amiodarone-treated patients are generally considered euthyroid. Over the long term, however, amiodarone therapy can lead to hypothyroidism or hyperthyroidism. Whereas hypothyroidism is more common in iodine-sufficient areas, patients are more likely to develop hyperthyroidism if they live in areas of iodine insufficiency.[58] This may occur because multinodular goiter with areas of autonomous function may be more common in areas of iodine deficiency.[59]

Amiodarone-induced hypothyroidism is more common in patients with underlying autoimmune thyroid disease, and may result in part from the failure to escape from the Wolff-Chaikoff effect. Some investigators have suggested that amiodarone may also lead to thyroid damage and release of thyroid autoantigens, leading to worsening autoimmune thyroid disease.[60] Patients with other thyroid abnormalities, such as dyshormonogenesis defects, are also likely to become hypothyroid during treatment with amiodarone.[52] Amiodarone-induced hypothyroidism is slightly more common in women than men, perhaps reflecting the increased incidence of autoimmune hypothyroidism in women. Hypothyroidism, when it occurs, usually develops between about 6 and 12 months of amiodarone therapy.[51] Patients with amiodarone-induced hypothyroidism can be treated with doses of levothyroxine to render the patient clinically euthyroid with a normal TSH level, although higher than usual doses of levothyroxine may be required.[61] There is no need to stop amiodarone under these circumstances. Certain clinicians aim for a TSH in the high-normal range.[52] If amiodarone is stopped, some patients become euthyroid but others remain hypothyroid. Patients with underlying thyroid disorders, particularly patients with evidence of thyroid autoimmunity, are most likely to develop permanent hypothyroidism.[62]

Patients with amiodarone-induced thyrotoxicosis are more difficult to treat. There are two types of amiodarone-induced thyrotoxicosis. In contrast to amiodarone-induced hypothyroidism, amiodarone-induced thyrotoxicosis may be more common in men than women. Hyperthyroidism can occur at any time during amiodarone therapy. In type 1 disease, the cause reflects the high iodine load resulting from amiodarone therapy, which leads to increased thyroid hormone synthesis and secretion. Patient with type 1 disease often have abnormalities on thyroid examination, with underlying thyroid nodular disease. These patients may be treated with high doses of thionamides. Amiodarone should be stopped if clinically reasonable, but this is not always feasible. If amiodarone is stopped, cardiac and thyroid function should be followed closely. Because amiodarone blocks deiodinase activity and interferes with thyroid hormone binding to its receptor, it is theoretically possible that stopping amiodarone could transiently increase symptoms of hyperthyroidism. Although high doses of thionamides (e.g., propylthiouracil and methimazole) are the mainstay of treatment, other agents have also been reported to be useful in the treatment of type 1 disease. Potassium perchlorate has been used to decrease iodine entry into the thyroid gland.[63] However, the usefulness of perchlorate is limited by side effects and limited availability. Lithium has been reported to be helpful by decreasing thyroid hormone release from the thyroid.[64] Radioactive iodine therapy usually cannot be used, because the high iodine load from amiodarone leads to low radioiodine uptake into the thyroid. This is particularly true in the United States and other iodine-sufficient areas. Ultimately, some patients require thyroidectomy, but such patients may be at high risk for surgery because of their underlying cardiac disease and thyrotoxicosis.

In type 2 disease, amiodarone causes a destructive thyroiditis. Pathologic evaluation of the thyroid glands in these patients reveals follicular damage.[65,66] In these patients, as in other patients with thyroiditis, thyrotoxicosis may be followed by hypothyroidism.[67] In patients with thyrotoxicosis caused by a destructive thyroiditis, even high doses of thionamides are generally ineffective. In contrast, these patients respond to glucocorticoid therapy. The usual starting dosage is about 40 to 60 mg/day of prednisone.

Although it is important to try to differentiate type 1 from type 2 amiodarone-induced thyrotoxicosis, the distinction can be difficult. IL-6 levels are generally higher in type 2 disease, but have not been as useful in clinical practice, as initially anticipated.[68] Radioiodine uptake measurements are low in both types of amiodarone-induced thyrotoxicosis, but may be lower in type 2 disease. One modality that has proven to be helpful is the use of color flow Doppler ultrasonography.[68] Vascularity is increased in type 1 disease and is normal or low in type 2 disease.[51] Some patients have a mixed clinical picture, and are treated with a combination of thionamides and glucocorticoids. Some clinicians treat with both types of agents if the distinction between types 1 and 2 disease cannot be made,[69] with an early effect favoring glucocorticoid treatment of type 2 disease.

Other Medications

Other medications have also been implicated in causing thyroid dysfunction. For example, a recent report has suggested that the novel chemotherapeutic agent sunitinib causes hypothyroidism, likely via a thyroiditis-like effect.[70] Case series have also implicated other medications in the development of hypothyroidism, including aminoglutethimide,[71] quetiapine,[72,73] thalidomide,[74] and St. John's wort.[75]

MEDICATIONS THAT AFFECT THYROID HORMONE–BINDING PROTEINS

Most thyroid hormones (both T_4 and T_3) are bound to proteins in plasma; these proteins include TBG, transthyretin (TTR), and albumin. There are two main ways that medications can affect TFTs via these proteins: (1) medications may directly affect binding protein levels (particularly TBG, which is quantitatively the most important binding protein); and (2) medications may instead displace thyroid hormones from these proteins (Table 23-3). Both these mechanisms do not generally cause long-term thyroid dysfunction. However, they

Table 23–3 Medications that Affect Serum-Binding Proteins or Thyroid Hormone Metabolism

Increase Thyroid Hormone-Binding Proteins
Estrogens and selective estrogen receptor modulators (SERMs)
Methadone
Fluorouracil
Decrease Thyroid Hormone-Binding Proteins
Androgens
Anabolic steroids
Glucocorticoids
Asparaginase
Nicotinic acid
Displace Thyroid Hormone from Binding Proteins
Aspirin and nonsteroidal anti-inflammatory drugs (to varying degrees)
Furosemide (high doses)
Heparin (generally considered an in vitro effect)
Increase Thyroid Hormone Metabolism
Phenobarbital
Phenytoin
Carbamazepine and oxcarbamazepine
Rifampin
Imatinib (mechanism not clearly defined)

can cause abnormalities in thyroid tests that can lead to inappropriate treatment. High TBG levels lead to elevated total T_4 and T_3 levels, even in the setting of normal free hormone levels. Thus, elevated TBG levels may lead to the inappropriate diagnosis of hyperthyroidism. Similarly, low TBG levels may be confused with hypothyroidism. In addition, replacement doses of levothyroxine may need to be altered when binding protein levels are significantly changed.

Drugs That Affect Binding Protein Levels

A number of medications increase or decrease TBG levels. Estradiol and other estrogens alter the glycosylation pattern of TBG, decreasing its breakdown.[76] Because of reduced clearance, TBG levels are elevated. These increased levels lead to high total thyroid hormone levels, but free thyroid hormone levels remain normal. In addition, because free thyroid hormone levels are normal, TSH level remain normal in euthyroid individuals. However, increased TBG levels may lead to increased levothyroxine requirements in postmenopausal hypothyroid women who initiate estrogen replacement therapy.[77] Women with hypothyroidism often require increased dosages of levothyroxine during pregnancy[78] and high TBG levels are one cause of this phenomenon.[79] In addition to estrogen, the newer selective estrogen receptor modulators (SERMs), such as tamoxifen and raloxifine, also increase TBG levels in postmenopausal women, although not to the same degree as with estrogen.[80,81] Other medications that increase TBG levels include methadone[82] and fluorouracil.[83,84]

In contrast to estrogen's effects, testosterone and the anabolic steroids decrease TBG levels and lead to low measured levels of total T_4 and total T_3. Again, free hormone levels remain normal. However, levothyroxine requirements may decrease in patients being treated for hypothyroidism.[85] Glucocorticoids, in addition to their other effects on thyroid hormone physiology, also decrease TBG levels.[8] As with other agents that decrease TBG levels, glucocorticoids lead to lower total T_4 and T_3 levels. However, the drop in T_3 is more pronounced than the decrease in T_4 in glucocorticoid-treated patients. This is because high doses of glucocorticoids also block the conversion of T_4 to T_3 (see later). Finally, asparaginase, a chemotherapeutic agent used in the treatment of acute leukemia, also dramatically lowers TBG levels.[86,87]

Drugs That Displace Thyroid Hormone from Binding Proteins

Various medications do not change binding proteins levels but instead displace thyroid hormone from these proteins. Salicylates compete with thyroid hormone to binding sites on TBG and transthyretin. One study has suggested that nonsteroidal anti-inflammatory drugs (NSAIDs) have this effect to varying degrees, and that salsalate is particularly likely to lead to abnormal TFT results.[88] The displacement of T_4 from TBG leads to a transient increase in free T_4 levels.[89] After a new equilibrium is reached, TSH levels are normal but total T_4 levels decline to maintain normal free T_4 levels. This pattern of TFTs can be confused with secondary hypothyroidism. Furosemide (at high doses) also interferes with thyroid hormone binding to TBG and can lead to abnormal thyroid hormone levels.[90,91]

Heparin causes an increase in measured free T_4 levels via an in vitro artifact related to the displacement of T_4 from TBG.[90,91] Heparin activates lipoprotein lipase, which in turn breaks down triglycerides to free fatty acids (FFAs). FFAs then displace T_4 from TBG. This is important mainly in the interpretation of TFT results, because heparin

Table 23–4 Medications that Impair Deiodinase Activity

Glucocorticoids
Amiodarone
Certain beta blockers (particularly propranolol)
Oral iodinated cholecystography contrast agents
Iopanoic acid
Ipodate
Propylthiouracil

treatment does not lead to thyrotoxicosis in vivo. This phenomenon is more apt to occur in the setting of high triglyceride levels.

MEDICATIONS THAT DECREASE CONVERSION OF THYROXINE TO TRIIODOTHYRONINE

The conversion of T_4 to T_3 is mediated by deiodinase enzymes.[92] There are three types of deiodinases; types 1 and 2 convert T_4 to T_3, whereas type 3 converts T_4 to the inactive molecule rT_3. Various medications interfere with deiodinase activity (Table 23-4). Some of these medications (e.g., amiodarone[93] and glucocorticoids[7]) have been discussed. Although amiodarone causes hypothyroidism and hyperthyroidism, even euthyroid amiodarone-treated patients generally have abnormalities in TFT results because of interference with deiodinase activity. These patients, like others treated with medications that block the conversion of T_4 to T_3, generally have high T_4 levels in the setting of a normal TSH (see earlier). This set of TFT results can be confused with secondary hyperthyroidism (or thyroid hormone resistance) if it is not known that the patient is receiving such medications. A subset of beta blockers, particularly propranolol at high doses, also block deiodinase enzymes.[94,95]

We have already discussed the effects of iodine on thyroid hormone production and the development of hyperthyroidism and hypothyroidism. However, iodine has additional effects on thyroid hormone physiology, including effects on deiodinase activity. In areas of iodine deficiency, these effects may help maintain T_3 levels.[96] The iodinated contrast agents sodium iopanoate and sodium ipodate dramatically block deiodinase activity and thus impair T_4 to T_3 conversion.[97] Therefore, these medications have been used successfully to treat hyperthyroidism; however, they are difficult to obtain at present, and their use has correspondingly diminished.

MEDICATIONS THAT INCREASE THYROID HORMONE METABOLISM

A number of anticonvulsant medications increase thyroid hormone metabolism by stimulating the hepatic P-450 system, including phenobarbital, phenytoin, and carbamezapine. The antituberculosis drug rifampin has a similar effect.[98] In addition to iodination, thyroid hormones are metabolized via glucuronidation and sulfation pathways. Medications such as phenobarbital increase the expression of glucuronosyltransferase (UGT) and sulfotransferase (SULT) enzymes.[99,100] Qatanani and colleagues[101] have shown that phenobarbital increases expression of these enzymes by activating an orphan nuclear receptor called constitutive androstane receptor (CAR). In the absence of an inducing signal, CAR is located in the cytoplasm of cells (e.g., hepatocytes). On stimulation, CAR is translocated to the nucleus, where it binds to gene promoter sequences and increases the transcription of these target genes.[102] Thus, CAR activation leads to the expression of genes involved in T_4 and T_3 metabolism. Some of these effects may also be mediated by the nuclear receptor pregnane X receptor (PXR).[103] In euthyroid patients treated with phenobarbital, compensation by the hypothalamic-pituitary-thyroid axis results in normal TSH levels and often even normal free T_4 levels.[104,105] However, patients with hypothyroidism treated with phenobarbital may require a higher dose of levothyroxine. In addition, patients with borderline hypothyroidism may develop frank hypothyroidism after initiation of phenobarbital therapy. Phenobarbital may also augment the effects of other medications, such as phenytoin or carbamezapine.

Treatment with phenytoin and carbamazepine results in more dramatic alterations in TFT results than phenobarbital, probably because they have more complex effects on thyroid hormone physiology. These medications, like phenobarbital, stimulate T_4 and T_3 metabolism via CAR.[106] However, phenytoin also interferes with T_4 and T_3 binding to TBG and may also have other effects.[107] The combination of reduced TBG binding and increased thyroid hormone metabolism results in decreased T_4 levels. Similar to phenobarbital, TSH levels remain normal in euthyroid patients and free T_4 levels, if measured by equilibrium dialysis methods, are generally normal as well. However, free T_4 estimations may not correct these abnormalities, and thus may be reported as decreased.[108] It is important not to confuse these TFT result abnormalities with secondary hypothyroidism. Normal TSH levels in patients taking phenytoin or carbamazepine generally indicate a euthyroid state.

Table 23–5 Medications that Decrease Levothyroxine Absorption

Calcium carbonate
Iron sulfate
Aluminum hydroxide
Sucralfate
Cholestyramine and colestipol
Soy products and formula
Omeprazole (via decreased gastric acidity)
Sevelamer
Chromium picolinate

Oxcarbazepine is a medication that is related to carbamazepine that has fewer effects on the hepatic P-450 enzyme system. However, oxcarbazepine has also been noted to decrease T_4 levels,[109,110] although another report has suggested that replacing carbamazepine with oxcarbazepine could help restore thyroid hormone levels to normal.[111]

Imatinib is novel chemotherapeutic agent that targets BLC-ABL and is used in the treatment of chronic myelogenous leukemia and gastrointestinal stromal tumors. One study has shown that hypothyroid patients taking imatinib require higher doses of levothyroxine, likely because of an increase in thyroid hormone metabolism.[112] In contrast, euthyroid control patients did not develop hypothyroidism under these circumstances.

MEDICATIONS THAT DECREASE THYROXINE ABSORPTION

There are various medications that decrease absorption of thyroid hormones in the gastrointestinal tract (Table 23-5). These do not cause TFT abnormalities in euthyroid patients. However, they can become clinically important in hypothyroid patients receiving levothyroxine replacement therapy, because levothyroxine requirements may increase. It is best if levothyroxine is ingested in the morning before any of these other medications is taken. The most clinically important of these medications are calcium carbonate,[113,114] ferrous sulfate,[115] aluminum,[116] sucralfate,[117] cholestyramine,[118] costipol,[119] and soy proteins.[120] Soy formula appears to decrease levothyroxine absorption in infants with congenital hypothyroidism.[121,122] A recent report has also suggested that omeprazole, a proton pump inhibitor (PPI) used in the treatment of peptic ulcer disease, interferes with levothyroxine absorption by decreasing gastric acidity.[123] It is likely that other PPIs also have this effect, and raises the possibility that other medications that decrease gastric acidity may interfere with levothyroxine absorption. Finally, case reports have also suggested that ciprofloxacin[124] and raloxifine[125,126] may decrease levothyroxine absorption.

CONCLUSIONS

Many medications alter thyroid hormone physiology and lead to abnormalities in TFT results. Some present problems only if these changes are misinterpreted as thyroid abnormalities; others can lead to frank thyroid dysfunction. Thus, it is of vital importance for the clinician to be aware of these effects. In addition, as novel medications continue to be introduced, it is likely that additional effects will continue to be discovered. It is imperative to consider medications when interpreting any set of abnormal TFT results.

References

1. Re RN, Kourides IA, Ridgway EC, et al: The effect of glucocorticoid administration on human pituitary secretion of thyrotropin and prolactin. J Clin Endocrinol Metab 43:338-346, 1976.
2. Ross DS, Ellis MF, Milbury P, et al: A comparison of changes in plasma thyrotropin beta- and alpha-subunits, and mouse thyrotropic tumor thyrotropin beta- and alpha-subunit mRNA concentrations after in vivo dexamethasone or T_3 administration. Metabolism 36:799-803, 1987.
3. John CD, Christian HC, Morris JF, et al: Kinase-dependent regulation of the secretion of thyrotrophin and luteinizing hormone by glucocorticoids and annexin 1 peptides. J Neuroendocrinol 15:946-957, 2003.
4. Adriaanse R, Brabant G, Endert E, et al: Pulsatile thyrotropin secretion in patients with Cushing's syndrome. Metabolism 43:782-786, 1994.
5. Topliss DJ, White EL, Stockigt JR: Significance of thyrotropin excess in untreated primary adrenal insufficiency. J Clin Endocrinol Metab 50:52-56, 1980.
6. Hangaard J, Andersen M, Grodum E, et al: The effects of endogenous opioids and cortisol on thyrotropin and prolactin secretion in patients with Addison's disease. J Clin Endocrinol Metab 84: 1595-1601, 1999.
7. Chopra IJ, Williams DE, Orgiazzi J, et al: Opposite effects of dexamethasone on serum concentrations of 3,3′,5′-triiodothyronine (reverse T_3) and 3,3′5-triiodothyronine (T_3). J Clin Endocrinol Metab 41:911-920, 1975.
8. Gamstedt A, Jarnerot G, Kagedal B, et al: Corticosteroids and thyroid function. Different effects on plasma volume, thyroid hormones and thyroid hormone-binding proteins after oral and intravenous administration. Acta Med Scand 205:379-383, 1979.
9. Weckbecker G, Lewis I, Albert R, et al: Opportunities in somatostatin research: Biological, chemical and therapeutic aspects. Nat Rev Drug Discov 2:999-1017, 2003.

10. Socin HV, Chanson P, Delemer B, et al: The changing spectrum of TSH-secreting pituitary adenomas: Diagnosis and management in 43 patients. Eur J Endocrinol 148:433-442, 2003.
11. Shupnik MA, Greenspan SL, Ridgway EC: Transcriptional regulation of thyrotropin subunit genes by thyrotropin-releasing hormone and dopamine in pituitary cell culture. J Biol Chem 261:12675-12679, 1986.
12. Cooper DS, Klibanski A, Ridgway EC: Dopaminergic modulation of TSH and its subunits: In vivo and in vitro studies. Clin Endocrinol (Oxf) 18:265-275, 1983.
13. Scanlon MF, Weightman DR, Mora B, et al: Evidence for dopaminergic control of thyrotrophin secretion in man. Lancet 2:421-423, 1977.
14. Scanlon MF, Weightman DR, Shale DJ, et al: Dopamine is a physiological regulator of thyrotrophin (TSH) secretion in normal man. Clin Endocrinol (Oxf) 10:7-15, 1979.
15. Giusti M, Lomeo A, Torre R, et al: Effect of subacute cabergoline treatment on prolactin, thyroid stimulating hormone and growth hormone response to simultaneous administration of thyrotrophin-releasing hormone and growth hormone-releasing hormone in hyperprolactinaemic women. Clin Endocrinol (Oxf) 30:315-321, 1989.
16. Kobberling J, Darragh A, Del Pozo E: Chronic dopamine receptor stimulation using bromocriptine: Failure to modify thyroid function. Clin Endocrinol (Oxf) 11:367-370, 1979.
17. Lee E, Chen P, Rao H, et al: Effect of acute high-dose dobutamine administration on serum thyrotrophin (TSH). Clin Endocrinol (Oxf) 50:487-492, 1999.
18. Mangelsdorf DJ, Thummel C, Beato M, et al: The nuclear receptor superfamily: The second decade. Cell 83:835-839, 1995.
19. Golden WM, Weber KB, Hernandez TL, et al: Single-dose rexinoid rapidly and specifically suppresses serum thyrotropin in normal subjects. J Clin Endocrinol Metab 92:124-130, 2007.
20. Sherman SI, Gopal J, Haugen BR, et al: Central hypothyroidism associated with retinoid X receptor–selective ligands. N Engl J Med 340:1075-1079, 1999.
21. Liu S, Ogilvie KM, Klausing K, et al: Mechanism of selective retinoid X receptor agonist-induced hypothyroidism in the rat. Endocrinology 143:2880-2885, 2002.
22. Desvergne B: RXR: From partnership to leadership in metabolic regulations. Vitam Horm 75: 1-32, 2007.
23. Ulloa ER, Zaninovich AA: Effects of histamine H1- and H2-receptor antagonists on thyrotrophin secretion in the rat. J Endocrinol 111:175-180, 1986.
24. Ogrin C, Schussler GC: Suppression of thyrotropin by morphine in a severely stressed patient. Endocr J 52:265-269, 2005.
25. Vigersky RA, Filmore-Nassar A, Glass AR: Thyrotropin suppression by metformin. J Clin Endocrinol Metab 91:225-227, 2006.
26. Roti E, Uberti ED: Iodine excess and hyperthyroidism. Thyroid 11:493-500, 2001.
27. Wolff J, Chaikoff IL: Plasma inorganic iodide as a homeostatic regulator of thyroid function. J Biol Chem 174:555-564, 1948.
28. Stanbury JB, Ermans AE, Bourdoux P, et al: Iodine-induced hyperthyroidism: Occurrence and epidemiology. Thyroid 8:83-100, 1998.
29. Eng PH, Cardona GR, Fang SL, et al: Escape from the acute Wolff-Chaikoff effect is associated with a decrease in thyroid sodium iodide symporter messenger ribonucleic acid and protein. Endocrinology 140:3404-3410, 1999.
30. Markou K, Georgopoulos N, Kyriazopoulou V, et al: Iodine-induced hypothyroidism. Thyroid 11:501-510, 2001.
31. Koh LK, Greenspan FS, Yeo PP: Interferon-alpha induced thyroid dysfunction: Three clinical presentations and a review of the literature. Thyroid 7:891-896, 1997.
32. Fernandez-Soto L, Gonzalez A, Escobar-Jimenez F, et al: Increased risk of autoimmune thyroid disease in hepatitis C vs hepatitis B before, during, and after discontinuing interferon therapy. Arch Intern Med 158:1445-1448, 1998.
33. Carella C, Mazziotti G, Amato G, et al: Clinical review 169: Interferon-alpha-related thyroid disease: pathophysiological, epidemiological, and clinical aspects. J Clin Endocrinol Metab 89:3656-3661, 2004.
34. Carella C, Mazziotti G, Morisco F, et al: The addition of ribavirin to interferon-alpha therapy in patients with hepatitis C virus-related chronic hepatitis does not modify the thyroid autoantibody pattern but increases the risk of developing hypothyroidism. Eur J Endocrinol 146:743-749, 2002.
35. Atkins MB, Mier JW, Parkinson DR, et al: Hypothyroidism after treatment with interleukin-2 and lymphokine-activated killer cells. N Engl J Med 318:1557-1563, 1988.
36. Krouse RS, Royal RE, Heywood G, et al: Thyroid dysfunction in 281 patients with metastatic melanoma or renal carcinoma treated with interleukin-2 alone. J Immunother Emphasis Tumor Immunol 18:272-278, 1995.
37. Vialettes B, Guillerand MA, Viens P, et al: Incidence rate and risk factors for thyroid dysfunction during recombinant interleukin-2 therapy in advanced malignancies. Acta Endocrinol (Copenh) 129:31-38, 1993.
38. Ghori F, Polder KD, Pinter-Brown LC, et al: Thyrotoxicosis after denileukin diftitox therapy in patients with mycosis fungoides. J Clin Endocrinol Metab 91:2205-2208, 2006.
39. Schou M, Amdisen A, Eskjaer Jensen S, et al: Occurrence of goitre during lithium treatment. Br Med J 3:710-713, 1968.

40. Berens SC, Bernstein RS, Robbins J, et al: Antithyroid effects of lithium. J Clin Invest 49:1357-1367, 1970.
41. Bocchetta A, Loviselli A: Lithium treatment and thyroid abnormalities. Clin Pract Epidemol Ment Health 2:23, 2006.
42. Kirov G, Tredget J, John R, et al: A cross-sectional and a prospective study of thyroid disorders in lithium-treated patients. J Affect Disord 87:313-317, 2005.
43. Myers DH, Carter RA, Burns BH, et al: A prospective study of the effects of lithium on thyroid function and on the prevalence of antithyroid antibodies. Psychol Med 15:55-61, 1985.
44. Wilson R, McKillop JH, Crocket GT, et al: The effect of lithium therapy on parameters thought to be involved in the development of autoimmune thyroid disease. Clin Endocrinol (Oxf) 34:357-361, 1991.
45. Perrild H, Hegedus L, Baastrup PC, et al: Thyroid function and ultrasonically determined thyroid size in patients receiving long-term lithium treatment. Am J Psychiatry 147:1518-1521, 1990.
46. Barclay ML, Brownlie BE, Turner JG, et al: Lithium associated thyrotoxicosis: A report of 14 cases, with statistical analysis of incidence. Clin Endocrinol (Oxf) 40:759-764, 1994.
47. Dang AH, Hershman JM: Lithium-associated thyroiditis. Endocr Pract 8:232-236, 2002.
48. Miller KK, Daniels GH: Association between lithium use and thyrotoxicosis caused by silent thyroiditis. Clin Endocrinol (Oxf) 55:501-508, 2001.
49. Bogazzi F, Bartalena L, Pinchera A, et al: Adjuvant effect of lithium on radioiodine treatment of hyperthyroidism. Thyroid 12:1153-1154, 2002.
50. Koong SS, Reynolds JC, Movius EG, et al: Lithium as a potential adjuvant to ^{131}I therapy of metastatic, well-differentiated thyroid carcinoma. J Clin Endocrinol Metab 84:912-916, 1999.
51. Basaria S, Cooper DS: Amiodarone and the thyroid. Am J Med 118:706-714, 2005.
52. Bogazzi F, Bartalena L, Gasperi M, et al: The various effects of amiodarone on thyroid function. Thyroid 11:511-519, 2001.
53. Martino E, Bartalena L, Bogazzi F, et al: The effects of amiodarone on the thyroid. Endocr Rev 22:240-254, 2001.
54. Burger A, Dinichert D, Nicod P, et al: Effect of amiodarone on serum triiodothyronine, reverse triiodothyronine, thyroxin, and thyrotropin. A drug influencing peripheral metabolism of thyroid hormones. J Clin Invest 58:255-259, 1976.
55. Iervasi G, Clerico A, Bonini R, et al: Acute effects of amiodarone administration on thyroid function in patients with cardiac arrhythmia. J Clin Endocrinol Metab 82:275-280, 1997.
56. Latham KR, Sellitti DF, Goldstein RE: Interaction of amiodarone and desethylamiodarone with solubilized nuclear thyroid hormone receptors. J Am Coll Cardiol 9:872-876, 1987.
57. Amico JA, Richardson V, Alpert B, et al: Clinical and chemical assessment of thyroid function during therapy with amiodarone. Arch Intern Med 144:487-490, 1984.
58. Martino E, Safran M, Aghini-Lombardi F, et al: Environmental iodine intake and thyroid dysfunction during chronic amiodarone therapy. Ann Intern Med 101:28-34, 1984.
59. Bonnema SJ, Bennedbaek FN, Ladenson PW, et al: Management of the nontoxic multinodular goiter: A North American survey. J Clin Endocrinol Metab 87:112-117, 2002.
60. Martino E, Aghini-Lombardi F, Bartalena L, et al: Enhanced susceptibility to amiodarone-induced hypothyroidism in patients with thyroid autoimmune disease. Arch Intern Med 154:2722-2726, 1994.
61. Albert SG, Alves LE, Rose EP: Thyroid dysfunction during chronic amiodarone therapy. J Am Coll Cardiol 9:175-183, 1987.
62. Martino E, Aghini-Lombardi F, Mariotti S, et al: Amiodarone iodine-induced hypothyroidism: Risk factors and follow-up in 28 cases. Clin Endocrinol (Oxf) 26:227-237, 1987.
63. Martino E, Aghini-Lombardi F, Mariotti S, et al: Treatment of amiodarone-associated thyrotoxicosis by simultaneous administration of potassium perchlorate and methimazole. J Endocrinol Invest 9:201-207, 1986.
64. Dickstein G, Shechner C, Adawi F, et al: Lithium treatment in amiodarone-induced thyrotoxicosis. Am J Med 102:454-458, 1997.
65. Brennan MD, Erickson DZ, Carney JA, et al: Nongoitrous (type I) amiodarone-associated thyrotoxicosis: Evidence of follicular disruption in vitro and in vivo. Thyroid 5:177-183, 1995.
66. Smyrk TC, Goellner JR, Brennan MD, et al: Pathology of the thyroid in amiodarone-associated thyrotoxicosis. Am J Surg Pathol 11:197-204, 1987.
67. Roti E, Minelli R, Gardini E, et al: Iodine-induced subclinical hypothyroidism in euthyroid subjects with a previous episode of amiodarone-induced thyrotoxicosis. J Clin Endocrinol Metab 75:1273-1277, 1992.
68. Eaton SE, Euinton HA, Newman CM, et al: Clinical experience of amiodarone-induced thyrotoxicosis over a 3-year period: Role of colour-flow Doppler sonography. Clin Endocrinol (Oxf) 56:33-38, 2002.
69. Daniels GH: Amiodarone-induced thyrotoxicosis. J Clin Endocrinol Metab 86:3-8, 2001.
70. Desai J, Yassa L, Marqusee E, et al: Hypothyroidism after sunitinib treatment for patients with gastrointestinal stromal tumors. Ann Intern Med 145:660-664, 2006.
71. Dowsett M, Mehta A, Cantwell BM, et al: Low-dose aminoglutethimide in postmenopausal breast cancer: Effects on adrenal and thyroid hormone secretion. Eur J Cancer 27:846-849, 1991.
72. Feret BM, Caley CF: Possible hypothyroidism associated with quetiapine. Ann Pharmacother 34:483-486, 2000.

73. Greenspan A, Gharabawi G, Kwentus J: Thyroid dysfunction during treatment with atypical antipsychotics. J Clin Psychiatry 66:1334-1335, 2005.
74. Dimopoulos MA, Eleutherakis-Papaiakovou V: Adverse effects of thalidomide administration in patients with neoplastic diseases. Am J Med 117: 508-515, 2004.
75. Ferko N and Levine MA: Evaluation of the association between St. John's wort and elevated thyroid-stimulating hormone. Pharmacotherapy 21:1574-1578, 2001.
76. Ain KB, Mori Y, Refetoff S: Reduced clearance rate of thyroxine-binding globulin (TBG) with increased sialylation: A mechanism for estrogen-induced elevation of serum TBG concentration. J Clin Endocrinol Metab 65:689-696, 1987.
77. Arafah BM: Increased need for thyroxine in women with hypothyroidism during estrogen therapy. N Engl J Med 344:1743-1749, 2001.
78. Alexander EK, Marqusee E, Lawrence J, et al: Timing and magnitude of increases in levothyroxine requirements during pregnancy in women with hypothyroidism. N Engl J Med 351:241-249, 2004.
79. Mandel SJ, Larsen PR, Seely EW, et al: Increased need for thyroxine during pregnancy in women with primary hypothyroidism. N Engl J Med 323:91-96, 1990.
80. Mamby CC, Love RR, Lee KE: Thyroid function test changes with adjuvant tamoxifen therapy in postmenopausal women with breast cancer. J Clin Oncol 13:854-857, 1995.
81. Marqusee E, Braverman LE, Lawrence JE, et al: The effect of droloxifene and estrogen on thyroid function in postmenopausal women. J Clin Endocrinol Metab 85:4407-4410, 2000.
82. English TN, Ruxton D, Eastman CJ: Abnormalities in thyroid function associated with chronic therapy with methadone. Clin Chem 34:2202-2204, 1988.
83. Ain KB, Refetoff S: Relationship of oligosaccharide modification to the cause of serum thyroxine-binding globulin excess. J Clin Endocrinol Metab 66:1037-1043, 1988.
84. Beex L, Ross A, Smals A, et al: 5-Fluorouracil–induced increase of total serum thyroxine and triiodothyronine. Cancer Treat Rep 61:1291-1295, 1977.
85. Arafah BM: Decreased levothyroxine requirement in women with hypothyroidism during androgen therapy for breast cancer. Ann Intern Med 121:247-251, 1994.
86. Ferster A, Glinoer D, Van Vliet G, et al: Thyroid function during L-asparaginase therapy in children with acute lymphoblastic leukemia: Difference between induction and late intensification. Am J Pediatr Hematol Oncol 14:192-196, 1992.
87. Garnick MB, Larsen PR: Acute deficiency of thyroxine-binding globulin during L-asparaginase therapy. N Engl J Med 301:252-253, 1979.
88. Bishnoi A, Carlson HE, Gruber BL, et al: Effects of commonly prescribed nonsteroidal anti-inflammatory drugs on thyroid hormone measurements. Am J Med 96:235-238, 1994.
89. Faber J, Waetjen I, Siersbaek-Nielsen K: Free thyroxine measured in undiluted serum by dialysis and ultrafiltration: Effects of non-thyroidal illness, and an acute load of salicylate or heparin. Clin Chim Acta 223:159-167, 1993.
90. Stockigt JR, Lim CF, Barlow JW, et al: High concentrations of furosemide inhibit serum binding of thyroxine. J Clin Endocrinol Metab 59:62-66, 1984.
91. Stockigt JR, Lim CF, Barlow JW, et al: Interaction of furosemide with serum thyroxine-binding sites: In vivo and in vitro studies and comparison with other inhibitors. J Clin Endocrinol Metab 60:1025-1031, 1985.
92. Bianco AC, Kim BW: Deiodinases: Implications of the local control of thyroid hormone action. J Clin Invest 116:2571-2579, 2006.
93. Sogol PB, Hershman JM, Reed AW, et al: The effects of amiodarone on serum thyroid hormones and hepatic thyroxine 5′-monodeiodination in rats. Endocrinology 113:1464-1469, 1983.
94. Cooper DS, Daniels GH, Ladenson PW, et al: Hyperthyroxinemia in patients treated with high-dose propranolol. Am J Med 73:867-871, 1982.
95. Perrild H, Hansen JM, Skovsted L, et al: Different effects of propranolol, alprenolol, sotalol, atenolol and metoprolol on serum T_3 and serum rT_3 in hyperthyroidism. Clin Endocrinol (Oxf) 18:139-142, 1983.
96. Obregon MJ, Escobar del Rey F, Morreale de Escobar G: The effects of iodine deficiency on thyroid hormone deiodination. Thyroid 15:917-929, 2005.
97. Braga M, Cooper DS: Clinical review 129: Oral cholecystographic agents and the thyroid. J Clin Endocrinol Metab 86:1853-1860, 2001.
98. Nolan SR, Self TH, Norwood JM: Interaction between rifampin and levothyroxine. South Med J 92:529-531, 1999.
99. Liu J, Liu Y, Barter RA, et al: Alteration of thyroid homeostasis by UDP-glucuronosyltransferase inducers in rats: A dose-response study. J Pharmacol Exp Ther 273:977-985, 1995.
100. McClain RM, Levin AA, Posch R, et al: The effect of phenobarbital on the metabolism and excretion of thyroxine in rats. Toxicol Appl Pharmacol 99:216-228, 1989.
101. Qatanani M, Zhang J, Moore DD: Role of the constitutive androstane receptor in xenobiotic-induced thyroid hormone metabolism. Endocrinology 146:995-1002, 2005.
102. Swales K, Negishi M: CAR, driving into the future. Mol Endocrinol 18:1589-1598, 2004.
103. Faucette SR, Zhang TC, Moore R, et al: Relative activation of human pregnane X receptor versus constitutive androstane receptor defines distinct classes of CYP2B6 and CYP3A4 inducers. J Pharmacol Exp Ther 320:72-80, 2007.

104. Rootwelt K, Ganes T, Johannessen SI: Effect of carbamazepine, phenytoin and phenobarbitone on serum levels of thyroid hormones and thyrotropin in humans. Scand J Clin Lab Invest 38:731-736, 1978.
105. Yeo PP, Bates D, Howe JG, et al: Anticonvulsants and thyroid function. Br Med J 1:1581-1583, 1978.
106. Wang H, Faucette S, Moore R, et al: Human constitutive androstane receptor mediates induction of CYP2B6 gene expression by phenytoin. J Biol Chem 279:29295-29301, 2004.
107. Smith PJ, Surks MI: Multiple effects of 5,5′-diphenylhydantoin on the thyroid hormone system. Endocr Rev 5:514-524, 1984.
108. Surks MI, DeFesi CR: Normal serum free thyroid hormone concentrations in patients treated with phenytoin or carbamazepine. A paradox resolved. JAMA 275:1495-1498, 1996.
109. Miller J, Carney P: Central hypothyroidism with oxcarbazepine therapy. Pediatr Neurol 34:242-244, 2006.
110. Vainionpaa LK, Mikkonen K, Rattya J, et al: Thyroid function in girls with epilepsy with carbamazepine, oxcarbazepine, or valproate monotherapy and after withdrawal of medication. Epilepsia 45:197-203, 2004.
111. Isojarvi JI, Airaksinen KE, Mustonen JN, et al: Thyroid and myocardial function after replacement of carbamazepine by oxcarbazepine. Epilepsia 36:810-816, 1995.
112. de Groot JW, Zonnenberg BA, Plukker JT, et al: Imatinib induces hypothyroidism in patients receiving levothyroxine. Clin Pharmacol Ther 78:433-438, 2005.
113. Singh N, Singh PN, Hershman JM: Effect of calcium carbonate on the absorption of levothyroxine. JAMA 283:2822-2825, 2000.
114. Singh N, Weisler SL, Hershman JM: The acute effect of calcium carbonate on the intestinal absorption of levothyroxine. Thyroid 11:967-971, 2001.
115. Campbell NR, Hasinoff BB, Stalts H, et al: Ferrous sulfate reduces thyroxine efficacy in patients with hypothyroidism. Ann Intern Med 117:1010-1013, 1992.
116. Liel Y, Sperber AD, Shany S: Nonspecific intestinal adsorption of levothyroxine by aluminum hydroxide. Am J Med 97:363-365, 1994.
117. Sherman SI, Tielens ET, Ladenson PW: Sucralfate causes malabsorption of L-thyroxine. Am J Med 96:531-535, 1994.
118. Harmon SM, Seifert CF: Levothyroxine-cholestyramine interaction reemphasized. Ann Intern Med 115:658-659, 1991.
119. Witztum JL, Jacobs LS, Schonfeld G: Thyroid hormone and thyrotropin levels in patients placed on colestipol hydrochloride. J Clin Endocrinol Metab 46:838-840, 1978.
120. Messina M, Redmond G: Effects of soy protein and soybean isoflavones on thyroid function in healthy adults and hypothyroid patients: A review of the relevant literature. Thyroid 16:249-258, 2006.
121. Conrad SC, Chiu H, Silverman BL: Soy formula complicates management of congenital hypothyroidism. Arch Dis Child 89:37-40, 2004.
122. Jabbar MA, Larrea J, Shaw RA: Abnormal thyroid function Tests in infants with congenital hypothyroidism: The influence of soy-based formula. J Am Coll Nutr 16:280-282, 1997.
123. Centanni M, Gargano L, Canettieri G, et al: Thyroxine in goiter, *Helicobacter pylori* infection, and chronic gastritis. N Engl J Med 354:1787-1795, 2006.
124. Cooper JG, Harboe K, Frost SK, et al: Ciprofloxacin interacts with thyroid replacement therapy. BMJ 330:1002, 2005.
125. Garwood CL, Van Schepen KA, McDonough RP, et al: Increased thyroid-stimulating hormone levels associated with concomitant administration of levothyroxine and raloxifene. Pharmacotherapy 26:881-885, 2006.
126. Siraj ES, Gupta MK, Reddy SS: Raloxifene causing malabsorption of levothyroxine. Arch Intern Med 163:1367-1370, 2003.

PART V

Structural Lesions

Chapter 24

Nontoxic Diffuse and Nodular Goiter

Joanna M. Peloquin and Fredric E. Wondisford

Key Points

- Nontoxic multinodular goiter represents the most common endocrine disorder worldwide, affecting 500 to 600 million people.
- Initial evaluation should begin with a focused history and physical, with particular attention to worrisome obstructive or malignant signs and symptoms. Initial studies should include a serum TSH and thyroid ultrasound.
- The risk of malignancy in a dominant nodule is estimated to be approximately 5%. Asymmetry of the gland, rapid enlargement or change in consistency of a nodule should lead to fine-needle aspiration biopsy.
- Treatment options for nontoxic multinodular goiter include thyroxine suppression, radioiodine, and surgery. Age of the patient, associated comorbidities, and symptomatology should guide treatment choice.

The word goiter is derived from the Latin word *guttrus,* meaning throat, and describes enlargement of the thyroid gland, encompassing a variety of thyroid pathologies. Simple nodular goiter encompasses a spectrum of disease from mild unilateral enlargement to diffuse, nodular, and multinodular enlargement of the thyroid gland. The terms *nontoxic goiter* or *sporadic goiter* may be used to describe focal or diffuse enlargement of the thyroid gland that is not associated with thyrotoxicosis or underlying autoimmune or inflammatory process. (Toxic goiter is discussed in Chapter 14.) In this chapter, the focus will be nontoxic goiter. The term *endemic goiter* is used when the prevalence of goiter surpasses 10% within a population. Worldwide, endemic goiter is most commonly caused by iodine deficiency.

Goiter is the most visible sign of iodine deficiency, but iodine deficiency is also associated with varying degrees of mental retardation and represents a significant cause of mental retardation worldwide that is potentially preventable. For centuries, seaweed has been used to prevent goiter in China, yet programs to mandate salt iodization in the United States did not begin until 1910 to 1920, after the revolutionary studies of Dr. David Marine demonstrated the reduction in goiter of adolescent girls in Ohio from 20% to 5% by iodine supplementation.[1,2] Salt iodization was chosen as the approach for iodine supplementation for the following reasons: (1) salt is consumed worldwide; (2) production is generally limited to a few geographic areas; (3) the implementation of salt iodization technology is easy and cost-effective (approximately $0.02 to $0.08/person/year); and (4) the quality of iodized salt can be effectively monitored at the time of production, retail, and consumption.[3]

In 1960, the World Health Organization published the first comprehensive report of the magnitude of iodine deficiency worldwide.[4] Over the intervening years, eliminating iodine deficiency, achieved by universal salt iodization of all salt used in agriculture, food processing, and households, now represents one of the great successes in public health efforts against noncommunicable diseases. In 1990, an estimated 1.572 billion people (28.9% of the world's population) were at risk for iodine deficiency disorders, and 655 million (12%) were affected by goiter. By 1999, of the 130 countries with the highest risk populations, 75% had salt iodization legislation and 68% of households had access to iodized salt (Table 24-1).[5] The elimination of iodine deficiency has greatly reduced the incidence of brain damage, mental retardation, goiter, impaired thyroid function, and perinatal mortality.[3] Adequate daily iodine

Table 24–1 Access of Households to Iodized Salt

WHO Region	Number of IDD-Affected Countries	Households Having Access to Iodized Salt (%)
Africa	44	63
North and South America	19	90
Southeast Asia	9	70
Eastern Mediterranean	17	66
Europe	32	27
Western Pacific	9	76

IDD, iodine deficiency disorder.
Adapted from WHO, UNICEF, IDD: Progress Towards the Elimination of Iodine Deficiency Disorders (IDD) (WHO Publ. WHO/NHD/99.4). Geneva, World Health Organization, 1999.

intake is now recommended by the National Health and Nutrition Examination Survey III (NHANES III) to be 145 μg.[6]

EPIDEMIOLOGY, RISK FACTORS, AND PATHOGENESIS

As the most common endocrine disorder, nontoxic goiter was estimated to affect 500 to 600 million people worldwide.[1] This number can be expected to decrease in the coming decade after the advent of worldwide salt iodination. However, despite iodine repletion, the prevalence of goiter in the United States remains at approximately 4% to 6%, highlighting that iodine deficiency is not the only cause of goiter formation.[7] Nontoxic goiter is more common in women than men. In a population-based study in England, palpable goiters were identified in 10% of adult women and 2% of adult men.[8] Goiter development in iodine-replete populations is typically a disease of adulthood, whereas goiter development in areas of iodine deficiency is typically a disease of prepubertal children. No epidemiologic studies have suggested a relationship between race and the prevalence of goiter.

Iodine deficiency is associated with goiter formation through activation of the hypothalamic-pituitary-thyroid axis. Because iodine is required for the organification of thyroglobulin, iodine deficiency results in upregulation of thyroid-stimulating hormone (TSH) in the setting of decreased thyroid hormone release. The increased TSH stimulation of the thyroid gland results in gland enlargement, or goiter. In iodine-replete populations, patients with nontoxic goiter are commonly euthyroid, thus suggesting additional causes for the development of goiter in addition to TSH stimulation. In these populations, the clinical phenotype of nontoxic goiter likely results from a number of genetic and environmental factors.

The role of genetic factors in the development of goiter has been suggested by the aggregation of goiter within families.[9,10] In 1999, Neumann and colleagues[11] first identified a genetic locus associated with nontoxic goiter on chromosome 14q. In a study of twins in a nonendemic region, Brix and associates[12] demonstrated a substantially higher heritability of goiter in monozygotic versus dizygotic twins. Multiple environmental factors have been identified as risk factors for goiter formation. Examples include ingestion of goitrogens in the diet (e.g., soybeans, cabbage, turnips, Brussels sprouts, rutabagas, seaweed), administration of goitrogenic drugs such as lithium, environmental agents such as phenolic and phthalate ester derivatives found downstream from coal mines, and cigarette smoking.[13,14] Nontoxic goiter can also be observed in patients with an inherited dyshormonogenesis, resulting in a defect in the thyroid hormone biosynthetic pathway. Finally, radiation exposure to the head and neck during childhood increases the likelihood of benign and malignant thyroid growth.

The natural history of goiter is characterized clinically by thyroid growth, nodule formation, and the development of functional autonomy. This has been demonstrated in cross-sectional studies of patients with nontoxic goiter by Vanderpump and coworkers[8] and Berghout and colleagues.[15]

Increased thyroid growth results from excessive cell replication, mainly of follicular cells. Whereas TSH stimulation contributes to the iodine-deficient goiter, in the euthyroid goiter additional growth factors, such as insulin-growth factor, epidermal growth factor, and fibroblast growth factor, are known to stimulate thyroid growth.[16] In addition to growth factors, growth inhibitors, released by the thyroid gland itself, are known to regulate thyroid mass size. The expression of transforming growth factor (TGF) was shown to be decreased in the nontoxic goiter compared with normal thyroid tissue.[17] In the setting of multiple growth factors and inhibitors, nodules are thought to arise because of heterogeneity of the growth responses among follicular cells.

Follicular cells with high growth potential are unequally distributed throughout a normal thyroid gland and, in the setting of replication, daughter cells remain clustered, causing nontoxic goiters to become increasingly nodular over time.[18] An additional mechanism contributing to nodule formation is hemorrhagic necrosis and subsequent fibrosis

Table 24–2 Clinical Signs, Symptoms, and Investigations in Multinodular Nontoxic Goiter Diagnosis

History

Often, family history of benign thyroid disease
Slowly growing anterior neck mass
Enlargement during pregnancy
Cosmetic complaints
Occasionally, upper airway obstruction, dyspnea, cough, dysphagia
Asymmetry, tracheal deviation, and/or compression
Uni- and multinodularity on examination with no lymphadenopathy
Sudden transient pain or enlargement secondary to hemorrhage
Gradually developing hyperthyroidism
Superior vena cava obstructive syndrome
Recurrent nerve palsy (rare)
Horner's syndrome (rare)

Investigations

Thyroid-stimulating hormone normal or decreased, free thyroxine and free triiodothyronine normal
Calcitonin normal
Thyroid autoantibodies negative in approximately 90% of cases
Scintigraphy with solitary or multiple hot and/or cold areas
Ultrasound finding of solitary or multiple nodules, with varying echogenicity
CT and MR imaging demonstrating solitary or multiple nodules, with varying echogenicity
Lung function testing—may demonstrate impaired inspiratory capacity
Fine-needle aspiration of nodule(s)—reveals benign cytology

Adapted from Hegedus L, Bonnema SJ, Bennedbaek FN: Management of simple nodular goiter: Current status and future perspectives. Endocr Rev 24:102-132, 2003.

within areas of rapid growth, with newly formed, fragile, and insufficient capillary networks. Within these populations of rapidly dividing follicular cells, it has also been observed that functional autonomy develops, because follicles have varying sensitivities to TSH stimulation for iodine metabolism.[19] Because of the greater number of follicular cells metabolizing iodine autonomously, patients with nontoxic goiter can progress to subclinical and then overt thyrotoxicosis, particularly in the setting of excessive amounts of iodine (e.g., iodinated contrast dye).[20]

Table 24–3 Signs and Symptoms Suggestive of Malignancy

High Suspicion	Moderate Suspicion
Family history of medullary thyroid cancer or multiple endocrine neoplasia	Age <20 or >60 yr
Rapid tumor growth	Male gender
Very firm nodule(s)	Solitary nodule
Fixation to adjacent structures	History of head and neck irradiation
Vocal cord paralysis	Firm texture, possible fixation
Regional lymphadenopathy	Nodule > 4 cm in diameter and partially cystic
Distant metastasis	Compressive symptoms

Adapted from Hegedus L, Bonnema SJ, Bennedbaek FN: Management of simple nodular goiter: Current status and future perspectives. Endocr Rev 24:102-132, 2003.

DIAGNOSIS

Patients typically present with diffuse or multinodular thyroid enlargement, as suggested by the pathogenesis of nontoxic goiter. In a patient with thyroid enlargement, a thorough history should be taken and physical examination carried out to guide diagnosis (Table 24-2).

The history should focus on determining the duration of the presence of the goiter, as well as any recent changes in its size or shape or the new onset of pain. Accelerated growth or the emergence of a dominant nodule should raise suspicion for malignancy or recent hemorrhage. Patients should be questioned regarding obstructive symptoms, such as dyspnea, stridor, solid food or pill dysphagia, and vocal cord dysfunction, developing in the setting of tracheal compression by an expanding goiter (Table 24-3). Often, these symptoms will be nocturnal or positional, particularly occurring when performing maneuvers that may obstruct the thoracic inlet, such as reaching. Patients should be asked about excessive iodine intake from diet and nutritional supplementation. Any personal history of head or neck radiation, particularly in childhood, should be noted, as well as any family history of thyroid disorders, including dyshormonogenesis or malignancy, as in the multiple endocrine neoplasia (MEN) disorders.

On examination, the neck and upper thorax should be inspected and palpated to determine the size, shape, asymmetry, and consistency of the goiter and any coincident lymphadenopathy. In general, nodules larger than 1 cm can be palpated. If the lower end of the thyroid is not palpable, intrathoracic extension of the thyroid gland should be considered.

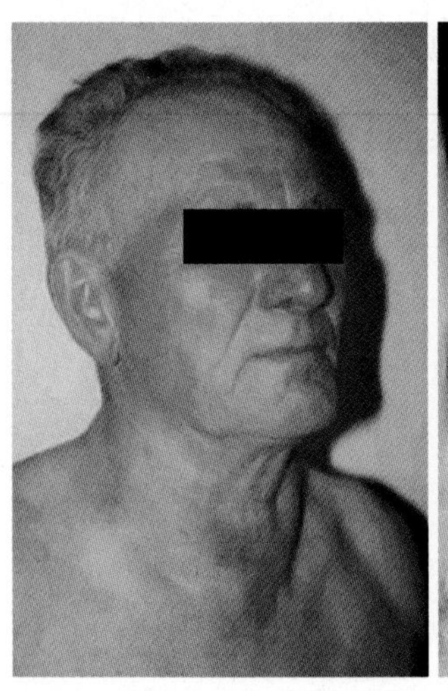
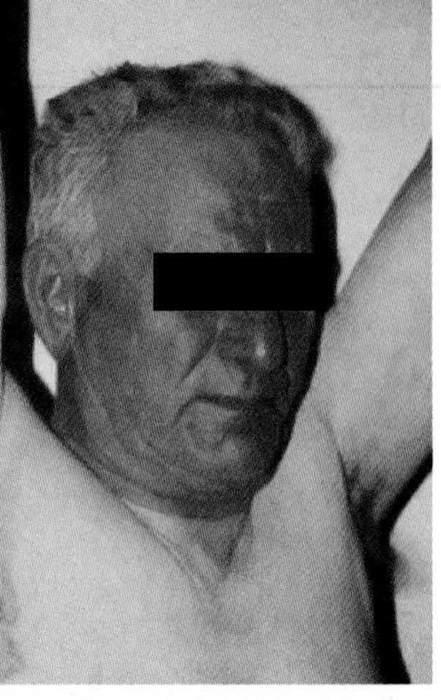

Figure 24–1 Pemberton maneuver. *(From Wallace C, Siminoski K: The Pemberton sign. Ann Intern Med 125: 568-569, 1996.)*

Table 24–4 Ultrasonographic Features Suggestive of Malignancy

Benign	Malignant
Normal echogenicity or hyperechogenicity	Hypoechogenicity
Coarse calcifications	Microcalcifications
Thin, well-defined halo	Thick, irregular, or absent halo
Regular margin	Irregular margin
Lack of invasive growth	Invasive growth
No regional lymphadenopathy	Regional lymphadenopathy
Low intranodular flow by Doppler	High intranodular flow by Doppler

Adapted from Hegedus L, Bonnema SJ, Bennedbaek FN: Management of simple nodular goiter: Current status and future perspectives. Endocr Rev 24:102-132, 2003.

Often, hyperextension of the patient's head will assist in elevating the inferior aspect of the gland.

Intrathoracic extension of the goiter is particularly important to recognize because compression symptoms by occlusion of the thoracic inlet (thoracic cork) may develop earlier in the course of the disease.[21] Symptoms and signs may arise from compression of the structures located within the bony confines of the thoracic inlet, including the trachea, esophagus, and vasculature.[22] Symptoms of tracheal narrowing generally develop slowly over time. However, emergency tracheal stenting or tracheostomy might be required in the setting of acute progression of the obstruction caused by hemorrhage into a nodule or cyst or upper respiratory infection. Because of the posterior position of the esophagus, esophageal compression is less common than tracheal compression. Hoarseness and, rarely, vocal cord paralysis can occur with compression of one or both of the recurrent laryngeal nerves. Phrenic nerve or Horner's syndrome can be seen because of compression of the cervical sympathetic chain.

Compression or thrombosis of the jugular or subclavian veins or superior cava causes facial swelling (plethora) and dilated neck and upper thoracic veins. Described by Pemberton in 1946, the Pemberton maneuver elicits the signs and symptoms of venous outflow obstruction. The maneuver involves "elevat[ing] both arms until they touch the sides of the head....[if the sign is present] after a minute or so, congestion of the face, some cyanosis, and lastly distress become apparent" (Fig. 24-1).[23] Evidence of venous obstruction is not uncommon in substernal goiters; distended veins over the neck and thorax have been reported in 8% to 18% of patients.[22]

Laboratory Studies

In patients with thyroid enlargement, the initial laboratory investigation should begin with measurement of the serum TSH level.[24,25] Elevated TSH concentrations suggest chronic autoimmune thyroiditis or ingestion of an antithyroid agent, such as lithium, resulting in hypothyroidism. If the serum concentration is low, measurement of serum free thyroxine (T_4) is indicated to exclude subclinical or overt hyperthyroidism. In the patient with low serum TSH and normal free T_4 levels, measurement of free triiodothyronine (T_3) can exclude T_3 thyrotoxicosis. To complete the laboratory evaluation, a thyroid antibody profile (antithyroid peroxidase, antimicrosomal, antithyroglobulin) is commonly also obtained. In a population of patients presenting with nontoxic goiter, Berghout and associates[15] showed that subclinical hyperthyroidism occurred in 27.5% of patients (low TSH, normal free T_3 and T_4), whereas only 2% to 3% presented with symptomatic thyrotoxicosis. Most patients with nontoxic goiter will be euthyroid at presentation, with typically absent to low autoantibodies.[26]

Imaging Studies

Historically, the routine use of ultrasonography or cross-sectional imaging was not favored in the initial management of nontoxic goiter.[27,28] However, palpation of the neck and thyroid gland has consistently been shown to identify thyroid gland morphology or size imprecisely.[29] For nontoxic goiter, the preferred imaging techniques include ultrasonography, computed tomography (CT), and magnetic resonance imaging (MRI). For cost, convenience, limited discomfort to the patient, and use of nonionizing radiation, ultrasonography has emerged as the first-line imaging modality (Table 24-4).[24,25,30] Ultrasonography improves detection and characterization of nodules and estimation of nodule size and goiter volume. Wiest and coworkers[31] have demonstrated that ultrasonography detects five times as many nodules as thyroid palpation and twice as many when only nodules larger than 2 cm are considered. Ultrasonography, however, insufficiently evaluates for compression of the trachea, esophagus, nerve, or vascular structures. In such cases, CT and MRI, although more costly, provide more sensitive cross-sectional imaging to detect tracheal compression and intrathoracic extension of a goiter and guide any further surgical intervention. Of note, when CT is used, iodinated contrast should not be administered because of the risk of inducing thyrotoxicosis. If clinically indicated, an antithyroid agent should be administered prior to the iodinated contrast exposure, and subsequent scintigraphy or radioiodine therapy should be held for 4 to 6 weeks.

Functional tracheal obstruction can be investigated with pulmonary function testing. In a study of patients referred with moderately enlarged goiter, Gittoes and coworkers demonstrated that flow volume loops revealed upper airway obstruction in a third of patients, correlating poorly with symptoms.[32] For patients presenting with dysphagia, a barium swallow may demonstrate an extrinsic esophageal compression as the cause.

Radionuclide thyroid scanning or scintigraphy is not indicated for the routine assessment of goiter size but such imaging is indicated if there is concern for malignancy, such as a rapidly enlarging dominant nodule. Radionuclide scanning (see later) demonstrates functional thyroid tissue. In nontoxic goiter, radionuclide scanning will most typically show variable uptake in numerous areas of the thyroid, rather than diffusely homogenous uptake or a single dominant nodule. If radioiodine therapy is being considered for treatment and thyroid mass reduction, radionuclide thyroid scanning is also useful to demonstrate uptake and predict effectiveness of the therapy.[26]

Fine-Needle Aspiration

In general, fine-needle aspiration (FNA) is not routinely indicated for patients presenting with a history and examination consistent with nontoxic goiter. Exceptions include patients presenting with an asymmetrical and rapidly enlarging nodule, dominant nodule, nodule of variable consistency when compared with other nodules within the gland, or a cold region on radionuclide thyroid scanning. For a further discussion of indications for FNA for management of a solitary nodule, see Chapter 25. In a study of 61 patients, Tollin and colleagues[33] have examined the risk of malignancy in thyroid nodules occurring in multinodular nontoxic goiter, demonstrating an overall malignancy rate of approximately 5%. Given the high prevalence of nontoxic goiter in the community, contrasted with the relatively low incidence of thyroid carcinoma, however, it is expected that the incidence of clinically relevant thyroid carcinomas is rare in the general multinodular goiter population.[34]

Table 24–5 Advantages and Disadvantages of Treatment Options for Nontoxic Multinodular Goiter

Treatment	Advantages	Disadvantages
Surgery	Rapid decompression of trachea; prompt relief of compressive symptoms; histologic diagnosis; cosmetic improvement	Surgical risk; high cost; inpatient; vocal cord paralysis, ~1%; hypoparathyroidism, ~1%; risk of hypothyroidism if total thyroidectomy
Radioiodine	Outpatient (when possible); generally well tolerated; goiter reduction—50% within 1 yr; can be repeated if necessary	Hypothyroidism (1-yr risk of 15% to 20%); risk of cancer induction; risk of thyroiditis; sudden worsening of obstructive symptoms
Thyroxine	Outpatient; goiter reduction—58% within 9 mo; may prevent new nodule formation	Lifelong treatment; low efficacy; high rate of recurrence with cessation of therapy; adverse effects (osteoporosis, cardiac arrhythmias)

Adapted from Hegedus L, Bonnema SJ, Bennedbaek FN: Management of simple nodular goiter: Current status and future perspectives. Endocr Rev 24:102-132, 2003.

TREATMENT

In patients with nontoxic multinodular goiter, the primary indications for treatment are tracheal or esophageal compression and venous-outflow obstruction. Additional indications for intervention include intrathoracic extension of goiter growth, neck discomfort, or cosmetic concerns. Treatment options are thyroxine, radioiodine, and surgery (Table 24-5).[35]

If iodine deficiency is suspected, iodine supplementation is not recommended because of the risk of inducing hyperthyroidism and an association with increased incidence of papillary thyroid cancers and lymphoid thyroiditis.[36,37]

Thyroxine Therapy

The hypothesis underlying thyroxine therapy is that thyroid tissue that has not undergone autonomous degeneration is dependent on TSH for growth. Thus, treatment with thyroxine will suppress TSH, prevent further goitrous tissue growth, and possibly decrease goiter size. In a placebo-controlled clinical trial of 78 patients with nontoxic goiter, thyroid volume decreased in 58% of the patients in the T_4 group as compared with 4% in the placebo group. After therapy was discontinued, goiter growth returned to baseline within 9 months of discontinuation of therapy, demonstrating the long-term need for thyroxine therapy to sustain the effect.[38] In a meta-analysis of seven nonrandomized trials of thyroxine therapy, 60% of 722 patients had a decrease in goiter size. The effect was most commonly seen within the first 3 months after initiating therapy, and a greater effect was observed in patients with diffuse goiters compared with those with nodule goiters.[39]

Although the data are convincing for the use of suppressive therapy in patients with nontoxic diffuse goiter, many patients with nontoxic multinodular goiter have autonomous thyroid hormone production resulting in TSH suppression and subclinical thyrotoxicosis. In these patients, no further benefit can be expected from thyroxine therapy. Therefore, prior to initiating suppressive therapy, the TSH level must be measured to avoid causing overt thyrotoxicosis. Because lifelong thyroxine therapy is required, resulting by definition in subclinical hyperthyroidism, the systemic effects on bone and cardiovascular system must be recognized.[40] Of those 60 years of age and older, a serum TSH level lower than 0.1 mU/L has been shown to be associated with a threefold higher risk for developing atrial fibrillation in the next decade.[41] Therefore, the use of suppressive therapy is limited in older patients at higher risk for atrial fibrillation and adverse cardiac effects, as well as postmenopausal women at risk for reduced bone density.[28] For patients with nontoxic goiter, the optimal level of TSH suppression has not been defined; some studies suggest suppression to between 0.1 and 0.5 mU/L.[34]

Radioiodine Therapy

Radioiodine (RAI; iodine-131) treatment has been demonstrated to reduce thyroid volume in many patients with nontoxic multinodular goiter.[42-46] In these patients, radioiodine therapy has been shown to have greater benefit than thyroxine therapy, with an decrease of goiter size of 46% in the RAI group compared with 22% in the thyroxine group.[46] In the reported studies, single doses of approximately 100 μCi of radioiodine/g of thyroid tissue were administered, resulting in a mean reduction in thyroid volume of approximately 40% after 1 year and 50% to 60% after 3 to 5 years. The decrease in goiter size after radioiodine treatment negatively correlated with pretreatment goiter size and presence of dominant nodules.[47] Importantly, most patients reported decreased compressive symptomatology, demonstrable on pulmonary function testing.[48]

In general, radioiodine therapy is well tolerated. Early side effects, including pain, radiation thyroiditis, increase in compressive symptoms, and esophagitis, are rare. If these occur, they are generally mild and transient. The most important side effect occurring several months after therapy is the development of autoimmune (Graves') hyperthyroidism, likely triggered by the release of thyroid antigens after radiation-induced damage to the gland. Graves' hyperthyroidism has been reported to occur in approximately 5% of patients. The incidence of post-treatment hypothyroidism is 20% to 50% at 5 years, and is more common in patients with small goiters, presence of thyroid peroxidase (TPO) antibodies, or a family history of thyroid disease.[47] Further studies have suggested that patients with normal pretreatment TSH have a significantly higher risk of developing hypothyroidism after RAI treatment than patients with suppressed baseline TSH.[46]

Little evidence is available to assess the risk of induction of carcinoma from large doses of radioiodine for nontoxic multinodular goiter. The lifetime risk of cancer induction depends on two factors: (1) dose of radioiodine administered; and (2) age at time of administration.[49] For patients with large multinodular goiters (>100 g), the estimated 1.6% lifetime risk of development of cancer outside the thyroid gland was calculated.[49] Therefore, historically, RAI treatment has been preferred for older patients over younger patients. However, more recent data have supported pretreatment with recombinant human TSH to create a more homogenous distribution of radioiodine and reduce the necessary therapeutic dose of ^{131}I by 50% to 60%.[50]

Surgery

For patients with large goiters or compressive symptoms, surgical management is indicated. Reportedly, approximately 10% to 15% of goiter patients will eventually require surgery.[51] In a study of approximately 500 patients with goiter referred for surgical intervention, Phitayakorn and associates[52] identified African American race, obesity, and increasing age as further risk factors for progression of simple nodular to large nodular goiter. Historically, there has been great debate regarding the appropriate extent of surgical excision to balance morbidity and benefit to the patient. Recent data have suggested that total thyroidectomy does not carry a significantly higher risk of operative morbidity or subsequent hypothyroidism as compared with subtotal thyroidectomy, and may offer the advantage of removing any tissue susceptible to recurrence or malignant transformation.[51,53] In a recent review of the literature, recurrence rates of benign multinodular goiter after total thyroidectomy were found to be essentially zero (range, 0% to 0.3%) compared with those after subtotal thyroidectomy (range, 2.5% to 42%) or more limited resections (range, 8% to 34%).[51]

Surgical intervention has the advantage of rapid decompression, relief of symptoms, and definite tissue diagnosis. Almost all goiters can be removed through a Kocher transverse collar incision, even if intrathoracic extension is anticipated or found on surgical exploration. Substernal goiter is defined as a thyroid mass of which more than 50% is located below the thoracic inlet; in a series of 59 patients undergoing surgery for substernal goiter, only 3% of patients required a thoracic approach.[54]

In general, the mortality after thyroidectomy for nontoxic goiter is low (less than 1%).[55] Specific complications of thyroid surgery for nontoxic goiter are tracheal obstruction caused by hemorrhage, tracheomalacia, temporary recurrent laryngeal nerve injury (1% to 10%), permanent recurrent laryngeal nerve injury (in 1% to 2% of cases when performed by a dedicated thyroid surgeon), hypoparathyroidism (0.5% to 5%), voice changes caused by laryngeal nerve damage, and hypothyroidism. Notably, total thyroidectomy is associated with a significantly higher rate of transient postoperative hypocalcemia than less extensive operations (9% to 35% vs. 0% to 18%, respectively).[35,51] Surgical morbidity remains the highest in those undergoing resection of very large goiters or reoperation.[51,56]

To prevent or delay recurrence, postoperative TSH suppression has been extensively studied, with varying results. Thyroxine is frequently prescribed, but there is insufficient evidence justifying this practice, and it could put the patient at risk for adverse effects of subclinical hyperthyroidism.[57]

PROGNOSIS

Multinodular nontoxic goiter may harbor occult malignancy at a rate of 4 to 12%, which is similar to the risk associated with solitary nodules.[58] These data support the practice of evaluating a dominant nodule in a multinodular goiter with the same standards of care applied to a single nodule.[33]

CONCLUSIONS

Multinodular nontoxic goiter is common in the general population. Evaluation should be guided by the risk of occult malignancy in dominant nodules. The age of the patient, associated comorbidities, and obstructive symptomatology must be considered to design a treatment plan.

References

1. Hetzel BS: The Story of Iodine Deficiency. Oxford, England, Oxford University Press, 1989.
2. Marine D, Kimball OP: Prevention of simple goiter in man. Arch Intern Med 25:661-672, 1920.
3. Delange F, de Benoist B, Pretell E, et al: Iodine deficiency in the world: Where do we stand at the turn of the century? Thyroid 11:437-47, 2001.
4. World Health Organization: Endemic Goitre. Geneva, World Health Organization, 1960.
5. WHO, UNICEF, IDD: Progress Towards the Elimination of Iodine Deficiency Disorders (IDD) (WHO Publ. WHO/NHD/99.4). Geneva, World Health Organization, 1999.
6. Hollowell JG, Staehling NW, Hannon WH, et al: Trends and public health implications: Iodine excretion data from National Health and Nutrition Examination Surveys I and III (1971-1974 and 1988-1994). J Clin Endocrinol Metab 83:3401-3408, 1998.
7. Daniels GH: Thyroid nodules and nodular thyroids: A clinical overview. Compr Ther 22:239-250, 1996.
8. Vanderpump MPJ, Tunbridge WMG, French JM, et al: The incidence of thyroid disorders in the community: A twenty-year follow-up of the Whickham Survey. Clin Endocrinol 43:55-68, 1995.
9. Sorensen EW: Thyroid diseases in a family. Acta Med Scand 162:123-127, 1958.
10. Heimann P: Familial incidence of thyroid disease and anamnestic incidence of pubertal struma in 449 consecutive struma patients. Acta Med Scand 179:113-119, 1966.
11. Neumann SE, Willgerodt H, Ackermann F, et al: Linkage of familial euthyroid goiter to the multinodular goiter-1 locus and exclusion of the candidate genes thyroglobulin, thyroperoxidase, and Na^+/I^- symporter. J Clin Endocrinol Metab 84:3750-3756, 1999.

12. Brix TH, Kyvik KO, Hegedus L: Major role of genes in the etiology of simple goiter in females: A population-based twin study. J Clin Endocrinol Metab 84:3071-3075, 1999.
13. Bertelsen JB, Hegedus L: Cigarette smoking and the thyroid. Thyroid 4:327-331, 1994.
14. Orenstein H, Peskind A, Raskind MA: Thyroid disorders in female psychiatric patients with panic disorder or agoraphobia. Am J Psychiatry 145:1428-1430, 1988.
15. Berghout A, Wiersinga WM, Smits NJ, et al: Interrelationships between age, thyroid volume, thyroid nodularity, and thyroid function in patients with sporadic nontoxic goiter. Am J Med 89:602-608, 1990.
16. Dumont JE, Maenhaut C, Pirson I, et al: Growth factors controlling the thyroid gland. Baillieres Clin Endocrinol Metab 5:727-754, 1992.
17. Grubeck-Loebenstein B, Buchan G, Sadeghi R, et al: Transforming growth factor beta regulates thyroid growth. Role in the pathogenesis of nontoxic goiter. J Clin Invest 83:764-770, 1989.
18. Peter HJ, Gerber H, Studer H, et al: Pathogenesis of heterogeneity in human multinodular goiter. J Clin Invest 76:1992-2002, 1985.
19. Studer H, Gerber H: Multinodular goiter. In DeGroot LJ (ed): Endocrinology, 3rd ed. Philadelphia, WB Saunders, 1995, pp 769-782.
20. Studer H, Peter JH, Gerber H: Natural heterogeneity of thyroid cells: The basis for understanding thyroid function and nodular goiter growth. Endocr Rev 10:125-135, 1989.
21. Blum M, Biller BL, Bergman DA: The thyroid cork. Obstruction of the thoracic inlet due to retroclavicular goiter. JAMA 227:189-191, 1974.
22. Wallace C, Siminoski K: The Pemberton Sign. Ann Intern Med 125:568-569, 1996.
23. Pemberton HS: Sign of submerged goitre [letter]. Lancet 251:509, 1946.
24. Bonnema SJ, Bennedbaek FN, Wiersinga WM, et al: Management of the nontoxic multinodular goitre: A European questionnaire study. Clin Endocrinol 53:5-12, 2000.
25. Bonnema SJ, Bennedbaek FN, Ladenson PW, et al: Management of the nontoxic multinodular goiter: A North American survey. J Clin Endocrinol Metab 87:112-117, 2002.
26. Day TA, Chu A, Hoang KG: Multinodular goiter. Otolaryngol Clin North Am 36:35-54, 2003.
27. Singer PA, Cooper DS, Daniels GH, et al: Treatment guidelines for patients with thyroid nodules and well-differentiated thyroid cancer. American Thyroid Association. Arch Intern Med 156:2165-2172, 1996.
28. Hegedus L, Bonnema SJ, Bennedbaek FN: Management of simple nodular goiter: Current status and future perspectives. Endocr Rev 24:102-132, 2003.
29. Jarlov AE, Nygaard B, Hegedus L, et al: Observer variation in the clinical and laboratory evaluation of patients with thyroid dysfunction and goiter. Thyroid 8:393-398, 1998.
30. Hegedus L: Thyroid ultrasound. Endocrinol Metab Clin North Am 30:339-360, 2001.
31. Wiest PW, Hartshorne MF, Inskip PD, et al: Thyroid palpation vs. high-resolution thyroid ultrasonography in the detection of nodules. J Ultrasound Med 17:487-496, 1998.
32. Gittoes NJ, Miller MR, Daykin J, et al: Upper airways obstruction in 153 consecutive patients presenting with thyroid enlargement. Br Med J 312:484, 1996.
33. Tollin SR, Mery GM, Jelveh N, et al: The use of fine-needle aspiration biopsy under ultrasound guidance to assess the risk of malignancy in patients with a multinodular goiter. Thyroid 10:235-241, 2000.
34. Hermus AR, Huysmans DA: Nontoxic diffuse and nodular goiter. In Braverman LE, Utiger RD (eds): Werner and Ingbar's The Thyroid: A Fundamental and Clinical Text. Philadelphia: Lippincott, Williams & Wilkins, 2000, pp 866-871.
35. Hermus AR, Huysmans DA: Treatment of benign nodular thyroid disease. N Engl J Med 338:1438-1447, 1998.
36. Roti E, Uberti ED: Iodine excess and hyperthyroidism. Thyroid 11:493-500, 2001.
37. Harach HR, Williams ED: Thyroid cancer and thyroiditis in the goitrous region of Salta, Argentina, before and after iodine prophylaxis. Clin Endocrinol (Oxf) 43:701-706, 1995.
38. Berghout A, Wiersinga WM, Drexhage HA, et al: Comparison of placebo with L-thyroxine alone or with carbimazole for treatment of sporadic nontoxic goitre. Lancet 336:193-197, 1990.
39. Ross DS: Thyroid hormone suppressive therapy of sporadic nontoxic goiter. Thyroid 2:263-269, 1992.
40. Toft AD: Clinical practice: Subclinical hyperthyroidism. N Engl J Med 345:512-516, 2001.
41. Sawin CT, Geller A, Wolf PA, et al: Low serum thyrotropin concentrations as a risk factor for atrial fibrillation in older persons. N Engl J Med 331:1249-1252, 1994.
42. Hegedus L, Hansen BM, Knudsen N, et al: Reduction of size of thyroid with radioactive iodine in multinodular non-toxic goitre. Br Med J 297:661-662, 1988.
43. Nygaard B, Hegedus L, Gervil M, et al: Radioiodine treatment of multinodular non-toxic goitre. Br Med J 307:828-832, 1993.
44. Huysmans DAKC, Hermus ARMM, Corstens FHM, et al: Large, compressive goiters treated with radioiodine. Ann Intern Med 120:757-762, 1994.
45. de Klerk JMH, van Isselt JW, van Dijk, et al: Iodine-131 therapy in sporadic nontoxic goiter. J Nucl Med 38:372-376, 1997.
46. Wesche MF, Tiel-Van Buul MM, Lips P, et al: A randomized trial comparing levothyroxine with radioactive iodine in the treatment of sporadic nontoxic goiter. J Clin Endocrinol Metab 86:994-9947, 2001.
47. Le Moli R, Wesche MF, Tiel-Van Buul MM, Wiersinga WM: Determinants of longterm outcome of radioiodine therapy of sporadic non-toxic goitre. Clin Endocrinol (Oxf) 50:783-789, 1999.

48. Nygaard B, Soes-Petersen U, Hoilund-Carlsen PF, et al: Improvement of upper airway obstruction after 131-I treatment of multinodular nontoxic goiter evaluated by flow volume loop curves. J Endocrinol Invest 19:71-75, 1996.
49. Huysmans DA, Buijs WC, van de Ven MT, et al: Dosimetry and risk estimates of radioiodine therapy for large, multinodular goiters. J Nucl Med 37:2072-2079, 1996.
50. Nieuwlaat WA, Hermus AR, Ross HA, et al: Dosimetry of radioiodine therapy in patients with nodular goiter after pretreatment with a single, low dose of recombinant human thyroid-stimulating hormone. J Nucl Med 45:626-633, 2004.
51. Moalem J, Suh I, Duh QY: Treatment and prevention of recurrence of multinodular goiter: An evidence-based review of the literature. World J Surg 32:1301-1312, 2008.
52. Phitayakorn R, Super DM, McHenry CR: An investigation of epidemiologic factors associated with large nodular goiter. J Surg Res 133:16-21, 2006.
53. Vaiman M, Nagibin A, Hagag P, et al: Subtotal and near total versus total thyroidectomy for the management of multinodular goiter. World J Surg 32:1546-1551, 2008.
54. Agha A, Glockzin G, Ghali N, et al: Surgical treatment of substernal goiter: An analysis of 59 patients. Surgery Today 38:505-511, 2008.
55. Kaplan EL, Shukla M, Hara H, et al: Surgery of the thyroid. In DeGroot LJ (ed): Endocrinology, 3rd ed. Philadelphia, WB Saunders, 1995, pp 900-914.
56. al Suliman NN, Ryttov NF, Qvist N, et al: Experience in a specialist thyroid surgery unit: A demographic study, surgical complications, and outcome. Eur J Surg 163:13-20, 1997.
57. Hegedus L, Nygaard B, Hansen JM: Is routine thyroxine treatment to hinder postoperative recurrence of nontoxic goiter justified? J Clin Endocrinol Metab 84:756-60, 1999.
58. Koh KBH, Chang KW: Carcinoma in multinodular goitre. Br J Surg 79:266-267, 1992.

Chapter 25

Solitary Thyroid Nodule

Bryan R. Haugen and Sherif Said

Key Points

- Thyroid sonography is an important tool to verify palpable thyroid nodules and guide biopsy decision making in patients with multiple nodules.
- Fine-needle aspirate cytology is generally classified as benign, malignant, neoplastic, suspicious, or inadequate.
- Integration of clinical assessment, serum TSH, ultrasound features, and cytology classification is currently the best way to assess malignancy risk in patients with thyroid nodules.

EPIDEMIOLOGY

Nodular thyroid disease is common and can be operationally defined in two primary ways, presentation and setting. The presentation of patients for nodular thyroid disease can be as symptomatic (uncommon), asymptomatic by palpation (prevalence), or asymptomatic by anatomic imaging or autopsy (prevalence). Furthermore, thyroid nodules can be defined as solitary or multiple by clinical examination, anatomic imaging, or autopsy.

Depending on the definition, age, and population studied, the prevalence of nodular thyroid disease can vary greatly.[1] Table 25-1 shows the prevalence of nodular thyroid disease based on definition in selected (representative) studies.[2-5]

Many more nodules are detected by sensitive neck ultrasound or careful autopsy (50% to 67%) than by palpation (4% to 20%). Furthermore, solitary nodules noted on palpation are commonly associated with other nodules identified by ultrasound imaging.[6]

RISK OF MALIGNANCY AND CLINICAL RISK FACTORS

The overall prevalence of malignancy in a patient population with thyroid nodules is approximately 4% to 7%. The risk of malignancy in a patient with a thyroid nodule is not different based on the method of detection (palpation, anatomic imaging) or presence of a solitary or multiple thyroid nodules.[7] The risk of malignancy in any one thyroid nodule in a patient with multiple nodules decreases based on the increasing number of nodules (larger than 10 mm) in the gland.[8]

Clinical presentation can alter the risk of malignancy in a patient presenting with a thyroid nodule. Table 25-2 shows clinical risk factors that can increase the chance that a patient with a thyroid nodule may harbor a malignancy.[9,10] In a study by Hamming and colleagues,[11] the clinical presence of rapid tumor growth, vocal cord paralysis, immobility, ipsilateral lymphadenopathy, or presence of metastatic thyroid cancer increased the risk of malignancy in a patient with a thyroid nodule to 71% based on clinical findings alone. All patients presenting with nodular thyroid disease should have a careful clinical evaluation for a history of radiation exposure (particularly as a child), family history of thyroid cancer (emphasis on first-degree relatives), symptoms of voice change, rapid growth, and pain and dysphagia, as well as examination for nodule mobility (swallowing), associated lymphadenopathy, and directed vocal cord evaluation for hoarseness.

LABORATORY AND RADIOLOGIC EVALUATION

Laboratory and Imaging Studies

There are a few laboratory tests that can help distinguish benign from malignant thyroid nodules in a given patient. Serum thyroglobulin, which is an excellent marker of disease in patients with differentiated thyroid cancer after thyroidectomy or ablation, cannot reliably distinguish benign from malignant nodules preoperatively. Measurement of a serum thyroglobulin level in patients with nodular thyroid disease is generally not recommended.[12-14]

The serum thyroid-stimulating hormone (TSH) level is valuable to distinguish the uncommon

Table 25–1 Population-based Prevalence of Thyroid Nodules Based on Method of Detection

Study	No. of Subjects	Detection Method	Nodule Prevalence (%)	Solitary (%)	Multiple (%)
Mortensen et al[2]	821	Autopsy	406/821 (49); >2 cm (17.5)	100/406 (25)	306/406 (75)
Ezzat et al[3]	100	Ultrasound	67/100 (67) >1 cm (25)	22/67 (33)	45/67 (67)
		Palpable	21/100 (21)	9/21 (43)	12/21 (57)
Brander et al[4]	253	Ultrasound	54/253 (21); >1 cm (30)	39/54 (72)	15/53 (28)
Vander et al[5]	5127	Palpable	218/5127 (4.2)	146/218 (67)	72/218 (33)

Table 25–2 Clinical Risk Factors for Thyroid Cancer in Patients with Thyroid Nodules

History, Symptoms
Head, neck irradiation (as a child)
Total body irradiation[9]
Exposure to radiation fallout (Chernobyl, <14 yr old)[10]
Family history of thyroid cancer (first-degree relative)
Cough, voice change
Hemoptysis
Rapid growth
Physical Examination, Signs
Size (modest risk factor)
Fixation to adjacent structures (immobility)
Ipsilateral lymphadenopathy
Vocal cord paresis

autonomous thyroid nodule (associated with low serum TSH, risk of malignancy rare) from the more common hypofunctioning thyroid nodule (associated with a normal serum TSH, 5% to 10% risk of malignancy). Most patients with a normal serum TSH can proceed directly to ultrasound and fine-needle biopsy, whereas patients with a low serum TSH should be considered for anatomic (ultrasound) and scintigraphic (^{123}I, $^{99}TcO_4$) imaging. A recent study has compared the serum TSH level with prevalence of malignancy in 1183 subjects with thyroid nodules.[15] Patients with thyroid nodules and a serum TSH in the lower end of the normal range (0.5 to 0.9 mU/L) had a 3.7% prevalence of malignancy, patients with a slightly higher TSH (1 to 1.7 mU/L) had approximately a twofold increased risk of malignancy (8.3% prevalence), and patients with a serum TSH in the upper half of the reference range (1.8 to 5 mU/L) had a threefold increased risk of malignancy (12.3% prevalence). Although these data need to be confirmed in other studies, serum TSH may be a useful tool for the overall assessment for risk of malignancy in patients with thyroid nodules.

Serum calcitonin may be helpful to identify patients with medullary thyroid carcinoma preoperatively. A patient with a serum calcitonin level > 100 pg/mL has a high likelihood of harboring medullary thyroid cancer or C-cell hyperplasia.[16] Lower levels of calcitonin are more difficult to interpret and pentagastrin (for stimulation testing) is not available in the United States, making it difficult to recommend serum calcitonin testing for all patients with thyroid nodules. We currently reserve calcitonin testing for patients with indeterminate or suspicious thyroid nodules, or those with a family history of thyroid cancer.

Thyroid sonography is now recommended for all patients with suspected thyroid nodules.[12] Thyroid ultrasound can determine whether the palpable nodule is a distinct thyroid nodule or just an irregular gland contour (15% to 20%), whether there are other nodules present (25%), or whether the nodule is posterior or more than 50% cystic, which could decrease the yield of a palpation-guided biopsy.[6,17] Modern sonography can also further characterize nodules for risk of malignancy based on various features (Table 25-3). Studies have shown that certain sonographic features increase the relative risk of malignancy in thyroid nodules: hypoechoic (relative risk [RR], 1.5 to 3.0), blurred margins (RR, 1.1 to 6.0), microcalcifications (RR, 2.0 to 5.0), increased intranodular vascularity (RR, 4.0 to 5.0), or wider than tall on transverse imaging (RR, 2.0 to 2.5).[8,18,19] No single feature accurately distinguishes benign from malignant nodules, but these features are useful to help direct biopsy of sonographically suspicious nodules in patients with multiple thyroid nodules; size alone is not a good criterion.

Table 25–3 Ultrasound (Sonographic) Characteristics of Thyroid Nodules

Sonographic Features Associated with Benign Nodules	Sonographic Features Associated with Malignant Nodules
Hyper-, isoechoic	Hypoechoic
No calcifications	Microcalcifications
Peripheral vascularity	Increased intranodular vascularity
Sharp margins	Blurred margins
Cystic	Solid
A/T ratio < 1	A/T ratio ≥ 1

A/T ratio, anteroposterior-to-transverse diameter ratio.

Table 25–4 Broad Categories of Fine-Needle Aspiration (FNA) Cytology of the Thyroid Gland

Group I (Lesions That Are Almost Certainly Benign)

Colloid nodule
Macrofollicular adenoma

Group II (Lesions That Can Be Benign or Neoplastic)

First subcategory:
- Adenomatoid (goitrous) nodule
- Follicular adenoma

Second subcategory:
- Follicular adenoma
- Follicular carcinoma
- Follicular variant of papillary thyroid carcinoma

Group III (Lesions Highly Suspicious for Malignancy or Accurately Diagnosed by FNA)

Papillary thyroid carcinoma
Medullary thyroid carcinoma
Anaplastic thyroid carcinoma
Lymphoma
Metastatic carcinoma
Chronic lymphocytic thyroiditis

Fine-Needle Aspiration Cytology and Correlation with Histology

Fine-needle aspiration (FNA) cytology of the thyroid gland has become the gold standard over the past few decades to distinguish benign from malignant thyroid nodules.[20-25] In this context, the findings of FNA of thyroid nodules fall into three major categories (Table 25-4).[26-28]

Group I: Lesions That Are Almost Certainly Benign

The possibility of neoplasia in this group is extremely low and, if neoplastic, will very likely be a benign neoplasm (benign macrofollicular adenoma).[27-31]

Group II: Lesions That Can Be Neoplastic

These fall broadly into two subcategories. In the first, the findings are indeterminate and differentiation between a benign cellular (adenomatoid) goitrous nodule and a follicular neoplasm cannot be easily made.[27,28] However, the vast majority of these lesions, if correctly interpreted, are benign non-neoplastic lesions; if neoplastic, they mostly represent benign follicular adenomas. In the second subcategory, the findings favor a follicular neoplasm.[31-35] In this group, histologic evaluation is required to confirm and ascertain the nature of the lesion (neoplastic vs. hyperplastic) by the determination of the presence or absence of a surrounding capsule to the nodule and, if neoplastic (follicular neoplasm), whether it exhibits benign or malignant behavior (capsular and vascular invasion).

The prevalence of a malignancy in the first subgroup is low and rises to approximately 10% to 20% in the second subgroup.[36,37] Studies have suggested that the reported incidence of follicular carcinomas diagnosed by FNA in this group is low.[38] Some of these aspirates diagnosed as follicular neoplasms also prove on surgical excision to be the follicular variant of papillary carcinoma and can be a diagnostic challenge.[36,37]

Group III: Lesions That Are Accurately Diagnosed

This group includes malignant lesions (papillary carcinoma, medullary carcinoma, lymphoma, anaplastic carcinoma, and metastatic thyroid disease) and inflammatory thyroid conditions (chronic lymphocytic thyroiditis, including Hashimoto's thyroiditis). Although the diagnosis of these lesions may at times pose a diagnostic challenge because of the cytomorphology presented to the cytopathologist or the complicated clinical picture, the entities in this category can usually be diagnosed reliably by a trained cytopathologist. We and many others prefer this grouping because the focus is put on the probability of neoplasia and the determination of the chance of being benign, as noted.

Some authors have suggested that the first two groups define the role of FNA as a screening tool, whereas the third group identifies its definitive diagnostic role.[28] Ideally, in an effective management setting, input from the ultrasound, clinical, and laboratory evaluations are integrated with the FNA findings in the final determination of surgical option versus follow-up and medical options. A close working relationship between the endocrinologist, surgeon, and cytopathologist is essential for optimal patient management.

In 2006, in an attempt to unify examination and reporting of thyroid fine needle aspirates similar to what is followed in the interpretations of Pap smears and breast pathology, the Papanicolaou Society of Cytopathology Task Force on Standards of Practice issued guidelines for the examination and reporting of FNA specimens from thyroid nodules.[39] Also in 2006, other terminology schemes were proposed by the American Thyroid Association[12] and the American Association of American Endocrinologists.[13] More recently, in 2008, a diagnostic terminology and morphologic criteria for the cytologic diagnosis of thyroid lesions was proposed by a working committee group of the National Cancer Institute.[40] Hopefully, these efforts will eventually lead to implementing unified thyroid FNA reporting that will be adopted by various groups.

CYTOLOGIC INTERPRETATION OF FINE-NEEDLE ASPIRATION OF SOLITARY THYROID NODULES

Before discussing the specific pathologic entities that a thyroid nodule can represent, evaluating a thyroid aspirate of a thyroid nodule must consider three important elements:

- Constituent cell types and cellularity of the aspirate
- Presence, quality, and quantity of colloid in the aspirate
- Patient history and clinical findings, including ultrasound and history of previous FNA and surgical intervention in the aspirate region

Cell Types

The major cell type seen is thyroid follicular cells. Normal follicular cells are small, uniform, and lymphocyte size,[41] and have round to slightly ovoid hyperchromatic nuclei. Their cytoplasm is usually pale and fragile. They often appear flat in a cohesive honeycomb-like arrangement,[33] as rounded follicular formations of different sizes, either intact or ruptured[34] or, less often, as single cells that may occasionally be in the form of naked nuclei without cytoplasm.[42] The nucleoli are invisible to inconspicuous. Reactive changes in follicular cells are often seen and may cause some nuclear pleomorphism, with more prominent nucleoli, but nevertheless the cells maintain their ordered appearance and cohesiveness.

Hürthle cells, also called oncocytes, oxyphils, or Ashkenazy cells, can also be seen in both neoplastic and non-neoplastic thyroid nodules. The cells are characterized by eccentrically placed nuclei, distinct prominent nucleoli, and granular, well-defined cytoplasm resulting from abundant abnormal mitochondrial content. Foci of metaplastic Hürthle cells are a usual benign finding in many thyroid gland aspirates and are usually seen in sheets or singly. Neoplasms consisting entirely of Hürthle cells (Hürthle cell adenoma, Hürthle cell carcinoma) are also seen.[43-45]

Other cell types can include chronic inflammatory cells (e.g., lymphocytes, plasma cells), parafollicular cells, which are not readily identifiable in aspirates, and others (e.g., fat, respiratory type, muscle).

In group III, which includes malignancies other than follicular carcinoma, the cancer cells usually exhibit special morphologic and immunocytochemical features that are characteristic for the individual cancer type, which makes them readily identifiable by an experienced cytopathologist. These will be discussed in more detail in the following sections.

Colloid

Thyroid hormones are stored in the thyroid gland in an acellular glycoprotein called colloid. Colloid is seen in various consistencies, from watery and pale to thick and dense forms, which consequently translates into a broad range of appearances in cytologic preparations. However, the cracking effect (stained glass, broken ice appearance) tends to be one of the more commonly identifiable features. In general terms, the more active the gland, the more watery and pale the colloid, and the less active it becomes the denser the colloid. The ratio of colloid to follicular cells in an aspirate is an important consideration in FNA interpretation. In this context, abundant colloid is more likely to be associated with benign nodules (large benign follicle formations that contain and extrude more colloid). A scant amount of colloid is seen in association with some follicular neoplasms (microfollicles with scant colloid).

A dense, bubblegum-like colloid consistency has been associated with papillary thyroid carcinoma. It is considered to be a helpful feature in assessing cytologic preparations suspicious for papillary thyroid carcinoma.

The other significant acellular material encountered in FNA aspirates is amyloid, which can be seen in association particularly with medullary carcinoma in addition to cases of plasmacytomas, goiter, and amyloidosis.

Clinical History and Findings

Knowledge of the clinical findings and history of the patient are important in FNA evaluation. A history of previous FNA or operative intervention will, for example, help elaborate some of the changes that may be encountered in the cells and tissues of the region (e.g., reactive, cystic, hemorrhagic). No FNA evaluation should be considered complete without thorough evaluation of the patient's history, physical examination, and imaging studies.

SPECIFIC CYTOLOGIC DIAGNOSIS

In making the final cytologic diagnosis of an FNA aspirate from a thyroid nodule, general and specific findings are integrated. Generally, a thyroid nodule aspirate should contain at least six groups of follicular cells (each group is composed of at least 10 cells) to be judged as cytologically adequate for interpretation.

Group I: Lesions That Are Almost Certainly Benign

In this group, the aspirate shows abundance of colloid, which may be watery to a thicker, honey-like consistency. Small bland follicular cells and occasional metaplastic Hürthle cells are also seen, usually in sheets. The amount of follicular cells is relatively small compared with colloid. Histiocytes are also seen and can have a pigmented cytoplasm. This cytomorphology is consistent with the formation of a goitrous colloid nodule. Rarely, some of these lesions will turn out to be benign macrofollicular adenomas.

Group II: Lesions That Can Be Neoplastic

In the first subcategory, the distinction between an adenomatoid or cellular nodule and a follicular neoplasm is not easily established. Adenomatoid nodules aspirates show a similar constellation of cytologic features as seen in group I lesions, but the cellularity is increased, together with a moderate amount of colloid. The presence of macrofollicular formations suggests that even if this lesion turns out to be neoplastic, it will probably represent a benign macrofollicular adenoma. Microfollicles can also be occasionally seen in these lesions. However, if they constitute a significant proportion of the follicular architecture seen (mixed macro- and microfollicular arrangement), the index of suspicion for neoplasm should increase, and some of these neoplasms can turn out to be the follicular variant of papillary carcinoma.

In the second subcategory, the aspirate morphology is hypercellular and can be dominated by microfollicular, trabecular, or solid architecture, with scant colloid formation. The likelihood of follicular adenoma in this group is approximately 80% to 90%. These lesions are found to be follicular thyroid carcinoma in approximately 15% to 20% of cases. Clinical and radiologic assessment is essential because in some cases the input of these parameters (e.g., radiation history) can raise the risk of an even higher percentage. As noted, the prevalence of follicular carcinoma in this group (20%) is challenged by a number of studies, which believes it to be much lower.

The recognition of follicular carcinoma in an aspirate can be difficult. Some cytopathologists, aware of the treacherous nature of this diagnosis, prefer only to express their inclination toward it in an explanatory note rather than give a definitive diagnostic statement. This may become more understandable because well-differentiated follicular carcinomas show no cytologic difference from adenomas on a cytologic smear; some cases that show marked nuclear atypia with concerning nuclear features turn out to be benign adenomas, with inconsequential nuclear atypia (follicular adenoma with bizarre nuclei). However, there are features that favor a diagnosis of malignancy, including irregular and disorganized follicles with significant cytologic atypia, pleomorphism, and increased numbers of single cells.

Group III: Lesions That Are Suspicious or Accurately Diagnosed

Fortunately, primary thyroid malignancies, other than follicular carcinoma, have specific cytomorphologic features that facilitate the recognition of the type of malignancy seen if the aspirate is a representative sample. However, on occasion, the features can be concerning enough but not conclusive for malignancy for a number of reasons, which that may vary from case to case. Two subcategories are seen in this category.

1. Suspicious for malignancy. Examples of diagnosis in this category include but not exclusive to some cases of the follicular variant of papillary carcinoma, medullary carcinoma where additional studies may be needed, metastatic lesions, or extensive necrosis of the tumor.
2. Malignant lesions. In the ensuing discussion, we will preview the cytologic features of the important entities in this group.

Papillary thyroid carcinoma (PTC). The most important diagnostic clue in PTC cytology rests with the nuclear features.[26-28,46-48] The aspirates are usually cellular with disorderly, crowded, and overlapping single-layer sheets and clusters in a syncytial arrangement. Occasionally, papillary and dome-shaped forms are seen in addition to two-dimensional flat sheets with finger-like projections. The nuclei are usually larger than normal follicular cells, ovoid, with fine powder-like chromatin and a small marginal nucleolus. Most importantly, the cells can focally exhibit longitudinal nuclear grooves and occasionally sharply demarcated intranuclear inclusions. The cellular cytoplasm is variable from pale and delicate to abundant, granular, and eosinophilic (squamoid), with sharply demarcated margins. Histiocytes can also be seen in aspirates from cystic papillary carcinoma.

The colloid in papillary carcinoma is usually dense, with a bubblegum-like appearance and consistency. Concentric calcifications (psammoma bodies) and giant cells can also be seen.

A number of variants of papillary thyroid carcinoma exist, including follicular, tall cell, columnar cell, diffuse sclerosing, Warthin's tumor–like, and cribriform-morular variant. The nuclear features are readily discernible in all these variants.[36,49-53] Aggressive variants of papillary thyroid carcinoma include tall cell, columnar cell, diffuse sclerosing, and Hürthle cell.[49]

One variant that frequently presents as a difficult cytologic diagnosis is the follicular variant of papillary carcinoma. The presence of follicle formations, lack of papillary forms, and absence of classic nuclear features, particularly pseudoinclusions, may lead to the cytologic diagnosis of a follicular neoplasm rather than papillary carcinoma.[36] Careful review of the nuclear features therefore is required when examining follicular lesions. Suspicion of the follicular variant of papillary thyroid carcinoma should be noted in cytologic reports if nuclear features raise the possibility of this variant.

Medullary thyroid carcinoma (MTC). Aspirates of medullary thyroid carcinoma are usually cellular and show a monotonous, dyscohesive population of neuroendocrine cells and amyloid.[54-57] The cells commonly exhibit three morphologies; spindle, epithelioid granular, and plasmacytoid. Other variants include oncocytic, clear cell, small cell, papillary, and giant cell (anaplastic).[58-61] The nuclear chromatin shows the characteristic salt-and-pepper appearance encountered in neuroendocrine tumors. Amyloid is seen in up to 80% of MTCs and appears as an acellular, amorphous, dense orange to pink material that is similar to thick colloid in many cases and can be differentiated by positive Congo red staining. Occasionally, medullary carcinoma contains nuclear pseudoinclusions, is multinucleated, and is similar to papillary carcinoma. If MTC is in the differential diagnosis, samples can be stained by immunocytochemistry for calcitonin or serum calcitonin levels can be measured.

Poorly differentiated (insular) carcinoma. These specimens are particularly cellular with monotonous small cells and high nuclear to cytoplasmic ratio and scant cytoplasm.[62-64] The cells usually have a small, bland, slightly hyperchromatic nuclei; however, some can be more pleomorphic and necrosis can be evident. The aspirates may be seen as trabeculae, in clusters or small cell aggregates.

Anaplastic thyroid carcinoma (ATC). Anaplastic carcinoma of the thyroid gland is an aggressive neoplasm that usually shows a cellular smear with frankly malignant cells with a background of necrosis and tumor diathesis. The cells vary in appearance, from squamoid, spindled, multinucleated giant cells to bizarre morphology.[65-67] A mixed morphology is usually seen. The nuclei, regardless of their morphology, show prominent malignant features with marked pleomorphism, chromatin clumping, prominent macronucleoli, focal pseudoinclusions, and irregular nuclear membrane. The specimens often contain abnormal mitotic figures.

Thyroid lymphoproliferative disorders. A number of lymphoproliferative disorders can be encountered in the thyroid gland, including plasmacytomas, and lymphomas. Many of these arise in the background of Hashimoto's thyroiditis. Lymphomas account for approximately 1% to 2% of primary thyroid malignancies.[68-70] The most common type of lymphoma seen in the thyroid gland is non-Hodgkin's lymphoma, particularly diffuse large B-cell lymphoma.[71]

Other tumors. Squamous cell carcinoma, mucoepidermoid carcinoma, and mucinous neoplasms are rarely encountered as primary thyroid tumors. The cytology of these tumors is well characterized and can be accurately interpreted. However, the poorly differentiated malignancies of these neoplasms can be difficult to subcategorize and occasionally can be confused with poorly differentiated or anaplastic thyroid cancer.

Other malignancies with metastases to the thyroid can present as a solitary nodule or multiple nodules.[72,73] Usually, with a history of a primary site, such as kidney, colon, lung, breast, or head and neck squamous cancer, lymphoma or melanoma is present. However, a prior history of malignancy may not be present, which poses diagnostic problems, particularly when considering that some metastatic tumors may appear cytologically similar to thyroid neoplasms (e.g., renal cell carcinoma). If doubt exists, however, careful history and patient examination, together with other laboratory and immunocytochemical studies on the aspirate, may be helpful in elaborating a definitive diagnosis.

CHRONIC THYROIDITIS

Chronic thyroiditis includes Hashimoto's thyroiditis, nonspecific thyroiditis, and Riedel's thyroiditis. Hashimoto's thyroiditis (chronic lymphocytic thyroiditis) is common and may present as a solitary

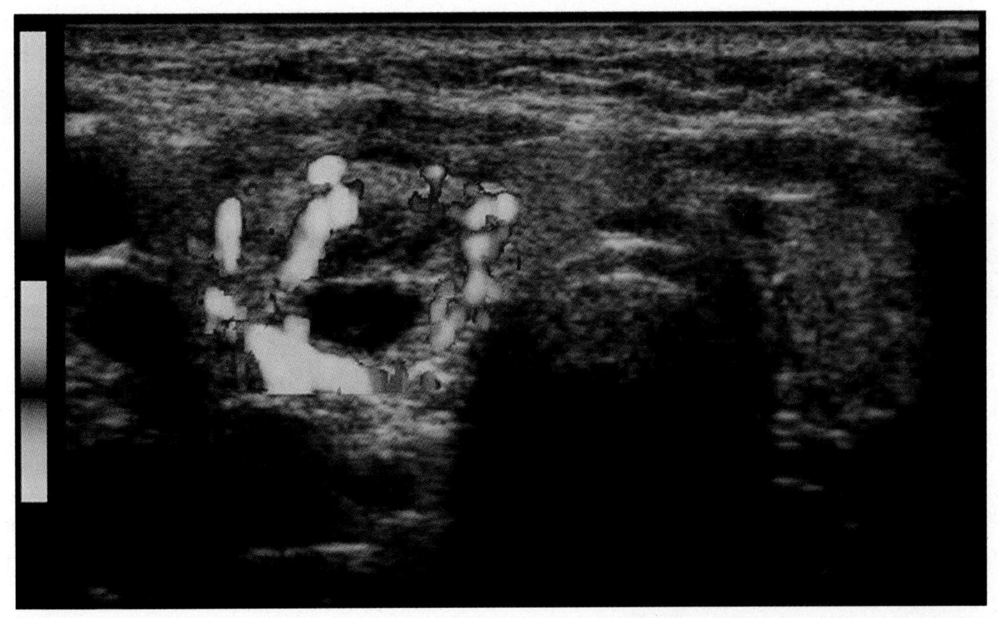

Figure 25–1 Thyroid ultrasound. A right-sided thyroid nodule with increased blood flow (Doppler imaging) is seen on transverse imaging.

thyroid nodule or as a dominant nodule in a diffusely enlarged thyroid gland.[74-76]

The cytologic diagnosis of Hashimoto's thyroiditis is usually straightforward. These aspirates typically show a lymphoplasmacytic population of cells with lymphoid tangles, lymphohistiocytic aggregates, and evidence of germinal center formation, with tangible body macrophages.[74] In addition, evidence of follicular cell degeneration in the form of Hürthle cell change is seen.[27,77] Nononcocytic follicular epithelium may show degenerative changes and foci of squamous metaplasia may be evident. As the disease progresses and fibrosis gradually replaces the normal gland, the aspirate may become scant, with fibrous tissue seen in addition to lymphocytes and Hürthle cells.

Triple Test

Evaluation and management of patients with thyroid nodules has traditionally been divided into two separate parts, clinical and ultrasound evaluation, to determine the need for FNA and independent results of the FNA to determine the need for surgical treatment. The results of these tests should not be considered in sequential isolation, but as a composite to help determine the best course of therapy. This approach has been used successfully for many years in the management of patients with breast masses and is called the triple test.[78,79] This approach combines results from clinical assessment, mammography, and biopsy to improve the accuracy of testing, primarily in patients with indeterminate or negative biopsies. Recently, investigators have replaced mammography with breast ultrasound to improve the accuracy of assessment further.[80]

Clinical assessment, thyroid ultrasound, and FNA may be combined into a thyroid triple test (T3) to improve the accuracy of FNA, especially for patients with indeterminate biopsies or the 1% to 4% of patients with false-negative benign biopsies. Clinical features may be less helpful in patients with thyroid nodules because most of these patients have no high risk features on history or physical examination.[11] The serum TSH level determination could be added to global testing (clinical assessment, serum TSH, ultrasound features, FNA cytology) for a combined quadruple thyroid test, or T4, and weighted scores could be applied to these factors to provide a T4 score reflecting the presurgical risk of malignancy in a thyroid nodule. This quantitative approach has been successfully applied to the evaluation of breast masses[79] and computer-based algorithms are being designed and applied to patients with thyroid nodules.

Patient Example

A 38-year-old woman was noted to have an asymptomatic, right-sided, mobile thyroid nodule on routine examination. There was no appreciable lymphadenopathy. She denied history of radiation exposure or family history of thyroid nodules or cancer. The serum TSH level was 2.7 mU/L. Thyroid ultrasound revealed a $1.6 \times 1.8 \times 3.0$-cm complex, hypoechoic, right-sided thyroid nodule with clear margins, no microcalcifications, and intranodular blood flow (Fig. 25-1). FNA biopsy showed multiple clusters of

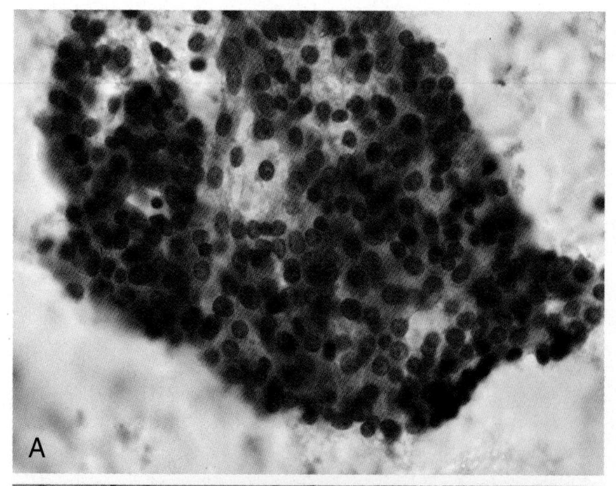

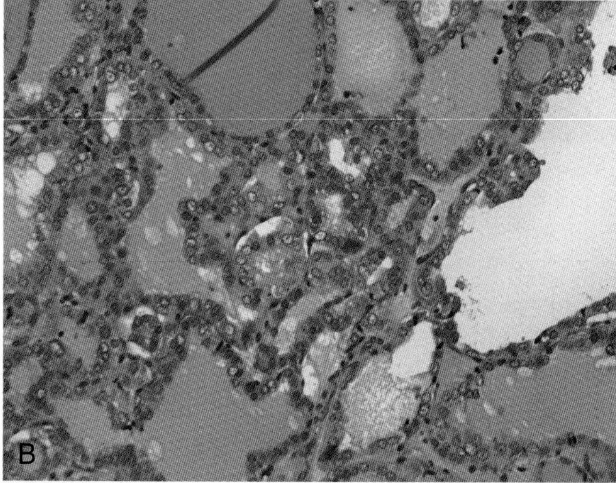

Figure 25–2 **A,** Fine-needle aspiration of a thyroid nodule showing mainly aggregates of microfollicle formations suggestive of follicular neoplasm. (Papanicolaou stain, ×6). **B,** The excised nodules show the follicular variant of papillary carcinoma. Note the nuclear crowding and clearing artifact of the nuclei seen in papillary carcinoma (H&E stain, ×40).

microfollicles with minimal atypia, scant colloid, and no intranuclear grooves or pseudoinclusions (Fig. 25-2). This was consistent with a follicular neoplasm. An ^{123}I thyroid scan showed a hypofunctioning right-sided thyroid nodule and 12% uptake.

Based on the indeterminate FNA, nodule size, and increased blood flow on ultrasound, the patient underwent a right hemithyroidectomy, which revealed a 3.0-cm follicular variant of papillary thyroid carcinoma (see Fig. 25-2). A completion thyroidectomy showed no additional malignancy.

This patient is an example of the usefulness of a composite evaluation using clinical evaluation (low risk; see Table 25-2), sonographic features (moderate risk; see Table 25-3), and FNA cytology (indeterminate) to help guide management. The patient's serum TSH level would also put her in a

Table 25–5 Features to Consider When Evaluating a Patient with a Thyroid Nodule

Clinical evaluation (see Table 25-2)
Ultrasound characteristics (Table 25-53)
Cytology features
Serum thyroid-stimulating hormone level*

*Based on one large study.[15]

moderate-risk category (threefold increased risk of malignancy over the same patient with a TSH < 1 mU/L) based on a large study.[15] Table 25-5 shows features to consider when evaluating a patient with a thyroid nodule.

FUTURE DIRECTIONS

FNA is an accurate assessment tool in patients with thyroid nodules. Patients with benign or malignant FNA cytology can be managed with this test alone, based on 97% sensitivity and 99% specificity.[3] Approximately 10% to 40% of FNA results yield an indeterminate or suspicious biopsy.[81-83] Although only 15% to 20% of these ultimately harbor a malignancy, many are subjected to surgery or close monitoring with multiple repeat FNA evaluations.

Novel imaging techniques and molecular markers have been studied in an attempt to define malignant potential of thyroid nodules in the 10% to 40% of patients with indeterminate or suspicious biopsies more accurately. Positron emission tomography (PET) using ^{18}F-fluorodeoxyglucose (FDG) has yielded mixed results and cannot yet be recommended as a diagnostic tool for patients with thyroid nodules and indeterminate biopsies.[84,85]

Molecular diagnostics is perceived as highly effective to discriminate malignant from benign thyroid nodules in patients with indeterminate or suspicious biopsies.[86,87] Markers, including galectin-3, thyroid peroxidase, mesothelioma antibody (HBME-1), and cytokeratin 19, have shown promise in different studies, but none of these are yet widely used in clinical practice. It appears that a panel of four to six complementary markers will be necessary to improve presurgical diagnostic sensitivity, specificity, and accuracy for patients with indeterminate or suspicious thyroid nodules. More recent studies have examined global approaches, including gene expression profiling[88,89] and proteomic profiling,[90,91] to define benign and malignant thyroid nodules more broadly. Novel panels of molecular markers will likely emerge from these powerful interactions between genomics, proteomics, statistics, and informatics.

References

1. Mazzaferri EL: Management of a solitary thyroid nodule. N Engl J Med 328:553-559, 1993.
2. Mortensen JD, Woolner LB, Bennett WA: Gross and microscopic findings in clinically normal thyroid glands. J Clin Endocrinol Metab 15:1270-1280, 1955.
3. Ezzat S, Sarti DA, Cain DR, Braunstein GD: Thyroid incidentalomas: Prevalence by palpation and ultrasonography. Arch Intern Med 154:1838-1840, 1994.
4. Brander A, Viikinkoski P, Nickels J, Kivisaari L: Thyroid gland: US screening in a random adult population. Radiology 181:683-687, 1991.
5. Vander JB, Gaston EA, Dawber TR: Significance of solitary nontoxic thyroid nodules: Preliminary report. N Engl J Med 251:970-973, 1954.
6. Marqusee E, Benson CB, Frates MC, et al: Usefulness of ultrasonography in the management of nodular thyroid disease. Ann Intern Med 133: 696-700, 2000.
7. Belfiore A, LaRosa GL, LaPorta GA, et al: Cancer risk in patients with cold thyroid nodules: Relevance of iodine intake, sex, age, and multinodularity. Am J Med 93:363-370, 1992.
8. Frates MC, Benson CB, Doubilet PM, et al: Prevalence and distribution of carcinoma in patients with solitary and multiple thyroid nodules on sonography. J Clin Endocrinol Metab 91:3411-3417, 2006.
9. Curtis RE, Rowlings PA, Deeg HJ, et al: Solid cancers after bone marrow transplantation. N Engl J Med 336:897-904, 1997.
10. Pacini F, Vorontsova T, Demidchik EP, et al: Post-Chernobyl thyroid carcinoma in Belarus children and adolescents: Comparison with naturally occurring thyroid carcinoma in Italy and France. J Clin Endocrinol Metab 82:3563-3569, 1997.
11. Hamming JF, Goslings BM, van Steenis GJ, et al: The value of fine-needle aspiration biopsy in patients with nodular thyroid disease divided into groups of suspicion of malignant neoplasms on clinical grounds. Arch Intern Med 150:113-116, 1990.
12. Cooper DS, Doherty GM, Haugen BR, et al: Management guidelines for patients with thyroid nodules and differentiated thyroid cancer. Thyroid 16:109-142, 2006.
13. AACE/AME Task Force on Thyroid Nodules: American Association of Clinical Endocrinologists and Associazione Medici Endocrinologi medical guidelines for clinical practice for the diagnosis and management of thyroid nodules. Endocr Pract 12:63-102, 2006.
14. Schlumberger M, Berg G, Cohen O, et al: Follow-up of low-risk patients with differentiated thyroid carcinoma: A European perspective. Eur J Endocrinol 150:105-112, 2004.
15. Boelaert K, Horacek J, Holder RL, et al: Serum thyrotropin concentration as a novel predictor of malignancy in thyroid nodules investigated by fine-needle aspiration. J Clin Endocrinol Metab 91:4295-4301, 2006.
16. Costante G, Meringolo D, Durante C, et al: Predictive value of serum calcitonin levels for preoperative diagnosis of medullary thyroid carcinoma in a cohort of 5817 consecutive patients with thyroid nodules. J Clin Endocrinol Metab 92:450-455, 2007.
17. Alexander EK, Heering JP, Benson CB, et al: Assessment of nondiagnostic ultrasound-guided fine-needle aspirations of thyroid nodules. J Clin Endocrinol Metab 87:4924-4927, 2002.
18. Cappelli C, Castellano M, Pirola I, et al: Thyroid nodule shape suggests malignancy. Eur J Endocrinol 155:27-31, 2006.
19. Papini E, Guglielmi R, Bianchini A, et al: Risk of malignancy in nonpalpable thyroid nodules: Predictive value of ultrasound and color-Doppler features. J Clin Endocrinol Metab 87:1941-1946, 2002.
20. Ashcraft MW, Van Herle AJ: Management of thyroid nodules. I: History and physical examination, blood tests, X-ray tests, and ultrasonography. Head Neck Surg 3:216-230, 1981.
21. Campbell JP, Pillsbury HC III: Management of the thyroid nodule. Head Neck 11:414-425, 1989.
22. VanHerle A, Rich P, Ljung BE, et al: The thyroid nodule. Ann Intern Med 96:221-232, 1982.
23. DeGroot LJ: Laboratory diagnosis of thyroid tumors. Ann Clin Lab Sci 13:77-82, 1983.
24. Griffin JE: Management of thyroid nodules. Am J Med Sci 296:336-347, 1988.
25. Baloch ZW, Hendreen S, Gupta PK, et al: Interinstitutional review of thyroid fine-needle aspirations: Impact on clinical management of thyroid nodules. Diagn Cytopathol 25:231-234, 2001.
26. Cibas ES: Thyroid gland. In Cibas ES, Ducatman BS, (eds): Cytology: Diagnostic Principles and Clinical Correlates. New York, WB Saunders, 1996, pp 217-242.
27. De May R: Thyroid. In De May R(ed): The Art and Science of Cytopathology. Chicago, ASCP Press, 1996, pp 704-778.
28. Clark D, Faquin WC: Thyroid Cytopathology. New York, Springer-Verlag, 2005.
29. Harach HR: Usefulness of fine-needle aspiration of the thyroid in an endemic goiter region. Acta Cytol 33:31-35, 1989.
30. Gharib H, Goellner JR, Johnson DA: Fine-needle aspiration cytology of the thyroid. A 12-year experience with 11,000 biopsies. Clin Lab Med 13:699-709, 1993.
31. Mazzaferri EL: Thyroid cancer in thyroid nodules: Finding a needle in the haystack. American Journal of Medicine 93:359-361, 1993.

32. Block MA, Dailey GE, Robb JA: Thyroid nodules indeterminate by needle biopsy. Am J Surg 146:72-78, 1983.
33. Kini SR, Miller JM, Hamburger JI, Smith-Purslow MJ: Cytopathology of follicular lesions of the thyroid gland. Diagn Cytopathol 1:123-132, 1985.
34. Klemi PJ, Joensuu H, Nylamo E: Fine-needle aspiration biopsy in the diagnosis of thyroid nodules. Acta Cytol 35:434-438, 1991.
35. La Rosa GL, Belfiore A, Giuffrida D, et al: Evaluation of the fine-needle aspiration biopsy in the preoperative selection of cold thyroid nodules. Cancer 67:2137-2141, 1991.
36. Baloch ZW, Gupta PK, Yu GH, et al: Follicular variant of papillary carcinoma. Cytologic and histologic correlation. Am J Clin Pathol 111:216-222, 1999.
37. Rosai J, Carcangiu ML, Delellis RA: Tumors of the thyroid gland. In Rosai J, Sobin LE (eds): Atlas of Tumor Pathology. Washington, DC, Armed Forces Institute of Pathology, 1992, pp 96-100.
38. DeMay RM: Follicular lesions of the thyroid. W(h)ither follicular carcinoma? Am J Clin Pathol 114:681-683, 2000.
39. The Papanicolaou Society of Cytopathology Task Force on Standards of Practice: Guidelines of the Papanicolaou Society of Cytopathology for the examination of fine-needle aspiration specimens from thyroid nodules. Diagn Cytopathol 15:84-89, 1996.
40. Baloch ZW, LiVolsi VA, Asa SL, et al: Diagnostic terminology and morphologic criteria for cytologic diagnosis of thyroid lesions: A synopsis of the Medical Cancer Institute Thyroid Fine-Needle Aspiration State of the Science conference. Diagn Cytopathol 36:425-437, 2008.
41. Soderstrom N: Puncture of goiters for aspiration biopsy. Acta Med Scand 144:237-244, 1952.
42. Nguyen GK, Ginsberg J, Crockford PM: Fine-needle aspiration biopsy cytology of the thyroid. Its value and limitations in the diagnosis and management of solitary thyroid nodules. Pathol Annu 26(Pt 1): 63-91, 1991.
43. Kini SR, Miller JM, Hamburger JI: Cytopathology of Hurthle cell lesions of the thyroid gland by fine needle aspiration. Acta Cytol 25:647-652, 1981.
44. Vodanovic S, Crepinko I, Smoje J: Morphologic diagnosis of Hurthle cell tumors of the thyroid gland. Acta Cytol 37:317-322, 1993.
45. Elliott DD, Pitman MB, Bloom L, Faquin WC: Fine-needle aspiration biopsy of Hurthle cell lesions of the thyroid gland: A cytomorphologic study of 139 cases with statistical analysis. Cancer 108:102-109, 2006.
46. Kini SR, Miller JM, Hamburger JI, Smith MJ: Cytopathology of papillary carcinoma of the thyroid by fine needle aspiration. Acta Cytol 24:511-521, 1980.
47. Akhtar M, Ali MA, Huq M, Bakry M: Fine-needle aspiration biopsy of papillary thyroid carcinoma: Cytologic, histologic, and ultrastructural correlations. Diagn Cytopathol 7:373-379, 1991.
48. Kaur A, Jayaram G: Thyroid tumors: Cytomorphology of papillary carcinoma. Diagn Cytopathol 7:462-468, 1991.
49. Livolsi VA: Papillary neoplasms of the thyroid. Pathologic and prognostic features. Am J Clin Pathol 97:426-434, 1992.
50. Evans HL: Columnar-cell carcinoma of the thyroid. A report of two cases of an aggressive variant of thyroid carcinoma. Am J Clin Pathol 85:77-80, 1986.
51. Harach HR, Zusman SB: Cytopathology of the tall cell variant of thyroid papillary carcinoma. Acta Cytol 36:895-899, 1992.
52. Caruso G, Tabarri B, Lucchi I, Tison V: Fine-needle aspiration cytology in a case of diffuse sclerosing carcinoma of the thyroid. Acta Cytol 34:352-354, 1990.
53. Dalal KM, Moraitis D, Iwamoto C, et al: Clinical curiosity: Cribriform-morular variant of papillary thyroid carcinoma. Head Neck 28:471-476, 2006.
54. Saad MF, Ordonez NG, Rashid RK, et al: Medullary carcinoma of the thyroid. A study of the clinical features and prognostic factors in 161 patients. Medicine (Baltimore) 63:319-342, 1984.
55. Kini SR, Miller JM, Hamburger JI, Smith MJ: Cytopathologic features of medullary carcinoma of the thyroid. Arch Pathol Lab Med 108:156-159, 1984.
56. Bose S, Kapila K, Verma K: Medullary carcinoma of the thyroid: A cytological, immunocytochemical, and ultrastructural study. Diagn Cytopathol 8:28-32, 1992.
57. Harach HR, Bergholm U: Medullary carcinoma of the thyroid with carcinoid-like features. J Clin Pathol 46:113-117, 1993.
58. Dominguez-Malagon H, Delgado-Chavez R, Torres-Najera M, et al: Oxyphil and squamous variants of medullary thyroid carcinoma. Cancer 63:1183-1188, 1989.
59. Landon G, Ordonez NG: Clear cell variant of medullary carcinoma of the thyroid. Hum Pathol 16:844-847, 1985.
60. Mendelsohn G, Baylin SB, Bigner SH, et al: Anaplastic variants of medullary thyroid carcinoma: A light-microscopic and immunohistochemical study. Am J Surg Pathol 4:333-341, 1980.
61. Albores-Saavedra J, Gorraez de la Mora T, de la Torre-Rendon F, Gould E: Mixed medullary-papillary carcinoma of the thyroid: A previously unrecognized variant of thyroid carcinoma. Hum Pathol 21:1151-1155, 1990.
62. Sakamoto A, Kasai N, Sugano H: Poorly differentiated carcinoma of the thyroid. A clinicopathologic entity for a high-risk group of papillary and follicular carcinomas. Cancer 52:1849-1855, 1983.
63. Pietribiasi F, Sapino A, Papotti M, Bussolati G: Cytologic features of poorly differentiated 'insular' carcinoma of the thyroid, as revealed by fine-needle aspiration biopsy. Am J Clin Pathol 94:687-692, 1990.
64. Sironi M, Collini P, Cantaboni A: Fine-needle aspiration cytology of insular thyroid carcinoma. A report of four cases. Acta Cytol 36:435-439, 1992.

65. Venkatesh YS, Ordonez NG, Schultz PN, et al: Anaplastic carcinoma of the thyroid. A clinicopathologic study of 121 cases. Cancer 66:321-330, 1990.
66. Guarda LA, Peterson CE, Hall W, Baskin HJ: Anaplastic thyroid carcinoma: Cytomorphology and clinical implications of fine-needle aspiration. Diagn Cytopathol 7:63-67, 1991.
67. Brooke PK, Hameed M, Zakowski MF: Fine-needle aspiration of anaplastic thyroid carcinoma with varied cytologic and histologic patterns: A case report. Diagn Cytopathol 11:60-63, 1994.
68. Aozasa K, Inoue A, Tajima K, et al: Malignant lymphomas of the thyroid gland. Analysis of 79 patients with emphasis on histologic prognostic factors. Cancer 58:100-104, 1986.
69. Samaan NA, Ordonez NG: Uncommon types of thyroid cancer. Endocrinol Metab Clin North Am 19:637-648, 1990.
70. Matsuzuka F, Miyauchi A, Katayama S, et al: Clinical aspects of primary thyroid lymphoma: Diagnosis and treatment based on our experience of 119 cases. Thyroid 3:93-99, 1993.
71. Jayaram G, Rani S, Raina V, et al: B cell lymphoma of the thyroid in Hashimoto's thyroiditis monitored by fine-needle aspiration cytology. Diagn Cytopathol 6:130-133, 1990.
72. Smith SA, Gharib H, Goellner JR: Fine-needle aspiration. Usefulness for diagnosis and management of metastatic carcinoma to the thyroid. Arch Intern Med 147:311-312, 1987.
73. Schmid KW, Hittmair A, Ofner C, et al: Metastatic tumors in fine-needle aspiration biopsy of the thyroid. Acta Cytol 35:722-724, 1991.
74. Friedman M, Shimaoka K, Rao U, et al: Diagnosis of chronic lymphocytic thyroiditis (nodular presentation) by needle aspiration. Acta Cytol 25:513-522, 1981.
75. Kini SR, Miller JM, Hamburger JI: Problems in the cytologic diagnosis of the "cold" thyroid nodule in patients with lymphocytic thyroiditis. Acta Cytol 25:506-512, 1981.
76. Gagneten CB, Roccatagliata G, Lowenstein A, et al: The role of fine-needle aspiration biopsy cytology in the evaluation of the clinically solitary thyroid nodule. Acta Cytol 31:595-598, 1987.
77. Tseleni-Balafouta S, Kyroudi-Voulgari A, Paizi-Biza P, Papacharalampous NX: Lymphocytic thyroiditis in fine-needle aspirates: Differential diagnostic aspects. Diagn Cytopathol 5:362-365, 1989.
78. Kaufman Z, Shpitz B, Shapiro M, et al: Triple approach in the diagnosis of dominant breast masses: Combined physical examination, mammography, and fine-needle aspiration. J Surg Oncol 56:254-257, 1994.
79. Morris A, Pommier RF, Schmidt WA, et al: Accurate evaluation of palpable breast masses by the triple test score. Arch Surg 133:930-934, 1998.
80. Dillon MF, Hill AD, Quinn CM, et al: The accuracy of ultrasound, stereotactic, and clinical core biopsies in the diagnosis of breast cancer, with an analysis of false-negative cases. Ann Surg 242:701-707, 2005.
81. Gharib H, Goellner JR: Fine-needle aspiration biopsy of the thyroid: An appraisal. Ann Intern Med 118:282-289, 1993.
82. Barroeta JE, Wang H, Shiina N, et al: Is fine-needle aspiration (FNA) of multiple thyroid nodules justified? Endocr Pathol 17:61-65, 2006.
83. Blansfield JA, Sack MJ, Kukora JS: Recent experience with preoperative fine-needle aspiration biopsy of thyroid nodules in a community hospital. Arch Surg 137:818-821, 2002.
84. Geus-Oei LF, Pieters GF, Bonenkamp JJ, et al: ^{18}F-FDG PET reduces unnecessary hemithyroidectomies for thyroid nodules with inconclusive cytologic results. J Nucl Med 47:770-775, 2006.
85. Kim JM, Ryu JS, Kim TY, et al: ^{18}F-fluorodeoxyglucose positron emission tomography does not predict malignancy in thyroid nodules cytologically diagnosed as follicular neoplasm. J Clin Endocrinol Metab 92:1630-1634, 2007.
86. Haugen BR, Woodmansee WW, McDermott MT: Towards improving the utility of fine-needle aspiration biopsy for the diagnosis of thyroid tumours. Clin Endocrinol (Oxf) 56:281-290, 2002.
87. Asa SL: The role of immunohistochemical markers in the diagnosis of follicular-patterned lesions of the thyroid. Endocr Pathol 16:295-309, 2005.
88. Cerutti JM, Delcelo R, Amadei MJ, et al: A preoperative diagnostic test that distinguishes benign from malignant thyroid carcinoma based on gene expression. J Clin Invest 113:1234-1242, 2004.
89. Eszlinger M, Krohn K, Kukulska A, et al: Perspectives and limitations of microarray-based gene expression profiling of thyroid tumors. Endocr Rev 28:322-338, 2007.
90. Brown LM, Helmke SM, Hunsucker SW, et al: Quantitative and qualitative differences in protein expression between papillary thyroid carcinoma and normal thyroid tissue. Mol Carcinog 45:613-626, 2006.
91. Krause K, Karger S, Schierhorn A, et al: Proteomic profiling of cold thyroid nodules. Endocrinology 148:1754-1763, 2007.

Section A

FOLLICULAR CELL THYROID CANCER

Chapter 26

Papillary Thyroid Carcinoma

Naifa L. Busaidy and Richard T. Kloos

Key Points

- Papillary thyroid carcinoma (PTC) is increasing in incidence.
- Initial treatment of PTC includes surgery, radioactive iodine, and thyroid hormone suppression.
- FDG PET-CT has a role in identifying metastatic or locoregional disease not found on routine imaging in patients with radioactive iodine negative, thyroglobulin positive patients.
- Clinical trials or off-label sorafenib should be considered for the treatment of metastatic disease not amenable to surgery.

INCIDENCE AND EPIDEMIOLOGY

Carcinoma of the thyroid gland is the most common endocrine malignancy, but it accounts for only 2.3% of all new malignancies.[1] It has a prevalence in the United States of 310,000 people, and approximately 37,340 new cases were diagnosed in 2008. Papillary thyroid carcinoma (PTC) is the most common type of thyroid carcinoma, especially in regions where dietary iodine is sufficient. Women are affected three times as often as men, although men have a higher risk of disease-specific mortality. Although the median age of diagnosis is 45 years, thyroid carcinoma affects both children and older adults. At MD Anderson Cancer Center, less than 10% of all patients with thyroid cancer were diagnosed before 20 years of age. Similarly, more than 90% of patients diagnosed with thyroid cancer were 20 to 79 years old at Ohio State University.

The incidence of thyroid cancer has increased more than twofold to 8.7 cases/100,000 in 2002, a rise attributable almost entirely to PTC.[2,3] Given that most of these tumors are small (smaller than 2 cm) and that the mortality rates have been stable, most have attributed the rising incidence to the increased detection of previously unrecognized cases resulting from heightened diagnostic scrutiny, including the increasing use of ultrasound (US) and fine-needle aspiration (FNA).[3] If the population prevalence of PTC is 5%, as suggested by autopsy series (5,000/100,000), then one may predict that the incidence would still need to rise significantly if all PTC cases were to be accounted for during life, an outcome that is not currently desirable.

OUTCOMES AND PROGNOSTIC FACTORS

Despite the generally good prognosis of thyroid carcinoma, an unfortunate 5% to 10% of patients die of the disease.[1,4,5] More specifically, PTC accounts for 80% of all thyroid carcinomas, and accounts for more than 50% of all thyroid cancer–related deaths, almost three times the number of thyroid cancer deaths compared with follicular thyroid cancer, and almost four times the number of thyroid cancer deaths compared with undifferentiated anaplastic thyroid carcinoma.[6] Five-year survival rates range from 94% to 98% across all ages and races.[1,7,8] Worse outcomes are seen with larger primary tumors, gross extrathyroidal tumor extension, aerodigestive invasion, older adult patients, distant metastatic disease at presentation, and other factors.[9]

Fortunately, current management strategies for patients with PTC yield good outcomes in most patients. The prolonged course of the disease, its relative rarity, and infrequent mortality have made it difficult to perform randomized controlled trials. Thus, much of information is derived from retrospective, observational cohort studies. However, reliable research to improve mortality and morbidity from this disease and its treatments is still needed.

Currently, optimal treatment of these patients requires a multidisciplinary team with expertise in endocrinology, radiology, pathology, nuclear medicine, surgery, radiation, and oncology.

CAUSATIVE FACTORS

External low-dose radiation therapy to the head and neck during childhood, used in the 1940s to 1960s to treat various benign diseases, has been shown to predispose to PTC. The average time from irradiation to recognition of the tumor is approximately 10 years but may be longer than 30 years.[10] Higher radiation doses (more than 2000 cGy) used in the treatment of malignant diseases has also been associated with an increased risk of PTC. The Chernobyl nuclear accident, which occurred on April 26, 1986, led to a 3- to 75-fold increase in the incidence of PTC in fallout regions, especially in younger children.[11]

Except for reports of radiation-induced thyroid cancer, there is little information about the cause of this malignancy.[12] There are a few uncommon familial syndromes associated with PTC, including familial adenomatous polyposis—Gardner's syndrome, Werner's syndrome, and Carney complex type 1. Cowden's syndrome (PTEN mutation [***p***hosphatase and ***ten***sin homologue, deleted on chromosome ***ten***]) is more commonly associated with follicular thyroid cancer (Fig. 26-1). Familial PTC cases have been reported in 5% of all patients with PTC[13,14] and may portend a more aggressive disease course,[15,16] but causative genes have not been identified to account for these families. In one study, the familial risk of PTC was 3.21 and 6.24 when a parent or sibling, respectively, was diagnosed with thyroid cancer. The risk was higher among sisters and for early-onset cancers. Conversely, thyroid adenocarcinoma was associated with other neoplasms such as melanoma and connective tissue tumors, and probably also schwannomas. PTC was also associated

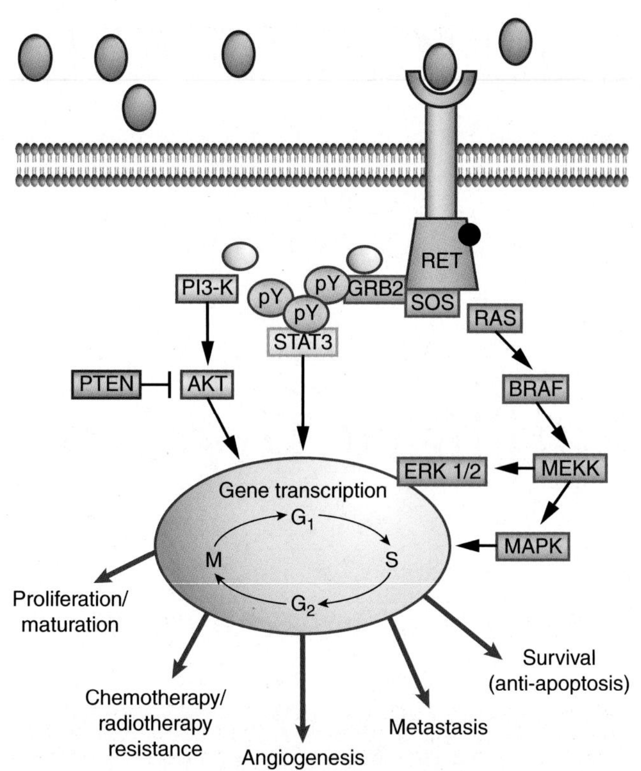

Figure 26–1 Pathway activation in papillary thyroid cancer. Constitutive activation of *RET, RAS, BRAF* (most commonly V600E) through gene rearrangements or mutations are found in most papillary thyroid carcinomas. Activation of the *RAS/RAF* cascade (shown in green) and other pathways regulate thyroid cancer formation and progression.

with right-sided colon, breast, ovarian, and kidney cancers.[17]

There is enthusiasm that understanding follicular cell tumorigenesis pathways may offer opportunities for targeted cancer therapy. Chromosomal rearrangements of the gene encoding the transmembrane tyrosine kinase receptors *ret* and *trk* have been implicated as an early step in the development of these tumors (see Fig. 26-1). *RET-PTC* genetic alterations have been found in 40% and 60% of papillary carcinomas in adults and children, respectively. Activating *ret* mutations may be the result of ionizing radiation[18] and is the most common mutation found in the Chernobyl-associated thyroid carcinomas.[19-21] Other potential causative factors include DNA hypermethylation of the promoter region of the sodium iodide symporter gene and constitutive activation of the MAP kinase cascade through activating mutations of *RAS*, although the latter are more common in follicular thyroid cancer.[18,22,23] *BRAF* mutations (see Fig. 26-1) have been identified in approximately 45% or more of clinically evident papillary carcinomas and 18% of microcarcinomas.[24] Tumors with *BRAF* mutations have been associated with more aggressive biologic behavior.[25,26]

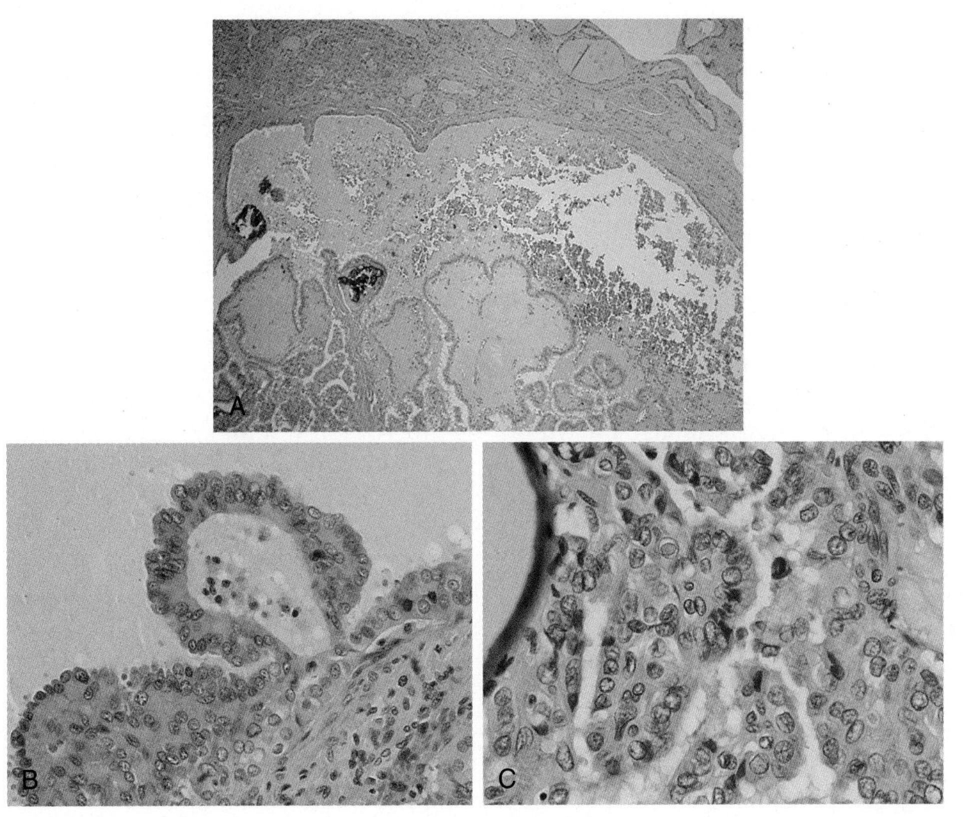

Figure 26–2 Histology of papillary thyroid carcinoma showing papillae **(A, B)** and typical nuclear features **(C)**.

PATHOLOGY

Papillary tumors arise from thyroid follicular cells. They vary in size from microscopic to large cancers that infiltrate contiguous structures. PTC tends to invade the lymphatics, with less tendency to invade the blood vessels. Psammoma bodies (calcified scarred remnants of tumor papillae that have presumably infarcted) are commonly seen in about half of papillary carcinomas (Fig. 26-2).

Many tumors have both papillary and follicular elements. Histologically, they are called follicular variants of PTC and are classified as papillary lesions because their clinical behavior is typically the same as that of conventional papillary cancer. Occasionally, both papillary and follicular tumors occur as small lesions surrounded by a dense fibrotic reaction; these are called occult sclerosing lesions and may be associated with lymph node metastases. Tall cell, columnar cell, and insular variants are histologic subtypes of PTC that portend a worse prognosis.

STAGING

Many clinicopathologic staging systems exist for differentiated thyroid carcinomas.[27-31] The American Joint Committee on Cancer (AJCC)–International Union Against Cancer (UICC) classification system based on TNM (***t***umor, ***n***ode, ***m***etastasis) has been recommended by the American Thyroid Association's (ATA's) most recent guidelines.[32] Although other staging systems have been developed to account for several additional prognostic variables with more accurate risk stratification, the usefulness of the AJCC classification system in predicting disease mortality and its requirement for many cancer registries make it a more favorable choice. Tumor size, multifocality, vascular invasion, extrathyroidal extension, incomplete tumor resection and/or positive surgical margins, tumor necrosis, lymph node metastases, extranodal extension, and histologic variants all carry prognostic importance, and their presence or absence should be included in every pathology report.

TREATMENT

Initial Therapy

Initial treatment modalities include imaging studies and surgery.

PREOPERATIVE IMAGING

It has become apparent in recent years that despite careful intraoperative palpation, malignant lymph nodes may still go undetected. Preoperative US of the thyroid and neck compartments II to VI are indicated to help identify nodal metastases; this helps with operative planning to decrease disease persistence and recurrence.[32,33] In a study from the Mayo Clinic, preoperative US detected nonpalpable lateral neck lymph node metastases in 14% of patients. In patients with palpable lymph node metastases, US still changed the operation in 41%.[34] US sensitivity is highly operator- dependent. The traditional imaging criterion for differentiating benign from malignant lymph nodes is a size cutoff of about 1 cm, but this misses most disease. Benign lymph nodes tend to be elongated (pancake-like) and show a linear, hyperechoic central structure (the hilum) with a central hilar-oriented blood flow pattern. Malignant lymph nodes have a rounded appearance in over 80% of cases and do not have a hilum. Cystic fluid, micro- or macrocalcifications, and irregular diffuse intranodal blood flow are all highly predictive of malignancy.[35] Relatively new is the use of sonoelastography. A recent study has examined the usefulness of gray-scale US, power Doppler US, and sonoelastography. An elastogram strain index higher than 1.5 was very useful for identifying metastatic lymph nodes, with 98% specificity, 85% sensitivity, and 92% overall accuracy. These results were significantly better than the best gray-scale criterion of a short to long axis diameter ratio higher than 0.5, which had 81% specificity, 75% sensitivity, and 79% overall accuracy.[36]

Chest X-rays may be helpful for routine preoperative screening of macronodular lung metastases, but their sensitivity for disease detection is low. Chest computed tomography (CT) is much more sensitive in the detection of thoracic lung or bone metastases, which should be suspected in patients with extensive lymph node metastases, vascular invasion within the primary tumor, a markedly elevated serum thyroglobulin (TG) level more than a few weeks postoperatively, or pathologic radioiodine uptake in the thorax. CT of the chest does not routinely require iodinated radiographic contrast agents and thus will not interfere with ^{131}I imaging.

CT or magnetic resonance imaging (MRI) of the neck yields high-resolution cross-sectional images of the thyroid bed and neck, but the sensitivity is typically less than that of skilled ultrasonography and is therefore not usually necessary. CT or MRI of the neck may be helpful for those with more advanced tumors with extensive local invasion for preoperative planning, especially in the setting of suspected aerodigestive invasion.[37] The iodinated radiographic contrast agents necessary for CT scans of the neck, mediastinum, and abdomen interfere with ^{131}I uptake for at least 6 to 12 weeks. If MRI imaging and local radiology expertise is available, this may prove more useful than CT for preoperative imaging because MRI contrast does not interfere with ^{131}I imaging.

SURGICAL MANAGEMENT

Total thyroidectomy is the preferred initial surgical procedure for most patients with PTC.[32,38] Arguments for total thyroidectomy rather than lobectomy include the fact that papillary foci are seen bilaterally in up to 60% to 85% of patients[39] and 5% to 10% of recurrences after a unilateral lobectomy arise from the contralateral lobe.[40] Of the 1685 low-risk patients reviewed in a retrospective analysis of patients with PTC at the Mayo Clinic, the recurrence rate at 20 years after total thyroidectomy was 8% versus 22% after unilateral lobectomy, although there was no difference in cause-specific mortality.[30,41,42] Other retrospective studies have supported these findings of lower recurrence and show only minimal improvement in survival.[43] A third argument for total thyroidectomy is that treatment with radioiodine and the specificity of serum TG concentrations as a tumor marker become more efficacious when minimal thyroid tissue remains. Furthermore, the routine use of TSH suppression therapy by levothyroxine diminishes the argument toward preserving normal thyroid tissue.

Some institutions still advocate unilateral surgery because of the lack of survival benefit with more extensive surgery and the lower risk of hypoparathyroidism and recurrent laryngeal nerve injury[44] although these complications occur in less than 1% of total thyroidectomies when done by an experienced surgeon. Most current management guidelines favor a total thyroidectomy in the setting of a primary tumor larger than 1 to 1.5 cm if there are contralateral thyroid nodules, extrathyroidal invasion, the tumor is multicentric, histologic variants with known aggressive behavior, or regional or distant metastases are present. Patients with a history of head and neck irradiation undergoing thyroid surgery should have a total thyroidectomy because they are at higher risk for multicentric disease. Increased extent of primary surgery may improve survival for high-risk patients.[43,45,46] Conversely, for patients whose primary tumor is smaller than 1 cm and who do not meet the previously mentioned criteria, a unilateral lobectomy may be sufficient.[7,30,47-49]

Regional nodal metastases are present in 20% to 90% of patients with PTC,[50,51] whereas 35% of patients will have grossly detectable nodal (cervical or mediastinal) metastases.[52] The presence of lymph node metastases increases the risk for disease recurrence. However, unlike other malignancies, it is only a minor risk factor for mortality, which is increased when metastases are present in the bilateral neck or mediastinum.[30]

Clinically, metastatic lymph nodes should be surgically removed, with current recommendations for functional compartmental neck dissections (e.g., ipsilateral central neck dissection [level VI] or modified neck dissection [levels II to V spare the spinal accessory nerve, internal jugular vein, and sternocleidomastoid muscle])[53-55] rather than selective lymph node resection ("berry picking").[56,57] Bilateral central node dissection may improve survival and reduce the risk for nodal recurrence in patients with clinically apparent disease.[58,59] However, controversy exists regarding routine central neck dissection in the absence of clinical disease because the modest reduction in tumor recurrence is partially offset by increased surgical complications, which emphasizes the importance of an experienced surgeon.

Postoperative Radioactive Iodine

Iodine 131 (^{131}I) is increasingly given as adjuvant therapy for PTC (remnant ablation), as well as for treatment of known disease. The principal behind this is that iodine is preferentially taken up and trapped by the thyroid follicular cells and their malignant counterparts. The beta particles of ^{131}I are largely responsible for its therapeutic effect and its gamma rays allow for scintigraphic imaging. The pure gamma-emitting radionuclide ^{123}I provides superior images but is without therapeutic effect.

Postoperative imaging with radioiodine (^{123}I or ^{131}I) permits the identification of residual regional or distant disease foci and ^{131}I can be used therapeutically to ablate these deposits. The emergence of fused single-photon emission computed tomography (SPECT)–CT technology may allow for greater accuracy in identifying and localizing these lesions.

Administration of cold (nonradioactive) iodine, such as that found in contrast material routinely used for CT imaging and various invasive procedures, should be avoided for at least 3 months prior to radioactive iodine imaging or therapy. This cold iodine will interfere with the uptake of radioactive iodine and can make the radioiodine scan falsely negative. Urinary concentrations of iodine can be measured to assess total body iodine content. The low-iodine diet should not be initiated until the ambient urinary level has dropped into the normal range of lower than 350 μg/L.

DIAGNOSTIC AND POST-THERAPY WHOLE BODY RADIOIODINE IMAGING

Using 2 to 5 mCi of ^{123}I or ^{131}I and imaging 24 or 24 to 72 hours later, respectively, a radioiodine scan for localization of uptake prior to ablation (diagnostic whole-body scan, DxWBS) is routinely done in some centers to evaluate the extent of residual disease or thyroidal tissue, which would then influence the subsequent therapeutic modality prescribed. Centers that do not alter therapy based on these findings omit the DxWBS, especially in low-risk patients who are clinically free of residual tumor.[60] Other centers use a low ^{131}I dose, such as 50 to 100 μCi, only to confirm thyroid bed activity prior to ablation.[61]

Controversy exists as to whether this DxWBS should be performed and whether ^{123}I or ^{131}I should be used. The disadvantage of ^{131}I is its potential for stunning, defined as when the low dose of ^{131}I for the DxWBS interferes with subsequent ^{131}I uptake for treatment.[62] This may be mediated by downregulation of the sodium iodide symporter.[63] However, more recent studies, have argued that stunning does not impair ^{131}I ablation, especially when a low activity is used and therapy is administered within 72 hours of the diagnostic procedure.[64,65] Although stunning does not occur with ^{123}I, the disadvantages can include expense and availability.

After thyroidectomy, most patients will demonstrate uptake of radioiodine near the midline in the thyroid bed (presumably normal residual tissue), ideally below 5% (Fig. 26-3). The thyroid bed may be identified using dual isotope imaging and radioactive markers placed on the thyroid cartilage and suprasternal notch. An uptake of more than approximately 5% on a whole-body scan indicates excessive thyroid tissue remaining and may warrant further surgical resection, especially if the patient is unable to achieve an elevated TSH level despite thyroid hormone withdrawal. If extensive locoregional disease is seen, additional surgery may also be considered. Unlike the DxWBS, there is widespread agreement on the need to obtain a post-treatment whole-body scan (RxWBS), usually 5 to 8 days after ^{131}I therapy. The RxWBS is more sensitive than the DxWBS to detect metastatic disease.[66]

Common erroneous interpretations of radioiodine images include the confusion of salivary, thyroglossal duct remnant, or thymic uptake (seen in young patients) for metastatic disease (see Fig. 26-3). Similarly, diffuse hepatic uptake on post-therapy images may be misinterpreted as metastases. Conversely, mild diffuse pulmonary metastases are commonly underappreciated, are best seen on the posterior whole-body images, and may not be associated with structural abnormalities on the chest CT scan.

IODINE-131 REMNANT ABLATION

Remnant ablation is ^{131}I given to destroy residual normal thyroid tissue present after thyroidectomy in the absence of known residual cancer (referred to as therapy rather than ablation). ^{131}I uptake is almost

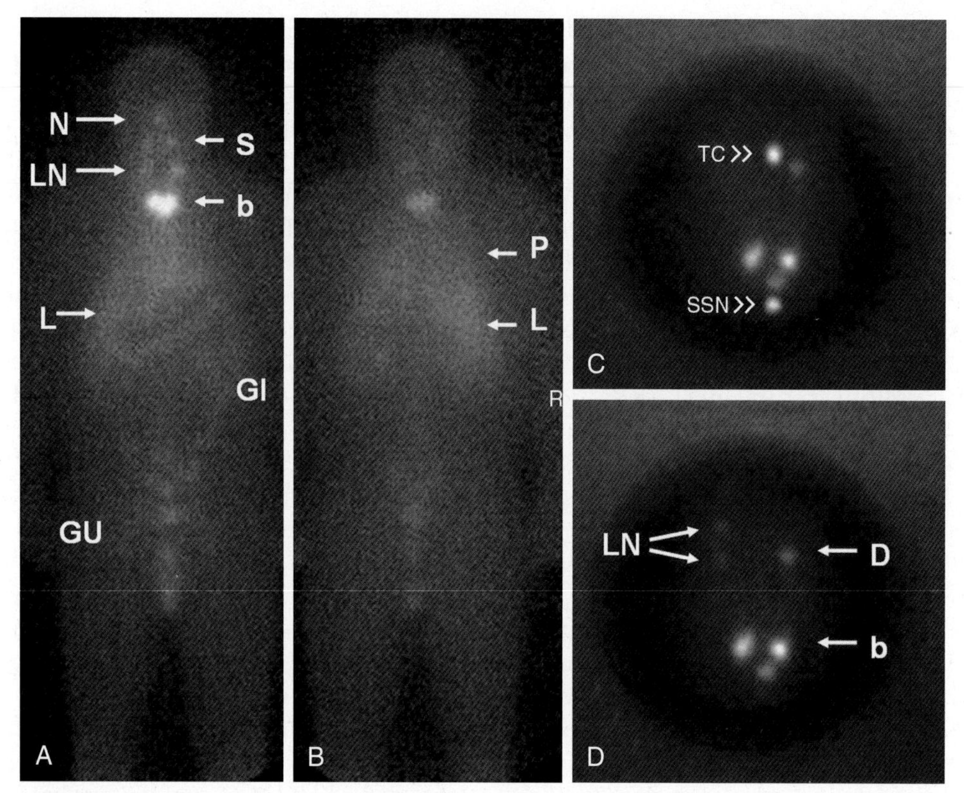

Figure 26–3 Post-therapy whole-body anterior **(A)** and posterior **(B)** images, and pinhole images of the neck with markers **(C)** at the thyroid cartilage (TC) and suprasternal notch (SSN), and without markers **(D).** The whole-body images show uptake in the thyroid bed (b) that is comprised of three foci seen on the pinhole images. Pathologic uptake is seen in the right upper lateral neck (LN) on the whole-body scan and faintly on the pinhole images, and diffuse uptake is present in the lungs (P). Neither were seen on neck or chest CT. Physiologic uptake is seen at the tip of the nose (N), salivary glands (S), liver (L), lower gastrointestinal system (GI), and lower genitourinary (GU) and skin contamination. Uptake just to the left of the TC is likely thyroglossal duct remnant tissue in this patient with disease confined to the right side of the neck at surgery.

universally present postoperatively in the thyroid bed because it is uncommon to remove all thyroid and thyroglossal duct remnant tissue during surgery (see Fig. 26-3). The rationale for using ^{131}I as adjuvant therapy is that it may destroy any residual undocumented microscopic foci of disease,[9] increase specificity of subsequent ^{131}I scanning for detection of disease by elimination of uptake by residual normal tissue,[67,68] and improve the specificity of serum TG as a tumor marker. Hence, any elevation in TG level would represent disease and not residual normal thyroid tissue.[7]

Combined retrospective data have suggest that remnant ablation reduces long-term, disease-specific mortality in patients with primary tumors 1cm in diameter or larger, those with multicentric disease, or those in whom there is evidence of soft tissue invasion at presentation.[30,46,69,70] A meta-analysis looking at the effectiveness of remnant ablation for patients with differentiated thyroid carcinoma has shown that the risk of 10-year locoregional recurrence was lowered from 10% to 4% (relative risk [RR], 0.31; 95% confidence interval [CI], 0.2 to 0.49) and the rate of distant metastases was decreased from 4% to 2% (absolute decrease in risk, 3%; 95% CI, risk decreases 1% to 4%) with ^{131}I remnant ablation.[71] In a recent prospective analysis of 2936 patients in the National Thyroid Cancer Treatment Cooperative Study Group (NTCTCSG),[72] postoperative radioiodine administration improved overall survival in patients NTCTCSG stage II and higher. Disease-specific survival was improved in high-risk patients, but not in stage II patients. Adjuvant radioactive iodine given to high-risk patients thought to be disease-free after initial surgery was also associated with improved disease-free survival. In this same study, however, NTCTCSG stage I patients did not benefit from remnant ablation, although follow-up was a median of only 3 years. Remnant ablation is not recommended for solitary primary tumors smaller than 1 cm that are confined to the thyroid in the absence of aggressive tumor histology.

IODINE-131 CANCER THERAPY

Patients with known residual disease have prolonged disease-free survival with postoperative ^{131}I treatment, which is conceptually different than remnant ablation. Although ^{131}I is the most effective systemic medical treatment for differentiated thyroid carcinoma, only about 50% to 80% of primary tumors and their metastases take up radioactive iodine.[73-77]

ENDOGENOUS AND EXOGENOUS THYROID-STIMULATING HORMONE STIMULATION FOR RADIOIODINE IMAGING AND THERAPY

The efficacy of radioiodine is dependent on tumor characteristics, including the distribution of radioiodine uptake and retention, patient preparation, and magnitude of radioiodine administered.[52] Uptake of iodine by follicular cells (both malignant and benign) is stimulated by TSH and is suppressed by increased iodide stores. For maximum uptake of radioiodine, elevated serum TSH concentrations must be achieved via recombinant human TSH (rhTSH) or endogenous TSH.

To generate an adequate endogenous TSH elevation, thyroid hormone concentrations should be lowered sufficiently to allow the TSH level to rise higher than 25 mU/L.[78] Postoperative hypothyroidism develops after 2 to 4 weeks in the absence of thyroid hormone therapy. To help alleviate symptoms of hypothyroidism, some prescribe only triiodothyronine (liothyronine; T_3) at 25 μg twice daily.[79] Lower T_3 doses are given to older adults and those with coronary artery disease. Two weeks prior to radioiodine scanning or treatment, the T_3 is stopped and a low-iodine diet is initiated.[80] Alternatively, T_3 therapy may be avoided and patients allowed to develop hypothyroidism after thyroidectomy or off levothyroxine (L-T_4) for 3 weeks. This can often be reduced to 2.5 weeks in healthy young individuals (e.g., younger than 30 years) who typically raise their TSH levels quickly.

Thyrotropin alfa, or rhTSH, may be used in lieu of standard thyroid hormone withdrawal to increase thyrotropin concentrations, which is needed for adequate stimulation of both radioiodine uptake for imaging and therapy and for sensitive serum TG assessment. The use of rhTSH is of particular benefit when endogenous TSH levels cannot rise because of hypopituitarism or when the clinician prefers to avoid prolonged hypothyroidism and its resultant complications because of concurrent medical problems.[81] A randomized, international, multicenter study has investigated the safety and efficacy of using rhTSH for 100 mCi ^{131}I remnant ablation compared with traditional hypothyroidism.[82] Successful remnant ablation with minimal (less than 0.1%) to no uptake on an rhTSH-mediated DxWBS at 8 months was achieved in all subjects in both groups. No visible uptake was achieved in 75% of the rhTSH group and 86% of the hypothyroid group. An rhTSH-stimulated TG level lower than 2 ng/mL was seen in 96% of the rhTSH ablation group and 86% of the hypothyroid ablation group, who had a significantly worse quality of life. Furthermore, the subjects in the rhTSH group had a one third lower radiation dosage to blood compared with hypothyroid subjects.[83] No comparable randomized study exists to evaluate the use of rhTSH in the setting of distant metastases, although retrospective cohort series have been described. In Europe, recombinant human TSH is approved for follow-up of thyroid cancer patients, remnant ablation, and treatment of metastatic disease. The U.S. Food and Drug Administration (FDA) has approved the diagnostic use of rhTSH for follow-up of thyroid cancer patients, but not treatment.

SELECTING THERAPEUTIC IODINE-131 ACTIVITY

Once the decision is made to administer radioactive iodine, there are three choices for selecting the ^{131}I activity. The most commonly used method is empirical, using 25 to 100 mCi for routine adjuvant ablation, approximately 150 mCi for nodal metastases, and 200 mCi or more for aggressive local or distant disease. The drawback of empirically chosen methods is that they do not take into account unique factors of the target tissue to ensure that the activity is high enough for adequate treatment, nor do they ensure that the activity is low enough to ensure patient safety. Tuttle and colleagues[84] have studied hypothyroid patients with normal renal function and used 200 cGy to the blood or bone marrow to define the maximum tolerable activity (MTA). The MTA was lower than 140 mCi in 3%, lower than 200 mCi in 8%, and lower than 250 mCi in 19%. However, an empirical dose of 200 mCi exceeded the MTA in 22% to 38% of patients 70 years or older.

A second method to determine the ^{131}I activity includes determination of an upper activity safety limit by blood and/or body dosimetry. This method determines the maximum safe limit of ^{131}I activity that can be given in one dose, and is usually limited by the activity that will deliver 200 rad to the whole blood.[85] If diffuse pulmonary metastases are present, the method also ensures that less than 80 mCi (compared with 120 to 150 mCi with no pulmonary metastases) of ^{131}I remains in the whole body 48 hours after therapy to decrease the risk of pulmonary fibrosis.[85-89] Traditionally, this method required determinations over multiple days, but a recent study has suggested that a single determination of whole-body retention at 24 to 72 hours can allow a reasonable approximation.[83]

A third method of determining ^{131}I activity is the use of quantitative tumor dosimetry. The ^{131}I activity is calculated to provide sufficient ^{131}I for the most efficacious therapy to the tumor while limiting systemic toxicity. This technique requires measurement of the target mass and aims to deliver 30,000 rad to the thyroid remnant or 8,000 to 12,000 rad to nodal or discrete soft tissue metastases.

In the United States, administration of radioiodine is done in a hospital or outpatient setting depending on state regulations by the Nuclear Regulatory Commission (NRC). In 1997, the NRC revised Title 10 of the Code of Federal Regulations (10 CFR 35.75) to allow NRC licensees to release patients on a dose-based basis. This ruling did not include agreement states, whose officials may adopt the NRC guidelines. The NRC change permitted a patient to be released from the hospital provided that the total effective dose equivalent to any individual (other than the patient) would not exceed 500 mrem. In a patient for whom the dose could exceed 100 mrem, the patient is provided with instructions on how to maintain doses to others as low as reasonably achievable (ALARA). In practical terms, for normal household environments, this often translates to an upper limit activity of about 178 or 217 mCi for small or normal-sized persons, respectively.

ADVERSE EFFECTS

Short-term acute complications include impaired taste (dysgeusia), which is common and lasts several weeks. Tender oral aphthae and stomatitis are seen with high ^{131}I dosage, whereas radiation thyroiditis and neck edema are seen when large thyroid remnants are treated. Acute sialoadenitis is seen in one third of patients treated with more than 100 mCi ^{131}I, and is dose-dependent.[90] Delayed salivary complications include obstructive sialoadenitis and salivary dysfunction (dry mouth [xerostomia]), which predispose to dental caries. Saliva induction has been presumed to be beneficial by increasing transit of radioactive saliva out of the glands. However, there is no evidence that this is true, and increased damage has not been excluded. Nakada and colleagues[91] have studied 116 consecutive patients who were instructed to suck one or two lemon candies every 2 to 3 hours during the day for 5 days, starting within 1 hour of ^{131}I therapy. Subsequently, 139 consecutive patients did the same, except that they waited until 24 hours after therapy to begin. Patients who sucked candies within 1 hour of therapy had significantly more acute sialoadenitis, taste dysfunction, dry mouth, and xerostomia. A possible explanation for this outcome is that active salivary stimulation increases salivary blood flow and, when radioiodine blood levels are elevated shortly after therapy, there is increased delivery of ^{131}I to the salivary tissue.

Additional long-term complications of ^{131}I, which tend to increase with the cumulative dose, include nasolacrimal duct obstruction,[92-95] pulmonary fibrosis (if diffuse functioning metastases are present and are treated with high dosages), oligospermia, transient ovarian failure, and early menopause.[96-98] Patients treated with ^{131}I may be at a small but increased risk for secondary malignancies, such as acute myelogenous leukemia, bladder cancer, salivary gland tumors, colon cancer, and female breast carcinomas.[99-101]

Although there is no evidence of congenital abnormalities in children conceived shortly after ^{131}I treatment, there is an increased risk of miscarriage, and it is recommended that women not conceive for at least 6 to 12 months after treatment.[32,98] Radioactive iodine should not be given to a pregnant women because of theoretical teratogenic effects in early gestation and known risks to the fetal thyroid after the first trimester. Thus, all women of childbearing age must have a negative pregnancy test prior to ^{131}I administration.

Thyroid Hormone Suppression Therapy

Patients are placed on thyroid hormone therapy after surgery and/or after receiving ^{131}I for PTC to treat iatrogenic hypothyroidism and to minimize potential TSH-stimulated growth of thyroid cancer cells. TSH has tropic effects on thyroid tissue; thyroid follicular cell proliferation and thyroid size are dependent on TSH. Differentiated thyroid carcinomas respond to TSH stimulation by increasing the expression of several thyroid-specific proteins, including thyroglobulin and the sodium iodide symporter, and by increasing the rate of cell growth. Pharmacologic suppression of TSH is a mainstay of therapy in the management of PTC.[32] Previous investigations have shown a benefit of TSH suppression to diminish disease recurrence, progression, and mortality.[30,102,103] In a large prospective study, thyroid hormone suppression therapy was associated with improved overall survival in NTCTCSG stage II and higher patients, but no advantage was seen for stage I patients.[72]

Suppression of TSH is often achieved with 2.11 µg/kg/day or more of L-T_4.[104,105] Thyroid function should be checked 6 to 8 weeks after initiation or change in dose. Brand name L-T_4 products are generally preferred and the patient should stay on the same brand of thyroid hormone, given the variability in TSH levels that can occur when switching from one product to another.[106]

The degree and length of TSH suppression are controversial. The NTCTCSG study[72] has recently shown that thyroid hormone suppression is associated with significantly improved overall survival in stages II, III, and IV differentiated thyroid cancer patients. In stage II patients, TSH levels of 0.1 to 0.5 mU/L were associated with improved overall survival, but no additional improvement was associated with further TSH suppression. With higher risk patients, each successive degree of TSH suppression was associated with additional improvement in overall survival, with the highest overall survival being associated with undetectable to subnormal TSH values. In general, it is recommended to keep the TSH suppressed below 0.1 mU/L in patients at high risk for morbidity and mortality and to keep the TSH minimally suppressed (from 0.1 to 0.5 mU/L) in low-risk patients, at least until it is clear that they are free of disease.[32,107,108]

Oversuppression of TSH can present morbid cardiac and bone consequences. The potential benefits of long-term suppression should be weighed against the potential risks of subclinical hyperthyroidism. Long-term thyroid hormone suppression may induce or worsen bone loss, particularly in postmenopausal women on no antiresorptive bone therapy.[109-111] Postmenopausal women with TSH levels lower than 0.1 mU/L have a threefold increase in hip fracture and fourfold increased risk for vertebral fracture compared with those with a normal TSH level.[112] Regarding the heart, a large study has shown a 3.1-fold increase in the development of atrial fibrillation in older patients with TSH concentrations lower than 0.1 mU/L.[113] In a population-based study of mortality in approximately 1200 patients older than 60 years, a low serum TSH level was associated with increased all-cause mortality, particularly because of circulatory and cardiovascular diseases.[114] Higher heart rates, increased cardiac contractility, and ventricular hypertrophy are also associated with subclinical thyrotoxicosis that may be ameliorated with beta blockade.[115-117]

External Beam Radiotherapy

External beam radiotherapy (EBRT) has a role in the treatment of selected PTC patients.[118,119] Although it is controversial, several retrospective studies have shown that it may be an effective adjuvant therapy after surgery to prevent locoregional recurrence in patients older than 45 years with locally invasive disease.[120,121] Ten-year local relapse free rates (93% vs. 78%) and disease-specific survival rates (100% vs. 95%) were significantly improved in patients with papillary histology and presumed microscopic disease (disease within 2-mm margin resections, tumor shaved off structures) treated with EBRT.[121] Often, this therapy is reserved for older patients with macroscopic residual disease or those with aerodigestive invasion and at least presumed microscopic residual disease, and patients with recurrent disease who cannot be satisfactorily managed with additional surgery and ^{131}I. Patients younger than 45 years are generally not treated with EBRT because of their good prognosis and the possible late side effects of therapy, including secondary malignancies.

Acute complications of EBRT include esophagitis and tracheitis. Long-term complications include neck fibrosis, xerostomia, dental decay, and the risk of esophageal or tracheal stenosis.[77] Newer three-dimensional conformal techniques to deliver radiation have been developed for cancer therapy, including intensity-modulated radiation therapy (IMRT). There are limited data in thyroid cancer, although short-term follow-up studies have suggested similar outcomes.[122]

LONG-TERM FOLLOW-UP

Imaging Studies

After total thyroidectomy and radioiodine ablation, lifelong monitoring includes clinical and radiographic data. Disease-free status in patients who have had near-total or total thyroidectomy and ablation includes the following: no clinical evidence of tumor; no imaging evidence of tumor (ultrasound of the neck in all patients, and some would include a negative diagnostic radioiodine WBS in high-risk patients); and undetectable serum thyroglobulin (suppressed and stimulated), with negative anti-TG antibodies.

ROLE OF DIAGNOSTIC WHOLE-BODY SCANNING

The ATA has suggested that after the first RxWBS following radioiodine remnant ablation, low-risk patients with negative TSH-stimulated TG levels and negative cervical ultrasound do not require routine DxWBS during follow-up.[32] However, DxWBS may be of value in the follow-up of patients with high or intermediate risk of persistent disease.[32,123]

ROLE OF ULTRASOUND

US of the neck (thyroid bed and cervical neck compartments) is used increasingly in the preoperative and postoperative follow-up of PTC patients, especially those with persistent anti-TG antibodies, detectable TG during TSH suppression (more than 0.2 ng/mL), or stimulated TG (more than 1 ng/mL). Recurrent PTC is most commonly found in the neck (thyroid bed and lymph nodes). US can be used to diagnose and identify lesions in the neck as small as 3 mm accurately. Although US can aid in distinguishing benign lesions from malignant lesions, FNA (US-guided) is most helpful to prove recurrent or persistent disease definitively. Measurement of TG in the needle wash specimen may complement the cytologic analysis.[124,125] Routine use of US in the 3- to 12-month monitoring of patients with extrathyroidal invasion or locoregional nodal metastases[76,126] is advocated in consensus guidelines.[32] Patients with

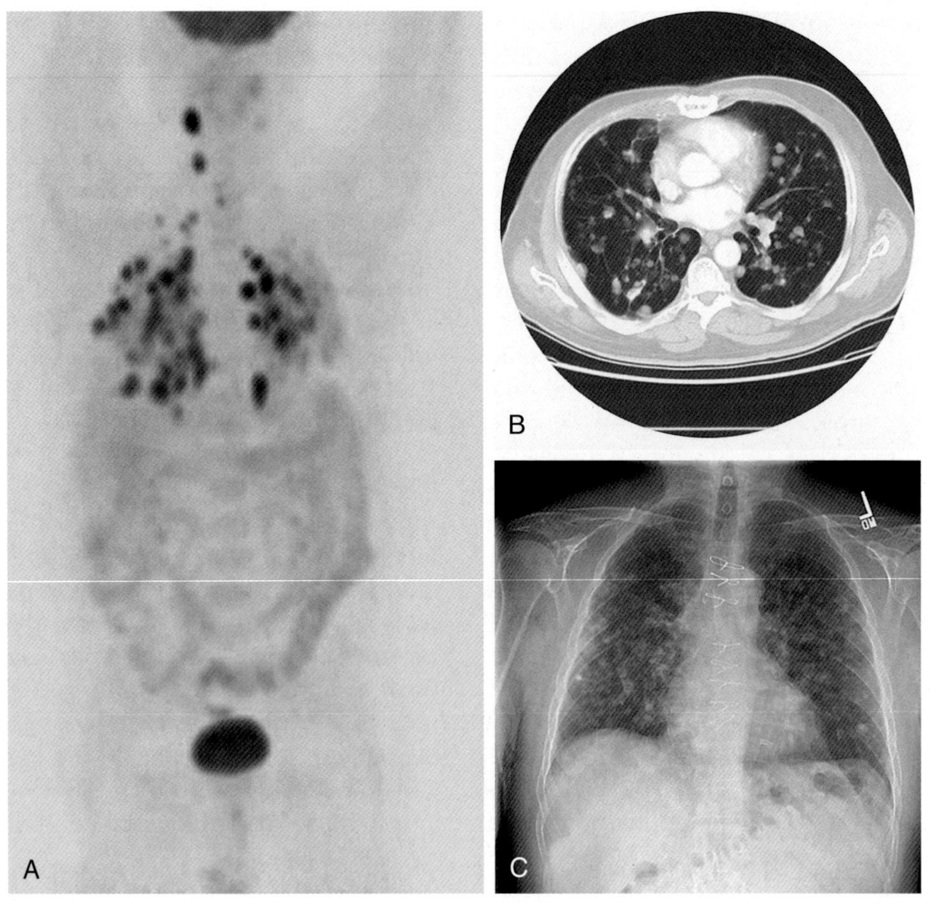

Figure 26–4 **A,** Fluorodeoxyglucose positron emission tomography (FDG PET) imaging with innumerable metastatic lesions in the lungs and a few in the neck in a patient with no pathologic uptake on radioiodine imaging. **B,** Chest CT scan with multiple pulmonary metastases of various sizes, with corresponding chest x-ray **(C).**

findings of recurrence on US commonly have no pathologic uptake on DxWBS, and often have an undetectable serum TG during TSH suppression.[127]

COMPUTED TOMOGRAPHY, X-RAY, AND MAGNETIC RESONANCE IMAGING

Other imaging techniques that can be used in individual cases of thyroid cancer follow-up include CT imaging of the neck and chest, chest radiography, and MRI. MRI and CT imaging of the neck can play important roles in the detection of recurrent disease. Although not as sensitive as US, they are much less operator-dependent and evaluate areas of the neck obscured by the trachea on US. The most common extracervical location for PTC to metastasize is the chest. Chest radiographs may show macronodular pulmonary metastases (Fig. 26-4) but they are less sensitive for micronodular metastases compared with CT (Fig. 26-5). Iodinated contrast is not necessary for CT imaging of the lungs or bones. Chest CT without contrast may be helpful before ^{131}I treatment in patients with vascular invasion, aggressive histology, gross extrathyroidal extension, or marked cervical lymphadenopathy. Otherwise, helical chest CT, with slice thickness less than 5 mm, is recommended in the following situations: when thoracic uptake is identified on the RxWBS; patients have persistent or recurrent cervical disease or anti-TG antibodies; or patients have detectable TG during TSH suppression (>0.2 ng/mL), or stimulation (>2 ng/mL). Chest CT is used in long-term follow-up when thoracic metastases are known, especially in the setting of a rising serum TG level.

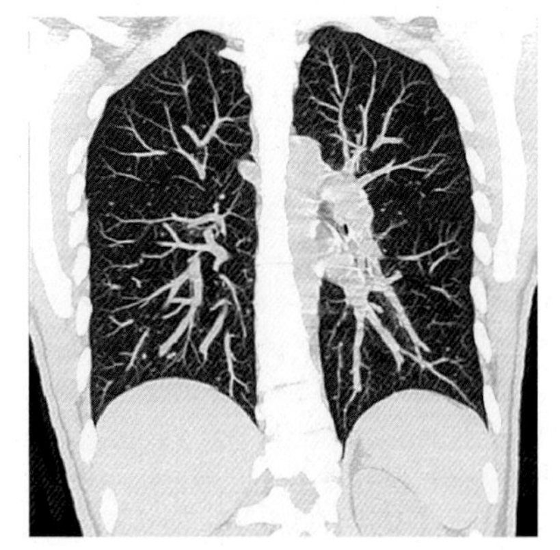

Figure 26–5 Chest CT scan with innumerable pulmonary metastases up to 4 mm in size.

FLUORODEOXYGLUCOSE POSITRON EMISSION TOMOGRAPHY

Fluorodeoxyglucose positron emission tomography (FDG PET) imaging is a reasonably sensitive and useful imaging tool for the staging and detection of oncologic disease. It is not specific for thyroid cancer, and caution should be exercised when searching for recurrent disease. False-positive imaging results has been reported to occur as often as in 11% to 25% of cases, suggesting that disease confirmation should be considered prior to altering therapy.[128-130] The recent fusion of PET and CT imaging, however, has probably improved sensitivity and specificity and provides for simultaneous anatomic investigation of suspicious areas.

Thyroid carcinomas with little to no iodine activity tend to have higher glucose metabolism and positive FDG PET imaging (see Fig. 26-4).[131-133] FDG avidity tends to be representative of tumor dedifferentiation, and tumors that take up radioactive iodine are less likely to yield positive FDG PET scans.[134] Systematic reviews of the use of FDG PET in differentiated thyroid cancer has found a beneficial role in the setting of non–iodine-avid disease.[133,135] FDG PET can aid in localization of the recurrent tumor (Fig. 26-6)[131,136,137] and in prognostication.[136] The overall sensitivity, specificity, and accuracy of ^{18}F-FDG PET–CT in a recent study of patients with radioiodine-negative, TG-positive recurrent disease were 68%, 82%, and 74%, respectively,[138] consistent with other studies, which yielded a sensitivity of 70% to 95% and specificity of 77% to 100%.[133,135] FDG PET is not sensitive enough to detect subcentimeter metastases reliably; these are common in metastatic PTC and FDG PET should therefore be used in conjunction with neck US and chest CT imaging. Patients with larger volumes of FDG-avid disease are much less likely to respond to radioiodine therapy and had a higher mortality over a 3-year follow-up compared with patients with no FDG uptake.[139,140] In a recent study of 400 thyroid cancer patients studied with FDG PET and followed for an average of 3 years, 45% of patients with a positive PET scan died of disease compared with less than 3% of those with a negative PET scan. A multivariate analysis has been performed; it included age at PET, AJCC stage, histopathology, gender, serum TG on T_4 suppression, radioiodine avidity, FDG avidity, number of FDG-avid lesions/patient, and site of metastases. Of these variables, only age, FDG status, number of FDG lesions, and standardized uptake value (SUV_{max}) were significant and correlated with survival.[141]

FDG PET imaging is not useful for initial diagnosis or routine follow-up of patients with thyroid cancer, but may play an important role in the subset of patients with radioiodine-negative, TG-positive disease (Fig. 26-7). Typically, it is used to identify surgically resectable disease or identify distant

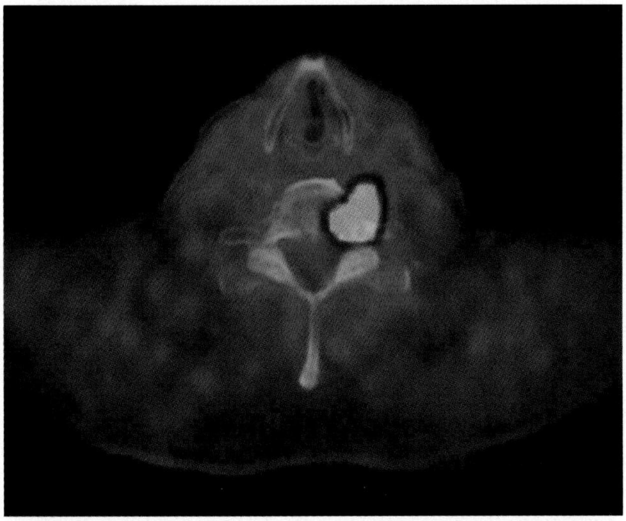

Figure 26–6 Thyroglobulin-positive, radioiodine scan–negative metastatic papillary thyroid carcinoma with positron emission tomography (PET)–CT identified lesion whose thyroglobulin level normalized after surgical resection.

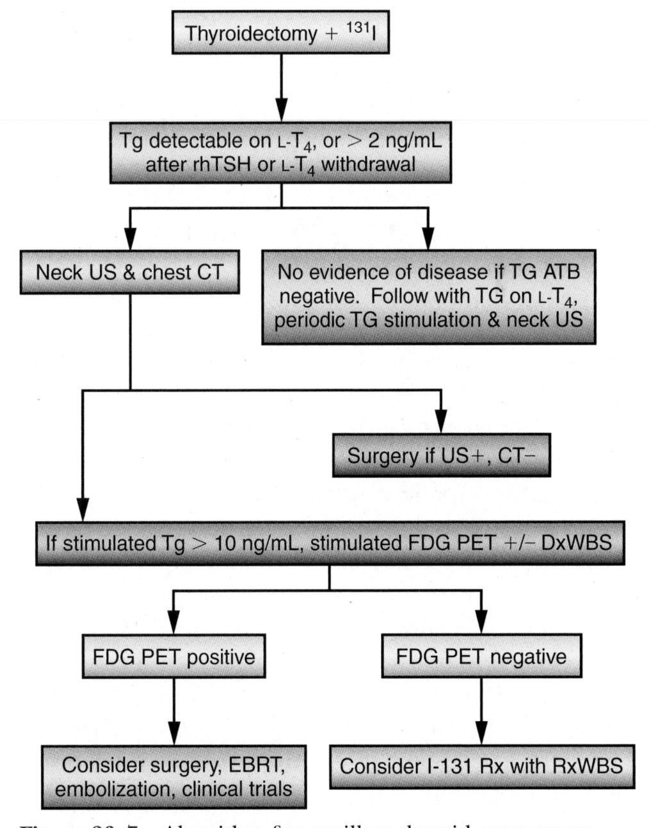

Figure 26–7 Algorithm for papillary thyroid cancer management after thyroidectomy and radioiodine ablation or therapy. ATB, antibody; DxWBS, diagnostic whole-body scan; EBRT, external beam radiotherapy; FDG PET, fluorodeoxyglucose positron emission tomography; L-T_4, levothyroxine; rhTSH, recombinant human TSH; RxWBS, post-treatment whole-body scan; TG, thyroglobulin; US, ultrasound.

metastases that may preclude surgery and necessitate other treatment. FDG PET has been approved by the Centers for Medicare and Medicaid Services for reimbursement in this setting when the serum TG level is higher than 10 ng/mL, which is associated with greater test sensitivity.

TSH stimulates FDG uptake by differentiated thyroid carcinoma, suggesting that PET scans may be more sensitive after TSH stimulation with rhTSH or thyroid hormone withdrawal.[142-144]

Monitoring Serum Thyroglobulin

TG is a protein synthesized only by the thyroid follicular cells—both benign and differentiated malignant tissue—and therefore is an excellent biochemical test to assess the presence of residual, recurrent, or metastatic disease.[145] After total thyroidectomy and ablation, the serum TG level should be undetectable. The nadir is often reached within 3 months post-treatment but may take as long as 1 to 2 years.[146] In exceptionally rare cases, the tumor may dedifferentiated and no longer secrete TG, making the serum TG level falsely low and unreliable for monitoring.

In the absence of interfering anti-TG antibodies, stimulated serum TG testing has the highest sensitivity of any single test to detect residual or recurrent PTC. Detectable serum TG during TSH suppression, or more than 2.0 ng/mL after TSH stimulation, is likely to indicate residual disease. The highest sensitivity to detect residual disease is the combination of stimulated TG and neck ultrasonography, because a small percentage of PTC patients have small malignant lymph nodes that are undetected by stimulated serum TG.[147-151] Similarly, some patients have interfering anti-TG antibodies, which may falsely lower serum TG levels in immunometric assays; worse, these antibodies may not be detected by all current anti-TG antibody assays. TG antibodies are present in approximately 25% of patients with thyroid cancer and 10% of the general population.[152] The presence of persistent antibodies in itself after total thyroidectomy and after ^{131}I administration may indicate the presence of cancer.[153] Sensitive methods to detect TG mRNA in serum remain under investigation; these have the potential to circumvent the problem of anti-TG antibodies. In patients with anti-TG antibodies, US may detect persistent disease long before it becomes clinically apparent.

TG should always be measured and recorded in the context of the TSH value because TG production is dependent on TSH secretion, and anti-TG antibodies should be measured with each TG determination. It is important that TG and anti-TG antibodies be serially monitored by the same assay, preferably in the same laboratory, to avoid problems of interassay variability that make comparisons over time nearly impossible.

The sensitivity of TG measurements to detect cancer is increased to 85% to 95% during TSH stimulation.[76,154-156] In an initial study of thyroid cancer patients who were clinically free of disease and had low or undetectable TG levels during TSH suppression, an rhTSH-stimulated TG level higher than 2 ng/mL had a sensitivity and negative predictive value of 100%. However, in 40% of patients with an rhTSH-stimulated TG level higher than 2 ng/mL, no disease could be immediately found.[156] In a follow-up study 3 years later, however, 81% of the original patients with a stimulated TG level higher than 2 ng/mL now were found to harbor disease, whereas only 5% demonstrated a spontaneous remission.[157] Furthermore, disease was found in 2% and 6% of patients with an initial stimulated TG lower than 0.5 and 0.6 to 2.0 ng/mL, respectively. These findings indicate that a single, undetectable, stimulated TG does not exclude the possibility of future disease recurrence, but patients with a TSH-stimulated TG level higher than 2 ng/mL are likely to have residual/recurrent disease.

Several recent studies have investigated the use of supersensitive TG assays with lower TG detection limits, raising the possibility that such assays could obviate the need for TSH stimulation testing. For example, one study[158] used a TG assay with a detection limit of 0.1 ng/mL. In these patients, with TSH-suppressed TG values lower than 0.1 ng/mL, only 2.5% had a stimulated TG higher than 2 ng/mL. However, in another study of assays with functional sensitivities of 0.02 to 0.9 ng/mL, specificity was poor in those with lower limits below 0.2 and 0.3 ng/mL, and it was concluded that TG determinations after TSH stimulation permit a more reliable assessment of cure.[159]

Therapy for Recurrent and Metastatic Disease

The thyroid bed or cervical lymph node is the most common site of PTC recurrence of neck disease. Typically, the highest rate of recurrence is within the first 5 years of diagnosis, although late recurrences do occur. In one study, over a 40-year period, 35% of patients with PTC recurred and two thirds of these were within the first decade after initial therapy.[9] Disease recurrence is higher in those younger than 20 and older than 60 years. Local disease comprised more than two thirds of all recurrences. Within the group of local recurrences, cancer-related mortality rates were higher in those with the recurrence in the soft tissues of the neck (30%) as compared with those with cervical lymph node or contralateral thyroid recurrence (16%). Metastases to distant sites occurred in 32% of recurrences; 50% of these patients died over the follow-up period. It is likely that most of these recurrences happened in patients who currently would be considered to have persistent disease based on TG testing and anatomic imaging. The increased use and sensitivity of these tests are likely to diminish the number of patients who recur after being declared free of disease by current assays. However, such recurrences still occur[157] and are a reminder that testing can yield imperfect results and long-term follow-up is still necessary.

RECURRENT NECK DISEASE

A patient with metastatic cervical disease identified by physical examination, US, or other imaging has typically survived ^{131}I therapy and should be considered for surgery, especially in the absence of distant metastases. Most thyroid cancer surgeons and clinical practice guidelines recommend complete ipsilateral compartmental dissection of involved areas, as opposed to selective lymph node resection procedures or ethanol ablation.[55,160] In the lateral neck, this would indicate a modified neck dissection, including levels II to V, and sparing the spinal accessory nerve, internal jugular vein, and sternocleidomastoid muscle. This compartment-oriented approach, rather than a selective approach, is indicated because microscopic lymph node metastases are commonly more extensive than can be identified on imaging studies.[56,57,161,162] Even then, however, although the serum TG level is significantly reduced with surgery, less than 25% of these patients can be biochemically cured when strictly defined by a completely undetectable TSH-stimulated serum TG. The option to follow patients with small cervical metastases that are non–iodine-avid may be elected, especially if the patient has failed one or more prior surgical attempts for biochemical cure. Theoretically, this delayed intervention may allow the serum TG level to rise, which has been associated with a decreased chance of subsequent biochemical cure, or may allow the disease to metastasize further. However, there has been no randomized study of intervention versus observation to address these issues. If observation is elected, then intervention would need to be revisited in the event of significant tumor growth.

In the setting of distant metastases, it is not evident that locoregional disease should be empirically resected, unless there is a clear risk to the airway, esophagus, recurrent laryngeal nerves, or other vital structures. From a practical standpoint, this may include central compartment disease larger than 1 cm or bulky lateral compartment disease. However, one may also elect to follow this disease as the rate of growth of distant metastases or response of disease to systemic therapy is determined.

In patients in whom the recurrence invades the aerodigestive tract, a combined treatment modality of surgery and ^{131}I and/or external beam radiotherapy is typically advised, with necessary resections and anastomoses of appropriate structures.[163-166]

DISTANT METASTASES

Distant metastases are evident in about 5% of patients at the time of initial diagnosis, but develop in another 5% during long-term follow-up. The most common sites of metastasis, in decreasing order of frequency, are the lungs, bones, and other soft tissues. Older patients are at higher risk for distant metastases.

Pulmonary Metastases

Pulmonary metastases in differentiated thyroid carcinoma are often classified radiographically as micronodular or macronodular disease (see Figs. 26-4 and 26-5). Micronodular metastases present a miliary, diffusely reticular pattern predominating in the lower lung fields, which tend to concentrate radioiodine diffusely. This is the pattern of distant metastasis seen most often in children.[167-171] Macronodular metastases are distinct nodular metastases, often between 0.5 cm and 3.0 cm in size. Radioiodine uptake is often heterogeneous but may be nil, especially in older patients and those with aggressive PTC variants.

In a review of 101 patients with differentiated thyroid carcinoma and pulmonary metastases, Samaan and colleagues[73] analyzed potential prognostic factors and the efficacy of radiodine (RAI) treatment over time. Uptake of ^{131}I by lung metastases conferred a favorable prognosis, especially in patients with negative chest x-rays. The probability of ^{131}I uptake was related to the degree of differentiation of the primary tumor. Patients younger than 40 years had a better prognosis (71% survival) than those older than 40 years (16% survival; $P < .01$). Patients with ^{131}I uptake in pulmonary metastases had 5- and 10-year survival rates of 61% and 31% compared with 29% and 7% in patients with no uptake, respectively.

High-dose ^{131}I treatments are typically used to treat pulmonary metastases. Dosimetric techniques are preferred to ensure delivery of less than 200 cGy to the red bone marrow in all patients, whole-body retention less than 80 mCi at 48 hours in those with diffuse iodine-avid pulmonary metastases to prevent pulmonary fibrosis, and less than 120 to 150 mCi in those with scattered or no pulmonary metastases.[85] Baseline and periodic pulmonary function tests should be performed in patients with diffuse pulmonary metastases, especially if fibrosis or pneumonitis is suspected or if repeated ^{131}I treatments are being considered.

Repeated doses of radioactive iodine every 6 to12 months are recommended for patient with pulmonary metastases as long as the disease continues to respond to this therapy, as shown by a reduction in serum TG levels and anatomic improvement. Long-term complete remissions may be seen in those with micronodular metastases, but those with macronodular metastases are highly unlikely to be cured.[32,77,172,173]

Macronodular pulmonary metastases that do not take up RAI on diagnostic imaging do not typically respond to radionuclide therapy; these patients are at high risk of death, especially if the metastases are FDG PET–avid.[141,174] Traditional cytotoxic chemotherapy such as doxorubicin, taxol, and cisplatin are associated with a 25% to 38% partial response rate, with rare complete remission.[175-177] These treatments are typically considered ineffective. Currently, patients who demonstrate progressive disease are optimally enrolled in an appropriate clinical trial. When clinical trials are not an option, these patients may be offered off-label empirical systemic therapy with targeted agents that have been FDA-approved for other malignancies and have demonstrated at least preliminary favorable activity against metastatic PTC.[178]

Central Nervous System Metastases

Brain metastases tend to occur in older adult patients with more advanced disease; they have an overall very poor prognosis,[179] but some patients are long-term survivors. The median survival of patients with one or more brain metastases is 22 months in those who undergo surgical resection, compared with 4 months in those who do not.[179] Current guidelines recommend surgical resection as first-line therapy, when feasible.[180] However, it is unclear whether the worse outcome in those not operated is caused by the lack of resection or by the factors that prohibited surgery. Nonsurgical treatment with ^{131}I therapy (if the tumors are iodine-avid) and/or external beam radiotherapy or a gamma knife procedure may be considered after surgical resection, especially if disease remains.[181] The use of concomitant glucocorticoids to minimize tumor swelling during ^{131}I therapy is recommended.[182] If central nervous system lesions are not amenable to surgical resection, nonsurgical approaches should be used.

Bone Metastases

Bone lesions that concentrate radioiodine may undergo ^{131}I therapy as described for pulmonary metastases. However, complete resolution is uncommon. Bone metastases may be found on anatomic imaging, such as CT, or on FDG PET. Unfortunately, some patients present with painful bone lesions, fracture, or spinal cord compression, with the latter requiring urgent glucocorticoid therapy and surgical treatment. Surgery is indicated for weight-bearing lesions with fracture or impending fracture, or lesions with impending neurologic compression. EBRT has also been used successfully to render bone lesions pain-free, and is indicated for clinically significant lesions that are not candidates for surgery, especially if they demonstrate disease progression or may threaten adjacent structures if they progress.[121,183] Arterial embolization has been used anecdotally with successful reduction in pain, but this therapy should typically be followed by surgery or EBRT. Small bone metastases that are non–iodine-avid, asymptomatic, and are not an immediate threat may be followed. Asymptomatic isolated bone metastases may be surgically resected, but it is extremely uncommon for these patients to be rendered free of disease in the setting of PTC. Intravenous bisphosphonates such as pamidronate or zoledronic acid have been prescribed for painful bony metastases, with some success. Whether bisphosphonate therapy reduces the risk of future pathologic fracture or osseous metastases in the setting of known bone metastases is unknown.

USE OF TRADITIONAL CYTOTOXIC CHEMOTHERAPEUTIC AGENTS

Systemic chemotherapies such as doxorubicin, epirubicin, taxol, and cisplatin have all been used in various combinations, with disappointing responses. They are no better than single-agent therapy but have increased toxicity.[177,184] Response rates have varied from 25% to 37%, with mostly partial best responses, rather than complete remissions. Doxorubicin has also been used as a radiation sensitizer,[185] with results not much different from radiation therapy alone.

CLINICAL TRIALS

The recent further understanding of the molecular and cellular pathogenesis of the development and progression of PTC is leading to the development of new molecules offering the possibility of targeted therapy. Some of the strategies currently under investigation include oncogene inhibitors, modulators of growth or apoptosis, angiogenic inhibitors, immunomodulators, and gene therapy. Furthermore, biologic response modifiers are under investigation to determine whether dedifferentiated PTC can be modified to increase ^{131}I uptake. Most clinical trials are currently directed toward patients with progressive disease that has failed conventional therapy.

Some of the most experience with these new compounds has been with sorafenib (Nexavar), an FDA-approved oral compound for the treatment of advanced renal cell carcinoma. Preliminary results of a study of 58 thyroid cancer patients have demonstrated more than a 50% reduction in serum TG level, decreased tumor perfusion by MRI, decreased FDG uptake on PET, and about 50% partial or minor tumor responses on anatomic imaging. No complete tumor responses were seen, and side effects of hand-foot syndrome, scalp itching, hypertension, and diarrhea were reasonably well tolerated.[178]

Axitinib, an investigational antiangiogenesis agent, is another oral compound with an initial favorable experience in thyroid cancer. Preliminary results have demonstrated a 30% partial response, 42% stable disease, and 17% tumor progression. Side effects have included hypertension, diarrhea, and nausea.[186]

Thalidomide's antiangiogenic effects have been studied in rapidly progressive thyroid carcinomas in a phase II trial.[187] Overall partial response or stabilization was seen in 50% of cases and that lasted 2 to 14 months. Fatigue was the most common side effect.

References

1. Jemal A, Siegel R, Ward E, et al: Cancer statistics, 2007. CA Cancer J Clin 57:43-66, 2007.
2. Burke JP, Hay ID, Dignan F, et al: Long-term trends in thyroid carcinoma: A population-based study in Olmsted County, Minnesota, 1935-1999. Mayo Clin Proc 80:753-758, 2005.
3. Davies L, Welch HG: Increasing incidence of thyroid cancer in the United States, 1973-2002. JAMA 295:2164-2167, 2006.
4. Robbins J, Merino MJ, Boice JD Jr, et al: Thyroid cancer: A lethal endocrine neoplasm. Ann Intern Med 115:133-147, 1991.
5. Gilliland FD, Hunt WC, Morris DM, Key CR: Prognostic factors for thyroid carcinoma. A population-based study of 15,698 cases from the Surveillance, Epidemiology and End Results (SEER) program 1973-1991. Cancer 79:564-573, 1997.
6. Hundahl SA, Fleming ID, Fremgen AM, Menck HR: A National Cancer Data Base report on 53,856 cases of thyroid carcinoma treated in the U.S., 1985-1995. Cancer 83:2638-2648, 1998.
7. Sherman SI: Thyroid carcinoma. Lancet 361:501-511, 2003.
8. Hayat MJ, Howlader N, Reichman ME, Edwards BK: Cancer statistics, trends, and multiple primary cancer analyses from the Surveillance, Epidemiology, and End Results (SEER) Program. Oncologist 12:20-37, 2007.
9. Mazzaferri EL, Kloos RT. Clinical review 128: Current approaches to primary therapy for papillary and follicular thyroid cancer. J Clin Endocrinol Metab 86:1447-1463, 2001.
10. DeGroot L, Paloyan E: Thyroid carcinoma and radiation. A Chicago endemic. JAMA 225:487-491, 1973.
11. Pacini F, Vorontsova T, Demidchik EP, et al: Post-Chernobyl thyroid carcinoma in Belarus children and adolescents: Comparison with naturally occurring thyroid carcinoma in Italy and France. J Clin Endocrinol Metab 82:3563-3569, 1997.
12. Spitz MR, Sider JG, Katz RL, et al: Ethnic patterns of thyroid cancer incidence in the United States, 1973-1981. Int J Cancer 42:549-553, 1988.
13. Grossman RF, Tu SH, Duh QY, et al: Familial nonmedullary thyroid cancer. An emerging entity that warrants aggressive treatment. Arch Surg 130:892-897, 1995.
14. Musholt TJ, Musholt PB, Petrich T, et al: Familial papillary thyroid carcinoma: Genetics, criteria for diagnosis, clinical features, and surgical treatment. World J Surg 24:1409-1417, 2000.
15. Alsanea O: Familial nonmedullary thyroid cancer. Curr Treat Options Oncol 1:345-351, 2000.
16. Alsanea O, Wada N, Ain K, et al: Is familial nonmedullary thyroid carcinoma more aggressive than sporadic thyroid cancer? A multicenter series. Surgery 128:1043-1050, 2000.
17. Hemminki K, Eng C, Chen B: Familial risks for nonmedullary thyroid cancer. J Clin Endocrinol Metab 90:5747-5753, 2005.
18. Bounacer A, Wicker R, Caillou B, et al: High prevalence of activating ret proto-oncogene rearrangements in thyroid tumors from patients who had received external radiation. Oncogene 15:1263-1273, 1997.
19. Jhiang SM, Sagartz JE, Tong Q, et al: Targeted expression of the ret/PTC1 oncogene induces papillary thyroid carcinomas. Endocrinology 137:375-378, 1996.
20. Jhiang SM: The RET proto-oncogene in human cancers. Oncogene 19:5590-5597, 2000.
21. Zafon C, Obiols G, Castellvi J, et al: Clinical significance of RET/PTC and p53 protein expression in sporadic papillary thyroid carcinoma. Histopathology 50:225-231, 2007.
22. Bongarzone I, Butti MG, Coronelli S, et al: Frequent activation of ret protooncogene by fusion with a new activating gene in papillary thyroid carcinomas. Cancer Res 54:2979-2985, 1994.
23. Specht MC, Barden CB, Fahey TJ 3rd: p44/p42-MAP kinase expression in papillary thyroid carcinomas. Surgery 130:936-940, 2001.
24. Ugolini C, Giannini R, Lupi C, et al: Presence of BRAF V600E in very early stages of papillary thyroid carcinoma. Thyroid 17:381-388, 2007.
25. Xing M, Westra WH, Tufano RP, et al: BRAF mutation predicts a poorer clinical prognosis for papillary thyroid cancer. J Clin Endocrinol Metab 90:6373-6379, 2005.

26. Kim TY, Kim WB, Rhee YS, et al: The BRAF mutation is useful for prediction of clinical recurrence in low-risk patients with conventional papillary thyroid carcinoma. Clin Endocrinol (Oxf) 65:364-368, 2006.
27. Byar DP, Green SB, Dor P, et al: A prognostic index for thyroid carcinoma. A study of the E.O.R.T.C. Thyroid Cancer Cooperative Group. Eur J Cancer 15:1033-1041, 1979.
28. Hay ID, Grant CS, Taylor WF, McConahey WM. Ipsilateral lobectomy versus bilateral lobar resection in papillary thyroid carcinoma: A retrospective analysis of surgical outcome using a novel prognostic scoring system. Surgery102:1088-1095, 1987.
29. Cady B, Rossi R. An expanded view of risk-group definition in differentiated thyroid carcinoma. Surgery 104:947-953, 1988.
30. Mazzaferri EL, Jhiang SM. Long-term impact of initial surgical and medical therapy on papillary and follicular thyroid cancer. Am J Med 97:418-428, 1994.
31. Sherman SI, Brierley JD, Sperling M, et al: Prospective multicenter study of thyroid carcinoma treatment: Initial analysis of staging and outcome. National Thyroid Cancer Treatment Cooperative Study Registry Group. Cancer 83:1012-1021, 1998.
32. Cooper DS, Doherty GM, Haugen BR, et al: Management guidelines for patients with thyroid nodules and differentiated thyroid cancer. Thyroid 16:109-142, 2006.
33. AACE/AME Task Force on Thyroid Nodules: American Association of Clinical Endocrinologists and Associazione Medici Endocrinologi medical guidelines for clinical practice for the diagnosis and management of thyroid nodules. Endocr Pract 12:63-102, 2006.
34. Stulak JM, Grant CS, Farley DR, et al: Value of preoperative ultrasonography in the surgical management of initial and reoperative papillary thyroid cancer. Arch Surg 141:489-494, 2006.
35. Gorges R, Eising EG, Fotescu D, et al: Diagnostic value of high-resolution B-mode and power-mode sonography in the follow-up of thyroid cancer. Eur J Ultrasound 16:191-206, 2003.
36. Lyshchik A, Higashi T, Asato R, et al: Cervical lymph node metastases: Diagnosis at sonoelastography—initial experience. Radiology 243:258-267, 2007.
37. Burman KD, Anderson JH, Wartofsky L, et al: Management of patients with thyroid carcinoma: Application of thallium-201 scintigraphy and magnetic resonance imaging. J Nucl Med 31:1958-1964, 1990.
38. Sherman SI, Angelos P, Ball DW, et al: Thyroid carcinoma. J Natl Compr Canc Netw 3:404-457, 2005.
39. Katoh R, Sasaki J, Kurihara H, et al: Multiple thyroid involvement (intraglandular metastasis) in papillary thyroid carcinoma. A clinicopathologic study of 105 consecutive patients. Cancer 70:1585-1590, 1992.
40. Silverberg SG, Hutter RV, Foote FW Jr. Fatal carcinoma of the thyroid: Histology, metastases, and causes of death. Cancer 25:792-802, 1970.
41. Hay ID, Grant CS, Bergstralh EJ, et al: Unilateral total lobectomy: Is it sufficient surgical treatment for patients with AMES low-risk papillary thyroid carcinoma? Surgery 124:958-964, 1998.
42. DeGroot LJ, Kaplan EL, Straus FH, Shukla MS: Does the method of management of papillary thyroid carcinoma make a difference in outcome? World J Surg 18:123-130, 1994.
43. Samaan NA, Schultz PN, Hickey RC, et al: The results of various modalities of treatment of well differentiated thyroid carcinomas: A retrospective review of 1599 patients. J Clin Endocrinol Metab 75:714-720, 1992.
44. Cady B: Papillary carcinoma of the thyroid gland: Treatment based on risk group definition. Surg Oncol Clin N Am 7:633-644, 1998.
45. Mazzaferri EL, Young RL: Papillary thyroid carcinoma: A 10-year follow-up report of the impact of therapy in 576 patients. Am J Med 70:511-518, 1981.
46. DeGroot LJ, Kaplan EL, McCormick M, Straus FH: Natural history, treatment, and course of papillary thyroid carcinoma. J Clin Endocrinol Metab71:414-424, 1990.
47. Baudin E, Travagli JP, Ropers J, et al: Microcarcinoma of the thyroid gland: The Gustave-Roussy Institute experience. Cancer 83:553-559, 1998.
48. Akslen LA, LiVolsi VA: Prognostic significance of histologic grading compared with subclassification of papillary thyroid carcinoma. Cancer 88:1902-1908, 2000.
49. Prendiville S, Burman KD, Ringel MD, et al: Tall cell variant: An aggressive form of papillary thyroid carcinoma. Otolaryngol Head Neck Surg 122:352-357, 2000.
50. Grebe SK, Hay ID: Thyroid cancer nodal metastases: Biologic significance and therapeutic considerations. Surg Oncol Clin North Am 5:43-63, 1996.
51. Kouvaraki MA, Shapiro SE, Fornage BD, et al: Role of preoperative ultrasonography in the surgical management of patients with thyroid cancer. Surgery 134:946-954, 2003.
52. Sherman SI, Gillenwater A: Neoplasms of the thyroid. In Bast RJ, Kufe D, Pollock R, et al (eds): Cancer Medicine. Hamilton, Ontario, Canada, BC Decker, 2000, pp 1105-1114.
53. Kouvaraki MA, Lee JE, Shapiro SE, et al: Preventable reoperations for persistent and recurrent papillary thyroid carcinoma. Surgery 136:1183-1191, 2004.
54. Kouvaraki MA, Shapiro SE, Lee JE, et al: Surgical management of thyroid carcinoma. J Natl Compr Canc Netw 3:458-466, 2005.
55. Uchino S, Noguchi S, Yamashita H, Watanabe S: Modified radical neck dissection for differentiated thyroid cancer: Operative technique. World J Surg 28:1199-1203, 2004.

56. Kupferman ME, Patterson DM, Mandel SJ, et al: Safety of modified radical neck dissection for differentiated thyroid carcinoma. Laryngoscope 114:403-406, 2004.
57. Kupferman ME, Patterson M, Mandel SJ, et al: Patterns of lateral neck metastasis in papillary thyroid carcinoma. Arch Otolaryngol Head Neck Surg 130:857-860, 2004.
58. Scheumann GF, Gimm O, Wegener G, et al: Prognostic significance and surgical management of locoregional lymph node metastases in papillary thyroid cancer. World J Surg 18:559-567, 1994.
59. Tisell LE, Nilsson B, Molne J, et al: Improved survival of patients with papillary thyroid cancer after surgical microdissection. World J Surg 20:854-859, 1996.
60. Pacini F, Schlumberger M, Dralle H, et al: European consensus for the management of patients with differentiated thyroid carcinoma of the follicular epithelium. Eur J Endocrinol 154:787-803, 2006.
61. Pacini F, Schlumberger M, Harmer C, et al: Postsurgical use of radioiodine (^{131}I) in patients with papillary and follicular thyroid cancer and the issue of remnant ablation: A consensus report. Eur J Endocrinol 153:651-659, 2005.
62. Muratet JP, Giraud P, Daver A, et al: Predicting the efficacy of first iodine-131 treatment in differentiated thyroid carcinoma. J Nucl Med 38:1362-1368, 1997.
63. Norden MM, Larsson F, Tedelind S, et al: Down-regulation of the sodium/iodide symporter explains ^{131}I-induced thyroid stunning. Cancer Res 67:7512-7517, 2007.
64. Morris LF, Waxman AD, Braunstein GD: Thyroid stunning. Thyroid 13:333-340, 2003.
65. Silberstein EB: Comparison of outcomes after (123)I versus (131)I pre-ablation imaging before radioiodine ablation in differentiated thyroid carcinoma. J Nucl Med 48:1043-1046, 2007.
66. Sherman SI, Tielens ET, Sostre S, et al: Clinical utility of posttreatment radioiodine scans in the management of patients with thyroid carcinoma. J Clin Endocrinol Metab 78:629-634, 1994.
67. Schlumberger M, Arcangioli O, Piekarski JD, et al: Detection and treatment of lung metastases of differentiated thyroid carcinoma in patients with normal chest X-rays. J Nucl Med 29:1790-1794, 1988.
68. Wartofsky L, Sherman SI, Gopal J, et al: Use of radioactive iodine in patients with papillary and follicular thyroid cancer. J Clin Endocrinol Metab 83:4195-4203, 1998.
69. Wong JB, Kaplan MM, Meyer KB, Pauker SG: Ablative radioactive iodine therapy for apparently localized thyroid carcinoma. A decision analytic perspective. Endocrinol Metab Clin North Am 19:741-760, 1990.
70. Taylor T, Specker B, Robbins J, et al: Outcome after treatment of high-risk papillary and non-Hurthle-cell follicular thyroid carcinoma. Ann Intern Med 129:622-627, 1998.
71. Sawka AM, Thephamongkhol K, Brouwers M, et al: Clinical review 170: A systematic review and meta-analysis of the effectiveness of radioactive iodine remnant ablation for well-differentiated thyroid cancer. J Clin Endocrinol Metab 89:3668-3676, 2004.
72. Jonklaas J, Sarlis NJ, Litofsky D, et al: Outcomes of patients with differentiated thyroid carcinoma following initial therapy. Thyroid 16:1229-1242, 2006.
73. Samaan NA, Schultz PN, Haynie TP, Ordonez NG: Pulmonary metastasis of differentiated thyroid carcinoma: Treatment results in 101 patients. J Clin Endocrinol Metab 60:376-380, 1985.
74. Ruegemer JJ, Hay ID, Bergstralh EJ, et al: Distant metastases in differentiated thyroid carcinoma: A multivariate analysis of prognostic variables. J Clin Endocrinol Metab 67:501-508.
75. Simpson WJ, Panzarella T, Carruthers JS, et al: Papillary and follicular thyroid cancer: Impact of treatment in 1578 patients. Int J Radiat Oncol Biol Phys 14:1063-1075, 1988.
76. Franceschi M, Kusic Z, Franceschi D, et al: Thyroglobulin determination, neck ultrasonography and iodine-131 whole-body scintigraphy in differentiated thyroid carcinoma. J Nucl Med 37:446-451, 1996.
77. Schlumberger M, Challeton C, De Vathaire F, et al: Radioactive iodine treatment and external radiotherapy for lung and bone metastases from thyroid carcinoma. J Nucl Med 37:598-605, 1996.
78. Schlumberger M, Tubiana M, De Vathaire F, et al: Long-term results of treatment of 283 patients with lung and bone metastases from differentiated thyroid carcinoma. J Clin Endocrinol Metab 63:960-967, 1986.
79. Goldman JM, Line BR, Aamodt RL, Robbins J: Influence of triiodothyronine withdrawal time on 131I uptake postthyroidectomy for thyroid cancer. J Clin Endocrinol Metab 50:734-739, 1980.
80. Lakshmanan M, Schaffer A, Robbins J, et al: A simplified low iodine diet in I-131 scanning and therapy of thyroid cancer. Clin Nucl Med 13:866-868, 1988.
81. Ladenson PW: Strategies for thyrotropin use to monitor patients with treated thyroid carcinoma. Thyroid 9:429-433, 1999.
82. Pacini F, Ladenson PW, Schlumberger M, et al: Radioiodine ablation of thyroid remnants after preparation with recombinant human thyrotropin in differentiated thyroid carcinoma: Results of an international, randomized, controlled study. J Clin Endocrinol Metab 91:926-932, 2006.
83. Hanscheid H, Lassmann M, Luster M, et al: Iodine biokinetics and dosimetry in radioiodine therapy of thyroid cancer: Procedures and results of a prospective international controlled study of ablation after rhTSH or hormone withdrawal. J Nucl Med 47:648-654, 2006.
84. Tuttle RM, Leboeuf R, Robbins RJ, et al: Empiric radioactive iodine dosing regimens frequently exceed maximum tolerated activity levels in elderly patients with thyroid cancer. J Nucl Med 47:1587-1591, 2006.

85. Benua RS, Cicale NR, Sonenberg M, Rawson RW: The relation of radioiodine dosimetry to results and complications in the treatment of metastatic thyroid cancer. Am J Roentgenol Radium Ther Nucl Med 87:171-182, 1962.
86. Leeper RD: The effect of ^{131}I therapy on survival of patients with metastatic papillary or follicular thyroid carcinoma. J Clin Endocrinol Metab 36:1143-1152, 1973.
87. Maxon HR 3rd, Smith HS: Radioiodine-131 in the diagnosis and treatment of metastatic well differentiated thyroid cancer. Endocrinol Metab Clin North Am 19:685-718, 1990.
88. Sgouros G, Song H, Ladenson PW, Wahl RL: Lung toxicity in radioiodine therapy of thyroid carcinoma: Development of a dose-rate method and dosimetric implications of the 80-mCi rule. J Nucl Med 47:1977-1984, 2006.
89. Song H, He B, Prideaux A, et al: Lung dosimetry for radioiodine treatment planning in the case of diffuse lung metastases. J Nucl Med 47:1985-1994, 2006.
90. Alexander C, Bader JB, Schaefer A, et al: Intermediate and long-term side effects of high-dose radioiodine therapy for thyroid carcinoma. J Nucl Med 39:1551-1554, 1998.
91. Nakada K, Ishibashi T, Takei T, et al: Does lemon candy decrease salivary gland damage after radioiodine therapy for thyroid cancer? J Nucl Med 46:261-266, 2005.
92. Shepler TR, Sherman SI, Faustina MM, et al: Nasolacrimal duct obstruction associated with radioactive iodine therapy for thyroid carcinoma. Ophthal Plast Reconstr Surg 19:479-481, 2003.
93. Morgenstern KE, Vadysirisack DD, Zhang Z, et al: Expression of sodium iodide symporter in the lacrimal drainage system: Implication for the mechanism underlying nasolacrimal duct obstruction in I(131)-treated patients. Ophthal Plast Reconstr Surg 21:337-344, 2005.
94. Burns JA, Morgenstern KE, Cahill KV, et al: Nasolacrimal obstruction secondary to I(131) therapy. Ophthal Plast Reconstr Surg 20:126-129, 2004.
95. Kloos RT, Duvuuri V, Jhiang SM, et al: Nasolacrimal drainage system obstruction from radioactive iodine therapy for thyroid carcinoma. J Clin Endocrinol Metab 87:5817-5820, 2002.
96. Ceccarelli C, Bencivelli W, Morciano D, et al: ^{131}I therapy for differentiated thyroid cancer leads to an earlier onset of menopause: Results of a retrospective study. J Clin Endocrinol Metab 86:3512-3515, 2001.
97. Hyer S, Vini L, O'Connell M, et al: Testicular dose and fertility in men following I(131) therapy for thyroid cancer. Clin Endocrinol (Oxf) 56:755-758, 2002.
98. Vini L, Hyer S, Al-Saadi A, et al: Prognosis for fertility and ovarian function after treatment with radioiodine for thyroid cancer. Postgrad Med J 78:92-93, 2002.
99. de Vathaire F, Schlumberger M, Delisle MJ, et al: Leukaemias and cancers following iodine-131 administration for thyroid cancer. Br J Cancer 75:734-739, 1997.
100. Vassilopoulou-Sellin R, Palmer L, Taylor S, Cooksley CS: Incidence of breast carcinoma in women with thyroid carcinoma. Cancer 85:696-705, 1999.
101. Chen AY, Levy L, Goepfert H, et al: The development of breast carcinoma in women with thyroid carcinoma. Cancer 92:225-231, 2001.
102. Pujol P, Daures JP, Nsakala N, et al: Degree of thyrotropin suppression as a prognostic determinant in differentiated thyroid cancer. J Clin Endocrinol Metab 81:4318-4323, 1996.
103. McGriff NJ, Csako G, Gourgiotis L, et al: Effects of thyroid hormone suppression therapy on adverse clinical outcomes in thyroid cancer. Ann Med 34:554-564, 2002.
104. Bartalena L, Martino E, Pacchiarotti A, et al: Factors affecting suppression of endogenous thyrotropin secretion by thyroxine treatment: Retrospective analysis in athyreotic and goitrous patients. J Clin Endocrinol Metab 64:849-855, 1987.
105. Burmeister LA, Goumaz MO, Mariash CN, Oppenheimer JH: Levothyroxine dose requirements for thyrotropin suppression in the treatment of differentiated thyroid cancer. J Clin Endocrinol Metab 75:344-350, 1992.
106. American Thyroid Association; Endocrine Society; American Association of Clinical Endocrinologists: Joint statement on the U.S. Food and Drug Administration's decision regarding bioequivalence of levothyroxine sodium. Thyroid 14:486, 2004.
107. Singer PA, Cooper DS, Daniels GH, et al: Treatment guidelines for patients with thyroid nodules and well-differentiated thyroid cancer. American Thyroid Association. Arch Intern Med 156:2165-2172, 1996.
108. Thyroid Carcinoma Task Force: AACE/AAES medical/surgical guidelines for clinical practice: Management of thyroid carcinoma. American Association of Clinical Endocrinologists. American College of Endocrinology. Endocr Pract 7:202-220, 2001.
109. Uzzan B, Campos J, Cucherat M, et al: Effects on bone mass of long term treatment with thyroid hormones: A meta-analysis. J Clin Endocrinol Metab 81:4278-4289, 1996.
110. Karner I, Hrgovic Z, Sijanovic S, et al: Bone mineral density changes and bone turnover in thyroid carcinoma patients treated with supraphysiologic doses of thyroxine. Eur J Med Res 10:480-488, 2005.
111. Sun L, Davies TF, Blair HC, et al: TSH and bone loss. Ann N Y Acad Sci 1068:309-318, 2006.
112. Bauer DC, Ettinger B, Nevitt MC, Stone KL: Risk for fracture in women with low serum levels of thyroid-stimulating hormone. Ann Intern Med 134:561-568, 2001.
113. Sawin CT, Geller A, Wolf PA, et al: Low serum thyrotropin concentrations as a risk factor for atrial fibrillation in older persons. N Engl J Med 331:1249-1252, 1994.
114. Parle JV, Maisonneuve P, Sheppard MC, et al: Prediction of all-cause and cardiovascular mortality in elderly people from one low serum thyrotropin result: A 10-year cohort study. Lancet 358:861-865, 2001.

115. Biondi B, Fazio S, Carella C, et al: Cardiac effects of long term thyrotropin-suppressive therapy with levothyroxine. J Clin Endocrinol Metab 77:334-338, 1993.
116. Biondi B, Fazio S, Cuocolo A, et al: Impaired cardiac reserve and exercise capacity in patients receiving long-term thyrotropin suppressive therapy with levothyroxine. J Clin Endocrinol Metab 81:4224-4228, 1996.
117. Fazio S, Biondi B, Carella C, et al: Diastolic dysfunction in patients on thyroid-stimulating hormone suppressive therapy with levothyroxine: Beneficial effect of beta-blockade. J Clin Endocrinol Metab 80:2222-2226, 1995.
118. Lee N, Tuttle M: The role of external beam radiotherapy in the treatment of papillary thyroid cancer. Endocr Relat Cancer 13:971-977, 2006.
119. Chow SM, Yau S, Kwan CK, et al: Local and regional control in patients with papillary thyroid carcinoma: Specific indications of external radiotherapy and radioactive iodine according to T and N categories in AJCC 6th edition. Endocr Relat Cancer 13:1159-1172, 2006.
120. Farahati J, Reiners C, Stuschke M, et al: Differentiated thyroid cancer. Impact of adjuvant external radiotherapy in patients with perithyroidal tumor infiltration (stage pT4). Cancer 77:172-180, 1996.
121. Tsang RW, Brierley JD, Simpson WJ, et al: The effects of surgery, radioiodine, and external radiation therapy on the clinical outcome of patients with differentiated thyroid carcinoma. Cancer 82:375-388, 1998.
122. Rosenbluth BD, Serrano V, Happersett L, et al: Intensity-modulated radiation therapy for the treatment of nonanaplastic thyroid cancer. Int J Radiat Oncol Biol Phys 63:1419-1426, 2005.
123. Grigsby PW, Baglan K, Siegel BA: Surveillance of patients to detect recurrent thyroid carcinoma. Cancer 85:945-951, 1999.
124. Snozek CL, Chambers EP, Reading CC, et al: Serum thyroglobulin, high-resolution ultrasound and lymph node thyroglobulin in diagnosis of differentiated thyroid carcinoma nodal metastases. J Clin Endocrinol Metab 92:4278-4281, 2007.
125. Cunha N, Rodrigues F, Curado F, et al: Thyroglobulin detection in fine-needle aspirates of cervical lymph nodes: A technique for the diagnosis of metastatic differentiated thyroid cancer. Eur J Endocrinol 157:101-107, 2007.
126. Frilling A, Gorges R, Tecklenborg K, et al: Value of preoperative diagnostic modalities in patients with recurrent thyroid carcinoma. Surgery 128:1067-1074, 2000.
127. Antonelli A, Miccoli P, Ferdeghini M, et al: Role of neck ultrasonography in the follow-up of patients operated on for thyroid cancer. Thyroid 5:25-28, 1995.
128. Helal BO, Merlet P, Toubert ME, et al: Clinical impact of (18)F-FDG PET in thyroid carcinoma patients with elevated thyroglobulin levels and negative (131)I scanning results after therapy. J Nucl Med 42:1464-1469, 2001.
129. Schluter B, Bohuslavizki KH, Beyer W, et al: Impact of FDG PET on patients with differentiated thyroid cancer who present with elevated thyroglobulin and negative 131I scan. J Nucl Med 42:71-76, 2001.
130. Zimmer LA, McCook B, Meltzer C, et al: Combined positron emission tomography/computed tomography imaging of recurrent thyroid cancer. Otolaryngol Head Neck Surg 128:178-184, 2003.
131. Chung JK, So Y, Lee JS, et al: Value of FDG PET in papillary thyroid carcinoma with negative ^{131}I whole-body scan. J Nucl Med 40:986-992, 1999.
132. Alnafisi NS, Driedger AA, Coates G, et al: FDG PET of recurrent or metastatic ^{131}I-negative papillary thyroid carcinoma. J Nucl Med 41:1010-1015, 2000.
133. Hooft L, Hoekstra OS, Deville W, et al: Diagnostic accuracy of ^{18}F-fluorodeoxyglucose positron emission tomography in the follow-up of papillary or follicular thyroid cancer. J Clin Endocrinol Metab 86:3779-3786, 2001.
134. Feine U, Lietzenmayer R, Hanke JP, et al: Fluorine-18-FDG and iodine-131-iodide uptake in thyroid cancer. J Nucl Med 37:1468-1472, 1996.
135. Khan N, Oriuchi N, Higuchi T, et al: PET in the follow-up of differentiated thyroid cancer. Br J Radiol 76:690-695, 2003.
136. Wang W, Macapinlac H, Larson SM, et al: [18F]-2-fluoro-2-deoxy-D-glucose positron emission tomography localizes residual thyroid cancer in patients with negative diagnostic (131)I whole body scans and elevated serum thyroglobulin levels. J Clin Endocrinol Metab 84:2291-2302, 1999.
137. Van den Bruel A, Maes A, De Potter T, et al: Clinical relevance of thyroid fluorodeoxyglucose-whole body positron emission tomography incidentaloma. J Clin Endocrinol Metab 87:1517-1520, 2002.
138. Shammas A, Degirmenci B, Mountz JM, et al: ^{18}F-FDG PET/CT in patients with suspected recurrent or metastatic well-differentiated thyroid cancer. J Nucl Med 48:221-226, 2007.
139. Wang W, Larson SM, Fazzari M, et al: Prognostic value of [18F]fluorodeoxyglucose positron emission tomographic scanning in patients with thyroid cancer. J Clin Endocrinol Metab 85:1107-1113, 2000.
140. Wang W, Larson SM, Tuttle RM, et al: Resistance of [18F]-fluorodeoxyglucose-avid metastatic thyroid cancer lesions to treatment with high-dose radioactive iodine. Thyroid 11:1169-1175, 2001.
141. Robbins RJ, Wan Q, Grewal RK, et al: Real-time prognosis for metastatic thyroid carcinoma based on 2-[18F]fluoro-2-deoxy-D-glucose-positron emission tomography scanning. J Clin Endocrinol Metab 91:498-505, 2006.
142. Petrich T, Borner AR, Otto D, et al: Influence of rhTSH on [(18)F]fluorodeoxyglucose uptake by differentiated thyroid carcinoma. Eur J Nucl Med Mol Imaging 29:641-647, 2002.
143. Moog F, Linke R, Manthey N, et al: Influence of thyroid-stimulating hormone levels on uptake of FDG in recurrent and metastatic differentiated thyroid carcinoma. J Nucl Med 41:1989-1995, 2000.

144. Chin BB, Patel P, Cohade C, et al: Recombinant human thyrotropin stimulation of fluoro-D-glucose positron emission tomography uptake in well-differentiated thyroid carcinoma. J Clin Endocrinol Metab 89:91-95, 2004.
145. Spencer CA, LoPresti JS, Fatemi S, Nicoloff JT: Detection of residual and recurrent differentiated thyroid carcinoma by serum thyroglobulin measurement. Thyroid 9:435-441, 1999.
146. Ozata M, Suzuki S, Miyamoto T, et al: Serum thyroglobulin in the follow-up of patients with treated differentiated thyroid cancer. J Clin Endocrinol Metab 79:98-105, 1994.
147. Baudin E, Do Cao C, Cailleux AF, et al: Positive predictive value of serum thyroglobulin levels, measured during the first year of follow-up after thyroid hormone withdrawal, in thyroid cancer patients. J Clin Endocrinol Metab 88:1107-1111, 2003.
148. Frasoldati A, Pesenti M, Gallo M, et al: Diagnosis of neck recurrences in patients with differentiated thyroid carcinoma. Cancer 97:90-96, 2003.
149. Pacini F, Molinaro E, Castagna MG, et al: Recombinant human thyrotropin-stimulated serum thyroglobulin combined with neck ultrasonography has the highest sensitivity in monitoring differentiated thyroid carcinoma. J Clin Endocrinol Metab 88:3668-3673, 2003.
150. Torlontano M, Attard M, Crocetti U, et al: Follow-up of low-risk patients with papillary thyroid cancer: Role of neck ultrasonography in detecting lymph node metastases. J Clin Endocrinol Metab 89:3402-3407, 2004.
151. Torlontano M, Crocetti U, D'Aloiso L, et al: Serum thyroglobulin and ^{131}I whole body scan after recombinant human TSH stimulation in the follow-up of low-risk patients with differentiated thyroid cancer. Eur J Endocrinol 148:19-24, 2003.
152. Spencer CA, Takeuchi M, Kazarosyan M, et al: Serum thyroglobulin autoantibodies: Prevalence, influence on serum thyroglobulin measurement, and prognostic significance in patients with differentiated thyroid carcinoma. J Clin Endocrinol Metab 83:1121-1127, 1998.
153. Chiovato L, Latrofa F, Braverman LE, et al: Disappearance of humoral thyroid autoimmunity after complete removal of thyroid antigens. Ann Intern Med 139(Pt 1):346-351, 2003.
154. Pacini F, Lari R, Mazzeo S, et al: Diagnostic value of a single serum thyroglobulin determination on and off thyroid suppressive therapy in the follow-up of patients with differentiated thyroid cancer. Clin Endocrinol (Oxf) 23:405-411, 1985.
155. Haugen BR, Pacini F, Reiners C, et al: A comparison of recombinant human thyrotropin and thyroid hormone withdrawal for the detection of thyroid remnant or cancer. J Clin Endocrinol Metab 84:3877-3885, 1999.
156. Mazzaferri EL, Kloos RT: Is diagnostic iodine-131 scanning with recombinant human TSH useful in the follow-up of differentiated thyroid cancer after thyroid ablation? J Clin Endocrinol Metab 87:1490-1498, 2002.
157. Kloos RT, Mazzaferri EL: A single recombinant human thyrotropin-stimulated serum thyroglobulin measurement predicts differentiated thyroid carcinoma metastases three to five years later. J Clin Endocrinol Metab 90:5047-5057, 2005.
158. Smallridge RC, Meek SE, Morgan MA, et al: Monitoring thyroglobulin in a sensitive immunoassay has comparable sensitivity to recombinant human TSH-stimulated thyroglobulin in follow-up of thyroid cancer patients. J Clin Endocrinol Metab 92:82-87, 2007.
159. Schlumberger M, Hitzel A, Toubert ME, et al: Comparison of seven serum thyroglobulin assays in the follow-up of papillary and follicular thyroid cancer patients. J Clin Endocrinol Metab 92:2487-2495, 2007.
160. Lewis BD, Hay ID, Charboneau JW, et al: Percutaneous ethanol injection for treatment of cervical lymph node metastases in patients with papillary thyroid carcinoma. AJR Am J Roentgenol 178:699-704, 2002.
161. Noguchi S, Yamashita H, Murakami N, et al: Small carcinomas of the thyroid. A long-term follow-up of 867 patients. Arch Surg 131:187-191, 1996.
162. Marchesi M, Biffoni M, Biancari F, et al: Predictors of outcome for patients with differentiated and aggressive thyroid carcinoma. Eur J Surg Suppl (588):46-50, 2003.
163. Czaja JM, McCaffrey TV: The surgical management of laryngotracheal invasion by well-differentiated papillary thyroid carcinoma. Arch Otolaryngol Head Neck Surg 123:484-490, 1997.
164. Musholt TJ, Musholt PB, Behrend M, et al: Invasive differentiated thyroid carcinoma: Tracheal resection and reconstruction procedures in the hands of the endocrine surgeon. Surgery 126:1078-1087, 1999.
165. McCaffrey JC: Evaluation and treatment of aerodigestive tract invasion by well-differentiated thyroid carcinoma. Cancer Control 7:246-252, 2000.
166. Avenia N, Ragusa M, Monacelli M, et al: Locally advanced thyroid cancer: Therapeutic options. Chir Ital 56:501-508, 2004.
167. Okada T, Sasaki F, Takahashi H, et al: Management of childhood and adolescent thyroid carcinoma: Long-term follow-up and clinical characteristics. Eur J Pediatr Surg 16:8-13, 2006.
168. Lau WF, Zacharin MR, Waters K, et al: Management of paediatric thyroid carcinoma: Recent experience with recombinant human thyroid stimulating hormone in preparation for radioiodine therapy. Intern Med J 36:564-570, 2006.
169. Pazaitou-Panayiotou K, Kaprara A, Boudina M, et al: Thyroid carcinoma in children and adolescents: Presentation, clinical course, and outcome of therapy in 23 children and adolescents in Northern Greece. Hormones (Athens) 4:213-220, 2005.

170. Jarzab B, Handkiewicz-Junak D, Wloch J: Juvenile differentiated thyroid carcinoma and the role of radioiodine in its treatment: A qualitative review. Endocr Relat Cancer 12:773-803, 2005.
171. Vermeer-Mens JC, Goemaere NN, Kuenen-Boumeester V, et al: Childhood papillary thyroid carcinoma with miliary pulmonary metastases. J Clin Oncol 24:5788-5789, 2006.
172. Ilgan S, Karacalioglu AO, Pabuscu Y, et al: Iodine-131 treatment and high-resolution CT: Results in patients with lung metastases from differentiated thyroid carcinoma. Eur J Nucl Med Mol Imaging 31:825-830, 2004.
173. Ronga G, Filesi M, Montesano T, et al: Lung metastases from differentiated thyroid carcinoma. A 40 years' experience. Q J Nucl Med Mol Imaging 48:12-19, 2004.
174. Fatourechi V, Hay ID, Javedan H, et al: Lack of impact of radioiodine therapy in TG-positive, diagnostic whole-body scan-negative patients with follicular cell-derived thyroid cancer. J Clin Endocrinol Metab 87:1521-1526, 2002.
175. Ahuja S, Ernst H: Chemotherapy of thyroid carcinoma. J Endocrinol Invest 10:303-310, 1987.
176. Droz JP, Schlumberger M, Rougier P, et al: Chemotherapy in metastatic nonanaplastic thyroid cancer: Experience at the Institut Gustave-Roussy. Tumori 76:480-483, 1990.
177. Santini F, Bottici V, Elisei R, et al: Cytotoxic effects of carboplatinum and epirubicin in the setting of an elevated serum thyrotropin for advanced poorly differentiated thyroid cancer. J Clin Endocrinol Metab 87:4160-4165, 2002.
178. Kloos R, Ringel M, Knopp M, et al: Significant clinical and biologic activity of RAF/VEGF-R kinase inhibitor BAY 43-9006 in patients with metastatic papillary thyroid carcinoma (PTC): Updated results of a phase II study. J Clin Oncol ASCO Annual Meeting Proceedings (Post-Meeting Edition) 24(18S):5534, 2006.
179. Chiu AC, Delpassand ES, Sherman SI: Prognosis and treatment of brain metastases in thyroid carcinoma. J Clin Endocrinol Metab 82:3637-3642, 1997.
180. NCCN Thyroid Carcinoma Panel: National Comprehensive Cancer Network Clinical Practice Guidelines-Thyroid Carcinoma, 2008. Available at http://www.nccn.org/professionals/physician_gls/PDF/thyroid.pdf.
181. McWilliams RR, Giannini C, Hay ID, et al: Management of brain metastases from thyroid carcinoma: A study of 16 pathologically confirmed cases over 25 years. Cancer 98:356-362, 2003.
182. Luster M, Lippi F, Jarzab B, et al: rhTSH-aided radioiodine ablation and treatment of differentiated thyroid carcinoma: A comprehensive review. Endocr Relat Cancer 12:49-64, 2005.
183. Brierley JD, Tsang RW: External-beam radiation therapy in the treatment of differentiated thyroid cancer. Semin Surg Oncol 16:42-49, 1999.
184. Haugen BR: Management of the patient with progressive radioiodine non-responsive disease. Semin Surg Oncol 16:34-41, 1999.
185. Kim JH, Leeper RD: Treatment of locally advanced thyroid carcinoma with combination doxorubicin and radiation therapy. Cancer 60:2372-2375, 1987.
186. Cohen EE, Vokes EE, Rosen LS, et al: A phase II study of axitinib (AG-013736 [AG]) in patients (pts) with advanced thyroid cancers. J Clin Oncol 2007 ASCO Annual Meeting Proceedings Part I 25(18S):6008, 2007.
187. Ain KB, Lee C, Williams KD: Phase II trial of thalidomide for therapy of radioiodine-unresponsive and rapidly progressive thyroid carcinomas. Thyroid 17:663-670, 2007.

Chapter 27

Follicular Carcinoma

Kenneth B. Ain

Key Points

- Discrimination between benign follicular adenoma and follicular carcinoma is a most difficult pathologic distinction; it may require additional pathologist consultation.
- Minimal appropriate thyroid surgery for follicular thyroid cancer is total thyroidectomy.
- Follicular thyroid cancers spread hematogenously to distant sites (e.g., lung, bone, liver, brain).
- Macroscopic (large) tumor metastases are best dealt with by surgical resection prior to radioiodine or external beam radiotherapy.
- Appropriate preparation for radioactive iodine scans or therapies involves sufficient elevation of thyroid-stimulating hormone and strict low-iodine diet.
- Follicular thyroid cancer is a chronic disease requiring lifelong follow-up evaluation and monitoring.

EPIDEMIOLOGY

Thyroid cancer is increasing in incidence in the United States more rapidly than any other cancer in men and women.[1] This is paralleled by global increases in thyroid cancer incidence.[2] The reasons for this increase are currently unknown. Approximately 10% of thyroid carcinomas are characterized as follicular cancers, including oxyphilic and insular variants. Over the past several decades, it appears that the incidence of follicular thyroid cancer has precipitously declined relative to papillary cancers. However, this is mostly because of the recognition that many cases previously classified as follicular cancers were actually follicular variants of papillary carcinoma and there was as an actual decrease in follicular cancers, thought to be consequent to iodine supplementation (particularly in Europe).[3] Data from the Florida Cancer Data System suggest that in the context of modern histologic classification, follicular carcinomas are reasonably stable in proportion to new thyroid cancer cases.[4] Despite an eightfold higher incidence of papillary carcinomas, there are only twice as many deaths from papillary carcinomas compared with follicular carcinomas, demonstrating a generally higher mortality of follicular carcinomas.[5]

Follicular thyroid cancers constitute a histologic category of epithelial carcinomas of the thyroid follicular cell that have distinct clinical features. Aggressive subtypes of this category include the oxyphilic (Hürthle cell) and insular carcinomas. A thyroid tumor is called follicular when it "totally or almost totally (more than 95%) displays a follicular growth pattern, or thyroid follicles with a central lumen containing variable amounts of colloid."[6] Distinguishing a follicular carcinoma distinct from the larger group of follicular tumors is sufficiently problematic that the World Health Organization classification of follicular thyroid cancer adroitly defines it as a "malignant epithelial tumor showing evidence of follicular cell differentiation but lacking the diagnostic features of thyroid papillary carcinoma."[7] Further discussion regarding the diagnostic criteria of follicular carcinoma, molecular genetics, clinical presentation, and therapy is presented in this chapter.

DIAGNOSTIC CLASSIFICATIONS

In the chapters on thyroid nodules (Chapters 24 and 25), the cytologic issue of follicular neoplasia within the context of fine-needle aspiration (FNA) biopsy is addressed. When thyroid nodules are biopsied and found to have evidence of follicular neoplasia, the appropriate response is to have a surgical resection of the complete ipsilateral thyroid lobe (and usually the isthmus). This is necessary to determine the nature of the neoplasm and the appropriate clinical direction. Further evaluation is based on the pathologist's analysis of the surgical specimen (see later).

Adenoma Versus Carcinoma

Determining whether a follicular neoplasm is a benign follicular adenoma or a follicular carcinoma—warranting total thyroidectomy and diligent follow-up care—is one of the most difficult tasks of a pathologist. Even excellent pathologists may disagree,[8] suggesting that second opinions are usually a good idea. In general, these two diagnoses cannot be distinguished by any cellular feature except for the presence of vascular and/or tumor capsular invasion; the presence of either reveals the tumor to be a carcinoma. This diagnosis by exclusion mandates that the pathologist, to advance the diagnosis of a benign follicular adenoma, has meticulously evaluated sufficient numbers of tissue blocks and slides. Misdiagnosis, in addition to resulting in inappropriate or inadequate medical care, may have significant medicolegal repercussions.[9]

Adding to the complexity is the diagnosis of atypical follicular adenoma, in which cellular and architectural atypia are evident despite the absence of capsular or vascular invasion. Studies that have shown *p53* mutations in atypical follicular adenomas suggests that these might be precursors to aggressive thyroid cancers.[10] In addition, it is likely that follicular carcinomas arise from preexisting follicular adenomas, so that some follicular adenomas may be carcinomas in situ. This adenoma to carcinoma pathogenesis[11] is reminiscent of the well-accepted colonic tubular polyp to colon cancer transition. Because diagnosis of a thyroid follicular adenoma requires complete excision of the entire lesion (most appropriately in the context of an ipsilateral total thyroid lobectomy), the failure to see residual or metastatic disease from such lesions is equally consistent with a benign adenoma or a carcinoma in situ. Unfortunately, this academic distinction becomes of concern regarding efforts to distinguish these tumors by FNA biopsy using gene profiling[12] or assessment of specific markers, such as telomerase,[13] to avoid thyroid surgery. If not resected, would such adenomas evolve into carcinomas?

For those follicular neoplasms demonstrating capsular and/or vascular invasion, the next distinction is between minimally invasive follicular thyroid carcinoma (MIFC) and widely invasive follicular carcinoma (WIFC). Although some pathologists differentiate between MIFC with only tumor capsular invasion and those that have vascular invasion (with or without capsular invasion), calling them "grossly encapsulated angioinvasive follicular carcinomas,"[6] grouping both as MIFC is usually sufficient. Follicular carcinomas are clearly more aggressive at presentation when there is diffuse infiltrative growth, either nonencapsulated or partly encapsulated, invading thyroidal and/or extrathyroidal tissues and blood vessels.[11,14] Molecular profiling using gene microarray analysis has shown distinct genetic profiles between follicular adenomas, MIFC and WIFC.[15] Similarly, there are distinct differences in the clinical course of MIFC and WIFC, with excellent survival in MIFC patients compared with a significant 10-year mortality of WIFC, although both varieties are associated with distant metastases to lung and bone.[16]

Subtypes: Hürthle Cell Carcinomas and Insular Carcinoma

Follicular thyroid carcinomas with predominantly oxyphilic cells caused by metaplastic changes, with overabundance of large mitochondria, are known as Hürthle cell, oncocytic, or Askanazy cell carcinomas (HCFCs),[17] although they are distinct from Hürthle cell variants of papillary carcinoma.[14] Hürthle cell adenomas are distinguished from carcinomas by noting the absence of capsular or vascular invasion in the same way as follicular adenomas are distinguished from carcinomas. HCFC is half as common as nonoxyphilic follicular carcinomas and is considered to be clinically more aggressive. This may be related to a higher rate of loss of radioiodine uptake in these tumors[18]; however, they seem to have the same prognosis as nonoxyphilic follicular cancers,[19] particularly when matched for extent of local invasion at presentation.[20]

Insular carcinoma has been also known as primordial cell carcinoma, solid variant of follicular carcinoma, poorly differentiated variant of papillary cancer, trabecular-insular-solid carcinoma, and the compact subtype of anaplastic carcinoma.[21-24] Ten or 20 years ago, such tumors were considered to be anaplastic carcinomas; however, they are now known usually to concentrate radioiodine[25] and have an aggressive clinical course, midway between typical follicular carcinoma and anaplastic carcinoma.[24,26,27] Insular carcinoma cells have poorly defined cytoplasm, are not oxyphilic, and have cytoplasmic vacuoles containing thyroglobulin. They grow as microfollicles in a generally solid, lobular background, with typical vascular and extrathyroidal invasion. Primary tumors are generally larger than other types of follicular carcinoma and have higher rates of distant metastases.[27,28] Unlike other follicular cancers, insular carcinomas frequently have lymph node metastases and spread distantly to additional sites in addition to bone and lung, such as liver, pleura, and brain.[16]

MOLECULAR EVENTS AND PATHOGENESIS

Cowden's syndrome is an autosomal dominant genetic disease (affecting 1 in 200,000 people) that is part of the PTEN (***p***hosphatase and ***ten***sin homologue, deleted on chromosome ***ten***) hamartoma tumor syndrome (PHTS), associated with benign and malignant tumors of the breast, thyroid, uterus, brain, and mucocutaneous tissues.[29] More than half of affected individuals have thyroid abnormalities, particularly follicular adenomas and carcinomas, with up to a 10% lifetime risk for follicular carcinoma.[30,31] Mutations of *PTEN*, a tumor suppressor gene, reduces apoptosis and prevents PTEN-mediated dephosphorylation of proteins in critical cell survival and proliferation pathways. Aside from Cowden's syndrome, there are no germline mutations specifically associated with follicular thyroid carcinomas. Analysis of the Swedish Family Cancer Database for familial associations of nonmedullary thyroid cancers has been most revealing of papillary carcinomas, not follicular cancers.[32]

Somatic thyroid tumor genetic changes can be associated with follicular thyroid carcinoma. The best characterized is a rearrangement involving a chromosomal translocation, t(2;3)(q13;p25). The consequence is a fusion of the *PAX8* and *PPARγ* (peroxisome proliferator-activated receptor gamma) genes, producing a fusion transcription factor protein, PPFP (PAX8-PPARγ fusion protein).[33] This inhibits activity of the wild-type PPARγ transcription factor in a dominant-negative fashion, producing increased cell growth and decreased apoptosis, apparently sufficient for tumorigenesis.[34] Between 30% to 50% of follicular carcinomas express this fusion protein.[35,36] There is a small subgroup of follicular adenomas that has this translocation, suggesting its role in later malignant transformation; however, few Hürthle cell carcinomas show this genetic change.[37] Recent studies have shown that the Ras effector, NORE1A (RASSF5A), a putative tumor suppressor that binds Ras proteins, is downregulated in the subset of follicular carcinomas harboring a PPARγ/PAX8 translocation, suggesting a mechanism for tumorogenesis.[38]

There are three cellular Ras genes (*H-*, *K-*, and *N-Ras*) that can be mutated in association with follicular neoplasms. They code for 21-kD guanosine triphosphate (GTP)–binding proteins that enhance follicular cell proliferation.[39] Ras proteins function to convey signals from tyrosine kinase membrane receptors to mitogen-activated protein kinases (MAPKs), resulting in transcriptional activation of specific target genes. Mutations in *N-Ras* codon 61 are most frequent, seen in 19% of follicular tumors. More specifically, this mutation is seen in 23.3% of atypical follicular adenomas and 17.6% of follicular carcinomas. In general, there are higher rates of *Ras* mutations in follicular carcinomas than in follicular adenomas, supporting a role in malignant transformation.[40]

The phosphoinositide 3-kinase (PI3K) pathway is frequently activated in follicular thyroid carcinomas and AKT (protein kinase B) is its central signaling molecule. AKT activity is enhanced by PI3K activation or by reduced PTEN activity, as seen in Cowden's syndrome. Of the three AKT isoforms cloned in humans, AKT 1 and AKT 2 predominate and both are elevated in sporadic follicular carcinomas.[41] Because reduced PTEN activity, activating *Ras* mutations, and *PPARγ/PAX8* gene rearrangements also result in AKT activation, this may be a common event in follicular carcinoma initiation for both sporadic and inherited disease.[42]

A distinct subset (less than 10%) of follicular carcinomas are found to have increased basal adenylate cyclase activity resulting from an activating mutation of the TSH receptor.[43] A similar mutation was also reported in an insular thyroid carcinoma.[44] In both situations, the tumors were unusual in that they appeared hyperfunctioning in regard to radioactive iodine uptake.

MicroRNAs (miRNAs) are small, noncoding RNA transcripts that appear to regulate expression of multiple target genes at both transcriptional and post-transcriptional levels.[45] Using high-density miRNA array chip analysis, Weber and colleagues[46] have found overexpression of specific miRNAs, miR-197 and miR-346, in follicular carcinomas. In addition, in vitro overexpression of either of these miRNAs induced proliferation of follicular carcinoma cell lines, whereas inhibition of these miRNAs inhibited growth. These findings suggest that miRNAs may be important in carcinogenesis and as potential therapeutic targets.

There are a host of tumor suppressor genes that may be found to play a role in the development of follicular carcinomas. For example, gene expression studies have revealed marked reductions in expression of the tumor suppressor gene aplasia Ras homologue I (ARHI) in follicular and Hürthle cell carcinomas, consequent to genomic deletion combined with hypermethylation.[47] Our understanding of the molecular events underlying follicular cell oncogenesis is still at a very early stage.

CLINICAL PRESENTATION

Evaluation of the Primary Tumor

Just as with other types of thyroid cancers, follicular carcinomas most often present as a thyroid nodule or mass. In the absence of thyrotoxicosis, there is no role for nuclear thyroid scans for evaluation of these nodules. Most benign nodules are hypofunctional on these scans, as are most malignant nodules; consequently, there is no clinical rationale for ascertaining the iodine avidity of these nodules. The only useful preoperative diagnostic study is an FNA biopsy. When a nodule is easily palpable, this can be performed using direct palpation; however, it has become a standard approach to perform thyroid biopsies using ultrasound guidance. Although efforts have been made to discriminate benign from malignant nodules based solely on ultrasonographic findings,[48] such efforts are insufficiently robust to dictate a patient's entire course of treatment. Cytologic findings of follicular neoplasia are sufficient to mandate surgical resection, with definitive diagnosis based on the surgical pathology.

Follicular thyroid cancer is typically a thyroid malignancy of adults. Children younger than 18 years most often have papillary thyroid cancers, although teenagers may occasionally have follicular cancers. For that reason, the discussion regarding therapy will not make distinctions between pediatric and adult patients.

Metastatic Disease

Follicular carcinomas can metastasize to local lymph nodes, although they are far less prone to do so in comparison to papillary carcinomas. Although all thyroid carcinomas can spread through the bloodstream, follicular carcinomas are noteworthy for their tendency to spread hematogenously. In that respect, it is not unusual for the first evidence of this cancer to be a metastasis to bone, lung, liver, or brain.

Often, there is no other evidence of a preexisting thyroid malignancy and a metastatic tumor site may not be sufficiently evaluated to delineate the proper pathology, sometimes designated as an adenocarcinoma of unknown origin, resulting in inappropriate chemotherapy. In such situations, immunohistochemical evidence of thyroglobulin will point to the proper diagnosis.[49]

It is not unusual to see a patient who presents with follicular thyroid cancer in distant metastatic sites who has previously undergone partial thyroidectomy for a benign follicular adenoma at some time in the past, sometimes as long as 2 or 3 decades ago. If slides from the distant surgery are available for review, it is often possible for pathologic review to discern the diagnostic criteria of follicular carcinoma that were missed. Conversely, there are a few cases in which extremely fastidious review again suggested the original tumor to be a benign follicular adenoma and no additional evidence of malignancy was present in the completion thyroidectomy. This underscores the difficulty in discriminating follicular adenomas from follicular carcinomas and infers that the distinction may sometimes reflect pathologic convention rather than tumor biology.

Prognostic Factors and Staging Systems

There are a number of clinical characteristics that have prognostic value in assessing a patient's follicular thyroid cancer. The older the patient, the greater the chance that the tumor will behave aggressively and fail to respond to radioiodine therapy.[50,51] Multivariate analyses in a number of studies demonstrate male gender as an independent prognostic risk factor for thyroid cancer–related mortality.[52] As would be expected, the larger the primary tumor, the greater the tendency for aggressive behavior.[53,54] Unlike papillary thyroid cancers, in which a minimum tumor size delineates subclinical (occult) disease,[55] there is no evidence that such a minimum exists with follicular thyroid cancers, requiring the clinician to address primary tumors of every size. Extrathyroidal invasion has proven to be a reliable indicator of aggressive tumor behavior, predictive of distant metastases, tumor recurrence, and disease-specific mortality.[53,56-58] Approximately 5% of follicular cancers metastasizes to lymph nodes in the neck, with questionable prognostic significance. On the other hand, distant metastases predict higher mortality, with one third of these metastases seen in lung, one third in bone, and one third in all other distant sites.[54,59]

Various tumor staging systems have been devised with the intent of predicting the risk of mortality and disease recurrence in thyroid cancer patients. Some clinicians propose to use such systems to discriminate between low-risk patients requiring less aggressive therapy to achieve desirable clinical outcomes and higher risk patients requiring the most aggressive treatments to avoid likely morbidity or mortality from their disease. Unfortunately, none of these systems is sufficiently robust to be of any value in predicting outcome in individual patients or to ration treatment and follow-up diagnostic resources reasonably. This is because there are patients—in each tumor staging system in the lowest respective risk groups—who die from their disease. Such systems are best suited for use in epidemiologic studies, statistical analyses of large patient populations, and as tools for stratification in designing prospective clinical trials.

The most widely used staging system, useful for communicating clinical features of thyroid cancer patients, is the TNM system, which uses assessment of the primary ***t***umor, associated regional metastatic nodes, and presence of distant metastases.[60] There is a wide selection of staging systems for thyroid cancer, but the TNM classification appears to be the most useful in terms of predictability,[61] although there is some disagreement.[62]

TREATMENT

The approach to therapy is often similar between papillary thyroid cancers (see Chapter 26) and follicular thyroid carcinomas. Thus, this overview of treatment will emphasize the aspects of therapy that differ from those for papillary thyroid cancers. There have been a number of consensus statements from professional organizations in Europe and the United States regarding thyroid cancer treatment[63-65]; however, there are significant disagreements regarding therapeutic approaches that are unresolved in such statements. This section will provide a treatment strategy consistent with my expertise.

Surgery

Although initial thyroid surgery for a suspicious follicular neoplasm may be a thyroid lobectomy, once there is surgical pathologic confirmation of a follicular carcinoma, it is imperative to complete the removal of the entire thyroid gland, usually at a second surgery. If this cancer first presents as a local or distant metastasis, the initial thyroid surgery should be nothing less than a total thyroidectomy. Efforts to use radioactive iodine to ablate residual intact thyroid lobes or substantial remnants of the thyroid (from partial thyroid resections) are rarely satisfactory. These are often associated with painful radiation thyroiditis or exposure to higher cumulative radioiodine doses to ablate remnant tissue than would have been needed with a more complete thyroidectomy. Advocates for lesser thyroid resections are concerned about complications from this procedure in the hands of inexperienced surgeons; however, the intention of treatment should always aim for optimal care with appropriate surgical expertise, usually obtainable with proper surgeon selection.[66]

Macroscopic metastases are best dealt with by surgical resection prior to radioablative measures, such as radioactive iodine or external beam radiotherapy (EBRT). An unfortunate and common error of management is to attempt to treat such sites with radiation techniques without resection.[67] Both radioactive iodine and EBRT work best with micrometastatic tumors and ultimately fail to control macroscopic tumors. In addition, specific sites (particularly skeletal metastases) may benefit by surgical resection and stabilization procedures to maintain structural integrity and to present the most effectively diminished target for radioablation. Follicular carcinoma metastases are notoriously vascular, making resection of large tumor sites problematic. Preoperative angiographic embolization of feeding vessels permits these tumors to be resected with greater safety[68]; however, it is necessary to delay any planned radioiodine therapy for several months while waiting for iodinated contrast dye to clear from the circulation.

Radioactive Iodine

Radioiodine (specifically ^{131}I) is an effective postsurgical adjuvant that has unique specificity and application to differentiated follicular thyroid carcinomas[69] capable of expressing the sodium iodide symporter[70] (NIS) responsible for concentrating iodine. Effective radioiodine therapy requires delivery of sufficient total radiation dosage at a dose rate sufficiently high to prevent tumor cell repair of sublethal radiation damage, about 0.6 to 3.0 Gy/hr.[71,72] For this reason, the efficacy of this treatment is related to the adequacy of each administered dose, rather than the total cumulative effect of small and insufficient doses. There are two types of radioactive iodine therapy. The initial treatment (ablation dose) after surgical thyroidectomy is intended to destroy the remnant of thyroid tissue left by the surgeon and any persistent thyroid cancer, whereas subsequent treatments are aimed solely at remaining or recurring thyroid cancer.

The minimal ablation dose, used when the primary tumor has not penetrated the thyroid capsule and there is no evidence for tumor sites outside the thyroid bed (based on diagnostic ^{131}I whole-body scanning, surgical findings, physical examination, and radiologic studies), is 100 mCi (3.7 GBq). That is because this dose provides sufficient confidence in the successful elimination of the thyroid remnant[73] that any local evidence of persistent thyroidal tissue can be reasonably assumed to be malignant. For evident tumor in the neck outside the thyroid bed or for any radioiodine therapies subsequent to the initial ablation, the typical empirical dose is 150 mCi (5.5 GBq); however, doses of 200 mCi (7.4 GBq) may be used for invasive local disease. If there is evidence for thyroid cancer metastases involving a vital local structure (e.g., tracheal or esophageal invasion) or spread to distant sites beyond the neck, higher doses provide greater effectiveness. Quantitative ^{131}I blood dosimetry, as developed by Benua and associates in the early 1960s,[74-76] provides excellent guidance as to maximum safe limits of radioiodine administration for any particular patient using red marrow exposure limits of 200 rad and specific radioiodine retention criteria in the context of pulmonary metastases. This permits use of single ^{131}I doses exceeding

600 mCi (22.2 GBq) in some patients. Unfortunately, although there is almost a half-century of experience with ^{131}I dosimetry, it is not widely available to most clinicians and lower empirical doses are more commonly used.

Proper preparation for radioiodine therapy is critical. There are two requisites for preparation: (1) sufficient elevation of thyroid-stimulating hormone (TSH [thyrotropin]) for maximal stimulation of remnant and tumor cell production of NIS (to concentrate radioiodine) and (2) sufficient depletion of stable (nonradioactive iodine) from the diet to avoid diluting the specific activity of the treatment dose. The traditional method of endogenous TSH elevation is through withdrawal of thyroid hormone therapy, with consequent hypothyroidism. Typically, after thyroidectomy or after discontinuing levothyroxine, the patient is placed on liothyronine (Cytomel) twice daily for 1 month and then discontinued for 2 weeks. This method serves as the gold standard preparation technique, providing an appropriate elevation of the TSH level above 30 mU/L[77,78] and a diminished renal glomerular filtration rate to prevent rapid clearance of the radioiodine from the circulation, and permitting sufficient opportunity for optimal tumor uptake. Unfortunately, the consequent hypothyroidism can be uncomfortable, prevents safe driving, and often requires time lost from work. In addition, patients with pituitary dysfunction may not be able to generate endogenous TSH, and frail older patients and patients at psychiatric risk from hypothyroidism cannot safely tolerate it. Recombinant human thyrotropin (rhTSH; Thyrogen [thyrotropin alfa]) provides a reasonable alternative preparation modality, permitting the levothyroxine level to be maintained while providing sufficient exogenous TSH stimulation.[79] Recently, the U.S. Food and Drug Administration has approved it for use in radioiodine therapy, in addition to its longer experience as preparation for diagnostic scanning. Currently, I still prefer the enhanced efficacy of hypothyroid preparation for radioiodine therapy, reserving rhTSH preparations for patients intolerant of hypothyroidism or who cannot produce sufficient endogenous TSH.

Reduction of stable iodine is an important and often unrecognized necessity for radioiodine therapy and scans.[80] I have well-documented cases of patients with diffuse pulmonary metastases appearing unable to concentrate radioiodine on diagnostic and post-therapy scans, solely because of stable iodine contamination, most often from CT intravenous contrast dye administration, which can persist for as long as 10 months.[81] Basic radiobiologic principles dictate that a low-iodine diet, reducing dietary daily iodine intake (typically ranging from 400 to 600 μg) to below 40 μg, will substantially increase the specific activity of an administered ^{131}I dose that contains less than 2 μg of iodide. An effective low-iodine diet, easily followed in most cultures,[82-85] is initiated 2 weeks before radioiodine administration and continued for 24 hours afterward.

Potential adverse consequences of radioiodine therapy include salivary dysfunction,[86] nasolacrimal duct obstruction,[87,88] and temporary dysgeusia. Most patients do not have these complications; however, roughly one third will have variable reductions in their salivary output, with 10% having severe xerostomia. Patients undergoing high-dose radioiodine therapy, particularly if approaching 200 rad of red marrow exposure, will have a temporary lowering of the platelets and leukocytes, which reaches a nadir at 4 weeks after therapy and recovers to baseline by 8 weeks. Radiation pneumonitis, although originally described in patients with lung metastases receiving high-dose radioiodine therapy, is so rare that it has not been seen in any such patients in more than 2 decades of providing this treatment in our practice. Although some studies, using population-based databases, have suggested that radioiodine therapy may increase the risk of leukemia or bladder cancer, these are sufficiently low risks (if present) that they do not constitute a clinical concern when considering treatment of an existing thyroid malignancy.

External Beam Radiotherapy

EBRT has specific usefulness in follicular thyroid cancer when radioiodine is no longer useful because of loss of uptake into the tumor. Toxicity to normal surrounding tissues limits the administered radiation dose to around 60 Gy, whereas effective radioiodine therapy can deliver doses exceeding 300 Gy with minimal or no toxicity,[89] making radioiodine the preferred method of radiotherapy, when possible. Forms of EBRT include gamma rays produced by cobalt decay, high-energy photons produced by a linear accelerator, and electron therapy. It is administered in daily treatments (fractions) given over 4 to 6 weeks. Variations of EBRT include intensity-modulated radiation therapy (IMRT) and various techniques to focus the radiation into smaller defined tumor volumes. EBRT cannot be directed against large areas of tumor involvement, such as for diffuse metastases in the lungs or liver, but is sometimes useful for the neck and thoracic inlet or for selected sites involving the skeleton. Focused beam radiation techniques, such as gamma knife procedures, are useful for intracranial metastases.

A common use of EBRT is for following resection of recurrent tumor in the neck that no longer concentrates radioiodine. Surgical removal of macroscopic tumors invariably leaves micrometastatic disease behind. EBRT has particular benefit in reducing local recurrence in this circumstance.[90] Similarly, after resection of distantly metastatic tumor, such as in vertebral sites (with installation of supportive hardware), EBRT is useful to consolidate the treatment effects and delay or prevent recurrence at such sites. One frequent management error is to use EBRT in place of surgery at macroscopic sites of tumor metastases to the spine, rather than as adjuvant treatment. The unfortunate consequences of this approach include inadequate tumor response to the EBRT, destabilization of the spine lacking supportive additions, fibrosis in the operative field if later surgery is attempted, and inability to provide additional adjuvant radiation if surgery is performed later.

Levothyroxine Suppression of Thyroid-Stimulating Hormone

It is obvious that athyrotic thyroid cancer patients must receive lifelong thyroid hormone therapy with levothyroxine (L-T_4). Unlike typical hypothyroid patients, patients with follicular thyroid carcinomas should receive L-T_4 doses sufficiently high to suppress TSH to levels at or beneath 0.10 mU/L. This is biologically justified by the well-documented stimulation of thyroid cancer cell proliferation by TSH.[91-96] Similarly, an assortment of clinical studies have demonstrated decreased recurrence rates and/or decreased cancer-related mortality in thyroid cancer patients with TSH suppression.[52,97-102] The typical dosage of L-T_4 sufficient for this purpose averages 2.0 μg/kg body weight/day[103] and is titrated by aiming for the lowest serum free thyroxine level that is associated with a TSH value at or beneath 0.1 mU/L, best evaluated using a trough serum sample.[104]

The degree of TSH suppression remains controversial, with a wide range of opinions from "experts" with an equally wide variance of expertise. The only clinical study that has provided applicable data, by Pujol and coworkers,[100] indicates 0.1 mU/L as the threshold of best clinical response. Despite this, a number of professional organizations and publications have suggested that patients be stratified into prognostic risk groups, with high-risk patients maintaining their TSH values beneath 0.1 mU/L and low-risk patients keeping TSH less suppressed or even normal.[63-65,105] However, the prognostic definitions of risk continue to evolve and, although reasonably predictive for large populations of patients, continue to have limited reliability regarding individual patient outcomes. In addition, the risks of well-adjusted L-T_4 suppression of TSH are far fewer and more easily managed than such proponents suggest.

The side effects of properly titrated suppressive L-T_4treatment are minimal, if any. Concerns regarding acceleration of bone mineral loss appear unfounded[106] or, at the very most, may be an issue in the subset of postmenopausal women.[107] The most common side effects stem from enhanced adrenergic stimulation, particularly tachycardia. In some cases, this may result in cardiac hypertrophy and diastolic dysfunction, all significantly improved or prevented by β-adrenergic blockade.[108] The use of a long-acting cardioselective β-adrenergic blocker mitigates almost all clinically relevant side effects of suppressive L-T_4 therapy.

Chemotherapy

There are no known effective systemic tumoricidal chemotherapeutic agents for follicular thyroid carcinomas. As long as radioiodine demonstrates its effectiveness and is well tolerated in a patient, it remains the only systemic tumoricidal agent with demonstrated usefulness. When radioiodine is no longer effective, demonstrated either by loss of radioiodine avidity or progression of disease despite aggressive ^{131}I treatments (approximately 20% of patients[109]), specific critical tumor sites should be targeted with the combined modalities of surgery and radiotherapy. Unfortunately, these therapies are not useful for widely disseminated tumors, particularly in the lungs and liver. Chemotherapeutic agents have been tried under such circumstances and are rarely of any clinical benefit. Based on historical and outdated literature,[110] doxorubicin has been the most common agent tried, singly or in combination therapy, but complete responses are not seen and even partial responses are rare. Disease stabilization is sometimes achievable with diverse chemotherapeutic combinations, but this is not an appropriate therapeutic end point for cytotoxic agents with considerable morbidity that are unsuitable for chronic long-term treatment. In contrast to these agents, a new class of drugs is under development, known as tumor-modifying agents. These drugs are designed as tumoristatic agents for chronic therapy and are discussed in the final section of this chapter.

LONG-TERM FOLLOW-UP

Follicular thyroid cancer is best thought of as a chronic disease. Although initial treatment with surgery and radioiodine ablation may eliminate evidence of disease by all available modalities, there is a persistent risk of disease recurrence and progression that lasts for the entire life of the patient. In addition, tumor dedifferentiation may render functional studies that rely on radioiodine uptake and thyroglobulin production useless, requiring corroboration with diverse diagnostic techniques to avoid the pitfalls of false-negative studies. Within this clinical context, the physician must stress the need for continued patient compliance with long-term follow-up studies.

Clinical Evaluation

The physician and patient should perform regular physical examinations. The patient should be instructed to perform monthly neck self-examinations, as well as breast self-examinations in women, because of a potentially increased incidence of breast cancer in female thyroid cancer patients.[111] Physician visits should document regional node evaluations and carefully assess cardiac status, with attention to evidence of resting tachycardia in the context of L-T_4 suppression therapy. Because of a propensity for hematogenous dissemination to bone, there should be a low threshold for full evaluation of arthritic-type symptoms to avoid missing bone metastases. Some endocrinologists have undergone training in ultrasonography and use this modality for regular office visits; however, this might be overused and the patient better served by less frequent ultrasound evaluations in the hands of a dedicated ultrasonographer.

Tumor Marker: Thyroglobulin

Thyroglobulin is a 670-kD protein dimer of two identical subunits, secreted exclusively by thyroid follicular cells and differentiated malignancies arising from these cells. As such, after total thyroidectomy and radioiodine ablation of the postsurgical thyroid remnant, it serves as a powerful and specific marker for the presence of residual or recurrent thyroid carcinoma.[112] Thyroid follicular cells and thyroid carcinoma cells are stimulated to secrete thyroglobulin by TSH, either produced by the pituitary in response to thyroid hormone withdrawal or provided exogenously by the injection of rhTSH. Thus, thyroglobulin levels are most sensitive when evaluated under those conditions. Similarly, undetectable thyroglobulin levels, in the context of TSH levels suppressed by L-T_4, do not indicate the absence of tumor.

Because thyroglobulin has significant antigenic variability, thyroglobulin assays are poorly standardized and have highly variable sensitivities; 25% of the thyroid carcinoma population has antithyroglobulin autoantibodies that interfere with the assay,[113] so it is one of the most difficult proteins to quantify reliably in human serum.[114] Despite this, thyroglobulin assay sensitivities have continued to improve over the past 2 decades, sometimes revealing evidence of persistent tumor when previous assays had failed to reveal detectable thyroglobulin levels. Even in the context of future supersensitive assays, designed to detect extremely low thyroglobulin concentrations despite L-T_4 suppression therapy, TSH stimulation would likely prove additionally informative, rivaling the ability of advanced imaging modalities to detect thyroid cancer and requiring evolving paradigms of clinical use.

Measurable thyroglobulin levels after thyroidectomy and radioiodine ablation denote residual or recurrent disease, despite the absence of evidence of tumor on other diagnostic studies.[115-118] This has been shown to provide sufficient justification for a trial of administration of a therapeutic dosage of radioiodine. A reasonable portion of such patients will have positive post-therapy whole-body scans (at 2 to 7 days after the therapy dose) revealing the sites of disease, reductions in thyroglobulin levels on follow-up evaluation, or later resolution of metastatic sites after repeat therapeutic radioiodine administration.[119-124] Conversely, the absence of such responses documents the absence of iodine avidity in those patients, permitting the clinician to focus on other diagnostic techniques to identify tumor sites.

Nuclear Scanning

Radioactive iodine scanning is an important diagnostic modality for evaluating patients with follicular thyroid carcinomas, providing a sensitive method for assessing disease status when these tumors are able to concentrate iodine. It assesses a differentiated function of the tumor cell, requiring an intact TSH receptor and signal transduction pathway, the ability to express the NIS, and the ability to retain iodine within the cell for a sufficient length of time. There are cases in which persistent thyroglobulin secretion indicates the presence of tumor despite the loss of iodine avidity of tumor cells, and there are others in which radioiodine scans reveal tumor, despite the absence of measurable serum thyroglobulin.[125-129] This emphasizes that these differentiated functional assessments, although often congruent, are ultimately independent from each other.

Radioiodine whole-body scans are used to assess for the presence of disease, planning of treatments, and assessment of response to prior therapy. There are two types of scans, diagnostic scans that use a scanning dose of 2 to 5 mCi ^{131}I and post-therapy scans performed 2 to 7 days after administration of a therapeutic dose of ^{131}I that sensitively assess the extent of iodine-avid tumor. A variety of techniques have been used for such studies. Although some nuclear medicine facilities use ^{123}I rather than ^{131}I for scanning, citing lower radiation dosage and better scanning resolution, I have found that ^{131}I provides superior signal sensitivity and permits the opportunity to perform dosimetry for treatment planning.

Patients are prepared by increasing TSH levels, using either hypothyroidism (withdrawal of L-T_4) or injections of rhTSH, as well as a strict low-iodine diet (see earlier). It is important to individualize the scanning technique to account for the method of TSH elevation. Using hypothyroid withdrawal, 5 mCi ^{131}I (after obtaining serum for TSH and thyroglobulin assessment) is usually administered and whole-body scans obtained at 24 and 48 hours. Comparison of these studies permits the assessment of rapid radioiodine turnover as a potential cause of treatment failure, dealt with through the use of a lithium carbonate adjuvant,[130] and provides an opportunity to evaluate results quickly and plan therapeutic radioiodine therapy, if indicated.

Scanning using rhTSH permits the patient to remain on L-T_4 but still requires a strict low-iodine diet. Because there is rapid renal clearance of ^{131}I in this euthyroid patient, proper use of rhTSH for scanning mandates an ^{131}I scan dose of at least 4 mCi and increased time for scan count acquisition, usually at least 30 minutes per image. The intramuscular injections of rhTSH (0.9 mg) are given on days 1 and 2, with ^{131}I tracer given on day 3 and imaging done on days 4 and 5 (thyroglobulin levels measured on day 5). Although more convenient and without the morbidity of a hypothyroid withdrawal preparation, scans performed with rhTSH are inherently less sensitive than those prepared using hypothyroid withdrawal, and thyroglobulin stimulation is similarly lower.[131] For that reason, hypothyroid withdrawal preparation is used for most of our patients who are higher risk for recurrent disease and in most patients until this study is clearly negative, with stimulated thyroglobulin levels lower than 0.4 ng/mL (in a sensitive assay, detection limit is 0.1 ng/mL). When both parameters are clearly negative, the patient is given the option to use rhTSH for subsequent studies. It is not appropriate for a physician to use only one scan preparation method for all patients. The range of clinical cases in a practice should allow for a variety of scan preparation methods, based on the individual features of each case.

When both ^{131}I whole-body scan and thyroglobulin assessments are negative at 6 months following a preceding radioiodine therapy, the next study is typically performed after a 1-year interval. For continued negative studies, the interval grows to 2 years, 3 years, and then 4 years between studies. The longest interval between scans is typically 5 years when using hypothyroid withdrawal or 4 years using rhTSH scan preparation.

Whole-body positron emission tomography (PET) imaging with ^{18}F-fluorodeoxyglucose (18-FDG), fused with a low-sensitivity computed tomography (CT) scan for anatomic localization, has been able to detect metastatic foci of follicular thyroid cancers independent of iodine avidity.[132,133] This is most useful for evaluating patients with elevated thyroglobulin values but negative post-therapy ^{131}I whole-body scans. Increased avidity for 18-FDG correlates with aggressive tumor progression and inversely with radioiodine avidity,[134] thus producing tumor localization and prognostic information.[135] The sensitivity of this study can be enhanced with hypothyroidism or injection of rhTSH.[136]

Anatomic Imaging

Although radioiodine scanning makes use of functional properties of iodine avidity unique to thyroid carcinomas, roughly 20% of follicular thyroid cancers and more than a third of Hürthle cell carcinomas lose this function consequent to loss of expression of the sodium-iodide symporter gene.[137-139] Thus functional imaging alone will not suffice for proper prospective evaluation of disease status. Anatomical imaging, using computerized axial tomographic (CT) scanning, magnetic resonance (MR) imaging, ultrasonography, and radiographic studies (best for surveying for skeletal metastases), provides the means to assess and localize macroscopic disease independent of functional scans. These studies should be rotated at reasonable intervals to adequately evaluate disease status. The lungs are well visualized using non-contrast CT scans, noting that intravenous CT contrast must be avoided if radioiodine scans or therapy will be undertaken within 6 to 10 months. For such situations, MR imaging with gadolinium contrast can be used for other body sites without risk of interfering with radioiodine use. Ultrasonography is well suited for evaluating for local disease in the neck and is most effective when combined with fine needle aspiration biopsy of suspicious sites.

FUTURE DIRECTIONS

One major problem in dealing with follicular thyroid carcinomas is the absence of any effective systemic therapy for non-iodine avid disease. There are three general directions that have been explored. First, there are a number of studies investigating causes of loss of iodine uptake[139,140] in thyroid cancers and efforts to restore this function.[141] Second, new chemotherapeutic agents are being evaluated for

Table 27–1 Follicular Carcinoma: Pitfalls, Complications, and Consequences

Pitfall or Complication	Consequence or Response
Misdiagnosis of follicular carcinoma as benign tumor	Did not treat with radioiodine and developed distant metastases
Inadequate resection of thyroid gland; intact thyroid lobe or remnant larger than 3 g	Inability to ablate remnant with radioiodine or painful radiation thyroiditis during treatment
Postoperative hypoparathyroidism	If persistent longer than 3 mo, will need lifelong treatment with calcitriol and calcium carbonate
Operative damage to recurrent laryngeal nerve	If unilateral, single vocal cord paralysis will have varying effects on voice; if bilateral, likely to need tracheostomy
Resection of metastatic tumor difficult because of extreme vascularity and consequent blood loss	Preoperative angiographic embolization of tumor vessels—will assist in safe surgical resection
Inadequate ^{131}I treatment doses fail to ablate metastatic disease	Maximal safe dose treatment dose—can be determined by performing ^{131}I dosimetry studies
Rapid turnover of radioactive iodine from metastatic tumor sites—prevents successful therapy	Lithium carbonate (600-mg loading dose, then 300 mg q8h, PO × 8 days, ^{131}I on day 3)—can increase ^{131}I retention in tumor
Chronic suppression of thyroid-stimulating hormone with levothyroxine can cause tachycardia	Side effects mitigated by concomitant treatment with beta-1–selective beta blocker
Antithyroglobulin autoantibodies interfere with valid assessment of thyroglobulin levels	Anti-TG antibodies can serve as surrogate marker for persistent thyroid cancer (if levels not gradually diminished over 2 to 3 yr)
Sole reliance on functional studies: ^{131}I scans and thyroglobulin assays may miss progression of nonfunctional tumor	Functional studies balanced with judicious use of anatomic imaging (CT scans, MRI, ultrasound)

potential activity against a variety of thyroid cancers. The most productive direction has been in the use of "tumor-modifying agents" that are not tumoricidal, but instead, halt or diminish the progression of metastatic disease. This can be direct, through altering cellular tyrosine kinases,[41,142,143] or indirect by means of antiangiogenesis agents.[144] The future holds great promise for improving the effectiveness and choices of therapy for recalcitrant disease.

PITFALLS, COMPLICATIONS, AND CONSEQUENCES

See Table 27-1.

CONTROVERSIES

- Some investigators use diagnostic tests to discriminate follicular adenomas from carcinomas prior to thyroidectomy, whereas others believe that some adenomas are premalignant lesions or carcinomas in situ that should be resected regardless of test results.
- Some clinicians fear morbidity from a thyroidectomy performed by inexperienced surgeons and suggest that a subtotal thyroidectomy be performed, whereas others prefer optimal surgical management using total or near-total thyroidectomy.
- There are disagreements over the optimal dosing and safety limits of ^{131}I therapy.
- Some clinicians use rhTSH for almost all ^{131}I scans and therapies, whereas others are selective, using rhTSH for patients with minimal local disease or intolerance to hypothyroidism and follow-up studies after prior negative hypothyroid withdrawal evaluations.
- The role and degree of TSH suppression using L-T_4 is a point of significant disagreement and controversy.

References

1. Edwards BK, Brown ML, Wingo PA, et al: Annual report to the nation on the status of cancer, 1975-2002, featuring population-based trends in cancer treatment. J Natl Cancer Inst 97:1407, 2005.
2. Parkin DM, Bray F, Ferlay J, et al: Global cancer statistics, 2002. CA Cancer J Clin 55:(74), 2005.
3. LiVolsi VA, Asa SL: The demise of follicular carcinoma of the thyroid gland. Thyroid 4:233, 1994.
4. Hodgson NC, Button J, Solorzano CC: Thyroid cancer: Is the incidence still increasing? Ann Surg Oncol 11:1093, 2004.
5. Robbins J, Merino MJ, Boice Jr JD, et al: Thyroid cancer: A lethal neoplasm. Ann Int Med 115:133, 1991.

6. Baloch ZW, Livolsi VA: Follicular-patterned lesions of the thyroid: The bane of the pathologist. Am J Clin Pathol 117:143, 2002.
7. DeLellis RA, Lloyd RV, Heitz PU, et al (eds): Pathology and Genetics of Tumours of Endocrine Organs (World Health Organization Classification of Tumours). Lyon, France, IARC Press, 2004, pp 1-320.
8. Franc B, de la Salmoniere P, Lange F, et al: Interobserver and intraobserver reproducibility in the histopathology of follicular thyroid carcinoma. Hum Pathol 34:1092, 2003.
9. Zeiger MA, Dackiw AP: Follicular thyroid lesions, elements that affect both diagnosis and prognosis. J Surg Oncol 89:108, 2005.
10. Tzen CY, Huang YW, Fu YS: Is atypical follicular adenoma of the thyroid a preinvasive malignancy? Hum Pathol 34:666, 2003.
11. Schmid KW, Farid NR: How to define follicular thyroid carcinoma. Virchows Arch 448:385, 2006.
12. Barden CB, Shister KW, Zhu B, et al: Classification of follicular thyroid tumors by molecular signature: Results of gene profiling. Clin Cancer Res 9:1792, 2003.
13. Umbricht CB, Saji M, Westra WH, et al: Telomerase activity: A marker to distinguish follicular thyroid adenoma from carcinoma. Cancer Res 57:2144, 1997.
14. LiVolsi VA: Surgical Pathology of the Thyroid. Philadelphia, WB Saunders, 1990.
15. Lubitz CC, Gallagher LA, Finley DJ, et al: Molecular analysis of minimally invasive follicular carcinomas by gene profiling. Surgery 138:1042, 2005.
16. Collini P, Sampietro G, Rosai J, et al: Minimally invasive (encapsulated) follicular carcinoma of the thyroid gland is the low-risk counterpart of widely invasive follicular carcinoma but not of insular carcinoma. Virchows Arch 442:71, 2003.
17. Maximo V, Sobrinho-Simoes M: Hürthle cell tumours of the thyroid. A review with emphasis on mitochondrial abnormalities with clinical relevance. Virchows Arch 437:107, 2000.
18. Har-El G, Hadar T, Segal K, et al: Hürthle cell carcinoma of the thyroid gland: A tumor of moderate malignancy. Cancer 57:1613, 1986.
19. Haigh PI, Urbach DR: The treatment and prognosis of Hürthle cell follicular thyroid carcinoma compared with its non-Hürthle cell counterpart. Surgery 138:1152, 2005.
20. Evans HL, Vassilopoulou-Sellin R: Follicular and Hürthle cell carcinomas of the thyroid: A comparative study. Am J Surg Pathol 22:1512, 1998.
21. Carcangiu ML, Zampi G, Rosai J: Poorly differentiated ("insular") thyroid carcinoma: A reinterpretation of Langhans' "wuchernde Struma." Am J Surg Pathol 8:655, 1984.
22. Papotti M, Micca FB, Favero A, et al: Poorly differentiated thyroid carcinomas with primordial cell component: A group of aggressive lesions sharing insular, trabecular, and solid patterns. Am J Surg Pathol 17:291, 1993.
23. Rosai J, Saxén EA, Woolner L: Session III: Undifferentiated and poorly differentiated carcinoma. Semin Diagn Pathol 2:123, 1985.
24. Volante M, Landolfi S, Chiusa L, et al: Poorly differentiated carcinomas of the thyroid with trabecular, insular, and solid patterns: A clinicopathologic study of 183 patients. Cancer 100:950, 2004.
25. Justin EP, Seabold JE, Robinson RA, et al: Insular carcinoma: A distinct thyroid carcinoma with associated iodine-131 localization. J Nucl Med 32:1358, 1991.
26. Luna-Ortiz K, Hurtado-Lopez LM, Dominguez-Malagon H, et al: Clinical course of insular thyroid carcinoma. Med Sci Monit 10:CR108, 2004.
27. Pellegriti G, Giuffrida D, Scollo C, et al: Long-term outcome of patients with insular carcinoma of the thyroid: The insular histotype is an independent predictor of poor prognosis. Cancer 95: 2076, 2002.
28. Machens A, Hinze R, Lautenschlager C, et al: Multivariate analysis of clinicopathologic parameters for the insular subtype of differentiated thyroid carcinoma. Arch Surg 136:941, 2001.
29. Waite KA, Eng C: Protean PTEN: Form and function. Am J Hum Genet 70:829, 2002.
30. Liaw D, Marsh DJ, Li J, et al: Germline mutations of the PTEN gene in Cowden disease, an inherited breast and thyroid cancer syndrome. Nat Genet 16:64, 1997.
31. Nagy R, Sweet K, Eng C: Highly penetrant hereditary cancer syndromes. Oncogene 23:6445, 2004.
32. Hemminki K, Eng C, Chen B: Familial risks for nonmedullary thyroid cancer. J Clin Endocrinol Metab 90:5747, 2005.
33. Kroll TG, Sarraf P, Pecciarini L, et al: PAX8-PPARgamma1 fusion oncogene in human thyroid carcinoma [corrected]. Science 289:1357, 2000.
34. McIver B, Grebe SK, Eberhardt NL: The PAX8/PPAR gamma fusion oncogene as a potential therapeutic target in follicular thyroid carcinoma. Curr Drug Targets Immune Endocr Metabol Disord 4:221, 2004.
35. Dwight T, Thoppe SR, Foukakis T, et al: Involvement of the PAX8/peroxisome proliferator-activated receptor gamma rearrangement in follicular thyroid tumors. J Clin Endocrinol Metab 88:4440, 2003.
36. Nikiforova MN, Biddinger PW, Caudill CM, et al: PAX8-PPARgamma rearrangement in thyroid tumors: RT-PCR and immunohistochemical analyses. Am J Surg Pathol 26:1016, 2002.
37. Sahin M, Allard BL, Yates M, et al: PPARgamma staining as a surrogate for PAX8/PPARgamma fusion oncogene expression in follicular neoplasms: Clinicopathological correlation and histopathological diagnostic value. J Clin Endocrinol Metab 90:463, 2005.
38. Foukakis T, Au AY, Wallin G, et al: The Ras effector NORE1A is suppressed in follicular thyroid carcinomas with a PAX8-PPARgamma fusion. J Clin Endocrinol Metab 91:1143, 2006.

39. Meinkoth JL: Biology of Ras in thyroid cells. In Farid NR (ed): Molecular Basis of Thyroid Cancer, vol 122. Boston, Kluwer Academic, 2004, pp 131-148.
40. Vasko V, Ferrand M, Di Cristofaro J, et al: Specific pattern of RAS oncogene mutations in follicular thyroid tumors. J Clin Endocrinol Metab 88:2745, 2003.
41. Ringel MD, Hayre N, Saito J, et al: Overexpression and overactivation of Akt in thyroid carcinoma. Cancer Res 61:6105, 2001.
42. Shinohara M, Chung YJ, Saji M, et al: AKT in thyroid tumorigenesis and progression. Endocrinology 148:942, 2007.
43. Russo D, Arturi F, Schlumberger M, et al: Activating mutations of the TSH receptor in differentiated thyroid carcinomas. Oncogene 11:1907, 1995.
44. Russo D, Tumino S, Arturi F, et al: Detection of an activating mutation of the thyrotropin receptor in a case of an autonomously hyperfunctioning thyroid insular carcinoma. J Clin Endocrinol Metab 82:735, 1997.
45. Miska EA: How microRNAs control cell division, differentiation and death. Curr Opin Genet Dev 15:563, 2005.
46. Weber F, Teresi RE, Broelsch CE, et al: A limited set of human microRNA is deregulated in follicular thyroid carcinoma. J Clin Endocrinol Metab 91:3584, 2006.
47. Weber F, Aldred MA, Morrison CD, et al: Silencing of the maternally imprinted tumor suppressor ARHI contributes to follicular thyroid carcinogenesis. J Clin Endocrinol Metab 90: 1149, 2005.
48. Miyakawa M, Onoda N, Etoh M, et al: Diagnosis of thyroid follicular carcinoma by the vascular pattern and velocimetric parameters using high resolution pulsed and power Doppler ultrasonography. Endocr J 52:207, 2005.
49. Mizukami Y, Michigishi T, Nonomura A, et al: Distant metastases in differentiated thyroid carcinomas: A clinical and pathologic study. Hum Pathol 21:283, 1990.
50. Casara D, Rubello D, Saladini G, et al: Differentiated thyroid carcinoma in the elderly. Aging Clin Exp Res 4:333, 1992.
51. Tubiana M, Schlumberger M, Rougier P, et al: Long-term results and prognostic factors in patients with differentiated thyroid carcinoma. Cancer 55:794, 1985.
52. Cunningham MP, Duda RB, Recant W, et al: Survival discriminants for differentiated thyroid cancer. Am J Surg 160:344, 1990.
53. Brennan MD, Bergstralh EJ, van Heerden JA, et al: Follicular thyroid cancer treated at the Mayo Clinic, 1946 through 1970: Initial manifestations, pathologic findings, therapy, and outcome. Mayo Clin Proc 66:11, 1991.
54. DeGroot LJ, Kaplan EL, Shukla MS, et al: Morbidity and mortality in follicular thyroid cancer. J Clin Endocrinol Metab 80:2946, 1995.
55. Hay ID, Grant CS, van Heerden JA, et al: Papillary thyroid microcarcinoma: A study of 535 cases observed in a 50-year period. Surgery 112:1139, 1992.
56. Cody III HS, Shah JP: Locally invasive, well-differentiated thyroid cancer: 22 years' experience at Memorial Sloan-Kettering Cancer Center. Am J Surg 142:480, 1981.
57. Emerick GT, Duh Q-Y, Siperstein AE, et al: Diagnosis, treatment, and outcome of follicular thyroid carcinoma. Cancer 72:3287, 1993.
58. Jorda M, Gonzalez-Campora R, Mora J, et al: Prognostic factors in follicular carcinoma of the thyroid. Arch Pathol Lab Med 117:631, 1993.
59. Grebe SKG, Hay ID: Follicular thyroid cancer. Endocrinol Metab Clin North Am 24:761, 1995.
60. Greene FL, American Joint Committee on Cancer, American Cancer Society: AJCC Cancer Staging Manual, 6th ed. New York, Springer-Verlag, 2002.
61. Lang BH, Lo CY, Chan WF, et al: Staging systems for follicular thyroid carcinoma: Application to 171 consecutive patients treated in a tertiary referral centre. Endocr Relat Cancer 14:29, 2007.
62. D'Avanzo A, Ituarte P, Treseler P, et al: Prognostic scoring systems in patients with follicular thyroid cancer: A comparison of different staging systems in predicting the patient outcome. Thyroid 14:453, 2004.
63. Watkinson JC: The British Thyroid Association guidelines for the management of thyroid cancer in adults. Nucl Med Commun 25:897, 2004.
64. Cooper DS, Doherty GM, Haugen BR, et al: Management guidelines for patients with thyroid nodules and differentiated thyroid cancer. Thyroid 16:109, 2006.
65. Pacini F, Schlumberger M, Dralle H, et al: European consensus for the management of patients with differentiated thyroid carcinoma of the follicular epithelium. Eur J Endocrinol 154:787, 2006.
66. Soh EY, Clark OH: Surgical considerations and approach to thyroid cancer. Endocrinol Metab Clin North Am 25:115, 1996.
67. Proye CAG, Dromer DHR, Carnaille BM, et al: Is it still worthwhile to treat bone metastases from differentiated thyroid carcinoma with radioactive iodine? World J Surg 16:640, 1992.
68. Smit JWA, Vielvoye GJ, Goslings BM: Embolization for vertebral metastases of follicular thyroid carcinoma. J Clin Endocrinol Metab 85:989, 2000.
69. Chow SM, Law SCK, Mendenhall WM, et al: Follicular thyroid carcinoma: Prognostic factors and the role of radioiodine. Cancer 95:488, 2002.
70. Dohan O, De la Vieja A, Paroder V, et al: The sodium/iodide symporter (NIS): Characterization, regulation, and medical significance. Endocr Rev 24:48, 2003.
71. Samuel AM, Rajashekharrao B: Radioiodine therapy for well-differentiated thyroid cancer: A quantitative dosimetric evaluation for remnant thyroid ablation after surgery. J Nucl Med 35:1944, 1994.

72. Schlesinger T, Flower MA, McCready VR: Radiation dose assessments in radioiodine (^{131}I) therapy. 1. The necessity for in vivo quantitation and dosimetry in the treatment of carcinoma of the thyroid. Radiother Oncol 14:35, 1989.
73. Maxon HR, Englaro EE, Thomas SR, et al: Radioiodine-131 therapy for well-differentiated thyroid cancer — a quantitative radiation dosimetric approach: Outcome and validation in 85 patients. J Nucl Med 33:1132, 1992.
74. Benua RS, Cicale NR, Sonenberg M, et al: The relation of radioiodine dosimetry to results and complications in the treatment of metastatic thyroid cancer. Am J Roentgenol Radiat Ther Nucl Med 87:171, 1962.
75. Benua RS, Leeper RD: A method and rationale for treating metastatic thyroid carcinoma with the largest safe dose of ^{131}I. In Medeiros-Neto G, Gaitan E (eds): Frontiers in Thyroidology, vol 2. New York, Plenum, 1986, pp 1317-1321.
76. Rall JE, Foster CG, Robbins J, et al: Dosimetric considerations in determining hematopoietic damage from radioactive iodine. Am J Roentgenol Radiat Ther Nucl Med 70:274, 1953.
77. Edmonds CJ, Hayes S, Kermode JC, et al: Measurement of serum TSH and thyroid hormones in the management of treatment of thyroid carcinoma with radioiodine. Br J Radiol 50:799, 1977.
78. Goldman JM, Line BR, Aamodt RL, et al: Influence of triiodothyronine withdrawal time on ^{131}I uptake postthyroidectomy for thyroid cancer. J Clin Endocrinol Metab 50:734, 1980.
79. Mazzaferri EL, Kloos RT: Using recombinant human TSH in the management of well-differentiated thyroid cancer: Current strategies and future directions. Thyroid 10:767, 2000.
80. Pluijmen MJ, Eustatia-Rutten C, Goslings BM, et al: Effects of low-iodide diet on postsurgical radioiodide ablation therapy in patients with differentiated thyroid carcinoma. Clin Endocrinol (Oxf) 58:428, 2003.
81. Spate VL, Morris JS, Nichols TA, et al: Longitudinal study of iodine in toenails following IV administration of an iodine-containing contrast agent. J Radioanalyt Nucl Chem 236:71, 1998.
82. Ain KB, DeWitt PA, Gardner TG, et al: Low-iodine tube-feeding diet for iodine-131 scanning and therapy. Clin Nucl Med 19:504, 1994.
83. Gilletz N: The Low Iodine Diet Cookbook. Toronto, Your Health Press, 2005.
84. Lakshmanan M, Schaffer A, Robbins J, et al: A simplified low-iodine diet in I-131 scanning and therapy of thyroid cancer. Clin Nucl Med 13:866, 1988.
85. Tomoda C, Uruno T, Takamura Y, et al: Reevaluation of stringent low iodine diet in outpatient preparation for radioiodine examination and therapy. Endocr J 52:237, 2005.
86. Mandel SJ, Mandel L: Radioactive iodine and the salivary glands. Thyroid 13:265, 2003.
87. Burns JA, Morgenstern KE, Cahill KV, et al: Nasolacrimal obstruction secondary to I(131) therapy. Ophthal Plast Reconstr Surg 20:126, 2004.
88. Morgenstern KE, Vadysirisack DD, Zhang Z, et al: Expression of sodium iodide symporter in the lacrimal drainage system: Implication for the mechanism underlying nasolacrimal duct obstruction in I(131)-treated patients. Ophthal Plast Reconstr Surg 21:337, 2005.
89. Maxon HR, Thomas SR, Hertzberg VS, et al: Relation between effective radiation dose and outcome of radioiodine therapy for thyroid cancer. N Engl J Med 309:937, 1983.
90. O'Connell MEA, A'Hern RP, Harmer CL: Results of external beam radiotherapy in differentiated thyroid carcinoma: A retrospective study from the Royal Marsden Hospital. Eur J Cancer 30A:733, 1994.
91. Brabant G, Maenhaut C, Köhrle J, et al: Human thyrotropin receptor gene: Expression in thyroid tumors and correlation to markers of thyroid differentiation and dedifferentiation. Mol Cell Endocrinol 82:R7, 1991.
92. Dumont JE, Lamy F, Roger P, et al: Physiological and pathological regulation of thyroid cell proliferation and differentiation by thyrotropin and other factors. Physiol Rev 72:667, 1992.
93. Edmonds CJ, Kermode JC: Thyrotrophin receptors, tumour radioiodine concentration and thyroglobulin secretion in differentiated thyroid cancers. Br J Cancer 52:537, 1985.
94. Filetti S, Bidart J-M, Arturi F, et al: Sodium/iodide symporter: A key transport system in thyroid cancer cell metabolism. Eur J Endocrinol 141:443, 1999.
95. Müller-Gärtner HW, Baisch H, Garn M, et al: Individually different proliferation responses of differentiated thyroid carcinomas to thyrotropin. In Goretzki PE, Röher HD (eds): Growth Regulation of Thyroid Gland and Thyroid Tumors, vol 18. Basel, Switzerland, Karger, 1989, pp 137-151.
96. Siperstein AE, Claasen HR, Miller R, et al: Thyroid-stimulating hormone growth-responsive, cyclic adenosine monophosphate–unresponsive poorly differentiated thyroid carcinoma of follicular cell origin. In Goretzki PE, Röher HD (eds): Growth Regulation of Thyroid Gland and Thyroid Tumors, vol 18. Basel, Karger, 1989, pp 81-87.
97. Cooper DS, Specker B, Ho M, et al: Thyrotropin suppression and disease progression in patients with differentiated thyroid cancer: Rsults from the National Thyroid Cancer Treatment Cooperative Registry. Thyroid 8:737, 1998.
98. Mazzaferri EL, Young RL: Papillary thyroid carcinoma: A 10-year follow-up report of the impact of therapy in 576 patients. Am J Med 70:511, 1981.
99. Mazzaferri EL, Jhiang SM: Long-term impact of initial surgical and medical therapy on papillary and follicular thyroid cancer. Am J Med 97:418, 1994.

100. Pujol P, Daures JP, Nsakala N, et al: Degree of thyrotropin suppression as a prognostic determinant in differentiated thyroid cancer. J Clin Endocrinol Metab 81:4318, 1996.
101. Rossi RL, Cady B, Silverman ML, et al: Surgically incurable well-differentiated thyroid carcinoma. Prognostic factors and results of therapy. Arch Surg 123:569, 1988.
102. Simpson WJ, Panzarella T, Carruthers JS, et al: Papillary and follicular thyroid cancer: Impact of treatment in 1,578 patients. Int J Rad Onc Biol Phys 14:1063, 1988.
103. Ain KB, Pucino F, Csako G, et al: Effects of restricting levothyroxine dosage strength availability. Pharmacotherapy 16:1103, 1996.
104. Ain KB, Pucino F, Shiver TM, et al: Thyroid hormone levels affected by time of blood sampling in thyroxine-treated patients. Thyroid 3:81, 1993.
105. Biondi B, Filetti S, Schlumberger M: Thyroid-hormone therapy and thyroid cancer: A reassessment. Nature Clin Pract Endocrinol Metab 1:32, 2005.
106. Reverter JL, Holgado S, Alonso N, et al: Lack of deleterious effect on bone mineral density of long-term thyroxine suppressive therapy for differentiated thyroid carcinoma. Endocr Relat Cancer 12:973, 2005.
107. Heemstra KA, Hamdy NA, Romijn JA, et al: The effects of thyrotropin-suppressive therapy on bone metabolism in patients with well-differentiated thyroid carcinoma. Thyroid 16:583, 2006.
108. Fazio S, Biondi B, Carella C, et al: Diastolic dysfunction in patients on thyroid-stimulating hormone suppressive therapy with levothyroxine: Beneficial effect of β-blockade. J Clin Endocrinol Metab 80:2222, 1995.
109. Links TP, van Tol KM, Jager PL, et al: Life expectancy in differentiated thyroid cancer: A novel approach to survival analysis. Endoc Relat Cancer 12:273, 2005.
110. Ahuja S, Ernst H: Chemotherapy of thyroid carcinoma. J Endocrinol Invest 10:303, 1987.
111. Vassilopoulou-Sellin R, Palmer L, Taylor S, et al: Incidence of breast carcinoma in women with thyroid carcinoma. Cancer 85:696, 1999.
112. Whitley RJ, Ain KB: Thyroglobulin: A specific serum marker for the management of thyroid carcinoma. Clin Lab Med 24:29, 2004.
113. Spencer CA, Takeuchi M, Kazarosyan M, et al: Serum thyroglobulin autoantibodies: Prevalence, influence on serum thyroglobulin measurement, and prognostic significance in patients with differentiated thyroid carcinoma. J Clin Endocrinol Metab 83:1121, 1998.
114. Spencer CA, Bergoglio LM, Kazarosyan M, et al: Clinical impact of thyroglobulin (Tg) and Tg autoantibody method differences on the management of patients with differentiated thyroid carcinomas. J Clin Endocrinol Metab 90:5566, 2005.
115. Hamy A, Mirallie E, Bennouna J, et al: Thyroglobulin monitoring after treatment of well-differentiated thyroid cancer. Eur J Surg Oncol 30:681, 2004.
116. Lima N, Cavaliere H, Tomimori E, et al: Prognostic value of serial serum thyroglobulin determinations after total thyroidectomy for differentiated thyroid cancer. J Endocrinol Invest 25: 110, 2002.
117. Lin JD, Huang MJ, Hsu BR, et al: Significance of postoperative serum thyroglobulin levels in patients with papillary and follicular thyroid carcinomas. J Surg Oncol 80:45, 2002.
118. Toubeau M, Touzery C, Arveux P, et al: Predictive value for disease progression of serum thyroglobulin levels measured in the postoperative period and after (131)I ablation therapy in patients with differentiated thyroid cancer. J Nucl Med 45:988, 2004.
119. de Geus-Oei LF, Oei HY, Hennemann G, et al: Sensitivity of 123I whole-body scan and thyroglobulin in the detection of metastases or recurrent differentiated thyroid cancer. Eur J Nucl Med Mol Imaging 29:768, 2002.
120. de Keizer B, Koppeschaar HP, Zelissen PM, et al: Efficacy of high therapeutic doses of iodine-131 in patients with differentiated thyroid cancer and detectable serum thyroglobulin. Eur J Nucl Med 28:198, 2001.
121. Koh JM, Kim ES, Ryu JS, et al: Effects of therapeutic doses of 131I in thyroid papillary carcinoma patients with elevated thyroglobulin level and negative 131I whole-body scan: Comparative study. Clin Endocrinol (Oxf) 58:421, 2003.
122. Mazzaferri EL: Empirically treating high serum thyroglobulin levels. J Nucl Med 46:1079, 2005.
123. Pacini F, Agate L, Elisei R, et al: Outcome of differentiated thyroid cancer with detectable serum Tg and negative diagnostic (131)I whole-body scan: Comparison of patients treated with high (131)I activities versus untreated patients. J Clin Endocrinol Metab 86:4092, 2001.
124. Pineda JD, Lee T, Ain KB, et al: Iodine-131 therapy for thyroid cancer patients with elevated thyroglobulin and negative diagnostic scan. J Clin Endocrinol Metab 80:1488, 1995.
125. Bachelot A, Cailleux AF, Klain M, et al: Relationship between tumor burden and serum thyroglobulin level in patients with papillary and follicular thyroid carcinoma. Thyroid 12:707, 2002.
126. Dralle H, Schwarzrock R, Lang W, et al: Comparison of histology and immunohistochemistry with thyroglobulin serum levels and radioiodine uptake in recurrences and metastases of differentiated thyroid carcinomas. Acta Endocrinol (Copenh) 108:504, 1985.
127. Mertens IJ, De Klerk JM, Zelissen PM, et al: Undetectable serum thyroglobulin in a patient with metastatic follicular thyroid cancer. Clin Nucl Med 24:346, 1999.
128. Müller-Gärtner HW, Schneider C: Clinical evaluation of tumor characteristics predisposing serum thyroglobulin to be undetectable in patients with differentiated thyroid cancer. Cancer 61:976, 1988.

129. Roelants V, De Nayer P, Bouckaert A, et al: The predictive value of serum thyroglobulin in the follow-up of differentiated thyroid cancer. Eur J Nucl Med 24:722, 1997.
130. Koong SS, Reynolds JC, Movius EG, et al: Lithium as a potential adjuvant to ^{131}I therapy of metastatic, well differentiated thyroid carcinoma. J Clin Endocrinol Metab 84:912, 1999.
131. Pellegriti G, Scollo C, Regalbuto C, et al: The diagnostic use of the rhTSH/thyroglobulin test in differentiated thyroid cancer patients with persistent disease and low thyroglobulin levels. Clin Endocrinol (Oxf) 58:556, 2003.
132. Lind P, Kohlfurst S: Respective roles of thyroglobulin, radioiodine imaging, and positron emission tomography in the assessment of thyroid cancer. Semin Nucl Med 36:194, 2006.
133. Salvatore B, Paone G, Klain M, et al: Fluorodeoxyglucose positron emission tomography/computed tomography in patients with differentiated thyroid cancer and elevated thyroglobulin after total thyroidectomy and (131)I ablation. Q J Nucl Med Mol Imaging, 2007.
134. Lazar V, Bidart JM, Caillou B, et al: Expression of the Na^+/I^- symporter gene in human thyroid tumors: A comparison study with other thyroid-specific genes. J Clin Endocrinol Metab 84:3228, 1999.
135. Robbins RJ, Wan Q, Grewal RK, et al: Real-time prognosis for metastatic thyroid carcinoma based on 2-[18F]fluoro-2-deoxy-D-glucose-positron emission tomography scanning. J Clin Endocrinol Metab 91:498, 2006.
136. Chin BB, Patel P, Cohade C, et al: Recombinant human thyrotropin stimulation of fluoro-D-glucose positron emission tomography uptake in well-differentiated thyroid carcinoma. J Clin Endocrinol Metab 89:91, 2004.
137. Ain KB: Management of undifferentiated thyroid cancer. Baillieres Best Pract Res Clin Endocrinol Metab 14:615, 2000.
138. Arturi F, Russo D, Schlumberger M, et al: Iodide symporter gene expression in human thyroid tumors. J Clin Endocrinol Metab 83:2493, 1998.
139. Venkataraman GM, Yatin M, Marcinek R, et al: Restoration of iodide uptake in dedifferentiated thyroid carcinoma: Relationship to human Na^+/I^- symporter gene methylation status. J Clin Endocrinol Metab 84:2449, 1999.
140. Li W, Venkataraman GM, Ain KB: Protein synthesis inhibitors, in synergy with 5-azacytidine, restore sodium/iodide symporter gene expression in human thyroid adenoma cell line, KAK-1, suggesting trans-active transcriptional repressor. J Clin Endocrinol Metab 92:1080, 2007.
141. Haugen BR: Redifferentiation therapy in advanced thyroid cancer. Curr Drug Targets Immune Endocr Metabol Disord 4:175, 2004.
142. Fagin JA: How thyroid tumors start and why it matters: Kinase mutants as targets for solid cancer pharmacotherapy. J Endocrinol 183:249, 2004.
143. Salvatore G, De Falco V, Salerno P, et al: BRAF is a therapeutic target in aggressive thyroid carcinoma. Clin Cancer Res 12:1623, 2006.
144. Ain KB, Lee C, Williams KD: Phase II trial of thalidomide for therapy of radioiodine-unresponsive and rapidly progressive thyroid carcinomas. Thyroid 17:663, 2007.

Section B

MEDULLARY THYROID CANCER

Chapter 28

Medullary Thyroid Cancer

Douglas W. Ball

Key Points

- Activating *ret* gene mutations cause inherited MTC, accounting for 25% of cases.
- Initial surgical management is influenced by a high rate of lymph node and distant metastases.
- Advanced clinical stage, rapid calcitonin doubling time, and somatic *ret* mutation (at codon 918) are associated with poorer prognosis.
- Patients with progressive, inoperable MTC should be considered for clinical trials.
- Investigational tyrosine kinase inhibitors targeting ret and vascular endothelial growth factor receptors have activity against MTC.

Medullary thyroid cancer (MTC) is an uncommon thyroid tumor accounting for 3% to 5% of thyroid cancer cases, derived from calcitonin-producing C cells. Although the detection of new thyroid cancer cases has increased approximately 2.5-fold since the 1970s, MTC incidence has remained stable over this interval. Distinct from differentiated thyroid cancer (DTC), MTC has a higher prevalence of familial disease (25%) as part of inherited multiple endocrine neoplasia type 2 (MEN 2) syndromes. As detailed in this chapter, characteristic activating mutations in the *ret* proto-oncogene cause MEN 2 and account for distinctive phenotypes. In addition, acquired *ret* mutations can be detected in a significant percentage of tumors in sporadic cases, associated with an adverse prognosis. The initial surgical treatment for MTC is typically more intensive than for DTC, making accurate diagnosis essential. Patients with persistent MTC after surgery have a heterogeneous course. Careful assessment of prognosis, based on imaging findings and evolution of biochemical markers, is critical to appropriate selection of patients for systemic therapy agents, currently available as investigational drugs in clinical trials. The molecular pathogenesis, clinical presentation, initial surgical treatment, clinical course, prognosis, and treatment of advanced disease will be detailed in this chapter.

MOLECULAR PATHOGENESIS

Detailed understanding of the molecular pathogenesis of MTC dates from the 1990s, when activating mutations in the *ret* proto-oncogene were first detected in germline DNA from patients with MEN 2. MEN 2 is a family of three syndromes, including FMTC (familial isolated MTC), MEN 2A (MTC plus pheochromocytoma in 50% and hyperparathyroidism in 15%), and MEN 2B (MTC, pheochromocytoma, enteric ganglioneuromas, marfanoid body habitus, corneal nerve proliferation, and additional manifestations). The *ret* gene encodes a receptor tyrosine kinase, most homologous to fibroblast growth factor (FGF) and vascular endothelial growth factor (VEGF) receptors. Ret binds a family of ligands, including glial-derived neurotropic factor (GDNF), neurturin, persephin, and artemin, along with accessory receptors that lack enzymatic activity.[1] Ligand binding results in receptor dimerization and activation of intrinsic tyrosine kinase activity. Key phosphorylated tyrosine residues in the intracellular domain of ret, including Y905, Y1015, Y1062, and Y1096, allow docking of adapter molecules for downstream signaling pathways, including Ras-ERK, PI3-K, PL-Cγ, and others.[1] The net impact of ret receptor activation is cell growth and resistance to apoptosis. Overexpression of ret in nontransformed cells promotes neoplastic transformation.[2] The importance of the Y1062 site is illustrated by a transgenic knock-in mouse model. Mice born with an amino acid substitution blocking phosphorylation at this site have a strong ret deficiency phenotype that includes enteric nervous system and renal and urinary tract abnormalities.[3] Interestingly, ret signaling also promotes calcitonin gene transcription.[4] A ret deficiency syndrome is seen in some subjects with familial Hirschsprung's disease.

Ret expression is normally limited to cells derived from the embryonic neural crest, including tissues subsequently involved in MEN 2. Ret is transiently expressed in facial cartilage derived from the neural crest. A birdlike elongated facies is a frequent characteristic of those with MEN 2B. Tumorigenesis in MEN 2 is initiated by activating point mutations in ret. To date, mutations in other genes have not been detected in hereditary MTC. Specific genotype-phenotype correlations are listed in Table 28-1, including most of the reported ret codon mutations. The most frequent and important *ret* gene mutations occur at codon 634, seen in 70% to 80% of cases of MEN 2A, and ret codon 918, seen in approximately 95% of cases of MEN 2B. Codon 918 mutations are the most frequent somatic mutation in sporadic MTC as well, occurring in 30% to 50% of cases.[5] This acquired genetic abnormality confers an adverse prognosis for overall and progression-free survival.[6,7]

Ret codon 634 encodes an extracellular cysteine residue in the juxtamembrane region. This residue and adjacent clustered extracellular cysteines help form a three-dimensional configuration that prevents receptor dimerization in the absence of ligand binding.[1] Disruption of these extracellular cysteines leads to constitutive dimerization and signaling in the absence of ligand. The phenotype of patients bearing a codon 634 mutation includes relatively early penetrance of MTC, with C-cell hyperplasia and cancer in the first or second decade of life, frequent pheochromocytoma, and hyperparathyroidism. A minority of patients also have a characteristic skin manifestation related to cutaneous nerve involvement, termed *cutaneous lichen amyloidosis.* Recommendations for prophylactic thyroidectomy in gene carriers have been extensively reviewed by an international consortium,[8] whose recommendations are summarized in Table 28-2. Compared with the 634 mutation, patients with more proximal extracellular cysteine mutations (codons 609, 611, 618, 620) may have later and less severe MTC, much lower frequency of pheochromocytoma, and no increase in hyperparathyroidism.

Table 28–1 ***Ret* Mutation Genotype-Phenotype Correlations in Inherited Medullary Thyroid Cancer (MTC)**

Codon	Exon	Phenotype	No. of Patients with MEN 2 (%)
609	10	MEN 2A, FMTC	0-1
611	10	MEN 2A, FMTC	2-3
618	10	MEN 2A, FMTC	3-5
620	10	MEN 2A, FMTC	6-8
630	11	MEN 2A, FMTC	0-1
634	11	MEN 2A	70-80
635	11	MEN 2A	Rare
637	11	MEN 2A	Rare
768	13	FMTC	Rare
790	13	MEN 2A, FMTC	Rare
791	13	FMTC	Rare
804	13	MEN 2A, FMTC	0-1
883	15	MEN 2B	Rare
891	15	FMTC	Rare
918	16	MEN 2B	3-5
922	16	MEN 2B	Rare

FMTC, familial isolated MTC; MEN 2, multiple endocrine neoplasia type 2.

Adapted from National Comprehensive Cancer Network (NCCN): Thyroid Cancer Guidelines, vol 1, 2008.

Ret codon 918 encodes a methionine residue in the substrate-binding pocket of the intracellular tyrosine kinase domain. Mutation of this site to encode a threonine is associated with enhanced signaling and altered substrate specificity.[9] Approximately 50% of MTC patients lack any known initiating mutations or other molecular events. Interestingly, a small number of MTC tumors apparently have inactivating mutations of the p18 tumor suppressor protein, which helps regulate Rb function and cell cycle progression.[10] This mutation may be complementary rather than an alternative to *ret* mutations. MTC tumors, like pheochromocytomas, frequently have large-scale deletions in chromosome 1p.[11] The relevant 1p genes for MTC pathogenesis are still not known. MTC tumors express significant levels of VEGF as part of their tumoral angiogenesis program.

Table 28–2 Consensus Recommendations for Prophylactic Thyroidectomy in Inherited Medullary Thyroid Cancer

Level	Risk	Codon	Recommendation
3	Highest	Ret codon 883, 918, or 922	First year of life, if possible
2	Intermediate	Ret codon 611, 618, 620, or 634	Age 5
1	Lowest	Ret codon 609, 768, 790, 791, 804, or 891	No consensus (age 5 or 10, or based on monitoring

Adapted from Brandi ML, Gagel RF, Angeli A, et al: Guidelines for diagnosis and therapy of MEN type 1 and type 2. J Clin Endocrinol Metab 86:5658-5671, 2001.

In addition to ret, VEGF receptors are the most common targets for systemic therapy of MTC (see later).

CLINICAL PRESENTATION

Sporadic medullary thyroid cancer may present as a palpable thyroid nodule or as a lymph nodal mass, as an incidental finding on neck imaging or, less commonly, with systemic symptoms, including diarrhea, flushing, bone pain, or rarely symptoms of hypercortisolism related to ectopic adrenocorticotropic hormone (ACTH) secretion.

The presentation of patients with familial MTC may vary significantly. Since the onset of organized DNA-based family screening in the 1990s, pediatric patients with mutations for MEN 2A and FMTC can be identified in an asymptomatic state and referred for prophylactic surgery, based on guidelines described later. Older affected individuals who were not genetically screened may present with palpable neck masses, simultaneous MTC and pheochromocytoma or, rarely, pheochromocytoma alone. In contrast to FMTC and MEN 2A, most MEN 2B cases represent as new mutations in the paternally-derived ret allele.[12] In the absence of a positive family history, children with MEN 2B can be recognized by characteristic elongated birdlike facies and the presence of ganglioneuromas of the lip and tongue. Although in retrospect these abnormalities often appeared by age 4 to 5, the median age of clinical identification is approximately 14 years.[13] In a large German study,[13] ocular manifestations and corneal nerve enlargement (conjunctivitis sicca) were found in 86% of patients at diagnosis, intestinal dysfunction, constipation, and cramping (colonic dilation) in 90%, musculoskeletal manifestations (marfanoid habitus, weak muscles, hip malformations, and scoliosis) in 74%, and pheochromocytoma in 19% at presentation. Early detection of MEN 2B is critical, with nodal involvement in 60% of patients younger than 6 years and local invasion in up to 40% in this age group.

Patients with thyroid nodules are recommended to have a fine-needle aspiration (FNA) biopsy either with direct palpation or, increasingly, with ultrasound guidance. The sensitivity of FNA for the diagnosis of MTC ranges from 50% to 80% and improves with the addition of calcitonin immunohistochemistry. Patients with suspicious nodules for MTC should have additional testing with a serum calcitonin level, which will be elevated in the vast majority of patients with a palpable MTC nodule. The routine application of calcitonin testing in all patients with thyroid nodules is controversial. The American Thyroid Association currently recommends against such testing based on cost-effectiveness and poor specificity of low-level calcitonin elevations.[14] The European Thyroid Association, however, recommends this test as an adjunct for nodule assessment. These testing issues have been reviewed in detail.[15] In the case of cytologically proven MTC, a more extensive biochemical and staging workup is recommended for most patients than for those with DTC. In addition to a detailed family history, ret proto-oncogene DNA analysis (including exons 10, 11, 13 to 16) is recommended to exclude hereditary MTC. The prevalence of occult germline ret mutation in patients without a family history is 5% to 7%. If ret testing is positive or unavailable, patients should be screened preoperatively for pheochromocytoma (e.g., plasma and/or 24-hour urine metanephrine levels) and hyperparathyroidism, with calcium and parathyroid hormone (PTH). All MTC patients should have testing for preoperative calcitonin and carcinoembryonic antigen (CEA) levels. A neck ultrasound is the most sensitive study to detect cervical lymph node involvement. Additional imaging workup includes neck CT or MRI, chest CT, liver MRI or CT with arterial and venous phase contrast, and bone imaging.

Approximately 75% of MTC patients with palpable primary tumors have lymph node metastases.[16] There is a significantly higher rate of nodal metastasis than in PTC. Cervical nodal involvement involves central and ipsilateral nodes more frequently than contralateral nodes.[17] Contralateral and mediastinal involvement becomes common (50% to 60%) when the primary tumor is locally invasive.[18] Both

Table 28–3 TNM Staging for Medullary Thyroid Cancer

Stage	Features
I	Tumors < 2 cm in diameter without evidence of disease outside the thyroid gland
II	Any tumor between 2 and 4 cm without evidence of extrathyroidal disease
III	Any tumor larger than 4 cm, level VI nodal metastases, or minimal extrathyroidal invasion, regardless of tumor size
IV	Any distant metastases or lymph node involvement outside level VI or gross soft tissue extension

Adapted from National Comprehensive Cancer Network (NCCN): Thyroid Cancer Guidelines, vol 1, 2008.

contralateral and mediastinal nodal disease appear to correlate with distant metastases. Thus, adenopathy at these sites is a marker of systemic involvement, reducing the chance of a surgical cure in most cases.[19]

In addition to cervical and mediastinal lymph nodes, the lung, liver, and abdominal lymph nodes and bone are the most frequent sites of distal involvement. Estimates of the prevalence of distant metastases are strongly influenced by the sensitivity of imaging techniques. Approximately 10% of patients have clinically detectable distant metastases at presentation. This estimate rises if invasive techniques for liver involvement are used, such as laparoscopic liver biopsy or hepatic arteriography. Occult distant metastases, especially involving the liver, are a leading explanation for failure to normalize the calcitonin level after surgery. TNM staging of MTC is illustrated in Table 28-3.

SURGICAL TREATMENT

The initial surgical management of MTC is more extensive than for DTC, highlighting the importance of obtaining an accurate preoperative diagnosis. In addition, it is critical to detect concurrent pheochromocytoma as well as hyperparathyroidism, when present. Thyroid C cells are concentrated in the upper thyroid lobes, which is where MTC tumors typically reside. Outside of familial disease, multifocal thyroid involvement appears to be less common in MTC than in DTC. Early nodal metastasis is frequent, and not excluded by a negative neck ultrasound.[20] In the United States, the most typical recommendation for sporadic MTC is total or near-total thyroidectomy, plus a careful central neck dissection (level VI bilaterally) and, frequently, ipsilateral modified dissection of lymph node levels II to V (NCCN Thyroid Cancer Guidelines, vol 1, 2008). Some European centers additionally recommend a contralateral levels II to V dissection. As an alternative, the presence of involvement in contralateral level VI nodes appears to be a sensitive predictor that contralateral levels II to V could be involved.[17] If the surgical specimens are appropriately labeled, the contralateral procedure may be performed at a later date in selected patients, avoiding the morbidity of bilateral neck dissection in the 60% to 70% of patients who lack contralateral involvement.

For asymptomatic patients detected to have a germline *ret* mutation in family screening, the recommended timing of surgery depends on the specific *ret* mutation. With the codon 634 mutation, 50% of children develop MTC by the age of 10 years and 40% develop nodal metastases by age 20.[21] Subjects with a codon 634 mutation have been assigned an intermediate risk category (see Table 28-2) with a consensus for prophylactic thyroidectomy by age 5. The codon 918 mutation seen in the vast majority of cases of MEN 2B confers a high risk of metastatic MTC as early as in the first years of life. This mutation, along with codons 883 and 922, is considered highest risk. If possible, prophylactic surgery should be performed, even in the first year of life. In contrast, patients who have one of several other *ret* mutations, including 609, 768, 790, 791, 804, and 891, have variably reduced penetrance and are assigned risk category 1 (seeTable 28-2).[8] Although the extent of surgery is somewhat controversial, most young pediatric subjects undergoing prophylactic surgery with normal calcitonin levels typically can be managed with thyroidectomy alone, and have an excellent chance of surgical remission.[8] Older familial patients, and those with significant calcitonin elevations, need to be evaluated for regional lymph node involvement and often undergo central and bilateral neck dissections.

In addition to imaging, the preoperative calcitonin level provides much useful information about the extent of disease. Calcitonin levels lower than 100 pg/mL are associated with a median tumor size of 3 mm, with 98% smaller than 1 cm. Levels higher than 1000 pg/mL correlate with a median tumor size of 2.5 cm.[22] If the preoperative basal calcitonin level exceeds 3000 pg/mL in node-positive patients, an undetectable postoperative calcitonin level is uncommon.[23]

Following surgery, levels of calcitonin and a second tumor marker, CEA, are tracked, typically beginning at 6 weeks, when calcitonin is expected to be at its lowest level. A surgical remission is defined as an undetectable calcitonin level basally or with pentagastrin stimulation, if available. Patients with detectable calcitonin levels at this point are considered to have persistent disease, even if the calcitonin level is in the normal range. Surgical outcomes are strongly influenced by the degree of lymph node involvement. Negative lymph node dissections are associated with an approximately 95% chance of an undetectable calcitonin level postoperatively. If there is any lymph node involvement, the chance of undetectable calcitonin declines to approximately 30%.[17] As noted, contralateral nodes reduce the chance of undetectable postoperative calcitonin even further.

CLINICAL COURSE AND MONITORING

In the postoperative setting, the rate of further progression of MTC is highly variable. Patients with undetectable calcitonin levels, especially after pentagastrin stimulation, are likely to remain in long-term, if not permanent, remission. Patients with low-level calcitonin elevations, typically lower than 100 pg/mL, and negative postoperative imaging also have a generally excellent prognosis. A typical clinical practice is to obtain a number of sets of calcitonin and CEA in the first 2 years following surgery. Because these markers typically follow a logarithmic pattern of increase, an approximate calcitonin doubling time can be computed. Barbet and colleagues[24] have shown that a calcitonin doubling time shorter than 6 months correlated with an almost 75% risk of death over 5 years. No patient with a doubling time longer than 2 years died from MTC during follow-up in this series. Calcitonin doubling time was a strong prognostic indicator in multivariate analyses, even when adjusted for clinical stage. These study results help identify high-risk patients, even at a relatively early point in their disease course, when postoperative imaging studies may be negative and the absolute calcitonin level still relatively low. A limitation to calcitonin-based prognosis is that many patients have a relatively chaotic pattern of calcitonin secretion, and assay problems, including the high-dose hook effect, also can limit accuracy.[25] Concurrent use of CEA is recommended to help mitigate the variability of calcitonin monitoring. Approximately 40% of MTC patients, including most patients with advanced disease, also have CEA elevations.

In addition to calcitonin doubling time, established prognostic markers for MTC include clinical stage, local invasion, extranodal invasion and, in some studies, poor differentiation status, indicated by heterogeneous calcitonin immunoreactivity. Clinical stage has a powerful impact on the natural history of MTC. Patients with stages I and II disease (see Table 28-3) have superb survival. Regional lymphadenopathy (T1 to T4, N1M0) is associated with a 10-year survival of 75%. In patients with distant metastases, 10-year survival drops to approximately 30%.[26] These data reflect an era in which metastasis detection was less advanced and nonsurgical treatments were limited. In other natural history studies, Bergholm and associates[27] have reported an overall 10-year survival of 70% in the entire Swedish national MTC cohort and 65% at 15 years. When familial cases were excluded, the 10-year survival was 61% and 54% at 15 years. An emerging prognostic marker is the presence of the *M918T* somatic mutation in MTC tumors. Two groups have now noted a significantly higher rate of progression and disease-specific mortality in sporadic patients whose tumors bear this mutation.[6,7] Although tumoral *ret* mutation analysis is not widely available at this time, the advent of *ret*-targeted therapies is likely to encourage more widespread adoption of this test.

Monitoring of patients with MTC seeks to provide prognostic information, detect significant progression, and identify patients in need of further therapy. A typical practice is to monitor calcitonin and CEA, along with thyroid function, at approximately 6-month intervals. The extent of imaging depends on the degree of calcitonin elevation and prior areas of known disease. Patients with calcitonin levels lower than 100 pg/mL are unlikely to have detectable disease, except conceivably by neck ultrasound. Patients with higher levels of calcitonin frequently undergo periodic imaging with neck ultrasound, chest CT, abdominal MRI or CT with arterial and venous phase contrast, and bone imaging. The relative sensitivity of different imaging modalities was compared in a comprehensive study by Giraudet and colleagues.[28] Interestingly, fluorodeoxyglucose positron emission tomography (FDG PET) imaging had a lower sensitivity in this study. Octreotide and metaiodobenzylguanidine (MIBG) scintigraphy are also less sensitive. For bone imaging, MRI of the axial skeleton, combined with technetium scintigraphy, appears to offer the best sensitivity.

Management of Persistent Disease

Appropriate management of persistent MTC requires an understanding of the highly heterogeneous course of the disease and appropriate use of prognostic markers. Many patients with low to moderate calcitonin levels, prolonged doubling times, and minimal or stable disease on imaging can be followed expectantly with no active interventions. Patients symptomatic with diarrhea can be treated with loperamide or diphenoxylate. Flushing may be difficult to treat, except by reducing the disease volume. Occasionally, palliative resections, including liver metastases, can relieve these symptoms. Results with octreotide have been inconsistent. Painful bone metastasis should be treated with external beam radiation. The role for radiation in treating soft tissue mass lesions is more controversial, however. Brierley and coworkers[29] have described indications for adjuvant radiation of the neck in patients without gross residual disease but at high risk for recurrence. There is no U.S. Food and Drug Administration (FDA)-approved chemotherapy for MTC and prior small-scale trials have provided only limited evidence of activity.[30]

Investigational systemic therapies targeted at ret and/or VEGFR2/KDR are now emerging for patients with progressive MTC. Several studies to date have shown encouraging radiographic responses. Currently, improvements in progression-free survival and overall survival have not yet been documented. Vandetanib is an oral multikinase inhibitor with moderate efficacy at inhibiting both ret and VEGFR2 (inhibitory concentration of 50% [IC_{50}] = 100 nM for ret, 40 nM for VEGFR2). In a phase 2 study of patients with progressive hereditary MTC, Wells and colleagues[31] have reported a 20% partial response rate (more than a 30% decrease in measurable tumors) and an additional 30% of patients experiencing prolonged stable disease. A larger international trial of vandetanib in hereditary and sporadic MTC is currently nearing completion. A pediatric MEN 2B trial is also under way. Reduced potency of vandetanib has been noted for some *ret* mutations, including V804M.[32] XL184 is a multikinase inhibitor with increased potency for both ret (IC_{50} = 4.5 nM) and VEGFR2 (IC_{50} = 0.035 nM). Preliminary results from an expanded phase 1 trial that included approximately 20 MTC patients (both sporadic and familial) revealed an approximately 50% partial response (PR) rate and an additional 40% with stable disease.[33] A large-scale phase 3 trial of XL184 is now under way. Side effects for both these agents are typical for the class, including fatigue, nausea, diarrhea, skin rash, and hypertension.

Treatment with ret kinase inhibitors frequently leads to declines in the calcitonin level out of proportion to radiographic response. Akeno-Stuart and colleagues[4] have reported that inhibition of ret signaling leads to decreased calcitonin gene transcription. Thus, in the setting of ret inhibitor treatment, declines in calcitonin may reflect drug action, but appear to be a poor surrogate marker for changes in tumor volume.

In addition to agents targeting both ret and VEGFR2, preliminary response data are also available for axitinib, a potent VEGFR2 inhibitor (IC_{50} = 0.25 nM) with no significant activity against ret.[34] Of 11 tested patients in this phase 2 trial, 2 had PR, 3 stable disease (SD), and 6 were considered indeterminate. Motesanib is a potent VEGFR2 inhibitor (IC_{50} = 4 nM),with moderate activity against ret (IC_{50} = 59 nM). Schlumberger and colleagues[35] have reported a high rate of SD but few partial responses to this drug. Limited data have been reported for the FDA-approved VEGFR2 inhibitors sorafenib and sunitinib in MTC, both of which also have moderate activity against ret. A variety of other approaches to systemic therapy of MTC are under investigation, including targeted radioimmunotherapy, cytotoxic chemotherapy, and combinations of tyrosine kinase inhibitors with chemotherapy.[36] In the absence of an FDA-approved systemic therapy, patients with progressive advanced MTC should be strongly considered for enrollment in a clinical trial.

The appropriate selection of patients for systemic therapy is still evolving. Currently available therapies have moderate to significant toxicities, which suggests that these agents should be targeted for patients with progressive MTC or those with significant symptoms that cannot be otherwise treated. Because even extensive MTC may sometimes follow an indolent course, these treatment decisions should be carefully individualized. In summary, this is a promising era in which new therapeutic advances can now be offered to many MTC patients.

References

1. Ichihara M, Murakumo Y, Takahashi M: RET and neuroendocrine tumors. Cancer Lett 204:197-211, 2004.
2. Santoro M, Carlomagno F, Romano A, et al: Activation of RET as a dominant transforming gene by germline mutations of MEN2A and MEN2B. Science 267:381-383, 1995.
3. Jijiwa M, Fukuda T, Kawai K, et al: A targeting mutation of tyrosine 1062 in Ret causes a marked decrease of enteric neurons and renal hypoplasia. Mol Cell Biol 24:8026-8036, 2004.
4. Akeno-Stuart N, Croyle M, Knauf JA, et al: The RET kinase inhibitor NVP-AST487 blocks growth and calcitonin gene expression through distinct mechanisms in medullary thyroid cancer cells. Cancer Res 67:6956-6964, 2007.
5. Blaugrund JE, Johns MM Jr, Eby YJ, et al: RET proto-oncogene mutations in inherited and sporadic medullary thyroid cancer. Hum Mol Genet 3:1895-1897, 1994.
6. Elisei R, Cosci B, Romei C, et al: Prognostic significance of somatic RET oncogene mutations in sporadic medullary thyroid cancer: A 10-year follow-up study. J Clin Endocrinol Metab 93:682-687, 2008.
7. Schilling T, Bürck J, Sinn HP, et al: Prognostic value of codon 918 (ATG → ACG) RET proto-oncogene mutations in sporadic medullary thyroid carcinoma. Int J Cancer 95:62-66, 2001.

8. Brandi ML, Gagel RF, Angeli A, et al: Guidelines for diagnosis and therapy of MEN type 1 and type 2. J Clin Endocrinol Metab 86:5658-5671, 2001.
9. Salvatore D, Melillo RM, Monaco C, et al: Increased in vivo phosphorylation of ret tyrosine 1062 is a potential pathogenetic mechanism of multiple endocrine neoplasia type 2B. Cancer Res 61:1426-1431, 2001.
10. van Veelen W, van Gasteren CJ, Acton DS, et al: Synergistic effect of oncogenic RET and loss of p18 on medullary thyroid carcinoma development. Cancer Res 68:1329-1337, 2008.
11. Marsh DJ, Theodosopoulos G, Martin-Schulte K, et al: Genome-wide copy number imbalances identified in familial and sporadic medullary thyroid carcinoma. J Clin Endocrinol Metab 88:1866-1872, 2003.
12. Carlson KM, Bracamontes J, Jackson CE, et al: Parent-of-origin effects in multiple endocrine neoplasia type 2B. Am J Hum Genet 55:1076-1082, 1994.
13. Brauckhoff M, Gimm O, Weiss CL, et al: Multiple endocrine neoplasia 2B syndrome due to codon 918 mutation: Clinical manifestation and course in early and late onset disease. World J Surg 28:1305-1311, 2004.
14. Cooper DS, Doherty GM, Haugen BR, et al: Management guidelines for patients with thyroid nodules and differentiated thyroid cancer. Thyroid 16:109-142, 2006.
15. Hodak SP, Burman KD: The calcitonin conundrum—is it time for routine measurement of serum calcitonin in patients with thyroid nodules? J Clin Endocrinol Metab 89:511-514, 2004.
16. Moley JF, DeBenedetti MK: Patterns of nodal metastases in palpable medullary thyroid carcinoma: Recommendations for extent of node dissection. Ann Surg 229:880-887, 1999.
17. Scollo C, Baudin E, Travagli JP, et al: Rationale for central and bilateral lymph node dissection in sporadic and hereditary medullary thyroid cancer. J Clin Endocrinol Metab 88:2070-2075, 2003.
18. Machens A, Hinze R, Thomusch O, Dralle H: Pattern of nodal metastasis for primary and reoperative thyroid cancer. World J Surg 26:22-28, 2002.
19. Machens A, Holzhausen HJ, Dralle H: Contralateral cervical and mediastinal lymph node metastasis in medullary thyroid cancer: Systemic disease? Surgery 139:28-32, 2006.
20. Kouvaraki MA, Shapiro SE, Fornage BD, et al: Role of preoperative ultrasonography in the surgical management of patients with thyroid cancer. Surgery 134:946-954, 2003.
21. Machens A, Niccoli-Sire P, Hoegel J, et al: Early malignant progression of hereditary medullary thyroid cancer. N Engl J Med 349:1517-1525, 2003.
22. Cohen R, Campos JM, Salaün C, et al: Preoperative calcitonin levels are predictive of tumor size and postoperative calcitonin normalization in medullary thyroid carcinoma. Groupe d'Etudes des Tumeurs a Calcitonine (GETC). J Clin Endocrinol Metab 85:919-922, 2000.
23. Machens A, Schneyer U, Holzhausen HJ, Dralle H: Prospects of remission in medullary thyroid carcinoma according to basal calcitonin level. J Clin Endocrinol Metab 90:2029-2034, 2005.
24. Barbet J, Campion L, Kraeber-Bodere F, Chatal JF: Prognostic impact of serum calcitonin and carcinoembryonic antigen doubling-times in patients with medullary thyroid carcinoma. J Clin Endocrinol Metab 90:6077-6084, 2005.
25. Leboeuf R, Langlois MF, Martin M, et al: "Hook effect" in calcitonin immunoradiometric assay in patients with metastatic medullary thyroid carcinoma: Case report and review of the literature. J Clin Endocrinol Metab 91:361-34, 2006.
26. Modigliani E, Cohen R, Campos JM, et al: Prognostic factors for survival and for biochemical cure in medullary thyroid carcinoma: Results in 899 patients. The GETC Study Group. Groupe d'etude des tumeurs a calcitonine. Clin Endocrinol (Oxf) 48:265-273, 1998.
27. Bergholm U, Bergstrom R, Ekbom A: Long-term follow-up of patients with medullary carcinoma of the thyroid. Cancer 79:132-138, 1997.
28. Giraudet AL, Vanel D, Leboulleux S, et al: Imaging medullary thyroid carcinoma with persistent elevated calcitonin levels. J Clin Endocrinol Metab 92:4185-4190, 2007.
29. Brierley J, Tsang R, Simpson WJ, et al: Medullary thyroid cancer: Analyses of survival and prognostic factors and the role of radiation therapy in local control. Thyroid 6:305-310, 1996.
30. Wu LT, Averbuch SD, Ball DW, et al: Treatment of advanced medullary thyroid carcinoma with a combination of cyclophosphamide, vincristine, and dacarbazine. Cancer 73:432-436, 1994.
31. Wells SA, Gosnell JE, Gagel RF, et al: Vandetanib in metastatic hereditary medullary thyroid cancer: Follow-up results of an open-label phase II trial. J Clin Oncol, 2007 ASCO Annual Meeting Proceedings. 25(suppl):6018, 2007.
32. Carlomagno F, Guida T, Anaganti S, et al: Disease associated mutations at valine 804 in the RET receptor tyrosine kinase confer resistance to selective kinase inhibitors. Oncogene 23:6056-6063, 2004.
33. Salgia R, Sherman S, Hong D, et al: Phase 1 study of XL184, a RET, VEGFR2 & MET inhibitor, administered orally to patients with solid tumors including medullary thyroid cancer. J Clin Oncol, 2008 ASCO Meeting Proceedings, 2008.
34. Cohen EE, Rosen LS, Vokes EE, et al: Axitinib is an active treatment for all histologic subtypes of advanced thyroid cancer: Results from a phase II study. J Clin Oncol 26:4708-4713, 2008.
35. Schlumberger MJ, Elisei R, Sherman SI, et al: Initial results from a phase 2 trial of motesanib diphosphate (AMG 706) in patients (pts) with medullary thyroid cancer (MTC). Proceedings of the 89th Annual Meeting of the Endocrine Society, Toronto, June 2007.
36. Schlumberger M, Carlomagno F, Baudin E, et al: New therapeutic approaches to treat medullary thyroid carcinoma. Nat Clin Pract Endocrinol Metab 4:22-32, 2008.

Index

Note: Page numbers followed by f or t refer to figures and tables, respectively.

H